BM

THE OXFORD HANDBOOK OF

REPRODUCTIVE ETHICS

THE OXFORD HANDBOOK OF

REPRODUCTIVE ETHICS

Edited by

LESLIE FRANCIS

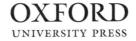

OXFORD

UNIVERSITY PRESS

OXFORD
UNIVERSITY PRESS

Oxford University Press is a department of the University of Oxford. It furthers
the University's objective of excellence in research, scholarship, and education
by publishing worldwide. Oxford is a registered trade mark of Oxford University
Press in the UK and certain other countries.

Published in the United States of America by Oxford University Press
198 Madison Avenue, New York, NY 10016, United States of America.

Library of Congress Cataloging-in-Publication Data
Names: Francis, Leslie, 1946- editor.
Title: The Oxford handbook of reproductive ethics / edited by Leslie Francis.
Other titles: Handbook of reproductive ethics
Description: New York, NY : Oxford University Press, [2017] |
Includes bibliographical references and index.
Identifiers: LCCN 2016028237 (print) | LCCN 2016037211 (ebook) |
ISBN 9780199981878 (cloth : alk. paper) | ISBN 9780199981885 (pdf) |
ISBN 9780190237684 (online course) | ISBN 9780190657796 (ebook)
Subjects: LCSH: Human reproduction—Moral and ethical aspects.
Classification: LCC QP251 .O93 2016 (print) | LCC QP251 (ebook) |
DDC 612.6—dc23
LC record available at https://lccn.loc.gov/2016028237

1 3 5 7 9 8 6 4 2

Printed by Sheridan Books, Inc., United States of America

CONTENTS

PART II PROVIDERS

PART III PARENTS

PART IV LAST BUT NOT LEAST: ZYGOTE, BLASTOCYST, EMBRYO, FETUS, NEWBORN

Biographical Sketches

Armand H. Matheny Antommaria earned his MD from Washington University School of Medicine and his PhD in religious ethics from the University of Chicago Divinity School. He is currently the Director of the Ethics Center and the Lee Ault Carter Chair of Pediatric Ethics at Cincinnati Children's Hospital Medical Center. He has served as a member of the American Academy of Pediatrics' Committee on Bioethics and is lead author of its policy on conscientious objection.

Margaret Pabst Battin, MFA, PhD, Distinguished Professor of philosophy and medical ethics at the University of Utah, has authored, coauthored, edited, or coedited some 20 books, including *Drugs and Justice* and *The Patient as Victim and Vector: Ethics and Infectious Disease*; two collections on end-of-life issues, *The Least Worst Death* and *Ending Life*; and a comprehensive sourcebook, *The Ethics of Suicide: Historical Sources*. She is currently working on the large-scale reproductive problems of the globe.

Jeffrey R. Botkin is a Professor of Pediatrics at the University of Utah and an Adjunct Professor of Human Genetics. He is Chief of the Division of Medical Ethics and Humanities and serves as the Associate Vice President for Research Integrity. Dr. Botkin is currently Chair of the DHHS Secretary's Advisory Committee on Human Research Protections and a former Chair of the Committee on Bioethics for the American Academy of Pediatrics.

I. Glenn Cohen is a Professor of Law at Harvard Law School and the Faculty Director of the Petrie-Flom Center for Health Law Policy and Biotechnology. He is the author of over 80 articles and book chapters and the author, editor, or coeditor of seven books.

Adam Cureton is an Assistant Professor of Philosophy at the University of Tennessee, having done his graduate work at Oxford and UNC Chapel Hill. He specializes in ethics, Kant, and disability. He is legally blind and is the founding president of the Society for Philosophy and Disability.

Judith Daar is a Professor at Whittier Law School and a Clinical Professor at the University of California, Irvine School of Medicine. She serves as a member of the UCI Medical Center Ethics Committee and is currently the Vice-Chair of the ABA Real Property, Trusts & Estates Bioethics Committee. She is the author of over 100 publications that focus on assisted reproductive technologies, including the forthcoming book, *The New Eugenics* (Yale University Press, 2017).

David DeGrazia is Senior Research Fellow in the Department of Bioethics, National Institutes of Health, and Professor in the Department of Philosophy, George Washington University. His seven books include *Creation Ethics: Reproduction, Genetics, and Quality of Life* (Oxford University Press, 2012).

Donna Dickenson is Emeritus Professor of Medical Ethics and Humanities at the University of London and Research Associate at the University of Oxford. In 2006 she became the first woman to win the International Spinoza Lens Award for contribution to public debate on ethics. Her books on commodification of the body include *Property in the Body: Feminist Perspectives* (Cambridge University Press, 2007, second edition, 2017) and *Body Shopping: Converting Body Parts to Profit* (Oneworld, 2009).

Leslie Francis is Distinguished Professor of Philosophy and Distinguished Alfred C. Emery Professor of Law at the University of Utah. She served as the President of the Pacific Division of the American Philosophical Association in 2015–2016. Her interests include privacy and disability rights, and she is currently completing *Privacy: What Everyone Needs to Know* (with John G. Francis, forthcoming from Oxford).

Sara Goering is Associate Professor of Philosophy, member of the Program on Values, and faculty for the Disability Studies Program at the University of Washington, Seattle. Her interests include medical ethics, philosophy of disability, and feminist philosophy. She leads the ethics thrust for the NSF-funded UW Center for Sensorimotor Neural Engineering.

Imogen Goold is Associate Professor in Law at the University of Oxford. She studied Law and Modern History at the University of Tasmania, receiving her PhD in 2005. She also received an MA in Bioethics from the University of Monash in the same year. She has previously held positions at the Centre for Law and Genetics, Tasmania and the Australian Law Reform Commission. Her research interests include reproductive medicine and the regulation of human biomaterials.

Christopher Gyngell is a Marie Skłodowska-Curie Fellow with the Uehiro Centre for Practical Ethics. His research interests lie primarily in bioethics, moral theory, and the philosophy of health and disease. He is currently working on a Marie Skłodowska-Curie Fellowship funded project titled "Selecting, Creating and Modifying Embryos," which will investigate the ethical and legal implications of new reproductive technologies, such as the gene-editing technique CRISPR.

Don Hubin is Professor Emeritus in the Philosophy Department at The Ohio State University and Founding Director of the Center for Ethics and Human Values. Don received his BA in philosophy from the University of California at Davis and his MA and PhD from the University of Arizona. He specializes in ethics, philosophy of law, and political philosophy.

Adam Kadlac is Associate Teaching Professor of Philosophy at Wake Forest University. He works broadly in ethics and political philosophy and has published papers in

American Philosophical Quarterly, Philosophical Studies, Ethical Theory and Moral Practice, Social Theory and Practice, Public Affairs Quarterly, and the *Southern Journal of Philosophy*.

Guy Kahane is Deputy Director of the Uehiro Centre for Practical Ethics. He is also Associate Professor at the Faculty of Philosophy, University of Oxford, and Fellow and Tutor in Philosophy at Pembroke College, Oxford.

Hilde Lindemann is Professor of Philosophy and Associate in the Center for Ethics and Humanities in the Life Sciences at Michigan State University, with ongoing research interests, including feminist bioethics and the social construction of persons and identities. Her books include *Holding and Letting Go: The Social Practice of Personal Identities* and *Damaged Identities, Narrative Repair*. She is a Fellow of the Hastings Center and past president of the American Society for Bioethics and Humanities.

Janet Malek is an Associate Professor in the Center for Medical Ethics and Health Policy at Baylor College of Medicine. She received her doctorate in philosophy from Rice University in 2004. Dr. Malek serves as an ethics consultant for the Houston Methodist Hospital System and teaches ethics and professionalism for Baylor medical students and residents. Her research focuses on ethics in pediatrics and obstetrics, particularly on issues at the intersection of genetic and reproductive technologies.

Lorna A. Marshall is a practicing reproductive endocrinologist and Director of the Center for Collaborative Reproduction at Pacific NW Fertility & IVF Specialists in Seattle. She is clinical professor of obstetrics and gynecology at University of Washington School of Medicine and has served on the ethics committees of the American Society for Reproductive Medicine and American College of Obstetrics and Gynecology.

Sheelagh McGuinness is Senior Lecturer in Law at the University of Bristol. She is interested in the fields of health law, law and reproduction, and law and gender. She has published across these areas in law, ethics, and health care journals. Sheelagh sits on the Research Ethics Committee of the British Pregnancy Advisory Service, the Independent Ethics and Governance Council of UK Biobank, and the Medical Ethics Committee of the Royal College of General Practitioners.

Diana Tietjens Meyers is Professor Emerita of Philosophy at the University of Connecticut, Storrs. Her new monograph, *Victims' Stories and the Advancement of Human Rights*, is now available. Her most recent edited collection is *Poverty, Agency, and Human Rights*. She currently works in three main areas of philosophy: philosophy of action, feminist ethics and aesthetics, and human rights.

Kimberly M. Mutcherson is a Professor of Law at Rutgers Law School in Camden, New Jersey, where she teaches courses in family law, bioethics, and health law policy. Her scholarly work focuses on law, families, and bioethics with a particular interest in assisted reproduction. She is a graduate of the University of Pennsylvania and Columbia Law School.

David Orentlicher is a Professor of Law and Medicine at Indiana University. He earned his MD and JD degrees at Harvard, and he has taught as a visiting or adjunct professor at Princeton, University of Chicago, and Northwestern. Orentlicher is author of *Matters of Life and Death* (Princeton) and coauthor of *Health Care Law and Ethics* (Wolters Kluwer). In *Two Presidents Are Better Than One* (NYU), he draws on his experiences as a state representative.

Amy Cabrera Rasmussen is an Associate Professor in the Department of Political Science at California State University, Long Beach. Her research uses interpretive methods to analyze the construction of meaning in public policy discourse and practice. Substantively, her research focuses on various aspects of public policy, including reproductive and sexual health, health disparities, and environmental health.

Rosamond Rhodes, PhD, is Professor of Medical Education and Director of Bioethics Education at Icahn School of Medicine at Mount Sinai, Professor of Philosophy at The Graduate Center, CUNY, and Professor of Bioethics and Associate Director of the Clarkson-Mount Sinai Bioethics Program. She writes on a broad array of issues in bioethics and has published more than 200 papers and chapters. She is coeditor of *The Human Microbiome: Ethical, Legal and Social Concerns* (Oxford University Press, 2013), *The Blackwell Guide to Medical Ethics* (Blackwell, 2007), *Medicine and Social Justice: Essays on the Distribution of Health Care* (Oxford University Press, first edition, 2002; second edition, 2012), and *Physician Assisted Suicide: Expanding the Debate* (Routledge, 1998).

Norvin Richards is Professor Emeritus at the University of Alabama. His published work includes "Life or Death Decisions in the NICU," *The Journal of Perinatology*, April, 2006, *The Ethics of Parenthood* (Oxford, 2010) and "Parental Love," in *The Philosophy of Love*, ed. Christopher Grau and Aaron Smutts (Oxford, forthcoming.)

Julian Savulescu is the Uehiro Chair in Practical Ethics, the Director of the Oxford Uehiro Centre for Practical Ethics, and the Oxford Centre for Neuroethics. He edits the *Journal of Medical Ethics* and the *Journal of Practical Ethics*. He is the Sir Louis Matheson Distinguished Visiting Professor at Monash University. He received an honorary doctorate from the University of Bucharest in 2014.

Michael J. Selgelid is Professor of Bioethics and Director of the Centre for Human Bioethics, and the World Health Organization (WHO) Collaborating Centre for Bioethics therein, at Monash University in Melbourne, Australia. He is a member of the Board of Directors of the International Association of Bioethics and serves on the Ethics Review Board of Médecins Sans Frontières. His main research focus is public health ethics—with emphasis on ethical issues associated with infectious disease and biotechnology. He edits a book series in Public Health Ethics Analysis for Springer and a book series in Practical Ethics and Public Policy for ANU Press. He is coeditor of *Monash Bioethics Review* and an associate editor of *Journal of Medical Ethics*. Michael earned a BS in biomedical engineering from Duke University and a PhD in philosophy from the University of California, San Diego.

Anita Silvers is Professor and Chair of Philosophy at San Francisco State University. She has been writing bioethics that is inclusive of disability perspectives for a quarter century. Silvers has been awarded the American Philosophical Association Quinn Prize for service to philosophy and philosophers and the Phi Beta Kappa Society Lebowitz Prize for excellence in philosophical thought. She is a longtime community representative on the San Francisco General Hospital Ethics Committee.

Bonnie Steinbock is Professor Emeritus of Philosophy at the University at Albany/ SUNY and professor of bioethics at Clarkson University. A Fellow of the Hastings Center, she is the author of *Life Before Birth: The Moral and Legal Status of Embryos and Fetuses*, 2nd edition (Oxford, 2011), 70 articles, and the editor or coeditor of several books, including the *Oxford Handbook of Bioethics* (Oxford, 2009) and *Ethical Issues in Modern Medicine*, 8th edition (McGraw-Hill, 2012).

David Wasserman is on the faculty of the Department of Bioethics at the National Institutes of Health. He works primarily on ethical issues in reproduction, disability, genetics, and neuroscience. He is coauthor of the recent *Debating Procreation* (with David Benatar) and coeditor of the forthcoming *Oxford Handbook of Philosophy and Disability* (with Adam Cureton).

Heather Widdows is Professor of Global Ethics in the Department of Philosophy at the University of Birmingham. She is the author of *Global Ethics* and *The Connected Self* and has coedited, with Herjeet Marway, *Women and Violence*, with Darrel Moellendorf, *The Routledge Handbook of Global Ethics*, with Nicola Smith, *Global Social Justice*, with Caroline Mullen, *The Governance of Genetic Information*, and with Itziar Alkorta Idiakez and Aitziber Emaldi Cirión, *Women's Reproductive Rights*.

THE OXFORD HANDBOOK OF

REPRODUCTIVE ETHICS

INTRODUCTION

LESLIE FRANCIS

THIS handbook of reproductive ethics brings together some of the very best scholars working on reproductive issues in the world today. Because I believe that full understanding of the ethical issues posed by reproduction must be embedded within the political and social contexts in which people lead their reproductive lives, I have attempted to go beyond some of the contemporary discussions of reproductive ethics to call on political philosophers, philosophers of science, legal philosophers, legal scholars and lawyers, physicians, and political scientists to contribute their analytic approaches to contemporary controversies. Reproduction is at once biological, technological, deeply personal, sometimes spiritual, heavily socially regulated, and—at least with the technologies available today—inevitably interpersonal. And it is an issue area in which ethics, law, politics, science, and perhaps even religion interact mutually to influence one other.

An edited collection is, perforce, limited by the editor's ability to entice people to write, by the availability of scholars in an area, by whether some important fields have nonetheless been well plowed, by the editor's own imagination, and by plans of a press to publish related volumes in a series or volumes dealing with related issues such as bioethics or religion and ethics. But an introduction is not so limited—so this will range over issues not treated in the volume in the effort to tie them together with the topics that are covered. Moreover, chapters in an edited volume may fit together in ways not originally anticipated but remarkably rich; thus, this introduction does not treat the chapters in the exact order in which they appear.

POLITICAL AND ETHICAL THEORY

Reproduction involves deeply difficult, conflicted, and conflictual personal choices: whether to have children at all, how to have these children, what to do with these children after birth, what is permissible in pregnancy or with a fetus, and whether to prevent pregnancy or birth. For some, responses are matters of bedrock faith: religious traditions such as Catholicism have rejected not only abortion but also contraception, whereas other religious groups such as the Shakers have insisted on celibacy in pursuit of spiritual purity. For some, reproductive activity is core to identity; being a father or mother may be perceived to be one, if not the most, important of life events. Reproductive decisions may have grave consequences for how societies develop and whether they flourish. Falling fertility rates in countries such as Italy raise fears of economic decline, while China now has ended its one-child policy in part to address the challenges of an aging population. Niger, Burundi, and Mali are still estimated to have fertility rates of over six children per woman, with concomitantly high rates of severe poverty.

Because views about reproduction rest for some people on fundamental theological, metaphysical, or ethical commitments, individual reproductive choice is frequently invoked by liberal theorists as an example of why the role of the state should be limited to preventing people from harming one another. This "harm principle," attributed to John Stuart Mill in *On Liberty* and developed by Joel Feinberg (1984) among others, thus insists that the sole justification for state coercion (and perhaps for the coercion of public opinion as well) is to prevent people from harming one another. State coercion may not be used to protect people from harming themselves or to make people do what is morally right or good.

The contested status of the fetus throws application of the harm principle into disarray, however. Is preventing abortion a proper application of the harm principle, or not? For those who see the fetus as having full moral status, abortion is nothing less than murder; for others, abortion may be a difficult personal choice but does not come within legitimate state protection of some from harm by others.

Reproduction also places pressure on the idea of harm: what is "harm"? Can it ever be a harm to be born? Conversely, is it a harm not to come into existence or continue in existence? Are differences or disabilities harms? Must harm attach to an existing individual? Can different modes of parenting be harms to offspring and when, if ever, should the state intervene? What kinds of psychological distress, if any, are of concern to the harm principle? Can altered identity be harm cognizable in liberal theory? And what about far-reaching changes in the nature or structure of society? For these and other reasons, reproduction is not an issue area that lends itself to easy resolution by application of liberalism's approach.

For those who reject the limits of the harm principle—perhaps because they believe that societies ought to be able to shape themselves according to values they cherish, or because they believe that pursuit of some value is so important as to warrant state intervention—reproduction may be of central concern. For societies, creation of the next generation is critical to survival; the structures within which this takes place (most likely the family) are basic social institutions. Social regulation of reproduction is thus not surprising despite its repressiveness when it conflicts with individuals' visions of the lives they hope to live.

Reproduction is also the locus of great vulnerability. There is the vulnerability of infertility, which may prove a lifelong disappointment or subject a supposedly infertile partner to rejection or even death. There is the vulnerability of pregnancy and child-birth: across the world today, about a third of a million women die each year from com-plications of pregnancy or birth (WHO 2015). There is the vulnerability of sex: women are raped at rates far higher than men; women experience the joys, travails, and con-sequences of pregnancy in ways men do not; and women who are caregivers for chil-dren all too frequently are unable to work, confined to domestic care roles, or consigned to poverty. Contraception has also been the locus of inequality, with women bearing primary responsibilities for control and men concomitantly disadvantaged by the lack of contraceptive alternatives available for them. These and other biological and social inequalities led radical feminists to explore possibilities for cybernetic or male repro-duction (e.g., Firestone 1970) as cornerstones for a postpatriarchal society.

Views of reproduction thus take many different forms, and this collection begins with an account of how such views may frame debates in both politics and philosophy. Amy Cabrera Rasmussen, a political scientist who studies the framing of public policy issues, especially in health and health care, leads off the volume with an account of the dis-cursive context of reproductive ethics. Discourse frames are cognitive maps that can be either subconscious or more purposefully utilized tools that convey perspectives and persuade others. In the politics of reproduction, frames are ubiquitous. Policies related to reproduction have been group specific, discouraging reproduction by the poor, the non-White, or people with disabilities. In the United States at least, abortion has become a political litmus test, particularly for Republicans. State legislatures have increasingly limited abortion rights and hope that the US Supreme Court will eviscerate or ulti-mately overrule *Roe v. Wade*, 410 U.S. 113, its 1973 decision implementing a constitu-tional right to reproductive liberty that includes most abortions. During its 2015 term, the US Supreme Court upheld a challenge to Texas's abortion law that required physi-cians performing abortions to have admitting privileges at a nearby hospital and clinics to be outfitted as surgical centers—a law that, if upheld, would have required all but a handful of clinics in a geographical area larger than France to close.[1]

To disentangle this controversy, Rasmussen outlines four ways of framing the abor-tion issue. The first is whether abortion is an appropriate target of governmental policy-making at all. The second is whether abortion should be categorized as an issue of health or of liberty, including the free exercise of religion. In US debates over coverage under the Affordable Care Act, reproduction is framed as a problem of health by those who would defend increased rights to the means of contraception or abortion, but as a matter of the free exercise of religion by those who believe employers should not be required to provide health care they oppose on religious grounds or even give notice to the govern-ment as a backup provider of the service.[2] Similarly, framing sexuality as a health issue legitimates sex education, including education about disease transmission, whereas opponents see sexual behavior as an ethical or religious matter. More broadly, abortion may serve as a synecdoche—a master issue standing in for resolution of related policy areas such as sex education, contraception, or health care funding. Finally, Rasmussen points out the complicating factor that reproductive technology is changing rapidly and that public understanding of the relevant scientific background is limited, with the result that elites and advocacy groups may play greater roles in influencing this highly contentious area of social policy.

It may seem unusual to have a volume on ethics begin with a discussion of how frames construct policy debates. I chose to do this not because I believe that ethical reasoning about sharply disputed issues such as reproduction should be seen as relativized to frames. Rather, as a practical matter of political debate, contested reproductive issues are framed as Rasmussen delineates. To understand how their views are likely to be perceived, discussed, criticized, and possibly even implemented, it is critical for moral and political philosophers to be aware of the contemporary frames that contextualize their work.

Starting Places: Reproduction and Justification in Moral and Political Philosophy

Sex, marriage, reproduction, childrearing, and abortion have been linchpins of controversy both within and about liberal political theory. One of John Stuart Mill's examples in his ringing defense of the harm principle was fornication, an act he saw as purely private and thus not appropriate for state interference. Pimping gave Mill more pause: on the one hand, he thought, people should be able to ask for advice about things that they would be free to do of their own choosing; on the other hand, economic gain from behavior regarded by society as evil lies on the boundary line of permissible state interference. Sir James Fitzjames Stephen's (1874) resounding critique objected to this vision of the role of the state and community as limited to protection from harm imposed by others. For Stephen, many of the examples of legitimate state interference involved sexuality and marriage. He cited a hypothetical example of an organization for the promotion of seduction and adultery as a legitimate subject of state interference (1874, 84). And he robustly criticized Mill's argument for the permissibility of fornication but the impermissibility of pimping, arguing that there is no clear line between vices that are private and vices that are injurious to others. Stephen thus rejected Mill's distinction between the public and the private along with Mill's view that sexuality is a matter of individual moral choice.

This disagreement between Mill and Stephen was reincarnated in the twentieth-century debate between H. L. A. Hart (1963) and Sir Patrick Devlin (1965) over the decriminalization of sexual offenses in the United Kingdom. Core to this debate was whether and why society might be said to have a right to protect itself from change or disintegration. Hart thought—in a statement of what would now be regarded as nonideal theory—that justification for the preservation of social institutions must take into account the type of society in question; racist societies would not have claims to perpetuation of their institutions, although ideal societies might (1963, 18–19).

Nonetheless, Hart did not see the full impact of nonideal social circumstances on sexual and reproductive issues. In his discussion of the specific examples under scrutiny in the debate—adultery, same-sex relationships, fornication, bestiality, incest, prostitution, bigamy or polygamy, and abortion (a mixed bag at best)—Hart treated them as matters of contested morality rather than social justice. For example, although his discussion of bigamy deploys the US Model Penal Code's argument for prohibition that it was particularly likely to result in women being left destitute, Hart develops instead the distinction between criminalizing bigamy because others find it offensive and a public nuisance and criminalizing it because it is believed to be immoral (43). Devlin interprets the possibility that prostitutes might be exploited as the moralistic concern that they might be enticed into moral weakness (12), not that they might be pressed by unjust economic circumstances into choices they might not otherwise make. Nowhere in their debate over the recommended liberalization of UK laws concerning sexual morality do either Hart or Devlin raise the risks of exploitation or links to trafficking that are at the center of contemporary discussions about the legalization of prostitution or some of the reproductive practices discussed in this volume.

The chapters in Part I develop approaches to problems in reproductive ethics in terms of human rights, civil rights, constructivism, commodification, and human improvement. These chapters develop theoretical tools that are critical to analyzing the complex issues of reproductive ethics in today's world where justice is at best unevenly achieved.

Many types of rights and rights holders appear in reproductive ethics. Rights to reproductive liberty, including the choice to procreate and the choice not to procreate, are pitted against rights of the embryo or fetus. Several chapters in Part I of the volume explore the nature and foundation of rights in reproduction. In Chapter 2, Sheelagh McGuinness and Heather Widdows argue for reproductive control as a basic human right. Without the ability to make choices about the number of children they have and the time of childbirth, women lack bodily integrity and may find pregnancy, childbirth, and motherhood imposed upon them against their will. Reproductive control, McGuinness and Widdows say, requires effective access to family planning services, particularly safe contraception and abortion. These basic reproductive rights are not only negative rights to noninterference as in the form of legal prohibitions. They also require an enabling environment, where women can readily access and pay for the services they need. Too often women across the world still lack effective access to basic reproductive services for religious, cultural, or economic reasons.

McGuinness and Widdows defend access to basic reproductive rights on grounds of equality. Reproductive rights are threshold rights, needed to bring women up to the control currently possessed by men. Without reproductive control, moreover, women may be unable to exercise other centrally important forms of agency, such as relationships or employment. Although related claims to rights such as parenting or accessing reproductive technologies may be important, McGuinness and Widdows contend, they are not basic rights that are critical to the realization of equality in the way that rights to reproductive control are. In this sense, these reproductive rights are human rights; without them, women are not fully human in the way that men are.

In their discussion, McGuinness and Widdows address reproduction in nonideal circumstances, detailing how commitments to reproductive rights in international law are imperfectly realized. The Universal Declaration of Human Rights does not make reproductive rights explicit, although it does specify the importance of bodily integrity (article 5) and the right to found a family (article 16). Later human rights instruments such as the Convention on the Elimination of All Forms of Discrimination Against Women (CEDAW) do specifically include rights in marriage, health, and family planning (articles 12 and 16) and have proved critical advocacy tools. Nonetheless, serious barriers remain. The US Helms Amendment prohibits US development aid from being used for abortions. It has been expanded to prohibit any recipient of US government funding from facilitating access to abortion services or advocating for liberalization of abortion policy—even when these activities are paid for from separate funding sources and US funds are spent only on activities such as family planning. Even research on the effects of the ban—such as whether lack of family planning results in increased abortion demand—is prohibited for recipients of US funds. Nongovernmental organizations such as the Gates Foundation also do not fund abortions.

Equality as a grounding for reproductive rights is also critical to Diana Meyers's argument in Chapter 4 for the reproductive rights of victims of trafficking. Her argument explores how sex trafficking systematically violates victims' human rights and thus presents them as ethically justified candidates for asylum and remedial health care. Her argument complements that of McGuinness and Widdows by contending that violations of other human rights that affect reproductive capability can also justify reproductive rights.

Sex trafficking presents a potential conundrum for liberal theory, however. On some views, trafficked women are seen as economic migrants making prudential choices in search of a better life. As such, they are not perceived as harmed and thus within the protection of the harm principle. These views explain why in some jurisdictions women trafficked internationally are not classified as refugees but as smuggled, illegal immigrants subject to criminal proceedings and deportation (Francis and Francis 2014).

Meyers, like McGuinness and Widdows, begins her argument with the ways in which human rights norms have grown to encompass rights to reproductive liberty. She then shows how this right is affected by violations of international prohibitions on forced sex work. Women trafficked into sex have very high rates of sexually transmitted diseases and abortion. They receive far less other medical care appropriate to their circumstances; their conditions and treatment may place their future fertility at risk. Thus, all too frequently, trafficked women are deprived of the right to reproductive liberty.

In light of the violation of human rights of trafficking victims, destination states have obligations to them, Meyers argues. Trafficking is lucrative and, despite increased vigilance, antitrafficking laws are imperfectly enforced. But criminal justice reform is only a first step. It must be accompanied by efforts to counteract implicit bias against trafficked women: condemning them as contaminated sex workers, stereotyping them as uneducated and likely to become welfare dependent, and perceiving them as lying to pursue economic advantage. Beyond asylum, Meyers contends, trafficking's victims should also receive health care needed to protect them against further deterioration in their ability to exercise their reproductive liberty rights. Such needed health care may include abortion of pregnancies conceived during coerced sex work.

McGuinness and Widdows and Meyers consider rights as human rights, grounding and interpreting them through the social institution of international human rights law. In Chapter 7, legal scholar Kimberly Mutcherson analyzes the rights to procreate and to parent as fundamental human and constitutional rights. In a postcoital world where reproduction can be achieved in ways that include pluralistic families and procreative pluralism, she contends, laws continue to privilege only certain types of families. Such limitations on access to reproductive technologies such as in vitro fertilization (IVF) violate reproductive rights, as the Inter-American Court of Human Rights recognized in a recent case. Reproductive injustice remains as well: race, income, sexual orientation, marital status, and disability may limit access to infertility care or adoption, as well as child custody decisions. Mutcherson concludes with a caution about regulation of assisted reproduction: individual decisions about procreation and parenting must be protected from unwarranted discrimination in a society that values equality and justice. Her chapter illustrates how tools of legal analysis can inform ethical analysis and why understanding what reproductive rights require cannot be detached from the underlying justice of social institutions.

In Chapter 8, Silvers and Francis also sound the theme of nondiscrimination, which, they believe, is best achieved by characterizing reproductive rights as civil rights. Silvers and Francis reject characterizing rights in the idealized and species-typical forms of some human rights views. Instead, they contend, rights may not be fully understood, developed, or instantiated at any particular point in time; what rights require should always be seen as critical tools for persons disfavored in obtaining opportunities needed for them to flourish. As such, rights need not be universalized or attached to all human beings in virtue of supposedly essential human-making properties, but deployed to expand possibilities for inclusion in particular configurations of social institutions.

Reproductive rights are such tools for inclusion, allowing persons to make decisions about whether and how to form families in the communities in which they live. Reproductive rights are part of the project of constructing justice through including outliers on terms of equality. Like Mutcherson, Silvers and Francis explain how institutions may present structural barriers to the exercise of these rights. They further contend that civil rights claims should not be cast purely as negative rights—that is, protections from interference—but also as the protections and resources required for inclusion in given social contexts. Abortion, for example, should not be seen simply in terms of the liberty of the woman to choose whether or not to have a child or the right to life of the fetus but against a background of whether social structures allow adequate support for persons with disabilities.

Rights-based accounts provide one set of tools for addressing reproductive issues. But there are theoretical alternatives to treating rights as initial starting places for analysis. Rosamond Rhodes, in Chapter 3, develops a constructivist account of the ethics of abortion. Constructivism as an approach to moral and political philosophy has garnered a great deal of recent interest (Rawls 1971, 1993; Korsgaard 1996; Scanlon 1999). Constructivists hold that morality is created based on reasons that reflect features of human nature and the social and natural circumstances in which we live. Moral principles are not derived from supposed facts (such as facts about fetal development) or postulated as a basic moral law (such as that all human beings have the right to life). Rather, on Rhodes's constructivist view, the moral task is to identify reasons that should govern the actions of similarly situated reflective individuals.

On Rhodes's version of constructivism, moral obligations may be either general or special. General obligations are duties that every reasonable person can be assumed to have undertaken, for example, not to threaten others' survival if others do not threaten theirs. Special obligations arise from commitments individuals make, for example a commitment to a charity such as Save the Children. Obligations thus are a matter of reciprocity or commitment; they arise for given individuals in given circumstances rather than as a matter of natural fact or law. Another way to put this point is that Rhodes reverses the direction of moral reasoning: it does not arise from natural fact or law, but from what we accept and the commitments we make. The right to life arises from a right-creating act—such as the decision to procreate. People who decide to conceive a child thus have obligations to that child such as to avoid actions that might cause harm. But there is no right to life possessed by the fetus absent such commitments. Rhodes concludes by applying her constructivist approach to some of the most difficult problems for her view: planned pregnancies that do not go as hoped, such as unexpected twin pregnancies or pregnancies where an unexpected diagnosis of a fetal anomaly is made far along in their course. In these cases, Rhodes considers what might be the limits of the commitment that the pregnant woman has made, and what might be the responsibilities of her community. Rhodes offers something of a voluntarist approach to constructivism: that obligations and any concomitant rights are built out of willing commitments and to what persons have reasons to accept. Other constructivist views may emphasize different aspects of how obligations are generated (for example, through trust-generating social practices) or what obligations are subject to construction (for example, primarily political obligations).

Technological developments in reproduction have introduced deep controversies about commercialization. Donna Dickenson, in Chapter 5, provides a powerful critique of commodification in reproduction based on an account of the intrinsic value of persons. Dickenson begins by carefully distinguishing objectification—the attribution of use value—from commodification, the attribution of both use value and exchange value. A donation such as blood that is useful is objectified but not commodified. Objectification is not intrinsically wrong; people must have things to satisfy their needs and thus objectify these things. But on a Kantian view, entities with intrinsic value, such as persons, should not be treated merely as objects.

How this analysis applies to body parts or use of the body to provide services is not immediately clear. Legal jurisdictions have developed very different answers, especially about commodification of gametes or reproductive services. Dickenson develops a nuanced account of objectification and commodification of reproductive tissues and reproduction itself. She presents reasons why gametes arguably should be subject to stricter limits on commodification than some other bodily tissues: they are not life-saving (unlike kidneys), oocytes are not renewable (unlike hair or sperm or blood), and donation of oocytes carries some risk. Gametes also exist in a social context; they carry linkages to ancestors and progeny in a way that other bodily tissues do not.

Dickenson applies this analysis of commodification to three reproduction-related areas of controversy: the sale of oocytes for IVF and research, the sale of umbilical cord blood, and commercial surrogacy. Dickenson points out a gendered anomaly in descriptions of the sale of gametes: whereas the sale of oocytes is often characterized as a "gift" or "donation," even when compensation is paid, the sale of sperm is frankly characterized as a commercial transaction. This characterization encourages women to buy into the illusion that what they are doing is helping others and masks the potential harms incentivized by commodification: unenforceability of professional guidelines on egg pricing, lack of incentives for clinics to follow up on the long-term health of donors, and the possibility that conflicts of interest might tempt providers to harvest more eggs than medically advisable or fail to assess fully any risks to donors. Similar issues attend commodification of oocytes for use in research, especially as research on techniques such as somatic cell nuclear transplant may require large numbers of oocytes.

The sale of umbilical cord blood is a fast-growing industry. These sales, like gamete sales, are often presented misleadingly. Cord blood is described as mere waste, taken from a discarded placenta, yet in some facilities it may be harvested by clamping the umbilical cord as part of the management of labor—an intervention that may lessen the blood flow available to the newborn. Sales may be characterized as donations to benefit the woman's own child or for another who might be saved by altruism, although units may instead be sold for commercial gain and not be available in case of later need.

In Dickenson's view, the most problematic area of commercialization in reproduction is surrogacy. She begins by inquiring what is commodified in surrogacy: services in the form of women's labor or the resulting child? Increasingly, she observes, surrogacy has become big business while still characterized in altruistic terms. Some jurisdictions that permit commercial surrogacy have drawn legal lines designed to prevent overt baby selling, such as the refusal to enforce contracts that require the gestational mother to give up rights to the child before it is born. Nonetheless, some jurisdictions have allowed practices such as permitting a surrogacy contract to be canceled if the newborn has a disability, increasing the contractual price for twins, or allowing a surrogacy contract to be enforced by the agreed-upon performance of transferring the child—practices that suggest that the contractual exchange is for the child rather than for gestational services. If we strip away the professed altruism of commodification of reproductive tissues or services, Dickenson concludes, we can see how it wrongs participants by treating them as though they lacked intrinsic value. We can also recognize the risk that these transactions will wrongfully exploit participants, even though they are portrayed as a matter of free choice. What kinds of entities have intrinsic value, and what recognition of this value requires will be a continuing theme throughout this volume.

Technological advances such as preimplantation genetic diagnosis, gamete selection, gene editing, and IVF bring new prospects for parents to influence the genetic makeup of their children. These new prospects may seem to echo earlier—and deeply morally problematic—eugenics movements. In Chapter 6, Christopher Gyngell and Michael Selgelid explore this concern, first offering a limited definition of eugenics and then considering whether moral arguments might be offered in favor of it.

"Eugenics," as defined by Gyngell and Selgelid, is "an attempt to improve heredity." Here, they distinguish between what might be regarded as public health efforts such as improved neonatal care and political movements primarily focused on controlling reproduction. They identify three problematic assumptions about heredity that led to the dark eugenics of earlier eras: the beliefs that complex behavioral traits or intelligence are heritable in a simple way, that the quality of the population was declining, and that there were significant genetic differences between races. Contemporary genetic technologies reject all three of these assumptions. Gyngell and Selgelid provide a rich description of the types of recent technologies that have been developed and are under development to that end, from prenatal diagnosis through amniocentesis with selective abortion to preimplantation genetic diagnosis to CRISPR and other gene-editing technologies. Attempts to improve heredity through these technologies, as well as attempts to understand and address conditions such as stress that have adverse epigenetic effects, they say, are forms of eugenics in the sense of efforts to improve heredity.

Understood in this way, Gyngell and Selgelid argue, eugenic efforts are not necessarily bad—indeed, eugenics thus defined would appear to have a positive normative slant. And it could do a great deal of good by implementing changes in the gene pool that attempt to avoid disease or to improve welfare. The difficulty then is to distinguish between practices that can be justified on this basis and practices that cannot be so justified. Here, Gyngell and Selgelid consider "liberal eugenics" that emphasizes state neutrality but permits individuals to engage in procreative beneficence (see Chapter 6). Noting the advantages of avoiding coercion, they also observe that widespread use of liberal eugenics might raise collective action problems creating overall social harms that might justify social intervention. Gyngell and Selgelid conclude by endorsing what they call "moderate eugenics": the view that gene pool improvement is not an overriding value but must be balanced against other values such as procreative liberty and social equality. Their conclusion suggests a final theoretical point that will appear throughout this volume: that the values at stake in reproduction are not absolute and their implementation may require complex weighing under different, often nonideal conditions.

INTERVENTIONS: THE ROLE OF PROFESSIONALS

Professional organizations play major roles in setting professional norms about conscience and many other issues. In addition to general medical organizations and organizations of providers for male or female reproductive systems, there are many more specialized organizations focused on specific aspects of reproduction. Examples include the American Society for Reproductive Medicine, the Society for Assisted Reproductive Technology, the European Society of Human Reproduction and Embryology, the National Association of Certified Professional Midwives, the American College of Nurse-Midwives, the Royal College of Midwives, and many others. These organizations typically provide codes of ethics for their members or provide ethical guidance; enforcement of these norms through persuasion, professional sanction, or legal rules remains controversial. Some commentators have also developed accounts of ethical conduct based on ideas of professionalization or professional norms (e.g., McCullough and Chervenak 1994).

Historically, many controversies in reproductive ethics emerged in concert with professionalization. In a fascinating history, John Riddle (1997) traces how herbal contraceptives and abortifacients were used before the nineteenth century. Figs and sage to induce menstruation and herbal pessaries were known in ancient and medieval times. A medical treatise published by Pope John XXI, before he was elevated to the papacy in 1276, contains practical information about birth control available to the poor (1997, 33). Opposition to birth control grew during the Middle Ages, however, with theologians such as St. Thomas Aquinas and the Catholic Church increasingly taking the stance that sexual intercourse was only for procreation within marriage (1997, 91). During the Inquisition, contraception and midwifery became associated with witchcraft (1997, 110) and persecution. Criminalization of abortion dates from 1791 in France and 1803 in Britain; the first statute criminalizing abortion in the United States was enacted in Connecticut in 1821 (1997, 206–209). Kristin Luker (2008, Chapter 2) details how the rise of antiabortion laws in nineteenth-century America—by 1900 every state prohibited abortion at any stage in pregnancy—was encouraged by physicians seeking to wrest control of reproduction from midwives. The American Medical Association, founded in 1847, resolved to condemn abortion in 1859 and thereafter began lobbying and educational efforts opposed to abortion (Luker 2008, 20).

Today, physicians' attitudes toward abortion are to some extent more favorable. One recent study in the United Kingdom indicates that the vast majority of general practitioners there consider themselves broadly supportive of women's choices about abortion (Francome and Freeman 2000). A recent US study indicated that about half of maternal fetal medicine fellowship trainees received opportunities for dilation and evacuation training in cases of pregnancy complications; an additional one-third of the fellows in programs not offering the training would welcome the opportunity. Receiving training is highly correlated with plans to provide the service in practice (Rosenstein et al. 2014). Nonetheless, there remain substantial numbers of physicians who are ethically opposed to at least some reproductive interventions, especially pregnancy terminations and some uses of reproductive technologies such as preimplantation genetic diagnosis for sex selection.

In a liberal society, the presence of divergent ethical views among physicians raises the problem of conscientious objection: under what circumstances is it permissible for a health care provider or institution to refuse to provide otherwise legal medical care that is desired by patients? May providers not only refuse to perform procedures themselves but also refuse to tell patients about these procedures or to refer patients to willing providers? Medical associations and the laws of many jurisdictions address these questions. For example, the British Medical Association guidance (2015) provides that physicians should have the right to conscientious objection when other providers are available and patients are not disadvantaged. Ethics Opinion 10.05 (2008) of the American Medical Association states that in nonemergency situations it may be ethically permissible for physicians to decline treatment incompatible with their personal, religious, or moral beliefs, as long as they are not engaged in invidious discrimination. Many jurisdictions specify a variety of conscientious objection legal rights for physicians, pharmacists, and sometimes other health care providers—although rights to conscientious objection may be less protected for salaried health care workers such as nurses and radiology technicians. The US Supreme Court has ruled that under the federal constitutional free exercise clause, corporations with religious owners cannot be required to pay for insurance coverage of contraception for their employees.[3]

In Chapter 9, Armand Antommaria takes up the ethical questions raised by conscientious objection, beginning by clarifying what conscience is. In Antommaria's view, conscience is a sense of moral integrity. Problems of conscientious objection arise when there is a lack of congruence between a professional's fundamental moral beliefs and expected actions, including cooperation with others. With respect to cooperation, theologians have argued that there is a difference between formal cooperation, when the cooperator shares the immoral intention, and material cooperation, in which the intention is not shared. Material cooperation may be immediate—participating in the act—or mediate, when the participation is remote. Antommaria argues that these distinctions are ethically relevant when considering the burden on the provider's fundamental beliefs: participating in an abortion, for example, is different from referring a patient to another provider for consultation about an abortion. On the other side, professionals have role responsibilities and responsibilities to their patients. The dominant approach to this tension is to identify systems that can accommodate both providers and their patients. Possible accommodations include providers making their limits clear to patients so that patients do not establish relationships with providers who may be unwilling to meet their needs. Accommodations might also include practicing within structures that make a service available from other providers. Accommodations should not place undue burdens on patients, however. Thus, providers should not blame or criticize their patients or behave in an obstructionist fashion (for example, by destroying prescriptions). Patients also should always be able to receive emergency care, care within a reasonable time, and care in an alternative manner that is reasonable. Providers must give patients adequate and unbiased information; referrals must be made when information is not otherwise readily available for patients; and providers must cooperate when patients choose to seek care elsewhere. Some of these obligations, Antommaria contends, also apply to institutions.

In Chapter 10, Judith Daar considers related questions about the role of providers in assisted reproduction technologies (ART). One problem in ART is that it may be unclear whether there is a provider–patient relationship at all between the ART physician and some participants in the process, such as gamete donors. Providers also may question whether to provide services to particular patients. In the United States at least, the standard legal view is that providers are free to choose whether or not to accept patients, unless their decisions would violate antidiscrimination laws or would be in violation of their contractual obligations. Difficult issues for physicians may include patients who are eager to receive care but who are at elevated risk from pregnancy complications, who are very unlikely to achieve a successful pregnancy with ART, who are carriers for serious genetic diseases, who are at risk for transmitting infectious diseases such as HIV, or who may seem unsuitable for parenthood. Since many of these patients may be able to reproduce without aid, others may ask why their need for ART services should be a barrier to their ability to achieve the important goal of having a child.

Guidance from professional organizations may be available to providers facing these dilemmas. For example, the American Society for Reproductive Medicine (ASRM) recommends special security practices for management of samples from HIV-positive gamete donors; the ASRM ethics committee judges that services should be offered if couples are willing to accept risk-reducing therapies and are fully informed. ASRM also states that providers may ethically refuse to provide services in cases of well-documented likelihood of risks to the child, for example cases in which the intended parents have a proven history of child abuse. By contrast, Daar argues, disability should not be a barrier to services; she is quite critical of the extent to which disability-based discrimination remains common in the fertility industry. As currently delivered, ART services are also disproportionately unavailable to minority women and poor women. Daar concludes her chapter with a discussion of some of the complex issues in the selection of embryos that face ART providers today: requests for sex selection, requests to implant more than two embryos in order to increase chances of achieving pregnancy, and requests for selection for or against particular genetic traits.

Reproductive physicians may also be involved in controversies over research ethics. In the United States, federal regulations governing human research apply strong protections to research involving pregnant women or fetuses. Surprisingly, these regulations even involve the father in some decisions. Among conditions that must be met for the research to be permissible[4] are as follows:

- to the extent appropriate, preclinical and clinical studies on nonpregnant women provide data for assessing risks to pregnant women and fetuses;
- the research must either hold out the prospect of direct benefit for the woman or fetus or, if there is no prospect of such benefit, the risk to the fetus may only be minimal and the purpose of the research must be the development of important biomedical knowledge that cannot be obtained by other means;
- if the research holds out the prospect of direct benefit solely to the fetus, then the consent of the pregnant woman and the father must be obtained, except that the father's consent need not be obtained if he is unable to consent because of unavailability, incompetence, or temporary incapacity; or the pregnancy resulted from rape or incest.

The US approach has been criticized for unduly limiting research with potentially important benefits for pregnant women and the children they bear (Macklin 2010). Some commentators have recommended that pregnant women not be regarded as a "vulnerable" population tagged with a presumption against inclusion in research, but instead be characterized as a scientifically complex population (Blehar et al. 2013). The Council for International Organizations of Medical Sciences (CIOMS) 2002 guideline presumes that pregnant women are eligible for participation in research, if it is relevant to the health needs of pregnant women and appropriate animal studies of teratogenicity or mutagenicity have occurred.[5] The European Parliament Directive governing research with human subjects within the European Union does not contain separate provisions for research with women or pregnant women.[6]

In the United States, research using fetal tissue is permitted under federal law, provided that the woman gives her fully informed consent and any decision about fetal tissue donation is made independently from a decision about abortion. Tissue sales are not permitted.[7] Federal funding for embryonic stem cell research is permitted under Presidential guidelines.[8] States impose a variety of additional restrictions on research involving fetal tissue or embryonic stem cells.[9] The European Commission funds stem cell and fetal tissue research.[10]

Screening of newborns for conditions that require intervention is an important public health measure. In the United Kingdom, screening using blood spots is strongly recommended for nine conditions, including congenital hypothyroidism, cystic fibrosis, sickle cell disease, and metabolic diseases such as phenylketonuria.[11] Blood spots are retained for public health and research, but some research may require parental consent. In the United States, all states require newborn screening for at least some inborn conditions; nearly all states screen for 31 core conditions and many others for at least some of 25 additional recommended conditions.[12] Controversy has erupted in Minnesota, Texas, and other states about retention and use of blood spot samples—despite their importance as a public health resource. As a result of litigation or protests, some states have destroyed their retained samples and others require affirmative parental consent for samples to be retained, with the result that far fewer of these samples will be available for research in the future.

In Chapter 11, Jeffrey Botkin reviews the history and purposes of newborn screening programs and their ethical implications for public health. One important feature of these programs in the United States is that they are provided for everyone regardless of ability to pay, with the costs typically either borne by the delivery facility or bundled into the delivery charge paid by insurance. As such, they are one of the few health care services with universal access in the United States. A second important feature is that they are "mandatory"—that is, presumed without the explicit consent of the parents, although opting out may be permitted if parents know to request it. In 2013, however, the American Academy of Pediatrics and the American College of Medical Genetics recommended requiring parental permission, in part because of the broadened range of conditions included in the screening in many states. Botkin argues that education about screening should be provided to expectant parents before delivery and that his study findings indicate this is likely to increase rather than decrease support for screening. He also points out that population screening can identify low-frequency conditions as well as individuals with biochemical abnormalities that are not apparent from clinical symptoms. Questions remain about the efficacy of newborn screening, especially as it is expanded beyond conditions such are PKU for which immediate interventions are available. Conducting research on the efficacy of screening may be difficult, because it may be unethical to randomize infants to groups that do not receive screening or to implement study designs that mask screening results until clinical symptoms become apparent. The result may be overestimation of the efficacy of screening because of ascertainment bias.

Botkin concludes by speculating about ethical problems that may arise if whole-genome sequencing for newborns becomes readily available. Questions include whether this testing should be universally available and issues of justice if it is not, risks that overemphasis may be placed on predictions of future health, and the role of parental education and choice.

PARENTS

Parents are the central actors in reproduction: without gametes, gestation, and caregivers, offspring would not come into being or survive for long. Despite parents' necessary involvement, the roles, responsibilities, and effects of parenting present diverse ethical challenges. These challenges include the justification for parental rights, what these rights include, what responsibilities parents have, whether there are connections between parental rights and parental responsibilities, how parental rights or responsibilities can be gained or lost, and what entities beyond parents have rights or responsibilities to care for children. These challenges are complicated by the fact that in today's world of reproductive technologies, many different people may be involved in creating a child: providers of gametes, providers of mitochondrial DNA (and perhaps also of DNA used in gene therapy if and when that becomes available), gestators and their partners or other providers of support, legally recognized parents, those intended to be legally recognized parents, and all those involved in treatment along the way. People may, of course, combine these roles: married couples desiring to become pregnant may be the genetic, gestational, actual legal, and intended legal parents of the child. But even here, roles may diverge: a legally married couple may decide that the woman will act as a surrogate gestator for another, or a couple intending to become legal parents may decide to use donated gametes or embryos.

Much reproduction is achieved through ordinary sexual encounters, but much is not; a fundamental question for this part of the volume is why the fact that copulation produces a child generates any special rights or responsibilities on the part of sexual partners toward the child they produce. A related set of questions is whether people who can reproduce in the ordinary way are any different than people who cannot. Should, for example, people who need infertility care or adoption be subject to any different scrutiny in becoming parents than those who do not? Is it justifiable for adoption to be treated differently than assisted reproduction using donated gametes or embryos? Than assisted reproduction itself?

For women and men who cannot conceive children on their own or through assisted reproductive technology, adoption and surrogacy are alternative routes to parenthood. It may come as a surprise to readers that adoption as a formal method of family formation is predominantly a modern phenomenon; before the nineteenth century, adoption was largely a method for legitimating inheritance (Haslanger and Witt 2005, 2–3). With the widespread availability of contraception and abortion, social acceptance of women keeping children conceived out of wedlock, and even social pressures for women not to relinquish children for adoption, numbers of infants available to adoptive parents in the United States have diminished markedly. There are also significant barriers to termination of parental rights; children may remain in foster care for years as a result. By comparison, prospective adoptive parents may face problematic judgments about their qualifications and their family structures—judgments that they would not face if they were able to conceive on their own. Changes in patterns of adoption toward adoption of older children, interracial adoption, adoption of children with what are termed "special needs," and international adoption raise further complex issues of identity and justice (Haslanger and Witt 2005; Javier et al. 2007). To take one illustration, concerns about exploitation, coercion, and child trafficking led the European Union to require Romania to ban intercountry adoptions as a condition of membership, a position the European Union has since reversed (Iusmen 2013). Legal trends against protection of the identity of the birth mother and in favor of open adoption raise questions of confidentiality and informed consent, especially when changes occur years after the original adoption decision. Although this volume does not include a chapter on adoption, many of these issues are explored in the chapters to follow.

Writers within liberal theory tend to argue that some kind of actual or reasonable, affirmative, or voluntary commitment is central to acquiring the rights or responsibilities of parents. Rosamond Rhodes's constructivist view presented in Chapter 3 of this volume, for example, holds that obligations stem from what people have or might reasonably be expected to have accepted. Judith Thomson's famous argument about abortion—that even if an entity has the right to life it doesn't follow that others have obligations to provide the means of life—concedes that certain voluntary actions might give rise to these obligations. Joseph Millum's (2010) desert-based approach attributes moral parenting rights to "the performance of parental work." Whether the connections are necessary conditions, sufficient conditions, necessary and sufficient conditions, prima facie considerations, or have some other looser linkage is an additional complication.

Norvin Richards leads off this section of the volume by asking what entitles parents to rights with respect to particular children from the beginning. Neither creation of the child nor sharing of genetic material with the child suffices, he contends. Nor does Millum's view that parental rights are earned by the parents' investment in the child. In each of these cases, problems arise about why there are rights at all and why these might take the particular form of parental rights. Many conceptions are unintentional. The amount of "investment" the parties producing a child can provide varies, of course with the work of pregnancy and birth being the greatest; but it would seem deeply unfair if advantages of biology or social location importantly affect rights of parents. Many other people invest substantially in children, without acquiring the rights of parents. Still others play important causal roles in a child's coming into being. Moreover, parties may participate in a joint project of creating a child, without one of the two gaining an upper hand on rights by means of larger contributions.

Instead, Richards locates parental rights in what procreators were doing: what they intended, whether they are continuing a morally innocent project they are at liberty to continue, and other aspects of the context within which they act. Promises to each other or expectations they have created matter, Richards argues, to the rights and responsibilities procreators subsequently have. Most difficult are cases in which the pregnancy was unintended or the woman became pregnant in a casual way. In such cases, she may choose to have the pregnancy continue, unless it is morally wrong for her to do so. She is entitled to have the man take on responsibilities of parenting if he promised or created expectations that he would do so if she conceived accidentally. Conversely, she is not free to conceal the pregnancy from him or to choose to shut him out as a parent, if she has created expectations that he would be the father to an otherwise unanticipated child. This does not require her to carry the pregnancy to term—the pregnancy is something she must choose to do with her body—but that it is a prima facie wrong for her to ignore the expectations that have been created. If there are no promises or background of expectations—as in a casual encounter—she may continue the pregnancy and he has no rights to expect to be considered a parent.

Equal causal roles in bringing a pregnancy about, however, may be the basis for responsibilities to deal with the costs, including the emotional costs, of pregnancy. Richards objects to the idea that the male partner has no responsibilities for a pregnancy if the woman decides to continue it, because they both played similar causal roles in bringing about the situation that presents the choice to her. On his view, what she does about being pregnant is not entirely independent of what they did together that resulted in the conception: she has been put in a position in which she must choose among difficult options. Richards then argues that they are equally responsible for the costs of the option it was reasonable to expect she would choose. This does not mean she may make any choice—only a reasonable one—but it does mean that they should share the costs of her choice of continued pregnancy and birth. Richards takes a different position about the costs of raising the child, however. Depending on expectations in the context— including social pressures on her about whether to keep the child and the availability of adoption—the sex that they had is not inevitably linked to the decision on her part to keep and raise the child. Richards's account is rooted in the voluntary actions of agents and the reasonable expectations they create; he concludes by applying this analysis to the expectations created with the use of assisted reproductive technologies.

In Chapter 14, Don Hubin considers sexual asymmetries in procreative duties to support and nurture children. His starting point is that those who voluntarily act in ways they know or should know will result in the creation of a dependent human being have the obligation to take reasonable steps to ensure its support and nurturance. The causal role in creation creates moral obligations, in the absence of special arrangements or justified conventions imposing these obligations on others and in the absence of wrongful actions by others. On Hubin's view, it is not necessary that the individual either intend or voluntarily accept the obligation—the voluntary causal role suffices. Hubin formulates a nuanced responsibility for dependent life principle that generates duties prima facie and then traces the implications of this principle through a variety of thought experiments designed to isolate factors that might diminish or remove the responsibility of one or both parties.

Hubin begins by rejecting a "copulator beware" principle to the effect that voluntary participation in sexual relations is sufficient for responsibility for any resulting dependent life. Such a strict liability approach is inconsistent with our views about responsibility for the consequences of action: for example, we do not hold people responsible for causal consequences when they acted as a result of wrongful deception if their reliance on the deception was reasonable. Lying by one partner about the use of reliable contraception (or sterilization) is an example; so is deception about whether a sexual act that could result in procreation is involved at all. The Frisard case—in which purloined sperm was used for insemination—should not have resulted in a finding of responsibility for child support, Hubin contends. But there may of course be circumstances in which it is not reasonable to rely on the representation of others, and Hubin also takes the position that individuals should bear some responsibility for their own fertility, a position explored more fully by Battin in Chapter 15. Asymmetries between the positions of men and women are relevant as well: Hubin would extend the moral authority of the pregnant woman to make decisions about termination to all cases and asks whether a woman's failure to have an abortion could ever be counted as the kind of wrongful conduct that would absolve a male of responsibility. He says that it does in the case in which she has promised that she will get an abortion if conception occurs and he has made it clear that this commitment is necessary for him to be involved in sexual relations.

That only women become pregnant is an obvious sexual asymmetry. Less discussed—but clearly important—is sexual asymmetry with respect to currently available contraception and abortifacient technologies. In Chapter 15, Margaret Battin presses the issues of justice these asymmetries present. The asymmetry with regard to after-the fact actions is clear-cut. Only women can take emergency contraception or obtain abortions, absent coercion; no one considers the science fiction possibility that men might be able to turn off sperm motility, other features of sperm, or efficacy of their contribution to fertilization after the fact. Perhaps the possibility seems altogether science fictional—or perhaps the explanation is that once sperm have entered the woman's body it seems to commentators that what happens must be up to the woman's control over her body or be judged unacceptably intrusive on her.

Battin describes the dismal picture with respect to the contraceptive options currently available to men—abstinence, condoms, or vasectomy—and the much better possibilities on the horizon for them. Available methods have grave disadvantages, including ineffectiveness, intrusiveness, and nonreversibility. Contraceptives available to women, by contrast, may be undetectable, effective, after the fact, safe, and long acting. Compounding these differences are social inequalities: male blaming and legal policies that hold the male financially responsible, even in the cases of fraud rejected by Richards and Hubin.

But, as Battin puts it, "help" may be on the way for men; many forms of male contraception are currently under development. Issues to consider about these contraceptives, in comparison to methods available to women, include safety, efficacy, impact on sexual drive and the experience of sex, mechanism of interference, and costs. There will be great advantages for men in having more methods available: sharing the responsibility of contraception, enhancing sexual freedom, and avoiding the need for political and legal controls, among others. Most important, Battin thinks, is the potential advantage of equality in the procreative decision. Battin concludes her chapter with a thought experiment: what if safe, effective, reversible, and long-acting contraception were routinely used by both men and women? With such double coverage, both parties would need to make affirmative decisions to try to achieve conception, rather than letting it happen accidentally. Battin argues that this would introduce a form of equality into contemporary sexual relations in many areas of the world today—although she also recognizes that there may be circumstances in which the male's ability to use contraception might subject women to coercion or deprive them of sources of power in contexts of social or economic inequality.

Two chapters in this section consider pregnancy and motherhood. It is perhaps an accident of editorial invitations that unlike the chapters considering the role of parents and fathers, both of these chapters draw on relational theories rather than liberal individualism as modes of analysis. Or perhaps it is not accidental, as motherhood and care have been central areas of interest for feminist theory (e.g., Noddings 1984; Ruddick 1989; Kittay 1999). These chapters consider two stages in the chronology of the narrative of becoming a mother—pregnancy and motherhood—and their implications for identity.

Pregnancy may alter women's self-conceptions in many ways. In Chapter 23, Hilde Lindemann unmasks three destructive narratives of pregnancy: the woman as fetal container, as good mother, and as public body. She then constructs counterstories against these damaging master narratives. Primary examples are stories that describe pregnant women as calling the fetuses they carry into personhood.

Even when it is wanted, but more so when it is undesired, pregnancy may force changes in self-conception, from feeling violated or inhabited by an alien, to not trusting a body's ability to keep a cherished other safe, to marveling at every moment of development. Master narratives shape these self-conceptions. The narrative of the fetal container, that the woman is entirely separate from the entity growing within, degrades the woman as a passive piece of equipment rather than an agent bringing a child into the world. It sees the interests of the woman-vessel as pitted against and subservient to those of the fetus-within. This narrative erases the woman and fails to understand the developing woman–fetus relationship, which is proleptic in the sense that it treats a future state of affairs (the presence of the child) as though it already had come into being.

The master narrative of the good mother is also destructive, treating the pregnant woman as obligated to submerge her interests to the best interests of her future child. Caregiver narratives may also be linked with cultural norms or discriminatory expectations about who should have children and provide support for them. Women may be blamed or even punished for their actions, such as working, refusing to accept unwanted medical care, allowing their children to take public transit or otherwise act independently, or failing to protect their children from abusers. Lindemann details how the good mother narrative subjects poor women and women of color to social policing in the name of fetal protection.

The third destructive master narrative is that of the public body subject outright to social control and policing. It treats the fetus as already a born child and supervises the mother so that the fetus will not come to harm from her actions. Total strangers may criticize women in public for drinking alcohol; health care providers may call in social authorities if she acts against medical advice.

In response, women must develop counterstories to these identity-destroying narratives. These counterstories must support the woman's agency in developing the relationship of the fetus becoming a child. Social institutions, policies, and practices must supplement stories that oppose these oppressive narratives of identity.

In Chapter 13, Sara Goering further develops themes of how motherhood and mothering affect autonomy. Mothering both makes us aware of the relational nature of our selves and can help to enhance the relational autonomy of mothers. Becoming a parent, she says, expands the self; deciding what to do is not simply a matter of self-assessment but must also take into account the needs and desires of a dependent being. Such transformations from "I" to "we" may expand to other relationships such as those with partners or spouses or families. This is not to say that the individual drops out but that the individual exists within units of shared goods in addition to individual goods. These units of sharing are not fixed in time; they grow and change as children become older and more independent. Our relationships, according to Goering, are both necessary for autonomy but also influence how autonomy is exercised. The difficulty is to ensure that relationality fosters rather than entraps autonomy's exercise.

Goering agrees with Lindemann that narratives play major roles in how identities are constructed. Such dependence on the recognition and responses of others leaves us vulnerable to devaluing or denial of important forms of identity, especially as we develop and change. Women who relished staying home with their children during infancy may be trapped by others' expectations that they continue in full-time caregiver roles. Children, too, need to develop independent identities, and Goering believes that these possibilities can be applied back to mothers themselves. The mothering relationship grows and develops in social contexts and must be supported not only by changing expectations but also communities of engagement in childrearing. Distributed responsibilities for child care, relational networks of support, family-friendly parks and workplaces are all necessary to ensure that motherhood is not a lonely activity and that the relational autonomy of mothers and others function together.

The dark side of fertility is infertility: the challenges facing those who very much wish to become parents but are unable to reproduce on their own. In Chapter 16, David Orentlicher argues that access to infertility care is a matter of social justice. He begins by noting the irony that despite the many family-friendly policies in the United States, there is little support for people who are infertile and are trying to become parents. Infertility is estimated to affect upwards of 15% of couples in the United States; rates are rising as people delay childbirth and as same-sex couples and single individuals increasingly seek parenthood. Orentlicher documents the lack of support for people in these situations by considering IVF, surrogate motherhood, and uterine transplantation.

In the United States, most couples seeking IVF must pay for this expensive treatment on their own; by contrast, insurance coverage for contraception and abortion is available far more widely. Particularly devastating for some people seeking care is the exclusion of IVF coverage from insurance available to disabled veterans, a limitation imposed by Congress in 1992 because of political opposition to the creation of frozen embryos that might never be implanted (PBS Newshour 2016). In the United Kingdom, although IVF is available through the National Health Service, it is only available for a limited number of cycles (three for women under 40; one for women over 40 with good ovarian reserve) (NICE 2013). In some other countries, health insurance covers IVF. Exclusions of IVF cannot be justified on the ground that it does not correct the underlying problem, as many forms of medical treatment compensate for lost function in this way. Nor can the exclusions be justified on cost–benefit analysis, as the treatment's effectiveness is much improved and data from areas where coverage is available indicate that it adds little to overall health care costs.

For people who seek to reproduce but cannot carry a pregnancy, surrogacy is an option. Many legal jurisdictions either prohibit or do not enforce contracts for what is termed "traditional" surrogacy, in which the pregnant woman is both the genetic and the gestational mother of the child. More jurisdictions will enforce contracts for gestational surrogacy, which employs an oocyte from either the intended parent or a donor, but even this technique is not permitted in many areas of the world. Orentlicher argues that despite the well-known objections to surrogacy, opposition to the practice discounts the interests of persons who are infertile. We do not, for example, expect otherwise fertile persons to adopt children rather than procreating themselves—yet this expectation is often suggested as a preferable alternative to surrogacy. And we overemphasize the interests of the surrogate to an extent not supported by the evidence.

Another possible intervention to enable pregnancy is uterus transplantation. Only a few of these procedures have been performed worldwide, and the situation about these transplants is changing quickly. Sweden reported the first live birth following a transplant in 2015 and has now reported five (Brannstrom et al. 2015; Grady 2016). The first in the United States occurred in a clinical trial at the Cleveland Clinic in February 2016 (NPR 2016) but failed shortly thereafter (Grady 2016). Critics of the procedure argue that it is not therapeutic, that it is a poor use of health care resources, and that its benefits do not justify its risks. Orentlicher contends that none of these justifications are persuasive; we support other health care interventions that make important contributions to quality of life even when they carry risks comparable to those of uterine transplantation. Even though women with oocyte reserve but uterine malfunction can achieve genetic parenthood through surrogacy, the experience of pregnancy itself (even without pelvic nerve connections) may be so valuable to these women that uterine transplantation should be a medically available option, Orentlicher contends.

Orentlicher concludes by arguing that infertility is not only a medical problem, with both physical and psychological implications, but also a disability. Protections from disability law are limited, however, and people with infertility too frequently find their interests trivialized or disparaged. These problems are especially severe for the socially infertile, same-sex couples, or individuals who cannot reproduce on their own. Some feminist writers even criticize the desire to reproduce as nonautonomous and a manifestation of patriarchy. Others see it as enabling women to lead free and fulfilling lives, despite the strong desires of many to become parents.

In Chapter 19, Imogen Goold develops these themes in the context of women delaying childbearing to their later years. Women who postpone childbearing until their late 30s or even later may be blamed for their inability to conceive, ridiculed if they are postmenopausal, or accused of being selfish and wanting to have it all. They may face legal or financial barriers to infertility care that include age cutoffs for access to treatment. They receive mixed messages that medical intervention may be able to help them conceive despite delay but that pregnancy may be difficult to achieve because of decreased ovarian reserve or risky because of medical conditions such as hypertension. These and other criticisms of women who delay childbearing, Goold contends, fail to take account of the many justifications women may have for postponing reproduction. Childbearing in later life should not be seen simplistically as a conflict between women's reproductive autonomy and risks of harm to self or others, but in the context of a complex set of questions about social justice.

Goold begins her discussion by addressing the argument that women who delay reproduction should bear the consequences of their decisions. Although fertility declines naturally with age, the distinction between such "natural" infertility and infertility due to disease or premature menopause cannot be sustained, she argues. Women delay childbearing for many reasons: lack of knowledge about infertility and especially childbearing risks at older ages, lack of stable partners, partners' desires to wait, pursuit of higher education and career goals, and economic instability. These decisions take place in social contexts in which women are expected disproportionately to perform carer roles, may receive limited support in so doing, and may suffer significant disadvantages in their careers from taking time to be with their children. The United States, for example, does not require employers to provide paid parental leave. As a general matter, we do not make receipt of health care dependent on whether individual choices about risks played a role in illness or functional limitations. This is especially so where the risks are reasonable, choices among them complex, and the consequences are not proportional to the risks. The harm of infertility may be significant, and it may be difficult to judge whose choices were such that they do not "deserve" help; on Goold's view, providing a social safety net of care when risks ensue helps people to lead more fulfilling lives and is thus justified as a matter of social justice.

The argument that later reproduction, and particularly postmenopausal reproduction, is "unnatural" is also flawed. Health care frequently addresses natural malfunctions to improve quality of life. Moreover, that something is "unnatural" does not mean that it is unethical; that conclusion would require further argument. The argument from nature, however, may rest on a more forceful concern: that risks of pregnancy to both mother and fetus do go up as women age. Miscarriage rates, hypertension rates, caesarean section rates, and rates of gestational diabetes are higher in older women. Goold argues that these increases do not mean that treatment is immoral: patient autonomy requires that people be able to choose the risks they are willing to run to achieve benefits that are important to them. Organizations such as the American Society for Reproductive Medicine take similar positions, arguing that if women are fully informed, it is ethical to provide treatment to them even though risks are elevated; ASRM also holds that if risks are too high, or if the likelihood of success is too low, physicians may ethically decline to provide treatment (ASRM 2012a, 2013a). Perhaps support for Goold's view that women of advanced age receive less favorable consideration, ASRM also holds that fertility treatment should be strongly discouraged for high-risk women of advanced age, but it does not similarly caution treatment that is unlikely to succeed or treatment of younger women who have become infertile due to treatment for cancer. (ASRM 2012a, 2013a, 2013b).

Risks of harm to offspring raise a more difficult set of questions that cannot be answered by invocation of the liberal harm principle that intervention is only justified to prevent harm to others. Concededly, there are greater risks to offspring of older mothers. Some of these risks can be mitigated by single embryo transfer in IVF (thus reducing risks of twin pregnancy) and by good prenatal care. Other risks, of fetal anomalies, miscarriage, low birth weight, or preterm labor will still remain elevated. But many younger women face these risks as well; it would seem arbitrary to make age the determining factor rather than individual assessments of risk. Concerns that parents will be unable to care for their children or may die before they reach adulthood must also be weighed against the benefits of older parents such as more time, greater maturity, or greater economic stability. Any discussion of these risks must pay careful attention to the evidence and must avoid arbitrary decisions to treat age as a limiting factor when these risks occur across the continuum of parental ages. A final caution is that the choice is between existence and nonexistence, not between better or worse lives for a particular child; this so-called nonidentity problem plays a major role in the chapters in Part IV of this volume.

Social harms are another objection raised to fertility treatment of older mothers. These potential harms include costs of the infertility care itself, costs of care for higher risk newborns, and costs of care if one or both parents become incompetent or die. Like Orentlicher, Goold believes that these costs must be weighed against the very real benefits of parenthood to people who would otherwise have been infertile. Goold also agrees that it is reasonable to consider probabilities of success in the allocation of limited state resources and to turn to oocyte donation when probabilities of pregnancy with the woman's own eggs are low. Goold concludes that far more social harm could be avoided by remedying social conditions that press women to delay, such as inadequate child care or workplace policies that discourage family leave.

For people who cannot become pregnant, surrogacy is a legal alternative in many jurisdictions. Surrogacy remains the target of significant criticism, however. The most developed criticisms attack commercial surrogacy, as baby selling, exploitation of the surrogate, risks to offspring, or even human trafficking. Donna Dickenson's Chapter 5 in Part I of this volume is a powerful illustration of these criticisms. In her chapter on surrogacy, Leslie Francis considers whether surrogacy might be ethically permissible if we set aside concerns about exploitation and trafficking. Even if much surrogacy is frankly or disguisedly exploitative, this is an important question, as many defenders of surrogacy would like to see the practice continue if abuses can be addressed. Francis counters three objections to surrogacy in any form: carrying a child is a type of bodily labor that it is impermissible for one person to perform for another, that surrogacy damages the identity of the resulting child, and that surrogacy fails to respect the relationship between the pregnant woman and the child-to-be. Francis's strategy is to argue that none of these claims can be sustained without rejecting other, clearly acceptable practices.

Francis begins with the distinction between traditional surrogacy—in which the surrogate is both gestational and genetic mother—and gestational surrogacy, in which she does not contribute the oocyte. Early legal challenges to surrogacy in the United States involved traditional surrogacy in exchange for payment and reasoned that it was impermissible because it violated state prohibitions on payment for adoption. Courts also believed it inevitably coercive to enforce contracts to relinquish the child entered into before its birth. This reasoning continued in some cases involving gestational surrogacy, although other courts characterized this practice as contracting for a service—childbearing—rather than contracting for the child. Francis points out that although courts characterize the practice as "natural" or "unnatural," they are really making legal choices about parentage. For example, some courts refusing to enforce prebirth agreements have nonetheless allowed issuance of the child's birth certificate to be delayed until the gestational mother agrees to relinquish her parental rights, so that the intended parents can be listed as the child's legal parents from birth.

Is surrogacy a permissible form of bodily labor? People are permitted to perform labor that uses their bodies for others, even when the use is invasive or risky. Organ donations, nursing, and home care are illustrations of risky uses of one individual's body for another; we allow these to happen and even regard them as praiseworthy in altruistic familial contexts. Commercial forms of nursing or care (but not organ "donation") are permissible, too; a problem with apparently altruistic surrogacy trenchantly observed by Dickenson is that what is described as altruistic may actually be commercialized in disguise. Francis agrees that the distinction between altruistic and compensated surrogacy may be difficult to draw. Pregnancy itself brings added expenses, significant opportunity costs, and even risks—and it would seem unfair to surrogates to expect them to bear all of these costs on their own. Although it may conceal exploitation to mislead-ingly characterize surrogacy as a gift, it may also be exploitative to insist that the practice be uncompensated.

A second type of objection to surrogacy in all forms is that it uses the gestating wom-an's body to serve the interests of intended parent(s). To this, Francis asks whether the physical use of a woman's body to produce a child for another necessarily fails to treat the pregnant woman as a subject of respect. She agrees that exploitative arrangements fail to show respect, but points out that it begs the question to stipulate that all surro-gacy arrangements are necessarily exploitative in this way. Arguments that the surrogate fails to demonstrate sufficient self-respect are similarly lacking. Francis also questions whether prebirth agreements should always be rejected: it is paternalistic to prohibit people from entering into contracts that they might later regret, and potentially stereo-typing to assume that any woman would develop feelings toward the child she carries that are so strong that it would be unconscionable to enforce a contract she has entered. Even conceding that enforcement of prebirth surrogacy agreements would be uncon-scionable, it remains possible to structure surrogacy contracts to permit the woman to change her mind for a period after birth, without introducing too much uncertainty into most surrogacy arrangements.

A final objection that Francis considers is that surrogacy alienates the parenting relationship and by so doing fails to respect the interests of the child. Here Francis asks why the parenting relationship should necessarily lie between the gestator and the resulting child and not between the intended parents and the resulting child. Answers that rely on the assumption that surrogacy is wrong or that genetic parent-age should take priority beg the question. If the intended parent(s) *are* the parents of the resulting child, then even commercial surrogacy is not selling the child, or even rights over the child; any pay for the surrogate goes for her bodily labor. To be sure, the child has rights to protection and to adequate parenting, but why these should be presumed for gestational or genetic parentage, but not intended legal parentage, is unclear.

People who require assistance to reproduce are dependent on their interaction with others. As several chapters in this volume discuss, people in disfavored groups may encounter significant barriers in accessing these services. Disability discrimination is a particularly pressing concern for those seeking assisted reproduction. Despite opinions of professional bodies to the contrary (ASRM 2013c) and laws prohibiting discrimina-tion against people with disabilities, people with disabilities report ongoing challenges to their efforts to become—as well as to remain—parents. Some of these challenges rest on problematic assumptions about the abilities of people with disabilities as parents. In Chapter 18, Adam Cureton dispels a number of myths about people with disabili-ties as parents. Himself a person with a visual impairment, Cureton details how people with disabilities may not be seen as sexual beings, romantic partners, or likely parents. General legal rules may not be sufficiently subtle to account for differing needs of peo-ple with disabilities. Importantly, moral and legal rights to parenting must be seen as separate questions; Cureton explores how the rights and well-being of children can be integrated with meaningful opportunities for people with disabilities to experience the values of having and raising children.

Multiple values are at stake when people decide to have and raise children: the value for people of having and raising children, the abilities of people to make important decisions about their own lives such as decisions about whether to reproduce, the well-being of vulnerable children, the importance of avoiding detrimental treatment based on stereotypes, and respect for dignity. Legal rules such as the ADA insist on individualized assessments when people are excluded from public services or public accommodations (such as medical clinics) because they are thought to pose risks to others. Reasonable accommodations are also required for persons who meet essential eligibility requirements for services or benefits. Cureton details how jurisdictions often fail to consider individual skills or provide effective accommodations in making decisions about custody or parental rights. Additional questions of justice arise when people with disabilities may lack the economic resources to seek reproductive assistance, to secure legal representation in custody proceedings, or to pay for adapting their homes to parenting or for other forms of parenting assistance. Cureton notes that people with disabilities may face disadvantages or forms of scrutiny, for example about fitness to parent, which are not imposed on others. Difficulties in specifying what kinds of resources should be socially available should not obscure the importance of avoiding these kinds of unfair disadvantages that are imposed on parents with disabilities. Moreover, a Rawlsian view about justice, under which liberties are given priority, fair equality of opportunity is provided for children, and economic resources are distributed fairly, may respond to concerns about resource allocations that enable people with disabilities to become parents.

A major portion of Cureton's chapter is devoted to discussion of how persons with disabilities may be good parents who serve the interests of the children they have. There is no single model of good parenting, Cureton claims, nor should we assume that one impairment automatically diminishes other skills or that reasonable accommodations will not be available and effective. Because parents with disabilities may require social services more frequently than other parents, and thus come under scrutiny, we should not assume that higher reported rates of deficiency reflect higher underlying rates overall. Fitness assessments must be conducted under conditions of accommodation and not in unfamiliar places such as public offices. Family and social supports matter, too. Most important, different forms of parenting by people with disabilities may yield values for their children: patience, self-reliance, compassion, and flexibility, among others.

Other issues about disability and parenting concern the social costs of having and raising children with disabilities. In Chapter 20, David Wasserman addresses an underexplored but often voiced objection to reproduction and disability: that having children with disabilities unjustly imposes increased costs on society. This concern may be raised because people with disabilities are thought more likely to have children with disabilities, because people with disabilities choose to have children like themselves, or because people without disabilities choose to parent despite known risks that they are likely or even almost certain to bear children with disabilities. This social costs argument may have been underexamined, Wasserman hypothesizes, because it echoes disfavored earlier eugenics movements. Yet social costs may be the most plausible objection to reproduction despite known disabilities, so Wasserman addresses the argument directly. In its most cautious form, the argument is for shared financing of prenatal diagnosis based on expected cost savings for society, perhaps also with increased responsibility for costs for parents who had reasonable opportunities to avoid the birth of a child with disabilities.

Wasserman's argument is that assumptions about increased costs are largely illusory. As a starting point, the luck egalitarian principle that people should be responsible for the costs of their voluntary choices but not for costs they do not control applies generally to people who voluntarily choose to become parents. If justice requires society to share the costs of raising children generally, there must be a special case for imposing the additional costs of disability on parents who could reasonably have chosen to avoid birth. What that case might be is unclear, however. The burdens of having and raising children with serious disabilities are often exaggerated and postulated without consideration of offsetting potential benefits of raising children with disabilities. As for exaggerated costs, Wasserman presents data that actual costs, while higher, may not be as high as many assume. Moreover, in assessing these costs, it is important to take into account background justice requirements of inclusion, although it might still be argued that parents are responsible for some of these costs if they could have avoided them easily. An additional point is that costs may stem from a background of injustice, for example, the failure to provide adequate child care, parental leave, or access to health care.

Finally, proposals to incentivize prenatal screening for and selection against disabilities must be consistent with other features of the distribution of social costs. In the United States, parents are positively encouraged by tax deductions and other benefits for having additional children. The only clear counterexamples to such encouragement are policies that cap welfare payments or reproductive assistance at a certain number of children. Discussions include how the costs of having and raising children with disabilities should be considered in light of the overall justice of social policies about support for children and families. They should also be considered in light of overall views about the role of the family in society. Wasserman's view is that there may be reasons to respect familial autonomy, despite its apparent conflicts at times with state interests, by adopting universal design measures that build inclusion and pursuing policies such as environmental protection that reduce overall disability risks.

Rounding out Part III are two chapters considering gamete donation. Lorna A. Marshall, a physician who provides fertility care, reviews the ethical issues in contemporary care involving egg donation in Chapter 21. Drawing on her extensive experience in patient care, Marshall details the particular issues raised by the complexity of obtaining donor eggs in comparison to donor sperm. Egg donation requires hormonal stimulation via injections and a surgical procedure for egg removal. Ovarian hyperstimulation syndrome is the most immediate complication; longer term risks of the procedure are simply unknown, although they are believed to be low. One difficulty is thus informed consent: patients who are providing eggs for others receive no direct benefits themselves and risks are not readily quantified. There is some evidence that clinics do an inadequate job of explaining risks and benefits. Although concerns have been raised that young adults are unable to independently assess risks and benefits, one study has shown adequate comprehension after an information session; education of participants is thus very important.

Commercialization poses other ethical problems for gamete use. Although "egg donation" is labeled altruistically, compensation is frequent and widely varied. The development of technologies for egg freezing, along with egg banking, has increased commodification of donor egg services. Increased egg costs may create incentives to overstimulate, thus raising risks of the procedure for women. High costs for eggs may also make IVF with donor eggs inaccessible for many women; markets in eggs may raise red flags about eugenics if participants' desires for traits perceived as particularly "valuable" were to become widespread. Increased payment for eggs may incentivize women to discount risks or discomfort of the procedure. Some jurisdictions now prohibit payment for eggs; on the other hand, it is arguably unfair to poorer women to deny compensation for the procedure. Additionally, although recommendations are that women undergo no more than six cycles of egg retrieval, there are no ways of tracing women who may provide services to multiple clinics. Privacy concerns must be addressed if adequate data are to be collected. Some donors may wish only to donate to married heterosexual couples; Marshall argues that it is problematic to honor discriminatory preferences. She also notes the increased concerns raised by cross-border reproductive care.

Donations by family members are popular because they may preserve at least some genetic linkage and because they may be less costly. The possibilities of intrafamilial pressure mean that special care is needed to ensure that consent is informed and voluntary. Donations among members of the same generation appear generally positive; concerns have been raised about intergenerational donation (daughter to mother, mother to daughter), but no reliable data exist about their implications for families.

The welfare of offspring is another concern about donor egg conception. Here, Marshall sides with the ASRM position that it is ethical to provide reproductive assistance unless there is a reasonable basis for thinking that a resulting child will suffer significant harm (ASRM 2013c). Marshall also thinks it is permissible to provide oocytes to older or postmenopausal women if risks are adequately evaluated and consent informed. In addition, she observes the importance of the procedure for same-sex couples and for single women or men, as well as the option for shared biological motherhood for lesbian couples when one donates the oocyte and the other carries the child. Indeed, one court in the United Kingdom has already considered the determination of parenthood in the case of a lesbian couple, one member of whom had carried embryos created from the other member's egg and donor sperm, requiring a detailed factual hearing on whether the estranged parties should share residential custody of the children, Re G (Children) [2014]EWCA Civ 336, http://www.familylawweek.co.uk/site.aspx?i=ed128566. A major future for egg donation may be women seeking to preserve their own eggs for later use; unfortunately, patients who seem to be using this procedure are older women, although the procedure is less likely to be beneficial for this group than for younger women.

Marshall also notes the variations among jurisdictions about donor anonymity and whether offspring should be informed about the circumstances of their conception, concluding that discussions may be trending toward greater openness. I. Glenn Cohen, in Chapter 22, considers the specific issue of donor anonymity in detail. He begins with the contrast between the United States, which still largely permits donor anonymity, and other jurisdictions across the globe where it is likely to be prohibited. In these jurisdictions, anonymity is "passive" in the sense that information about donors is available to children at the requisite age if they request it; later in the chapter Cohen questions whether arguments for disclosure can be limited to passive rather than active methods. Countries prohibiting anonymity have experienced short and possibly longer term declines in donor participation, although the data are unclear. A particular interpretive difficulty is that many jurisdictions that prohibit anonymity also prohibit or limit compensation; Cohen's empirical work suggests that donors would require a premium (in the $30–$40 range for sperm) to permit disclosure of donor information.

Cohen then discusses the situation in the United States, where there have been limited chinks in the legal armor of anonymity. More effective than legal changes has been use of the Internet by donors and children seeking to find one another. When physicians are involved in the donation, rather than private parties working with one another, courts are unlikely to assign paternity to the genetic father. This has been important in assuring the supply and use of donor sperm; donors may not want additional obligations, and recipients may not want unexpected intrusions into their family structures. Cohen, however, thinks that these arguments may not be entirely convincing and that there should be room to open up questions about the possibility of establishing legal relationships when the parties desire them.

The primary legal debate, however, has been whether the United States is wrong in largely permitting sperm donor anonymity, and Cohen contends that it is not. Cohen enters this debate by observing that although it may be important for children to have health information from their genetic parents, this information can be obtained without releasing identifying information and is often incomplete even when identifying information is available. Moreover, this information may be less relevant in a future of whole-genome sequencing and the use of large-scale databases to ascertain the significance of genetic variants. Cohen also questions the relevance of adoption as an analogy to gamete donation; data suggest that adoption and gamete donation may be quite different for those involved in them.

Cohen then turns to arguments in favor of prohibiting anonymity based on the interests of donors and rearing parents. If, surprisingly, interests of sperm donors favor disclosure, this consideration may be accounted for by differential pricing in market terms. There is also no reason to think that if preferences change after donation agreements, the most likely change is to be in the direction of preferring disclosure.

Nor is there an argument favoring disclosure based on the interests of the children: children available for adoption already exist, whereas donor-conceived offspring would not exist without the donation. This is called the "nonidentity" problem, which will reappear in Part IV—that because different children are involved, comparisons do not lie between states of affairs for the same person but between different people. Because of this problem there is no case to be made that the interests of a particular child favor disclosure, if the only alternative for that child would have been nonexistence. Cohen also questions whether disclosure would be better for the population as a whole. Such harms to offspring or others are consequentialist considerations; Cohen concludes the chapter by criticizing a variety of nonconsequentialist arguments for required disclosure.

Last but Not Least: Zygote, Blastocyst, Embryo, Fetus, Newborn

As outlined earlier, the status of fertilized oocytes, at whatever stage, is hotly contested. It cannot be handled by any simple application of the liberal harm principle, because at issue is whether the entity in question—zygote, blastocyst, embryo, fetus, or even newborn—has the kind of status to come under the purview of that principle.

A complex problem that runs through the chapters in this part is the "nonidentity problem" identified by Derek Parfit. Suppose someone contemplating pregnancy has a choice: she can stop taking contraceptives now, knowing that she has an upcoming trip with her partner to an area of the world where Zika virus infections are common, or she can wait to stop taking contraceptives until their return. If she stops before the trip, she may conceive a child who will suffer the effects of the virus; if she waits, she will conceive a child who will not. But they will not be the same child: hence, their "nonidentity." Thus, a child she conceives during her trip cannot complain that s/he could have been born without the effects of the virus, had her mother only waited. The only way to argue she would have been better off if her mother had not stopped contraception when she did, would be that on balance her life is not worth living at all. The world overall might have been better had the woman waited to conceive, but this is not to say that it would have been better for any particular person had she done so.

In Chapter 24, Adam Kadlac addresses an apparent paradox posed by this problem: people who have had children at a time when it might have been better for them to have waited both recognize that it would have been better for them to have waited but be unwilling to trade the situation of parenthood that they are actually experiencing. Acknowledging the burdens of their choices, they still would not have had it any other way. While other commentators have dissolved this tension as a change in values, Kadlac's solution is a deeper appeal to an account of our identity as the particular persons we are: that our identity varies and becomes increasingly fixed by our historical circumstances. Our identities are constituted by shared histories with others: as parents, children, or siblings. We become who we are through these interactions and this exerts "normative pull" on us.

But what if things don't work out and the relationship does not develop? People may regard decisions to have children at particular points in time as wronging others such as their partners or their own parents who share in caregiving responsibilities. Or she may care for the child poorly. She may thus experience regret about her decision to have the child when she did and even believe that she has wronged her child by deciding to raise her—even if she continues to value her relationship with the child. At the time children are born, their identities are radically underdetermined; our complex reactions to these situations reflect how identities develop in relationship.

Janet Malek, in this volume and in other writings (Malek and Daar 2012), has discerned a different issue with the nonidentity problem: it is thought to undermine objections to duties to use preimplantation genetic diagnosis to avoid harm to offspring, such as being born with genetic diseases. From the perspective of the nonidentity problem, it seems, the most plausible way to view coming into existence as harm to the resulting child is the rare case in which the child's life contains on balance more harm than good. Malek thinks this analysis is mistaken, and she devotes her chapter to explaining how conception can be seen to harm the resulting child. She begins with the concept of harm: harm occurs when a person is made worse off in a way that sets back his or her interests and constitutes a violation of others' obligations.

Malek then distinguished three ways in which people might be harmed by their conception:

- they are sometimes harmed by the fact that they are brought into existence.
- they are sometimes harmed by the way in which they are brought into existence.
- they are always harmed by being brought into existence.

The first possibility, that people are sometimes harmed by the fact of being brought into existence, poses a "different number" case in which an individual is brought into existence who otherwise would not have been. A reply is that it only applies in the rare circumstance in which a child's condition is so severe that it would have been better never to have lived at all. Malek characterizes this reply as relying on what she calls the "Life Worth Living Premise": that a child's interest level cannot have been lowered by his conception if his life on balance contains more harm than good, even if only marginally so. Coupled with the "Worse-Off Condition," that a child is worse off as a result of conception decisions only if his interest level is lowered by them, this entails that parents who bring children into the world whose lives are worth living do not harm them. But, Malek contends, both of these assumptions are false. The Life Worth Living Premise, as Benatar (2006) points out, trades on an ambiguity between a life being worth continuing and a life being worth conceiving. There is an asymmetry between the two, with the latter having a higher threshold than the former; thus, some children may have lives worth continuing but not lives worth conceiving, so the Life Worth Living Premise is false.

The Worse-Off Condition, Malek contends, is also false. Here, the problem is that when parents decide to conceive a child, they take on the obligation to assure that the child's interests are protected at least to a minimal degree; this obligation is reflected in the future child's interest baseline. The parent can compromise this interest baseline—that is, fail to protect the child to a minimal degree—even though the child's interests are not lowered because otherwise she would not have existed. Malek then replies to several objections to her view, including that it makes problematic assumptions in construing the obligations of parents in conceiving. Malek sums up the problem with both premises: each relies on problematic assumptions about the possible worlds and interest baselines that are to be used in drawing comparisons.

Similar problems attend the comparisons at stake in determining whether individuals are sometimes harmed by the way in which they are brought into existence. Here, the nonidentity problem is raised directly; the comparison is a "same number" comparison between a child conceived now and a child conceived later (e.g., after the risk of Zika exposure has passed). Malek argues that the nonidentity problem rests on confusion in how a child is identified: by a rigid designator (which always refers to a particular child in any possible world) or by a nonrigid designator such as "my first child" (which may refer to different children depending on what is true of the circumstances of conception). In Malek's view, the context of choosing to conceive requires nonrigid designators; at the time a conception choice is made, the exact identity of any resulting child is unknown. So a woman can harm her first child—understood nonrigidly—by conception choices made under unfavorable circumstances such as Zika exposure. After conception and birth, of course, the child will be referred to rigidly, as discussions such as Kadlac's clearly illustrate.

Finally, Malek considers David Benatar's (2006) extreme view that coming into existence is always harm. On Benatar's view, there is an asymmetry between absence of pain (it is good) and absence of pleasure (it is not bad unless there is someone who is deprived). This asymmetry can be used to show that existence does not have an advantage over nonexistence: if existence involves pain, nonexistence would involve the absence of pain and would thus have the advantage. If existence involves pleasure, nonexistence would be not bad (because no one is deprived), so there is no comparative advantage to existence. Malek thinks that the asymmetry reflects an insight but only in cases of lives with overwhelming pain: we do compare the overall balance of pleasures and pains in ordinary lives and in lives of great pleasure; it is only in lives of great suffering that we set aside the possibility of offsetting pleasures.

In a number of writings, Julian Savulescu has defended a view called "procreative beneficence" (PB): that reproducers should select the child (of the possible children they could have) who is expected to have the best life, or at least as good a life as the others, based on relevant and available information. This view has been understood and much criticized as the absolute duty to create the best overall child. In Chapter 26, Savulescu and Guy Kahane argue that PB is a far more nuanced approach. They begin with a German measles case much like the Zika virus case described earlier and a parallel case in which by taking vitamins for a month before conceiving a woman might increase the likelihood of higher intelligence in a child she bears.

Savulescu and Kahane first discuss the sense in which PB should be viewed as an obligation. They see it as a prima facie obligation, perhaps similar in strength to the obligation to give children nutritious food. Risks, costs (including costs of acquiring information), and other downsides must be weighed against PB. In their view, PB is a significant moral reason, but it is one reason among others, including parental health and social justice. Its strength as a reason depends on the confidence we have in it, including any empirical uncertainty and normative uncertainty about the value itself. Savulescu and Kahane also emphasize at the outset that PB is an ethical position, not a position about social or legal sanctions. They believe legal barriers to PB should be removed, that it should be advised and encouraged, that any relevant testing should be cheap and easily accessible, and that relevant information should be readily available. They also believe that there should be some limits on the use of state resources: their example is selecting for anencephaly, and they make clear that they believe shared resources should be available for people seeking selection for deafness. Thus limited, they say, PB is common sense and should not draw the vociferous critique it has received.

Critics of PB have attacked the idea that lives can differ in well-being. A preliminary point in addressing these criticisms is the distinction between the value of a life and the value in a life in the sense of well-being within a life. Savulescu and Kahane say that it is preferable to increase value within a life no matter what the source of the improvement, other factors being equal. Theirs is not a position about the value of lives.

In considering value within a life, Savulescu and Kahane develop a theme that emerges in many of the chapters in the volume: the interplay between subjective and objective conceptions of the good or of well-being. Subjective conceptions hold that individuals themselves are the judges of what is good for them. This is most plausibly a position about ends; most subjectivists agree that individuals might be wrong about what means will most effectively contribute to their ends, with the important caution to avoid bias in such assessments. Objective conceptions hold that some things are good for people, or contribute to their well-being, whatever their beliefs or preferences. More plausible objective conceptions adjust for context: how objective goods are best realized may vary with social and natural circumstances. Savulescu and Kahane hold a mixed theory on which there are good reasons for including objective elements along with subjective elements in accounts of well-being. They also think that we can predict that certain features of our biology or our societies are more conducive to possessing what is objectively good. Their example is that the capacity to form deep personal relationships is objectively good, and thus we should try to preserve and protect human capacities that further this good.

An aspect of their view that remains controversial is that some characteristics—for example, deafness—are disadvantages in most contexts, even when prejudice is removed. Another objection is that PB may seem to require unjust actions in unjust social circumstances, such as selecting a lighter skinned child in a racist world, because that child will predictably have a better life. To this, Savulescu and Kahane reply that PB is only one reason among many; the importance of making a statement about equality in such an unjust world might readily overwhelm any weight PB might otherwise have as a moral reason. Not all differences are unjust, however; Savulescu and Kahane argue that PB provides a moral reason to favor traits such as affability or attractiveness that are likely to lead to better lives. They are clear, however, about the uncertainty that attends any enhancement decisions: some goods (such as height) are in part positional goods and what is a disadvantage will vary widely and unpredictably with social context. These uncertainties would count against the weight any PB-based reason would have.

As Savulescu and Kahane develop it, PB provides impersonal reasons—reasons about what would be a better world—rather than person-affecting reasons, reasons about what would be better for any particular individuals. Such non-person-affecting reasons are in play in judgments about population health or environmental policy and future generations. Savulescu and Kahane discuss the possibility that impersonal reasons might be systematically weaker than person-affecting reasons. They see reasons to think this might be true: a manipulation that affects a particular individual might be weightier than a social policy with the same impact on an unidentified individual, and an environmental policy that harms identifiable individuals today might be more problematic than a comparable policy that affects future generations. Conceding this point, however, does not imply that impersonal reasons are always weaker than person-affecting reasons.

Savulescu and Kahane conclude by criticizing two kinds of reasons that are common in conservative criticisms of ART: it is unnatural and it imposes the will of those using it on those conceived by it, thus subjecting offspring to wrongful coercion. The upshot of their discussion is that the two best concerns about PB are that it relies on an objective account of well-being and on impersonal reasons. PB is, however, only a position about what we have prima facie reason to do, not about what we must do or about what we must make others do.

A practical question in some ART pregnancies is the occurrence of multiples. In the effort to increase chances of achieving a pregnancy, both ART providers and their patients may have incentives to use technologies that risk twin, triplet, or even higher order multiples. These technologies include ovarian hyperstimulation used for women with low ovarian reserve, intracytoplasmic sperm injection to achieve fertilization, or multiple embryo transfer. Some people who want to have two children may try to achieve twin pregnancies for reasons such as convenience or expense. Yet multiples are risky for both children and pregnant woman. Practice guidelines are increasingly recommending single embryo transfer (SET), especially for women at higher risk, but higher risks of multiples remain with most forms of ART (ASRM 2012b).

In Chapter 27, Bonnie Steinbock develops a view of procreative responsibility on which it is ethically wrong to attempt to achieve multiple pregnancies. Her focus is twin pregnancies, which are far more common in ART and which draw less criticism, perhaps because they also occur with some frequency in ordinary pregnancies. She begins with reasons why women might prefer double embryo transfer (DET) in IVF. Perhaps the most important reason is that women believe it increases their chances of achieving a pregnancy. Other reasons include reducing risks and expense by completing a two-child family in one pregnancy and, among older women, completing a two-child family before age catches up with them. In her evaluation, Steinbock sets aside risks to the pregnant woman—who may choose to take these on—and economic costs to society such as the costs of prematurity. Health risks to offspring are her predominant concern; these include infant mortality, prematurity, and cerebral palsy.

Because achieving pregnancy is a paramount reason for DET, Steinbock presents an overview of the data on whether comparable pregnancy rates can be achieved with SET. The data suggest that an initial trial of SET in favorable prognosis patients and the ability to identify good-quality embryos can achieve near parity between SET and DET in pregnancy rates. But this is only for good prognosis patients, and only for an initial transfer cycle. For many, achieving pregnancy might outweigh any risks, and having a child with a disability might be better than having no child at all.

A critique of urging SET to avoid birth of children with disabilities is that it might express morally problematic attitudes toward persons with disabilities. This critique would seem to have more force against interventions to avoid disability risks—for example, selective abortion—than against preventive strategies such as SET. Writers such as Adrienne Asch and David Wasserman have taken the position that selective abortion for disability expresses disrespect for persons with disabilities (Asch and Wasserman 2005). Steinbock rejects this analysis, first because it underestimates the difficulties involved in having and raising a child with intellectual disabilities—a position in tension with Wasserman's discussion in Chapter 20. She also takes issue with the view that it is not wrong to eschew preventive strategies such as SET: like Savulescu and Kahane, she thinks it is wrong to avoid preventable harm unless there are pressing countervailing moral considerations. Procreative liberty, she argues, must be coupled with procreative responsibility; parents have an obligation to prevent avoidable harm to offspring.

Moreover, with frozen embryo technologies, SET may not even pose nonidentity problems: the choice is not necessarily between transferring this embryo now and a different embryo at a later date, but potentially between transferring this embryo now and waiting to transfer it at a later time when it would be a singleton pregnancy. If waiting is not an option, procreative liberty might permit DET, but SET remains the preferable choice in other cases. Steinbock concludes by emphasizing the importance of addressing correctable factors that encourage DET, such as the fact that patients typically bear the high costs of ART and that clinics have incentives to keep up pregnancy rates by encouraging DET.

Procreative responsibility is the central question in the final chapter of the volume, by David DeGrazia. DeGrazia asks under what conditions is it morally responsible to procreate with the intention of parenting, in view of what parents owe their children. He argues that three conditions are necessary and sufficient to answer this question: worthwhile life, doing more, and basic needs. The worthwhile-life condition holds that the child must be reasonably expected to have a life worth living in the sense that it is worth starting. Here, DeGrazia distinguishes between terminating pregnancy and starting pregnancy. In the former, if there is a time in which a being exists in a preconscious state, it arguably wrongs that being to allow it to come to a conscious state in which it will experience only unremitting suffering. This analysis does not apply, however, to bringing a being into existence in the first place: the being is not worse off by being brought into existence than it would otherwise have been, because the only comparison is to nonexistence. DeGrazia handles this problem by pointing out that a being can be wronged without being harmed if it is brought into an existence that is noncomparatively bad for it. This does not have the implication some have drawn, that bringing any being into existence is wrongful if the being will suffer harm. Procreative choices expose children to harm; they do not impose such harms on them. So, DeGrazia says, the benefits of life can be considered to offset life's harms; lives that are overall worthwhile are not wrongful, even though there may be harms within them.

The doing-more condition holds that parents have obligations to do more for their children than just provide them with lives on balance worth living. It is too strong to say that parents are obligated to provide their children with whatever advantages they can afford. But parents are obligated to address their children's most important and legitimate interests and to do more if they can without undue sacrifice. (Here, DeGrazia agrees with Malek.) The most difficult cases for his view, DeGrazia thinks, are prospective parents in circumstances of grave injustice: they want to procreate but cannot be sure that they will be able to meet the basic needs of their child. DeGrazia believes that it may be responsible to procreate in such circumstances, where disadvantages are due to external circumstances beyond their control. But it is not responsible to procreate if one is incapable of being a kind, attentive, and reasonably competent parent.

The chapters in this section of the volume address in a variety of ways the responsibilities of procreators to their offspring and the morality of bringing offspring into existence. None address directly whether, when, and why an entity such as a fetus might have a right to life in that it is wrong to interfere with its continuing development or not to provide it with the ongoing means to life. Among the many explanations for this gap is that grounding the right to life is orthogonal to liberal theory's efforts to accommodate different fundamental moral positions. But perhaps most important is that there is so much else to say about reproducers' responsibilities to the beings they create beyond life itself.

WHAT IS ON THE HORIZON FOR REPRODUCTIVE ETHICS? BIOLOGY AND TECHNOLOGY—BRAVE NEW WORLD, AND NEWER WORLDS STILL

When I was born, and when many (but not all) of the authors in this volume were born, reproduction was quite different. Technological developments have radically changed what we can see, what we can know, and what we can do. Imagine just some of what's happened just in the past 50 years or so:

> 1965: US Supreme Court declares that it is unconstitutional for states to prohibit the use of contraceptives, *Griswold v. Connecticut*, 381 U.S. 479 (1965).

1966: First successful culture of fetal cells obtained from amniocentesis, the technique allowing for diagnosis of aneuploidies such as trisomy 21 (The Embryo Project Encyclopedia 2016).

1973: US Supreme Court issues its decision striking down state laws prohibiting abortions, *Roe v. Wade*, 410 U.S. 113 (1973).

1975: Ultrasound deployed widely in the British hospital system for use in pregnancy (Nicolson and Fleming 2013, Ch. 8).

1978: First successful IVF procedure in Oldham General Hospital, UK.

1988: First state appellate court case dealing with traditional surrogacy, *In re Baby M*, 537 A.2d 1227, 109 N.J. 396 (N.J. 1988).

1989–1990: First use of preimplantation genetic diagnosis to identify genetic disease (Center for Genetics and Society 2016).

1998: First reports of derivation of human embryonic stem cells (Thomson et al. 1998).

2001: First report of live births following mitochondrial transplantation 2(Barritt et al. 2001).

2014: First report of live birth following uterine transplant, in Sweden (NPR 2016).

And imagine what might be on the horizon shortly: male contraceptives, widespread mitochondrial transplantation, widespread uterine transplants, gene therapy, male pregnancy, or even extracorporeal pregnancy or autologous reproduction. Imagining such technologies has been the stuff of science fiction and utopian writing from myths about Amazonia to Charlotte Perkins Gilman's *Herland* to Margaret Atwood's *The Handmaid's Tale*. If developed and in widespread use, they may utterly change our experiences of pregnancy, gender roles, and the creation of offspring. Understandably, even speculation about what might be on the close, if not the far, horizon is highly controversial. Take just the emerging technology of mitochondrial replacement therapy; objections to this procedure include concerns about its safety, about the inappropriate use of maternal genetic material, about implications for the identity of any resulting children, and about "genetic engineering," among many others (e.g., Baylis 2013; Wrigley, Wilkinson, and Appleby 2015). And like other reproductive technologies, it raises questions of social justice: whether it will be available only to the better off, whether it risks creating social divisions between those who are better off due to reproductive technology (and not just due to the social circumstances of their birth), and whether it might be used to entrench disadvantage among those who are already worse off.

CONCLUSION: REPRODUCTION FOR AN UNJUST WORLD

Setting science fiction aside for the present, reproduction is how a species is perpetuated. To the extent that reproduction by individuals is under their control, or that social patterns of reproduction are subject to social influence (or more), reproductive choices may shape the ongoing future of a species. Thus, reproductive choices and policies affect who reproduces and how frequently, whether certain subpopulations grow or shrink, whether traits are increasingly represented in a given population, and whether species numbers overall rise or fall.

Each of these problem areas raises a host of questions in ethics and political philosophy that are treated only peripherally in this volume. Several writers—Mutcherson, Daar, and Orentlicher, for example—address injustices in access to reproductive technologies. DeGrazia considers the responsibilities of parents deciding to reproduce in circumstances of severe social injustice where they may not be able to provide even minimally adequate health care for their children. Savulescu and Kahane discuss the role of impersonal reasons such as those involved in assessing policies affecting unknown future generations. And Battin's chapter observes gender injustice in the availability of contraception and asks whether universal contraceptive use by both men and women, except when both affirmatively choose the possibility of reproduction, would lead to a more just world.

So this is largely a book about reproductive ethics in comparatively well-off societies. It leaves the lack of any prenatal care in so much of the world, the endemic rates of maternal–fetal transmission of HIV, and high infant and maternal mortality rates to volumes about global justice. It leaves the population pressures that contribute to these problems and that will continue to stress earth's resources to volumes about environmental ethics and policy. But these problems should not be ignored or set aside: they are the imperfect contexts within which everyone's reproductive decisions are made.

NOTES

1. Whole Woman's Health v. Hellerstedt, No. 15-274, https://www.supremecourt.gov/opinions/15pdf/15-274_new_e18f.pdf.
2. The US Supreme Court heard a consolidated set of cases in 2016 on whether filing a form requesting alternative contraceptive coverage for their employees unduly burdens employers' religious liberties. *Little Sisters of the Poor v. Burwell*, no. 15–105, cert. granted November 6, 2015.
3. Burwell v. Hobby Lobby Stores, Inc., 573 U.S. ___, 134 S.Ct. 678 (2014).
4. 45 C.F.R. § 46.204 (2015).
5. CIOMS (2002), *International Ethical Guidelines for Biomedical Research Involving Human Subjects*, Guideline 17, http://cioms.ch/publications/layout_guide2002.pdf (accessed February 7, 2016).
6. Directive 2001/20/EC (April 4, 2001). CELEX_32001L0020_en_TXT.pdf (accessed February 7, 2016).
7. 42 U.S.C. § 289 et seq. (2015).
8. White House, "Memorandum from the President for the Heads of Executive Departments and Agencies Regarding Guidelines for Human Stem Cell Research" (July 30, 2009), https://www.whitehouse.gov/the-press-office/memorandum-president-heads-executive-departments-and-agencies-regarding-guidelines

9. National Conference of State Legislatures, "Embryonic and Fetal Research Laws" (January 1, 2016), http://www.ncsl.org/research/health/embryonic-and-fetal-research-laws.aspx (accessed February 6, 2016).

10. European Commission, "Building Europe's Leading Information Source for Stem Cell Research" (September 26, 2014), https://ec.europa.eu/programmes/horizon2020/en/news/building-europe's-leading-information-source-stem-cell-research. See also Christian Lenk, Nils Hoppe, Katharina Beier, and Clausia Wiesemann, eds., *Human Tissue Research: A European Perspective on the Ethical and Legal Challenges* (Oxford: Oxford University Press, 2011).

11. National Health Service, "NHS Choices: Newborn Blood Spot Test," http://www.nhs.uk/conditions/pregnancy-and-baby/pages/newborn-blood-spot-test.aspx (accessed February 6, 2016).

12. National Newborn Screening and Genetics Research Center, "National Newborn Screening Status Report" (November 2, 2014), http://genes-r-us.uthscsa.edu/sites/genes-r-us/files/nbsdisorders.pdf (accessed February 6, 2016).

BIBLIOGRAPHY

American Medical Association. 2008. Opinion 10.05—Potential patients. http://www.ama-assn.org/ama/pub/physician-resources/medical-ethics/code-medical-ethics/opinion1005.page?. Accessed February 4, 2016.

Asch, Adrienne, and David Wasserman. 2005. Where is the sin in synecdoche? Prenatal testing and the parent-child relationship. In *Quality of life and human difference: Genetic testing, health care, and disability*, ed. David Wasserman, Jerome Bickenbach, and Robert Wachbroit. Cambridge: Cambridge University Press.

ASRM. 2012a. Fertility treatment when the prognosis is very poor or futile: A committee opinion. *Fertility and Sterility* 98, no. 1: e6–e9, http://www.asrm.org/uploadedFiles/ASRM_Content/News_and_Publications/Ethics_Committee_Reports_and_Statements/futility.pdf. Accessed February 28, 2016.

ASRM. 2012b. Multiple gestation associated with infertility therapy: An American Society for Reproductive Medicine Practice Committee opinion. *Fertility & Sterility* 97, no. 4: 825–834.

ASRM. 2013a. Oocyte or embryo donation to women of advanced age: a committee opinion. *Fertility and Sterility* 100, no. 2: 337–340, http://www.asrm.org/uploadedFiles/ASRM_Content/News_and_Publications/Ethics_Committee_Reports_and_Statements/postmeno.pdf. Accessed February 28, 2016.

ASRM. 2013b. Fertility preservation and reproduction in patients facing gonadotoxic therapies: A committee opinion. *Fertility and Sterility* 100, no. 5: 1224–1231.

ASRM. 2013c. Child-rearing ability and the provision of fertility services: A committee opinion. *Fertility and Sterility* 100, no. 1: 50–53.

Barritt, Jason A., Carol A. Brenner, Henry E. Malter, and Jacques Cohen. 2001. Mitochondria in human offspring derived from ooplasmic transplantation: Brief communication *Human Reproduction* 16, no. 3: 513–516.

Baylis, Françoise. 2013. The ethics of creating children with three genetic parents. *Reproductive BioMedicine Online* 26, no. 6: 531–534.

Benatar, David. 2006. *Better never to have been: The harm of coming into existence*. Oxford: Oxford University Press.

Blehar, Mary C., Catherine Spong, Christine Grady, Sara F. Goldkind, Leyla Sahin, and Janine A. Clayton. 2013. Enrolling pregnant women: Issues in clinical research. *Womens Health Issues* 23, no. 1: e39–45.

Brännström, Mats, Liza Johannesson, Hans Bokström, Niclas Kvarnström, Johan Mölne, Pernilla Dahm-Kähler, Anders Enskog, Milan Milenkovic, Jana Ekberg, Cesar Diaz-Garcia, Markus Gäbel, Ash Hanafy, Henrik Hagberg, Michael Olausson, and Lars Nilsson. 2015. Livebirth after uterus transplantation. *The Lancet* 385, no. 9968: 607–616.

British Medical Association. 2015. Conscientious objection guidance for doctors and medical students. http://www.bma.org.uk/support-at-work/ethics/expressions-of-doctors-beliefs. Accessed February 4, 2016.

Center for Genetics and Society. 2016. About genetic selection. http://www.geneticsandsociety.org/section.php?id=82. Accessed March 4, 2016.

Devlin, Sir Patrick. 1965. *The enforcement of morals.* Oxford: Oxford University Press.

Embryo Project Encyclopedia. 2016. Amniocentesis prior to 1980. https://embryo.asu.edu/pages/amniocentesis-prior-1980. Accessed March 4, 2016.

Feinberg, Joel. 1984. *The moral limits of the criminal law*, vol. 1. New York: Oxford University Press.

Firestone, Shulamith. 1970. *The dialectic of sex.* New York: Morrow.

Francis, Leslie P., and Francis, John G. 2014. Trafficking in human beings: Partial compliance theory, enforcement failure, and obligations to victims, In *Poverty, agency, and human rights*, ed. Diana Meyers, 171–205, New York: Oxford University Press.

Francome, Colin, and Edward Freeman. 2000. British general practitioners' attitudes toward abortion. *Family Planning Perspectives* 32, no. 4: 189–191.

Grady, Denise. 2016. First uterus transplant in U.S. has failed. *New York Times* (March 9), http://www.nytimes.com/2016/03/10/health/first-uterus-transplant-in-us-has-failed.html?emc=edit_au_20160309&nl=afternoonupdate&nlid=54733654. Accessed March 10, 2016.

Hart, H. L. A. 1963. *Law, liberty, and morality.* Stanford, CA: Stanford University Press.

Haslanger, Sally, and Charlotte Witt. 2005. *Adoption matters: Philosophical and feminist essays.* Ithaca, NY: Cornell University Press.

Iusmen, Ingi. 2013. The EU and international adoption from Romania. *International Journal of Law, Policy and the Family* 27, no. 1: 1–27.

Javier, Rafael A., Amanda L. Baden, Frank A. Biafora, & Alina Camacho-Gingerich, eds. 2007. *Handbook of adoption: Implications for researchers, practitioners, and families.* Thousand Oaks, CA: Sage Publications.

Kittay, Eva Feder. 1999. *Love's labor: Essays on women, equality and dependency.* New York: Routledge.

Korsgaard, Christine. 1996. *Creating the kingdom of ends.* Cambridge: Cambridge University Press.

Luker, Kristin. 2008. *Abortion and the politics of motherhood*, 2d ed. Berkeley: University of California Press.

Macklin, Ruth. 2010. Enrolling pregnant women in biomedical research. *Lancet* 375, no. 9715: 632–633.

Malek, Janet, and Judith Daar. 2012. The case for a parental duty to use preimplantation genetic diagnosis for medical benefit. *American Journal of Bioethics* 12, no. 4: 3–11.

McCullough, Laurence B., and Frank A. Chervenak. 1994. *Ethics in obstetrics and gynecology.* New York: Oxford University Press.

Mill, John Stuart. 1869. *The subjection of women*. London: Longmans, Green, Reader, and Dyer. http://www.gutenberg.org/files/27083/27083-h/27083-h.htm. Accessed December 14, 2015.

Millum, Joseph. 2010. How do we acquire parental rights? *Social Theory & Practice* 36, no. 1: 112–132.

National Institute for Healthcare Excellence (NICE). 2013. Fertility problems: Assessment and treatment 1.11, http://www.nice.org.uk/guidance/cg156/chapter/1-recommendations. Accessed February 28, 2016.

National Public Radio (NPR). 2016. Cleveland clinic performs first successful uterus transplant in the U.S. http://www.npr.org/sections/thetwo-way/2016/02/26/468283774/cleveland-clinic-performs-first-successful-uterus-transplant-in-the-u-s. Accessed February 28, 2016.

Nicolson, Malcolm, and John E. E. Fleming. 2013. *Imaging and imagining the fetus: The development of obstetric ultrasound*. Baltimore, MD: The Johns Hopkins University Press.

Noddings, Nel. 1984. *Caring: A feminine approach to ethics and morality*. Berkeley: University of California Press.

PBS Newshour. 2016. Wounded vets can't get help with in vitro fertilization costs (January 4). http://www.pbs.org/newshour/bb/wounded-vets-cant-get-help-with-in-vitro-fertilization-costs/. Accessed February 28, 2016.

Rawls, John. 1971. *A theory of justice*. Cambridge, MA: Harvard University Press.

Rawls, John. 1993. *Political liberalism*. New York: Columbia University Press.

Riddle, John. 1997. *Eve's herbs: A history of contraception and abortion in the West*. Cambridge, MA: Harvard University Press.

Rosenstein, M. G., J. K. Turk, A. B. Caughey, J. E. Steinauer, and J. L. Kerns. 2014. Dilation and evacuation training in maternal-fetal medicine fellowships. *American Journal of Obstetrics & Gynecology* 210, no. 6: 569.e1–569.e5.

Ruddick, Sara. 1989. *Maternal thinking: Toward a politics of peace*. Boston: Beacon Press.

Scanlon, T. M. 1999. *What we owe to each other*. Cambridge, MA: Harvard University Press.

Stephen, Sir James Fitzjames. 1874. *Liberty, equality, fraternity*, ed. Stuart D. Warner. Indianapolis: Liberty Fund. http://oll.libertyfund.org/titles/572#Stephen_0021_117. Accessed December 14, 2015.

Thomson, James A., Joseph Itskovitz-Eldor, Sander S. Shapiro, Michelle A. Waknitz, Jennifer J. Swiegriel, Vivinne S. Marshall, and Jeffrey M. Jones. 1998. Embryonic stem cell lines derived from human blastocysts. *Science* 282, no. 5391: 1145–1147.

World Health Organization (WHO). 2015. Maternal mortality. http://www.who.int/mediacentre/factsheets/fs348/en/.

Wrigley, Anthony, Stephen Wilkinson, and John B. Appleby. 2015. Mitochondrial replacement: Ethics and identity. *Bioethics* 29, no. 9: 631–638.

PART I

SOCIETY

CHAPTER 1

....

THE DISCURSIVE CONTEXT
OF REPRODUCTIVE ETHICS

....

AMY CABRERA RASMUSSEN

ETHICS, discourse, and policy are inextricably linked and often highly divisive. This chapter presents an analysis of the contours of the contemporary US policy discourse on reproduction, with the goal to help illuminate the social and political context within which ethical arguments about reproduction are made. Such ethical discussions do not occur in a vacuum; instead, they take place within a given set of policy discourses and narratives. Such discourses vary in different policy contexts; in the US context, in particular, reproductive discourse and policymaking display four contours: *reproduction as an appropriate target of governmental policymaking, contested issue categorization, abortion as master subcategory and synecdoche*, and the *importance of medical and technological factors*.

Examining policy discourse—and, in particular, issue framing and categorization processes—throws into sharp relief the underlying value differences and ethical positions that guide policymaking. Despite the prevailing view that facts guide policymaking, the role of discourse has been shown to be increasingly significant. Discourse provides a lens through which we can understand the construction and communication of meaning (Yanow 2000). Discourse, then, allows us to better illuminate what is at stake for various social and political actors and comprehend their complex perspectives on whether and how government and individuals ought to act. All sorts of social and political actors use discursive means to persuade government decision-makers to adopt their particular policy perspectives, and this is certainly the case with regard to reproduction. Succeeding in having one's value and ethical positions codified into law is a significant victory because of the scope of governmental activities in the contemporary United States; government is heavily engaged in policymaking on reproduction. In addition, successful persuasion of governmental actors to adopt legislation or craft legal rulings that reflect one's values is particularly powerful because governmental authority plays a key role in setting and enforcing norms. Therefore, we must also view the outcomes and contours of past policy debates as influencing the present day, for existing policy (including even its absence or inadequacy) is the terrain on which ethical arguments are crafted.

Policy discourse can be said to consist of multiple devices, ranging from stories and narratives to metaphors and frames, categories and synecdoche. Each device, sometimes evidenced singly, other times operating in tandem, allows for the simplification and translation of complex real-life circumstances and value positions. In the intricate and conflict-laden arena of reproduction, such devices are particularly well wrought and can be thought of as supplying a basic "architecture" within which persuasive argumentation exists and can be built. Framing, in particular, stands at the center of this discursive structure. Frames are cognitive maps that can be either subconscious or more purposefully utilized tools that convey perspectives and persuade others (Schön and Rein 1994; Lakoff 2009). There is no singular frame for a given policy issue. Instead, policy actors construct anew, select among, and deploy frames that they believe will lead to the policy outcomes they prefer. When disputes arise between competing policy actors, framing conflicts ensue. Such conflicts are not resolved by an assessment of facts (Schön and Rein 1994). Frames do not require all facts to be taken into consideration or validated; new or contrary evidence can be simply excluded, reinterpreted, or incorporated into a given frame. There is much evidence that public understanding, attitudes, and positions on policy issues are influenced by elite framing (Iyengar 1990; Nelson and Oxley 1999; Jacoby 2000; Haider-Markel and Joslyn 2001). In any policy issue context, a set of cognitive frames and discursive structures exists, having many implications for the argumentation that follows.

This chapter provides a theoretically and substantively grounded overview and analysis of the four features of this "architecture" of policy framing and discourse on reproduction, coupled with carefully selected examples from contemporary American reproductive policy history and informed by the theoretical lessons regarding policy discourse in each case. Such an approach does not attempt to supply a comprehensive summary or a chronological listing of reproductive discourse over time, but instead it highlights the key contours of recent decades' framing, concluding with a brief discussion of the implications of this framing context for ethical argumentation to come.

Contours of Reproductive Discourse and Framing

Reproduction as an Appropriate Target of Governmental Policymaking

Throughout American history, but particularly in the late twentieth and early twenty-first centuries, reproduction has been framed as a topic of particular policymaking concern. This is primarily due to the link between reproduction and gender, as well as additional and intersecting axes of identity and difference such as race, class, sexuality, and immigrant status. Policymaking elites and powerful societal actors have often framed themselves and government as having a legitimate role in increasing, decreasing, or otherwise modifying the reproduction of various groups in American society. This has led to many reproduction-related policies, the bulk of which are group-specific rather than generally applicable. Going back in US history, this can include practices of breeding and family separation utilized during slavery; sterilization of those deemed unworthy to be parents because of race, mental health, or class; or in more recent years, educational programs meant to discourage young and single women's sexual activity and childbearing. Because government is not a neutral arbiter of contending viewpoints, power differences can be thrown into sharp relief through policy debates and their outcomes.

Indeed, those targeted by governmental policies related to reproduction have also framed modified or alternative policies as essential to achieving broader goals of autonomy and citizenship for themselves and those similarly singled out by policymakers. For instance, it is for this reason that reproductive rights have been and remain at the center of women's movements—albeit with the caveat that what is meant by "reproductive rights" is not always defined in the same way by different groups of women. For some, reproductive rights might prioritize the choice not to procreate, whether through the use of abortion or contraception; governmental policies might then be required to secure these rights. For others, reproductive rights might be most centrally about being able to bear children, particularly when one's procreation is not valued; discriminatory or exclusionary governmental policies might need to be overturned to secure such rights. In both cases, arguments crafted by the targets of policy are often framed as having to do with rights to individual privacy and autonomy or the necessity of group-based protections. Because the groups targeted by policy often lack political representation and power and can be attempting to unsettle established policy, these arguments can face an uphill battle of persuasion, and so are difficult to craft and sustain.

In the last several decades, reproduction has come to be an issue that serves as a touchstone for policy actors and the public on both sides of the political aisle, and so it is framed as standing in for a larger set of value stances. For instance, an elected official's position on abortion has become a common shorthand for his or her partisan affiliation, even as parties are otherwise coalitions of individuals and groups that may have diverse views on a range of policy issues (Carmines, Gerrity, and Wagner 2010). Yet, within the American system, the partisanship of elected officials is closely linked to reproduction; those opposed to abortion rights are almost assuredly Republican, and those supportive of abortion rights are nearly always Democratic (it is worth noting that nonelite partisanship and stances on abortion are more complicated). Likewise, when a candidate or elected official varies from this existing schema, it is seen as a significant norm deviation and one's alteration of views over time can be viewed as reason to doubt his or her bona fide membership within his or her respective political party. In a time of divisive national politics, policymakers' stances and votes taken on reproduction garner "score cards" from major national advocacy organizations that are made available to the media and voters alike. In addition, a small but significant subset of voters highlights reproduction—specifically abortion—as a key issue in their support of candidates for elected office. In 2012, for example, Gallup found that for one in six Americans, the decision whether to vote for a candidate for a major elected office relied upon the candidate's expressed position on abortion matching the individual's own view (2012). Roughly similar percentages have asserted this opinion over the last two decades (ranging from 13% to 17%) and across issue positions (in 2012: 21% pro-life, 15% pro-choice). Because reproduction is an issue that can activate or influence the political participation of the most strident and committed participants on both sides, such a situation creates incentives for policy elites to act when they have the power to do so, even when such action is unreflective of the broader public's views or level of concern for such matters.

Perhaps the clearest manifestation of this phenomenon of substantial government action on reproduction is also the most recent: the proliferation of abortion restrictions in the states. States, and Congress to a lesser extent, have created a host of policies related to abortion since the *Roe v. Wade* decision in 1973. Such policies generally attempt to reduce the utilization and access to abortion through measures aimed at modifying abortion funding—whether via public monies or private insurance provision, altering the conditions that must be met to procure an abortion, such as mandating counseling or waiting periods, limiting the method or timing of abortion procedures, or delineating operating requirements of providers and/or facilities. However, such measures have dramatically increased in the years following the 2010 midterm election. The moral nature of such policy and the unified partisan control of key representative branches of state government have been shown to be predictors of such antiabortion policies in the post-*Roe* era (Kreitzer 2015). In the years 2011–2014, this pattern holds; Republican control of more state governments saw 231 individual restrictions passed (Guttmacher 2015a, 2015b). This exceeds the number of restrictions enacted during the entire prior decade and means that many states now have multiple restrictions in effect that have dramatic effects on the accessibility of abortion, particularly for the most vulnerable women—those disadvantaged by race, income, education, age, immigration status, or geography (Boonstra and Nash 2014). While studies do not yet exist that systematically delineate, sift through, or evaluate policymakers' motivations for the passage of such recent restrictions, the proliferation of policymaking is quite clear and is part of the larger trend wherein matters of reproduction solicit particular attention from policymakers. Americans United for Life, an advocacy group that has produced sample legislation utilized in this policymaking trend, has argued that "[T]he states remain a key battleground in the defense of life. State legislatures across the country continue to break new ground protecting women from the negative consequences of abortion and ensuring that the abortion industry is subject to medically appropriate regulation and oversight" (2015). Here, the active role of the (state) governments is argued to be legitimate and necessary. The framing of opposition to such measures, as in the text of a NARAL Pro-Choice America petition for the Women's Health Protection Act (a national law to preempt such state-level actions), is quite distinct. "We're seeing an enormous number of attacks on a woman's fundamental freedoms across the country today … But the fact is, the more roadblocks politicians put in front of legal abortion, the more they put women's lives at risk" (2015). In this framing, one sees the appeal to gender-based rights as well as a call for (national) policy to alter the existing (state) policy landscape. Beyond this, part of the strategy of those opposed to the laws is to increase public awareness, as advocates assert that the public is not always aware of such policies being passed (Sussman 2015). The lack of such knowledge and awareness can be an obstacle to framing, but the manner in which such awareness is provided can provide an opportunity for framing as well, especially in circumstances in which policymaking is prevalent.

Contested Issue Categorization: Reproduction as a Matter of Health?

A second key aspect of the discourse of reproduction is how framing can be used to construct the issue category in which reproduction is placed. Categorization can be utilized in regard to groups of people, types of issues, and understandings of causality, and each category has its concomitant membership and logic (Lakoff 1990; Schneider and Ingram 1993; Yanow 1996, 2003; Keeler 2007; Cabrera Rasmussen 2011; van Hulst and Yanow 2014). Like all categories, the policy issue categorizations one sees in operation may seem commonsensical or inevitable. However, in practice, issues are incredibly complex in cause and circumstance and so social and political actors must select or occlude aspects to frame the issue into one or another broader issue category. It is also rarely the case that all agree on which issue categorization is legitimate. Such categorizations, then, are political, and the result of framing contests undertaken by advocacy groups, elected officials, administrators, and more. It makes a difference whether an issue such as prenatal exposure to chemicals is deemed a matter of education, health, or environmental policy. While it is true that categorizations are most often contested, it is also true that issues become more associated with one broader policy category over another. The categorization that becomes dominant for a given issue brings with it a host of practical matters—ranging from the public's understanding and prioritization, the availability of funding streams, legislative committee oversight and governmental agency assignments, and more.

Reproduction is most often categorized as a health issue, but because there is no necessary equality among members of a given category (Lakoff 1990; Yanow 2003; Cabrera Rasmussen 2011), reproduction takes on the position of a marginal member of the category of health. Reproduction is far less central than something such as neurology, pediatric asthma care, or cancer treatment. This marginal position is largely because of the association of reproduction with gender and/or sexuality and also due to the frequent contestation of this categorization by religious-based framing. Advocates using such religious-based framing have been largely successful in advancing a view of reproduction as at least partially, if not wholly a matter of freedom of conscience or religious expression. Even advocates of more gender-based categorizations of procreation as a matter of health often concede that religious argumentation has some legitimacy, resulting in "conscience clause" exemptions to many otherwise health-focused policies. The most thoroughly elaborated ethical viewpoints present within policymaking are often based within religious notions of morality, rather than on other philosophical foundations. As a "special type" or nonprototypical member of the health issue category, reproduction therefore is subject to distinct ethical standards and, as noted earlier, framed as requiring relatively greater degrees of governmental policymaking. This marginal standing can affect governmental decisions about whether to provide and how to regulate certain types of reproductive medical services, decisions that create inequities of access among differently positioned Americans.

In the 1990s, a debate began over the appropriateness of comprehensive sex education and condom availability programs; this debate highlights the manner in which issue categorization conflicts operate. While initially provoked by the growing awareness of the impact of HIV/AIDS on youth, these debates inherently grappled with questions related to procreation. Should young people outside of marital relationships engage in sexual activity? Did types of sexual activity that did not relate to procreation require particularly strenuous governmental intervention? Did the provision of information—and in some cases methods—of preventing HIV/AIDS transmission go beyond the function of appropriate health education and infringe upon the religious beliefs of parents and their school-age youth? Fundamental to these questions was a determination of what type of issue this was—if it was successfully framed as solely a matter of health, then urgent and thoroughgoing public health interventions seemed appropriate, including comprehensive information and the provision of potentially life-saving disease prevention measures. If, however, one argued this was a special type of health matter, one that could be constructed as less clearly within the arena of health due to concerns about religious freedom, then the public schools' and other government agencies' actions could be framed in turn as far less appropriate and needing greater deference to parental morality.

While HIV/AIDS was the immediate impetus for expanded sex education and condom availability programs in public schools, such efforts were not a new or fleeting phenomenon. For nearly 100 years, various state agencies had sought to provide information and resources about sexual behavior to young people and other subsets of the American population in situations where health and behavioral trends were seen as societal problems (Moran 2000). Like the broader reproductive policies related earlier, such educational interventions were often group-specific and aimed at engendering modifications to the reproduction of these groups. During World War II, American military men were admonished to refrain from sexual activity or use condoms as a means to ensure a healthy fighting force; but civilian American women's sexual activity was discouraged with a moralistic campaign against promiscuity (Moran 2000). Decreasing the likelihood of out-of-wedlock or teen pregnancies was also about asserting that only particular types of relationships ought to produce children. Abstinence-only education, a more recent form of sex education, seeks to deter youth sexual behavior, again for the purpose of "protecting" norms of marriage and appropriate childbearing; in this case, norms based within the Christian tradition.

In the 1990s debate, proponents of providing public school students with a more comprehensive and frank sexual education curriculum framed HIV/AIDS as a full-blown public health emergency. Public health data began to show that the teen years were a key locus of infection, from which AIDS would proceed to develop (New York City Department of Health 1990). Advocates framed the issue, then, as urgent, life-threatening, and requiring extraordinary measures. Such framing did not invoke the recipients of this information and resources as children, but rather as adolescents with burgeoning agency who ought to be assisted in making more responsible health decisions. That such programs were part of the schools' health education curriculum and health education mission more broadly was a common assertion; sex education was *health* education. The framing of sex education as part of the issue category of health, then, was reaffirmed.

For opponents, the reverse was true. Those opposed to comprehensive sex education and condom availability sought to unsettle the health categorization, and instead frame the issue as one that engaged what they argued to be more fundamental or primary issues of religious freedom. On the matter of HIV/AIDS infection, instead of endorsing school-based educational curricula or free provision of condoms, their solution was based within families and communities. For them, premarital sexual activity itself was the cause of the AIDS crisis, and so efforts must focus upon discouraging youth sexual behavior, not educating them in the methods for engaging in "safe" but in their minds, morally unacceptable sex. Such framing, then, seeks to move the issue of sex education out of the center of the category of health and to its margins, if not out of the category entirely.

Abortion as Master Subissue and Synecdoche

Matters of reproduction constitute a many and varied list: from fertility treatments, to surrogacy practices, to maternal–fetal conflicts, and to contraception and well beyond. Yet among this always-expanding issue inventory, one plays a unique and outsized role in reproductive discourse: abortion. Abortion operates discursively in two main ways. First, other issues are often linked to abortion and, when linked, abortion can have a determinative impact on the trajectory of policymaking. Second, in many ways abortion acts as a "stand-in" for the broader array of reproduction-related issues.

In the first case, then, abortion can be seen as a "master" member or subissue within the category of reproduction, having a more powerful discursive impact than other issues. As noted earlier, a feature of discursive and cognitive categories is that not all members of a given category need be equal. In many cases, one or more members of the category are framed as more central or prototypical while others may be constructed as marginal, deviant, or less significant (Lakoff 1990). Abortion, as the controversial wedge issue that it has become in the United States, plays the role of "master" issue within the arena of reproduction. This is partly due to the fact that abortion occupies a space temporally preceding most of the other issues of reproduction, many of which have only emerged as a result of more recent technological and medical advancements. Early policy debates often structure future debates on the same and related issues (Rochefort and Cobb 1994); for this reason, issues of reproduction are often seen through the lens of abortion, rather than on their own terms. In addition, in some cases, the impact of abortion may be inadvertent or unintended, as when government regulations regarding abortion have an impact on other issues, reproductive and more general health issues alike.

Yet, regardless of temporality, the extent to which another reproductive issue does or does not "activate" the abortion frame is likely to affect levels of governmental and advocacy action on the issue. The less an issue is framed as connected to abortion, the less likely it is to be subject to policy-related controversy; the more it is, the more likely such a situation will result. Whether by explicit strategy or practical proximity, whenever it occurs, connection to abortion draws in a specific set of ethical and moral concerns that are difficult to transcend. Such ethical concerns include definitions of what life is, when it begins, and what responsibilities follow. They also include significant questions of women's bodily autonomy, women's roles, and to what extent the state or others have an interest in burgeoning life. These sorts of questions are not easily resolved and advocates' positions tend to lie firmly entrenched within disparate value systems. Connection to the master issue of abortion also contributes to the marginality of reproduction within the category of health policy (this is a key reason why this circumstance exists, as noted earlier).

The second significant way that abortion functions within reproductive discourse is that it is often treated as a stand-in for the broader issue of reproduction. Such a depiction of part of an issue as the whole is an example of the discursive device of synecdoche (Burke 1969). We regularly use such discursive constructions in our everyday speech; a frequently cited example is the phrase "all hands on deck," which is easily understood to mean that all *persons* are needed, not simply that singular body part. In policy discourse, a part is selected to stand in for the whole as a way to make the complex and abstract nature of a policy question clearer for others (Stone 2002). Greater or lesser fidelity to making the part a microcosm of the original whole can allow policy actors to define the issue in a favorable manner and potentially occlude unfavorable aspects. Both of these can help them to alter public knowledge and understanding of an issue and alter incentives for policymakers.

In all cases, the selection of a particular object or issue as a synecdoche bears the imprint of power. Those with power define issues. In the case of abortion, there are influential interests on both sides of the issue that help to create and reinforce its role as synecdoche. On the one hand, abortion plays a central role for those opposed to its legality and utilization. Pro-life or anti-abortion advocates see this as a fundamental issue of faith and life. For them, abortion is an issue upon which compromise is not possible, and other issues such as contraception are not readily treated as something separate but instead are seen as forms of abortion or inherently connected to abortion. On the other hand, pro-choice or abortion rights supporters see the issue as bearing the greatest significance to women's bodily autonomy and so as a fundamental measure of gender equality. The class and racial composition of the pro-choice advocacy coalition has meant that abortion has historically been emphasized vis-à-vis the reproductive issues that have a disproportionate impact upon less privileged women. Such issues receiving less attention might include sterilization policies aimed at certain racial or ethnic women or exposure to toxins that might have a disproportionate impact on working-class women's fertility.

The 2010 Patient Protection and Affordable Care Act (ACA) highlights how an issue that is generally framed as closer to abortion can be impacted by its omnipresence in the discourse and, in particular, its role as master subissue within the category of reproduction. While state-level policies had previously determined whether or not insurers would be required to cover contraception within their benefit packages, the passage of the ACA provided the possibility that national-level policymaking would mandate greater uniformity. Early contentious debates during the drafting of the ACA made policymakers take heed of the powerful role of abortion; abortion was singled out for restricted governmental funding, treatment within benefit packages, and insurance accounting practices (Herszenhorn and Pear 2010; Salganicoff, Beamesderfer, Kurani, and Sobel 2014). Policymakers also made special arrangements for the treatment of contraception, delegating responsibility for determining how that issue would be handled to bureaucratic entities, at a distance temporally and structurally from the policymaking process. However, the issue of contraception remained tethered to that of abortion. A contraceptive benefit requirement was deemed appropriate by the Department of Health and Human Services, and this administrative regulation produced strong opposition. Those against the mandate argued in both congressional and legal venues that the exemption that was provided to houses of worship was too narrow and that the range of medications termed "contraception" was too broad. Religious-affiliated institutions such as universities and businesses argued that they ought to be exempted from the mandate, and they argued that certain devices and medications, including emergency contraception, were in fact abortifacients. Supporters of the mandate argued that contraception and abortion were distinct, and the exclusion of abortion coverage was intact in Health and Human Services's mandate, with necessary religious exemptions adequate. The dispute would be taken to the Supreme Court, which, in June 2014, ruled in *Burwell v. Hobby Lobby Stores* (13-354, 571 U.S. ___ (2014)) that the administration's contraceptive mandate violated the religious exercise rights of closely held for-profit corporations. Dozens of other cases are working their way through the federal courts concerning various types of religiously affiliated and for-profit enterprises (Becket Fund 2013), showing how the connection to abortion can alter the trajectory of other types of reproductive policymaking.

The Role of Medical and Technological Factors in Reproductive Discourse

Generally speaking, Americans' knowledge regarding the intricate aspects of policy issues and the policymaking process is low. While public opinion data are relatively sparse on the subject of reproduction, public understanding of many aspects of fertility, including prevalence, diagnosis, and treatment costs, was relatively low when measured in 1998–1999—with variations depending upon the national context (Adashi et al. 2000). Matters of reproduction are complex, often medically technical, and ever-changing, and often even policymakers can find themselves without the requisite understanding or the ability to keep pace with technological advances. Certain experiential factors are understood by the individuals who are involved in the processes of reproduction, of course, but those frequently targeted by policymakers—women—are underrepresented in most policymaking contexts. What scientific and medical knowledge of reproductive processes exists is largely restricted to experts in those fields, and so many in the public may lack either awareness or firm and informed policy stances on the issues, leaving policymakers with little popular accountability for their actions regarding reproduction. Because framing has a significant impact on policy knowledge and understanding of causality—factors that contribute to the creation of public will to advance policymaking (Entman 1993)—reproduction is a subject for which framing can be particularly important. Framing gives advocates a shorthand through which values and policy positions can be articulated, without the need to fully address lack of knowledge among the public or policymakers. And, as noted earlier, framing need not rely exclusively upon facts and evidence.

In addition, technological and medical advances create a continually "moving target" for policymakers. Understanding the mechanics of a newly invented procedure or the safety evidence regarding a new medication, or studying a biological phenomena still incompletely understood by scientific experts, makes contemplating and devising ethical standards that are then translated into laws, judicial rulings, or administrative guidelines (or all of these) a difficult process. Even more, rules that are successfully established may become moot quickly if new techniques or medical admixtures to avoid such regulatory ensnarement are developed. Norms change as well: What might have been thought of as an experimental or superfluous intervention may become commonplace and expected, rather than extraordinary. Such norm changes can have the effect of drawing policy toward such new realities. Technological advance and social response are thus always at least a step ahead of policymaking.

In such circumstances of low knowledge and seemingly ever-changing facts, issues may avoid governmental action, or if acted upon, policies may be the result of the outsized influence of well-organized interests, such as professional associations of researchers and doctors, the health industry, or alternatively, religious or gender-driven advocates. Assisted reproduction is one area where the role of medical and technological factors can be clearly seen.

Methods to increase or decrease the likelihood of pregnancy have been long part of cultural traditions, and moderately involved medical procedures such as artificial insemination have been practiced in some forms since the late 1800s. However, it is with the professionalization of medicine and improved scientific understanding of reproduction that processes such as in vitro fertilization were created. The twentieth century history of usually independent trial and error by a host of independent research physicians highlights that it is difficult for government or other institutions to fully control processes of scientific development. The setting of guidelines, the withholding of funding, or religious dictates were inadequate to prevent the development of such technologies. In more recent times when acceptance of such technologies is more widespread, the public is still less likely to have a direct impact on policymaking on these issues. The framing of the issue by advocates, then, has a great influence. Scholars point to the prominence of the Catholic Church, physicians, and feminists among the groups who are able to frame and influence assisted reproduction policymaking. In the United States, national regulations are quite limited, leaving some states to make their own policies, but most often fertility specialists are left with wide discretion as to standards of operation (Storrow 2011; Heidt-Forsythe 2013). While the reasons for the relative absence of government regulation of assisted reproduction in the US context (versus other industrialized nations) have not been fully substantiated, a contributing factor is likely to be the role of medicine and technology. In some ways, policymakers' inaction can be seen as a successful framing of such matters as positive developments and the domain of the medical and scientific professions. Deviations into policymaking on assisted reproduction are largely the result of links made to the master subissue of abortion.

Concluding Thoughts: Implications

Interaction of the discursive features mentioned earlier creates additional patterns in discourse and policy. While presented as discrete features, there are, in reality, complicated interactions between all of these. For example, that abortion is an issue of primacy within matters of reproduction affects the incentives that policymakers have to earn their "bona fides" through taking a firm stance on these issues as well as its standing on the margins of health care. The fact that technology complicates the policymaking process on matters of reproduction makes it more likely that policymakers will "fall back" on familiar framing of the issue (related to abortion) rather than being able to deal with an issue's unique complexities.

For all of these reasons, the creation and successful deployment of ethical standards on these issues is fraught with a level of difficulty considerably greater than many other policy issues. That said, the creation of persuasive alternative framing of the issue for the public and for policymakers grounded in ethical considerations can go far toward improving both discourse and policy on reproduction in the American context and beyond, as the *mechanisms* of discourse—if not always their content—are present in any national or other context.

Bibliography

Adashi, E. Y., J. Cohen, L. Hamberger, H. W. Jones, Jr, D. W. de Kretser, B. Lunenfeld, Z. Rosenwaks, A. Van Steirteghem, and C. de Bellevue. 2000. Public perception on infertility and its treatment: An international survey. The Bertarelli Foundation Scientific Board. *Human Reproduction* 15, no. 2: 330–334.

Americans United for Life. 2015. 2015 State legislative sessions mid-session report. http://www. aul.org/wp-content/uploads/2015/04/2015-Mid-Session-Report-04-22.pdf

The Becket Fund. 2013. HHS mandate information central website. http://www.becketfund. org/hhsinformationcentral/

Boonstra, H. D., and E. Nash. 2014. A surge of state abortion restrictions puts providers—and the women they serve—in the crosshairs. *Guttmacher Policy Review* 17, no. 1: 9–14, 28. http:// www.guttmacher.org/pubs/gpr/17/1/gpr170109.html

Burke, K. 1969. *A grammar of motives*. Berkeley: University of California Press.

Carmines, E. G., J. C. Gerrity, & M. W. Wagner. 2010. How abortion became a partisan issue: Media coverage of the interest group–political party connection. *Politics & Policy* 38, no. 6: 1135–1158.

Entman, R. M. 1993. Framing: Toward clarification of a fractured paradigm. *Journal of Communication* 43, no. 4: 51–58.

Gallup. 2012. Abortion is threshold issue for one in six U.S. voters. http://www.gallup.com/ poll/157886/abortion-threshold-issue-one-six-voters.aspx

Guttmacher Institute. 2015a. In just the last four years, states have enacted 231 abortion restrictions. http://www.guttmacher.org/media/inthenews/2015/01/05/

Guttmacher Institute. 2015b. State policies in brief: An overview of abortion laws. http://www. guttmacher.org/statecenter/spibs/spib_OAL.pdf

Haider-Markel, D. P., and M. R. Joslyn. 2001. Gun policy, opinion, tragedy, and blame attribution: The conditional influence of issue frames. *Journal of Politics* 63, no. 2: 520–543.

Heidt-Forsythe, E. A. 2013. Reconceiving the state: Morals, markets, and state regulation of assisted reproductive technologies. Doctoral diss., Rutgers University.

Herszenhorn, D. M., and R. Pear. 2010. Democrats woo abortion foes in push for health bill. *The New York Times*, March 19.

Iyengar, S. 1990. Framing responsibility for political issues: The case of poverty. *Political Behavior* 12, no. 1: 19–40.

Jacoby, W. G. 2000. Issue framing and public opinion on government spending. *American Journal of Political Science* 44, no. 4: 750–767.

Lakoff, G. 1990. *Women, fire, and dangerous things: What categories reveal about the mind.* Chicago: University of Chicago Press.

Lakoff, G. 2009. *The political mind: A cognitive scientist's guide to your brain and its politics.* New York: Penguin.

Keeler, R. 2007. Analysis of logic: Categories of people in U.S. HIV/AIDS policy. *Administration & Society* 39, no. 5: 612–630.

Kreitzer, R. J. 2015. Politics and morality in state abortion policy. *State Politics & Policy Quarterly* 15, no. 1: 41–66.

Moran, J. 2000. *Teaching sex: The shaping of adolescence in the 20th century.* Cambridge, MA: Harvard University Press.

NARAL Pro-Choice America. 2015. Urge your members of Congress to cosponsor the Women's Health Protection Act. http://actnow.prochoiceamerica.org/letter/150324_ WHPA/?source=website#.VWej8OchDIU

Nelson, T. E., & Z. M. Oxley. 1999. Issue framing effects on belief importance and opinion. *Journal of Politics* 61, no. 4: 1040–1067.

New York City Department of Health. 1990. Fact sheet: Adolescent sexuality in New York City: HIV, STDs and pregnancy. Luis O. Reyes Papers (Box 38). Municipal Archives, New York.

Rasmussen, A. C. 2011. Contraception as health? The framing of issue categories in contemporary policy making. *Administration & Society* 43, no. 8: 930–953.

Rochefort, D. A., and R. W. Cobb. 1994. Problem definition: An emerging perspective. In *The politics of problem definition: Shaping the policy agenda*, ed. D. A. Rochefort and R. W. Cobb, 1–31. Armonk, NY: M.E. Sharpe.

Salganicoff, A., A. Beamesderfer, N. Kurani, and L. Sobel. 2014. Coverage for abortion services and the ACA. Kaiser Family Foundation. http://files.kff.org/attachment/coverage-for-abortion-services-and-the-aca-issue-brief

Schneider, A., and H. Ingram. 1993. Social construction of target populations: Implications for politics and policy. *American Political Science Review* 87, no. 2: 334–347.

Schön, D. A., and M. Rein. 1994. *Frame reflection: Toward the resolution of intractable policy controversies*. New York: Basic Books.

Stone, D. 2002. *Policy paradox: The art of political decision making*. Rev. ed. New York: W.W. Norton & Company.

Storrow, R. F. 2011. Religion, feminism and abortion: The regulation of assisted reproduction in two Catholic countries. *Rutgers Law Journal* 42, no. 3: 725–764.

Sussman, R. 2015. The landscape of state anti-abortion legislation. *Columbia Journal of Gender and the Law* 29, no. 1: 229–235.

Van Hulst, M. J., and D. Yanow. 2014. The political/process promise of policy framing. *Sociological Review* 10, no. 1–2: 87–113.

Yanow, D. 1996. American ethnogenesis and public administration. *Administration & Society* 24, no. 4: 483–509.

Yanow, D. 2000. *Conducting interpretive policy analysis*. Thousand Oaks, CA: Sage.

Yanow, D. 2003. *Constructing "race" and "ethnicity" in America: Category making in public policy and administration*. Armonk, NY: M.E. Sharpe.

....

CHAPTER 2

ACCESS TO BASIC REPRODUCTIVE RIGHTS

Global Challenges

....

SHEELAGH MCGUINNESS AND HEATHER WIDDOWS

IT has long been recognized that if women are to have true equality with men, they must be able to control the number of children they have and the time of childbirth. There are many factors that impact on this ability, but key are access to family planning services, particularly safe contraception and abortion. That is the focus of this chapter. The central premise of our analysis is that access to contraception and abortion is properly understood as *basic* reproductive rights. Our claim is that to disallow such access is effectively to bar women from attaining equality with men by denying minimal standards of bodily integrity. We argue for access to contraception and abortion as *basic* reproductive rights because they are necessary for controlling fertility and childbirth and as such necessary to make women equal to men. *Basic* reproductive rights should not be "trumped" by other rights or sacrificed or compromised to attain other goods.

The chapter is divided into three distinct parts. In the first section we provide the philosophical foundation which grounds our claim that women must be able to access contraception and abortion if they are to be truly equal to men. We move from this to provide a very brief overview of the evolution of how reproductive rights are conceptualized in international human rights norms. The final part of the chapter is focused on current threats to access to abortion and contraception. We provide an overview of one of the biggest impediments to family planning services on a global scale—the Global Gag Rule (GGGR). We describe the emergence of this rule and its impact. Looking forward, we consider the importance of continued improvements in women's reproductive rights "post 2015"; and we argue that restrictions on development aid funding of particular aspects of family planning services, for instance, safe abortion care, constitute a retrograde step and should be resisted.

Given the basic nature of rights to access contraception, it is not enough to protect these rights in a "negative" or "noninterference" form; rather, we must ensure an "enabling environment" such that both abortion and contraception are accessible to women (Cohen 2012). Our approach echoes that of reproductive justice scholars who "simultaneously demand a negative right of freedom from undue government interference and a positive right to government action in creating conditions of social justice and human flourishing for all" (Luna and Luker 2013, 328). Access to contraception and abortion is key to women and girls' ability to achieve equality because in the words of Sen and Batiwala:

> The control of women's and girls' sexuality and reproduction is at the heart of unequal gender relations, and is central to the denial of equality and self-determination to women. (as quoted in Baird 2004, 142)

We argue that these rights are basic on the grounds that such rights are assumed and taken for granted by men; because there is no parallel threat to which men are subject, men cannot be invaded in a similar way. Accordingly, if women are to be equal to men, then such basic rights are required for women to attain the same minimal standard of bodily control that all men automatically have. Moreover, such rights are basic in that they are necessary for the exercise of all other (human) rights, as basic bodily integrity and control is a prerequisite for the exercising of other rights.

CONCEPTUALIZING BASIC HUMAN RIGHTS

What Are Reproductive Rights?

Following Catherine MacKinnon, we ground our arguments about the importance of reproductive control as a basic right (the ability to actually access contraception and abortion and correspondingly the ability to refuse to undergo such procedures) in arguments from sex equality (MacKinnon 1991).

The nature of reproductive rights is highly contested, in terms of what they are and what they should be. In this chapter we separate "basic" reproductive rights from other possible understandings of reproductive rights, and we justify our position on a gendered basis using equality arguments. Reva Siegel summarizes some of the key features of a sex equality approach to reproductive rights as follows:

> [T]he sex equality approach to reproductive rights views control over the timing of motherhood as crucial to the status and welfare of women, individually and as a class. Arguments from the sex equality standpoint appreciate that there is both practical and dignitary significance to the decisional control that reproductive rights afford women, and that such control matters more to women who are status marked by reason of class, race, age, or marriage. Control over whether and when to give birth is practically important to women for reasons inflected with gender-justice concern: It crucially affects women's health and sexual freedom, their ability to enter and end

relationships, their education and job training, their ability to provide for their families, and their ability to negotiate work-family conflicts in institutions organized on the basis of traditional sex-role assumptions that this society no longer believes fair to enforce, yet is unwilling institutionally to redress. (Siegel 2007, 818–819)

Other arguments could be used, and philosophically and legally there is no consensus around what reproductive rights are. Moreover, the topic is highly contested, both in conceptual terms of what reproductive rights could and should amount to, and in practical terms about how such rights should be provided. The global picture is one of complexity and confusion. For instance, the Universal Declaration of Human Rights (UDHR) does not explicitly mention reproductive rights, although they are implied in the right to found a family (article 16), and the importance of bodily integrity, which forbids torture and cruel or inhuman treatment and punishment (article 5). Taken together, these rights can be used to claim that no one should be physically prevented from conceiving and bearing children; or conversely that no one should be forced to carry a child. Given there is so little clarity about what reproductive rights are, it is not surprising that what is available in practice varies widely both within localities and globally. In the second section of this chapter, we will track the evolution of human rights discourse on reproductive rights and note some of the key changes in how such rights are conceptualized.

The Importance of "Gender" Back in the Reproductive Rights Debate

Debates about reproductive rights touch on many controversial and sensitive issues. Perhaps one of the most contested issues relates to the moral status of the embryo/fetus. It is this way of framing the debate that is typical of "pro-choice," "pro-life" categories which beset much of the polarized political debate (Widdows 2011, 201–204). Such arguments "against abortion" are often made on religious grounds or on claims regarding the necessary features for moral personhood (Steinbock 1992). Those who wish to restrict access to abortion assert the "personhood" or "sanctity" of the embryo at various stages, including conception, quickening, and viability, and many who are not religious also share such views (George and Tollefsen 2008). Fetal-centric arguments often assume a complete separation between the pregnant woman and the fetus, elevating the latter to the status of the individual of equal moral worth to the woman. Such arguments are evident in the growing legal trend to afford protection to the fetus through the constitutionalization of fetal rights (DeLondras 2015). These arguments construct maternal/fetal conflict and acknowledge the embodied nature of pregnancy only to the extent that the pregnant woman is viewed as a threat to the fetus. The argument posits the woman as an aggressor and the fetus as an innocent bystander rather than a dependent. As Susan Bordo summarizes: "as the personhood of the pregnant woman has been drained from her and her function as fetal incubator activated, the subjectivity of the fetus has been elevated" (Bordo 1993, 85). These arguments have been used to justify restrictions on both abortion and contraception, although ironically they have sometimes had the perverse consequence of increasing the number of abortions rather than decreasing them (Cohen 2012).

Fetal-centric arguments are also often constructed in ways that fail to take account of the gendered nature of reproduction. In this chapter our approach is fundamentally gendered and highlights the gender injustice involved in failure to grant access to contraception and abortion. In adopting a gendered lens, our intention is to highlight that not only are women suffering from lack of access to contraception and abortion but also to show that this injustice is partly an injustice which women suffer as women. Failure to protect women from disadvantages and injustices they experience solely because of their gender undermines the universality of "rights" (Cook 1993). Women's reproductive rights are not just controversial in the abortion debate, but in other debates about family and social structures, and often these issues share commonality with the abortion debate in that they are essentially about controlling women's bodies. In the words of Alison Jaggar, "because women are typically seen as the symbols or bearers of culture, conflicts among cultural groups are often fought on the terrain of women's bodies" (Jaggar 2005, 46). Attempts to control women's bodies, particularly their sexual and reproductive functions, have a long and global history. Ways in which such control has been manifested in the family include practices of female genital mutilation, chastity belts, chaperoning women, and restricting freedom by denying movement or employment outside the home (to prevent opportunities for nonapproved sexual encounters) (Chavkin and Chesler 2005). In addition, blame for sexual and reproductive "mistakes" or what is deemed inappropriate behavior usually, and across cultures, falls disproportionally upon women. Such disparities raise equality questions as such attempts to control reproduction do not apply to men, and rarely to boys. Patriarchal norms have shaped many aspects of the world we inhabit and are mirrored at the policy level in marriage and divorce laws, employment laws, and perhaps most obviously in policies of population control. To neglect the gendered aspect of reproductive rights is to neglect key features of the injustices involved and to fail to accord these rights the respect they deserve. Hence, in the next section we develop an argument for access to contraception and abortion that is gender sensitive and grounds these basic reproductive rights in an argument from equality.

Basic Reproductive Rights From Equality

In this section we argue that in order for women to achieve equality with men, to be human, basic reproductive rights—including access to contraception and abortion—must be accessible to all women. From this argument follow claims about the importance of basic reproductive rights and the necessity of granting these over and before other rights—including, but not only, other reproductive rights. However, it is not necessary to agree with our argument to agree with our conclusion that these rights are basic for women to function effectively. For instance, one could argue from a perspective of autonomy that women should have access to these rights in order to be able to exercise their autonomy and make choices for their own lives, or that such rights follow from arguments based on negative rights of noninterference.[1] Moreover, some of these arguments complement and supplement our claims. Given this, it is possible to accept our conclusion that these basic rights are necessary, and to endorse the claims made in the latter part of the chapter about the global need to grant these basic rights to women, without endorsing the philosophical foundational argument regarding how to ground and construct such rights.

We argue that these rights are basic and are necessary for women to be human and equal to men. We argue that these rights are basic not because they are negative rights, nor because they are autonomy rights, but on grounds of equality. This then is a threshold concept. Only by guaranteeing bodily control, by the means of contraception and abortion, can women attain a comparable standard of bodily integrity to men and thus can the requirements of equality be met.[2]

To make this argument, we introduce the debate about whether "women's rights" amount to "human rights." We endorse the view that where there is a gap between the rights which women hold and the rights which men hold this should be closed if women are to be said to enjoy "human rights." If this gap is not closed, then women cannot be considered human, but are effectively subhuman, and treated as inferior to men. This approach draws on the seminal work by Catharine MacKinnon, who asks, "Are women human?" (MacKinnon 2006).[3] Her work considers women's rights taken as a whole, and not simply reproductive rights, and she is especially concerned with rape and violence in the context of conflict. But the structure, assumptions, and implications of her argument can be applied equally to reproductive rights. She states:

> If women were human, would we be a cash crop shipped from Thailand in containers into New York's brothels? Would be we sexual and reproductive slaves? Would we be bred, worked without pay our whole lives, burned when our dowry money wasn't enough or when men tired of us, starved as widows when our husbands died (if we survived his funeral pyre), sold for sex because we are not valued for anything else? Would we be sold into marriage to priests to atone for our family's sins or to improve our earthly prospects? Would we, when allowed to work for pay, be made to work at the most menial jobs and exploited at barely starvation level? Would we have our genitals sliced out to "cleanse" us (our body parts are dirt?) to control us, to mark us and define our cultures? Would we be trafficked as things for sexual use and entertainment worldwide in whatever form current technology makes possible? Would we be kept from learning to read and write? . . . Would we be sexually molested in our families? Would we be raped in genocide to terrorize and eject and destroy our ethnic communities, and raped again in that undeclared war that goes on every day in every country in the world in what is called peacetime? If women were human, would our violation be *enjoyed* by our violators? And, if we were human, when these things happened, would virtually nothing be done about it?" (MacKinnon 2006, 41)

MacKinnon's language is deliberately rhetorical and dramatic and intentionally controversial. Yet her point is simple: that many of the injustices to which women are subjected are gendered. The type of injustices that are often done to women happen only to women; they do not happen to men. That many of the injustices which MacKinnon lists are connected to sex and reproduction is not surprising, given the asymmetrical way they are experienced by women and men. Sex and reproduction are sites in which women's experience and men's experience are divergent, and as MacKinnon states, "nowhere is sexuality not central to keeping women down" (MacKinnon 2006, 13). It is this divergence which MacKinnon focuses on to explain why such gendered injustices are so widely perpetrated and why comparatively little is done to address them, and certainly less than would be done to address them if they were nongendered injustices. If we reframe MacKinnon's argument slightly so that it directly maps the argument we are making about basic reproductive rights, and why access to contraception and abortion are required if women are to be equal to men, then it would run something like this:

> If women were human, would they be denied the right to prevent the invasion of their bodies and involuntary impregnation? Would a foreign body be allowed to feed from them, to grow inside them, and to transform the shape of their body? Would they be required to adapt their lifestyles, eating, drinking, and physical activities to accommodate another? Would their wombs be treated as separate from themselves and regarded as the property of others? Would others—husbands, family, religious and cultural leaders, NGOs, and policymakers—be able to determine whether or not they put their lives at risk through childbearing? If women were human, would they not be granted the same minimum expectation of bodily integrity as men?

This is just an example of how such an argument could run, and we are not committed to any particular clause. We are merely introducing it as a hypothetical exercise that is useful in highlighting the gendered nature of reproductive rights. Putting the argument this way is, like MacKinnon's, rhetorical and confrontational and designed to be so. The style can be objected to on the grounds that such aggressive language obscures because of its highly political and polemical nature. However, such an approach is useful as a device to show the gender differential that is fundamental to claims about reproductive rights. When one formulates the claims to basic rights in this way, and makes women overtly the focus of the argument, and women as human beings *qua* human being, then the gender injustice emerges clearly. Formulated in this way, focusing on how women are treated when compared to men—or women as compared to "full humans"—then the extent of what is denied to women when they are denied contraception and abortion is clear. Thinking of reproductive rights in this framework helps us identify why such rights are basic—because they are threshold rights that allow women to be equal to men. It also provides reasons for prioritizing such rights over other rights, and for not simply regarding these as "negative rights" (rights to be left alone, rather than positive rights to actually have access). Such rights are basic, because they are threshold rights, assuring women's equality to men.

MacKinnon's approach highlights that often "human rights" means "men's rights," as "men" are the archetypal "human": the human rights system is structured and constructed according to male priorities rather than female priorities. For instance, MacKinnon suggests that it is likely that women would prioritize rights differently than men. Thus, she states, "lacking effective guarantees of economic and social rights, women have found political and civil rights, however crucial, to be largely inaccessible and superficial" (MacKinnon 2006, 5–6).[4] MacKinnon's critique suggests that women's rights initiatives have done little to address the gendered nature of human rights. For instance, she argues that the Convention on the Elimination of All Forms of Discrimination Against Women (CEDAW) says little about the evils of sexism and the inferiority of women.[5] However, one does not need to endorse all of MacKinnon's wider claims about the failures of human rights as women's rights to think that there are gendered injustices which must be addressed if women are to be equal to men and to think that MacKinnon's style of argumentation is useful for revealing these. With regard to basic reproductive rights, rights that raise women up to the same status and standard as men, her gendered analysis is revealing. Only if these basic reproductive rights are attained can women take for granted certain aspects of bodily integrity that men automatically have. Without the rights to avoid pregnancy or to end pregnancy (using the means of contraception and abortion services) women lack both bodily integrity and basic control of their reproductive functions. These are functions that men do not lack (men cannot suffer similar breaches in bodily integrity), and furthermore these rights are basic in that without them women are unable to exercise agency in other fields, including those of relationships and employment. Such control is a necessary aspect of not only furthering women's emancipation and equality in general, but importantly as threshold rights that allow women to experience the basic bodily integrity and control which men experience. Accordingly, if women are to be granted human rights, these basic reproductive rights must be granted, not just as formal rights of access. It is not enough for such rights to be formally available—not prohibited—but they must be actually available. Given this, these services are not, we argue, supplementary or mere parts of health care packages that can be reasonably sacrificed in order for women to gain other goods.

BEYOND BASIC RIGHTS

In this chapter we are not denying that there are, or may be, other reproductive rights, for instance, rights to parent. However, we are claiming that there are no other *basic* reproductive rights, at least such rights cannot be constructed from or grounded in equality claims. Furthermore, while we argue that access to contraception and abortion is a basic right—and one which is currently conspicuously lacking for a large number of women globally—the parallel rights not to be coerced into abortion and sterilization are also basic, as these too can be grounded in equality. The debate about basic reproductive rights does not exhaust the reproductive rights debate, and there are many other issues that are pertinent to the reproductive rights debate. In particular, there are questions about whether there is a right to access reproductive technologies. This right is particularly claimed from the "right to found a family." However, rights to reproductive technology are not basic rights in the way we have argued the case, as they do not contravene the gender equality criteria and as such are not threshold rights and thus are not our concern in this chapter. Before going on to consider specific case studies on access to contraception and abortion, we will provide a brief overview of how human rights discourses on reproductive rights and how we conceptualize them have evolved.

WHERE HUMAN RIGHTS BEGIN— THE SMALL PLACES

In this part of the chapter we consider the emergence and development of reproductive rights within human rights discourse. In doing so, we are mindful of the limitations of international human rights documents and wary of the criticisms of scholars like MacKinnon, as discussed earlier. However, consideration of the development of human rights gives us some cause to be hopeful, particularly the way in which human rights have empowered grassroots advocates by providing a rhetorical frame that they can use to ground claims against the state (Cook and Dickens 2009). International human rights are also being used as a mechanism for improving access to abortion services in countries like Poland and Ireland, where such services are highly restricted (Erdman 2014). As such, it is increasingly becoming evident to both scholars and activists who are advocating for improved reproductive futures for women in a variety of contexts that the incorporation of human rights within reproductive justice frameworks can be an important tool of empowerment (Luna 2009). In the 20 years since the International Conference on Population and Development (ICPD) in Cairo, we have witnessed some huge improvements to women's health worldwide, so while there is still much to do, it is clear that human rights discourses have been a useful political tool for activists worldwide.

In considering the question of where human rights begin, Eleanor Roosevelt posited "the small places." Here Roosevelt is hinting to the fact that human rights are important in all aspects of our lives—for only through achieving justice and equality in these spaces is it possible to achieve justice and equality in bigger, more public spaces. The full quote is as follows:

> Where, after all, do universal human rights begin? In small places, close to home—
> so close and so small that they cannot be seen on any maps of the world. Yet they
> are the world of the individual person; the neighbourhood he lives in; the school
> or college he attends; the factory, farm or office where he works. Such are the places

where every man, woman and child seeks equal justice, equal opportunity, equal dignity without discrimination. Unless these rights have meaning there, they have little meaning anywhere. Without concerned citizen action to uphold them close to home, we shall look in vain for progress in the larger world.[6]

Roosevelt was speaking in 1958, a decade after the creation of the UDHR. Roosevelt's sentiment holds to this day and is particularly apt in considering the importance and necessity of controlling sexual and reproductive activity if women are to have equality with men, or in MacKinnon's words, to be "truly human." In this section we provide a brief overview of *women's* human rights, paying specific attention to changing discourses around sexual and reproductive health. We do not aim here to be comprehensive in our account but rather to highlight some key shifts in emphasis.

The UDHR explicitly challenges the oppression of women in what was traditionally deemed the "private sphere." In so doing, it steps into the small places and transcends the traditional dichotomy of public and private spaces—a dichotomy feminist scholars have long rejected (see, for example, Pateman 1983). The UDHR recognizes that in order to fully advance women's rights the state must advance not just "public" rights, for example, employment but also "private" rights, for example, consent to marriage and education. Reproductive rights have long been recognized at the international level as a subset of human rights. At the United Nations (UN) Conference on Human Rights in Tehran in 1968, Resolution XVIII on the Human Rights Aspects of Family Planning was adopted. This resolution states that "couples have a basic human right to decide freely and responsibly on the number and spacing of their children and a right to adequate education and information in this respect."[7] This was adopted by a resolution of the UN General Assembly in 1969 and provides the basis upon which current Declarations regarding sexual and reproductive health rights are based.

CEDAW was adopted by the UN General Assembly in 1979. This Convention is important in providing protection for a broad range of rights; those specifically important in the context of our analysis include rights in marriage, health, and family planning. The Convention specifically aims to redress the systemic discrimination against women evident in society, and with its adoption "UN emphasis turned to moving women to the center of development strategies" (Chesler 2005, 15). It is beyond the scope of the chapter to map the trajectory of women's rights from this point forward (see, for example, Bunch 1990; Cook 1993), but it is clear that human rights instruments developed as an important tool in the global enfranchisement of women. Importantly in 1993, in Vienna, the World Conference on Human Rights reaffirmed that the protection of women's rights was integral to the protection of human rights, calling for an end to discrimination against women and women's enfranchisement in all aspects of political and social life (World Conference on Human Rights, Vienna, 1993). Attention to the importance of protecting sexual and reproductive health rights as part of this has become the focus of increasingly levels of attention since the early 1990s with calls for "maternal and reproductive health policies" to be "understood as a basic obligation of the state's positive social responsibility to protect women's right to life, liberty, and security" (Chesler 2005, 17).

The International Conference on Population and Development (ICPD) in Cairo in 1994 was a UN-led gathering that focused on the legitimacy and success of global population policies. The Cairo Programme of Action (ICPD 1994) produced a 20-year roadmap (1995–2015) for how human rights could be used to protect women's rights to bodily integrity and in particular their ability to control the timing and number of their children. Importantly this roadmap is concerned not just with the needs of adults but also those of adolescent children. The framing of these protections is not just individual; also emphasized is that these protections are necessary for the good of society generally. A key feature of the Programme was to increase investment and expenditure on sexual and reproductive health in a broad range of areas, including access to health care, education, and family planning. It aimed to reduce maternal child mortality rates and incidence of sexually transmitted disease globally. The ICPD in 1994 was the first time that safe abortion care was recognized as a necessary feature of reducing maternal morbidity and mortality globally. It draws on public health rhetoric and arguments from harm reduction to emphasis the importance in reducing the incidence of unsafe abortions (Hessini 2005).

Dixon Mueller explains a fundamental tension that exists in the development of family planning policies and the subsequent emergence of sexual and reproductive rights (Dixon Mueller, 1993). The first strand is that of population control. Family planning policies emerged in order to enable governments to deal with excessive population growth. The second strand to these policies is the protection of individual human rights. Family planning policies have developed to enable individual, and in particular women's, expression of rights of bodily control and bodily integrity. However, it is often the case that population control policies have infringed on individual human rights.

Population control policies include education, the provision of contraception and abortion, and sterilization; at times such measures have been forced. A controversial aspect of population control policies, forced sterilization, has a long history in Europe and the United States. In the early twentieth century it was widely practiced as part of public health measures supposed to improve population health (WHO 2014). There have also been instances of sterilization being linked with the criminal justice process; women from a variety of groups were forcibly sterilized in order to ensure that they did not pass on their "deviancy" to the next generation; women who were sterilized include those suffering from mental disabilities, the "feeble minded," the "sexually deviant" (which could be interpreted to include promiscuity, lesbianism, and adultery), and those from undesirable ethnic groups, particularly "gypsies"(see, for example, Trombley 1988). "Gypsies" was a general term to include many Roma ethnic groups, usually from central and eastern Europe.[8] Although campaigners and nongovernmental organizations (NGOs) acknowledged the importance of these policies in addressing increased global birth rates and the funding they provided to sexual and reproductive health services, they called for a shift in emphasis "to reflect a fundamental commitment to reproductive and sexual rights as fundamental human rights" (Chesler 2005, 19). Such a strategy was in keeping with an approach that acknowledged the importance of the role of women in society rather than being solely concerned with restricting women's reproductive freedom through control of their fertility.

An oft-cited example of a population policy that clearly infringes reproductive rights is China's "Family Planning Policy," often called the "one-child policy." This policy was established in 1979 as part of a broader program of population control being instituted by the Chinese government in the late 1970s with an aim of reducing China's rapidly increasing population (Hesketh and Wei Xing 2005). The main substance of the policy is a restriction on the ability of couples, particularly those from urban areas, to have more than one child. However, there were exemptions from the policy for those living in rural areas, particularly if their first child was a girl, and for ethnic minorities (Hesketh and Wei Xing 2005). The policy was implemented somewhat unevenly, as much power and discretion lie in the hands of local officials. Broadly the policy has been implemented through a series of monetary fines for those who breach it. More controversially, it has been reported that the policy has led to women who have an "unapproved" pregnancy being forced to have an abortion or avoiding antenatal health care for fear they would be made to undergo an abortion. As recently as 2010, Amnesty International reported that thousands of women in China were at risk of forced sterilization (Amnesty International 2010). It has also been reported that because women avoid antenatal care and deliver at home, usually without access to appropriate health care, they face much higher rates of maternal deaths (Hesketh and Wei Xing 2005). This highlights a number of ways in which the policy breaches basic reproductive rights. Although extreme, this policy is not isolated, and there is evidence of similarly coercive population control measures in other countries. Forced sterilization continues in many parts of the world today, as does "induced consent," when women are encouraged to undergo sterilization and even given payment or other forms of inducement as part of population control measures.

Cairo was quickly followed in 1995 by the Fourth World Conference in Beijing. The Beijing Platform for Action states:

> The human rights of women include their right to have control over and decide freely and responsibly on matters related to their sexuality, including sexual and reproductive health, free of coercion, discrimination and violence. Equal relationships between women and men in matters of sexual relations and reproduction, including full respect for the integrity of the person, require mutual respect, consent and shared responsibility for sexual behaviour and its consequences. (Beijing Platform for Action 1995)

The Platform for Action again reaffirms the importance of women's human rights, emphasizing the importance of women's emancipation as part of the development process. However, in addition to the broader aims of development, the platform moves beyond this position and also emphasizes the intrinsic importance of women's rights. Women's ability to control their reproductive futures is a necessary feature of their emancipation and a human right deserving of protection.

The move from "control" to "freedom," as emphasized in the Cairo Programme, has met with mixed success, and as detailed earlier, many human rights violations in this area are continuing. However, it is clear from the earlier discussion that international human rights documents have come to recognize that to respect women's bodily integrity and agency, it is necessary to protect a range of sexual and reproductive health rights that aim to facilitate women and girls' ability to control the timing and number of their children. These protections are necessary if women are to be able to enter society as equal to men. Specifically, family planning and contraception are mentioned as being important to this process. While abortion has proven to be more controversial, since Cairo it is clear that public health ethics arguments, particularly those regarding harm reduction, are becoming increasingly important as a means for advocating for abortion care (Erdman 2011; Colletti, IPAS, 2013). It has also been recognized across a range of human rights documents that access to safe and legal abortion care is necessary and expected in a number of cases (e.g., where the life of the pregnant woman is threatened or where the woman is pregnant as a result of rape). Furthermore, the WHO recognizes "safe abortion care" as one of the seven packages necessary to improve maternal morbidity and mortality worldwide (WHO 2010). This serves to highlight the important and necessary role of safe abortion care within holistic family planning programs. Although abortion is often subject to moral controversy, it is clear that unsafe abortions have serious negative consequences for maternal health on a global scale (Singh 2010; WHO 2007). It is also clear that legal restrictions on the availability of abortion do not decrease the incidence of abortion but rather increase the incidence of unsafe abortions—unsafe abortions are defined by the WHO as those that involve "inadequacy of the provider's skills and use of hazardous techniques and unsanitary facilities" (WHO 2007, 1). No method of contraception is 100% reliable and all are subject to the foibles of human use. Access to safe abortion care is therefore a necessary tool in family planning programs aimed at reducing maternal morbidity and mortality globally.

In tracing the emergence of reproductive rights on a global scale, it becomes clear that a holistic understanding of family planning services is necessary in order to improve maternal morbidity and mortality worldwide. Having argued, therefore, that access to contraception and abortion is a basic reproductive right necessary for all women, we spend the final part of this chapter examining what is arguably one of the most controversial aspects of global reproductive health policy: restrictions on development aid that aim to decouple safe abortion care from family planning services.

ACCESSING BASIC REPRODUCTIVE RIGHTS— RESTRICTIONS ON DEVELOPMENT AID

The most prominent example of a restriction on development aid being used to fund abortion services is the "Helms Amendment" and its subsequent extension through the

GGGR (Crane and Dusenberry 2004). Moving on from this example of US restrictions on development aid, we consider some emerging examples in other regions, specifically at the European Union (EU) level. Therefore, it is important to note that although the United States is the most prominent example of restrictions on development aid of this kind, it is not unique. Toward the end of the section we detail similar restrictions in NGOs. Restricting funding for abortion services is often considered as a compromise between opposing views on the permissibility of the procedure (see, for example, DeGrazia 2012). In this part of the chapter we consider the legitimacy of such a position. Far from being an example of a compromise, it is clear that such restrictions on a global scale often serve to skew domestic policy on abortion. By this, we mean that restrictions on development aid often serve to restrict access to contraception and abortion services in countries where they are legal and as such undermine official laws on the issue. The GGR applies to countries where access to abortion and contraception is legal and has the effect of blocking access to these services in ways that contravene international human rights norms (Barot 2013).

The GGR was introduced by Ronald Reagan, then president of the United States, in 1984. The GGR was an executive order that expanded on the Helms Amendment to the Foreign Assistance Act introduced by Sen. Jesse Helms in 1973. The Helms Amendment prohibited the use of US Foreign Aid for "the performance of abortions as a method of family planning" and for use to "motivate or coerce any person to practice abortions." At the time the Amendment was introduced, USAID, the government agency responsible for international development, strongly objected, stating that it contradicted the core principle of the organization that:

> [E]xplicitly acknowledges that every nation is and should be free to determine its own policies and procedures with respect to population growth and family planning. In contradiction of this principle, the amendment would place U.S. restrictions on both developing country governments and individuals in the matter of free choice among the means of fertility control . . . that are legal in the U.S. (As quoted in Barot 2013, 9)

Notwithstanding these objections, the Amendment was passed. It was then expanded with the introduction of the GGR almost 10 years later. The GGR prohibits any organizations that receive US government funding from facilitating access to abortion services or any advocates for the liberalisation of domestic abortion policy; and importantly it applies even if the organization provides a broad range of sexual and reproductive health services and obtains its funding for abortion services from another source (Center for Reproductive Rights 2000). As such, it amounts to a restriction on both US and non-US funding:

> While the Helms amendment limits the use of U.S. foreign aid dollars directly, the gag rule went far beyond that by disqualifying foreign NGOs from eligibility for U.S. family planning aid entirely by virtue of their support for abortion-related activities subsidized by non-U.S. funds. (Barot 2013, 10)

A version of the GGR has been endorsed by every Republican president since Reagan and rescinded by every Democrat president. The Helms Amendment has remained in place since its introduction in 1973. This muddled picture has had a "chilling effect" on a range of sexual and reproductive health services on a global scale (Barot 2013). It is important to note that the gag applies in countries where abortion is legal; US development aid has never been used to fund access to abortion where the procedure is illegal (Skuster 2004).

The impact of the GGR has been assessed by several organizations, including the Guttmacher Institute (Cohen 2006), Population Action International (2015), and the Center for Reproductive Rights (2010). All have highlighted the clear negative impact of this restriction on maternal and reproductive health measures in affected countries. Negative impacts include increased maternal morbidity and mortality, an increased number of unplanned pregnancies, an increased number of unsafe abortions, and a subsequent increase in deaths from unsafe abortion. The consequence of the GGR is therefore not a decrease in the number of abortions but rather an interference with family planning services generally with a subsequent increase in the number of unsafe abortions. There are three clear reasons for these negative impacts. First, there is confusion over what exactly is prohibited under Helms and what is prohibited under the GGR (Barot 2011, 2013). This is what has led to the "chilling effect" that encourages overly conservative practice as organizations do not want to be found in contravention of either policy. Second, the GGR extends the impact on the restrictions so that it applies not just to US Development Aid but to funds received through other avenues (Cohen 2006). And finally, and in some ways most worrying, the GGR results in a situation in which those experts who might otherwise be called upon by governments to provide evidence of the negative impact of unsafe abortion are restricted from speaking to these issues as this would constitute "abortion advocacy" (Skuster 2004). An example of the impact of the GGR is detailed by Karen Baird: in Nepal, family planning services lost $250,000 as a result of the GGR when they advocated for improved reproductive health care in the face of a maternal health crisis in that country (Baird 2004). The following quote from the Director of Family Planning Association of Nepal (FPAN) is stark:

> This is the challenge: do I listen to my own government that has asked FPAN to save women's lives or do I listen to the US government? (as quoted in Baird 2004)

It is important to note that such a restriction would not be permissible were it to impact on US NGOs, as detailed by Patty Skuster:

> The Global Gag Rule would be unconstitutional if applied to U.S. organizations. The restrictions that make up the order apply only to foreign NGOs—which do not have U.S. constitutional protection over free speech and free association. Federal courts have prohibited restrictions placed on U.S. NGOs similar to those of the GGR. The Constitution does not permit Congress to enact legislation that restricts a U.S.-based organization's constitutional rights by dictating how a grantee spends funds not provided by U.S. government sources. The U.S. government may not use funding restrictions to impinge upon a U.S.-based NGO's ability to exercise its rights to free speech or to lobby using its own private funds. (Skuster 2004, 100–101)

Therefore, as argued by USAID, it is clear that GGR has the potential to disrupt the democratic processes of the countries that it impacts on. The GGR has had significant negative impacts on the lives of real women in countries where access to safe abortion is a legal and necessary aspect of family planning services. Like all attempts to impose restrictions on development aid in this way, the impact is on countries where maternal mortality and morbidity are higher than those considered acceptable in the United States, and where access to safe and legal abortion is a basic health need (ICPD 1994).

Other governments, including Canada, have introduced similar restrictions.[9] In 2010 the Harper Government pledged increased levels of funding to reduce maternal mortality and morbidity worldwide; however, this policy was not to include increased funding for safe abortion care. At the EU level there was a failed attempt between 2012 and 2014 to use the newly introduced mechanism of a European Citizens' Initiative (ECI) to restrict EU development aid. The Citizenship Initiative is a mechanism introduced by the European Commission allowing citizens to propose legislation for consideration by the European Commission on any issue within its power if they gather 1 million signatures from at least seven of the 27 EU Member States. An ECI entitled "One of Us" aimed to provide human embryos with "dignity and integrity," and as a consequence of this "the EU should establish a ban and end the financing of activities which presuppose the destruction of human embryos, in particular in the areas of research, *development aid* and public health" (One of Us 2012). The initiative was introduced subsequent to a report by a conservative European think tank, European Dignity Watch, entitled "The Funding of Abortion Through EU Development Aid: An Analysis of EU's Sexual and Reproductive Health Policy," which argued that funding of abortion services was outside EU competence and as such should not be included within the development aid budget (European Dignity Watch 2012). If successful, "One of Us" would have severely restricted EU development aid with a worrying negative health impact on the lives of women in countries in receipt of such aid. It would also have directly challenged fundamental rights of women and been in direct conflict with the aims of UN Millennium Development Goal five: to improve maternal health (UN MDG 2000).

It is not just in the policies of national government that we are witnessing GGR style restrictions. In June 2014, Melinda Gates announced that the Gates Foundation would no longer fund abortions. Gates states that abortion is too controversial and ultimately harmful to helping women worldwide. In her explanation of this decision, Gates highlights the fact that the Foundation will continue to advocate for family planning and the ability of women worldwide to space their children. However, she thinks that abortion should be dealt with separately. Specifically, she says:

> The question of abortion should be dealt with separately. Both in the United States and around the world the emotional and personal debate about abortion is threatening to get in the way of the lifesaving consensus regarding basic family planning.[10]

Gates's rhetoric in justifying the position with regard to funding implies that they have chosen to stop funding abortions in order to promote the greater good overall. One of the global development goals of the Bill & Melinda Gates Foundation is improvement in family planning:

> OUR GOAL: to bring access to high-quality contraceptive information, services, and supplies to an additional 120 million women and girls in the poorest countries by 2020 without coercion or discrimination, with the longer-term goal of universal access to voluntary family planning.[11]

The tension between this goal and the refusal to fund abortion services contributes to the exceptionalisation of abortion care despite the clear evidence that such services are a necessary part of global family planning strategies and an important part of any strategy that aims to reduce maternal morbidity and mortality (WHO 2007). This approach also propagates the idea that contraception is the only tool necessary to combat family planning; this is despite the fact that there is much evidence to suggest that access to abortion and contraception should not be viewed as mutually exclusive but rather both should form part of holistic family planning strategies. In the words of Marge Berer:

> [I] feel . . . worried about the Gates Foundation's effects on things, because I think theirs is such a retrograde approach. Ideologically, it's supposedly prochoice, but it's very, very antichoice on many levels. (Berer 2014)

Restrictions on development aid of the sort outlined in this section are worrying for many reasons. They skew democratic processes and create negative health consequences of a sort that would not be acceptable in the country where they originate. Furthermore, the attempt to break down family planning policies into component parts ignores the reality of the necessity of both access to contraception and safe abortion care if we are to protect and promote basic reproductive rights. Restrictions that exceptionalize abortion are counter to the accepted principle of most international health bodies that such care is a necessary basic health need. It is for this reason that we suggest that those who are interested in protecting basic reproductive rights should challenge the legitimacy of such restrictions.

Conclusion

In this chapter we have argued on grounds of gender equality that access to contraception and abortion is a basic reproductive right. Consequently, we argued that such rights should be prioritized and not sacrificed in order to attain other goods. We have also emphasized the importance of these rights not being sacrificed as part of some effort at compromise for those who wish to restrict access to abortion domestically but have been unsuccessful in this aim.

International human rights norms have increasingly come to reflect and acknowledge the importance of access to abortion and contraception as integral to women's ability to control the number and timing of their children. These norms reflect our view that such rights are basic reproductive rights and should be protected as such.

Globally we found that these rights are often not delivered, and the most vulnerable women are too often denied them; we discussed some policies and practices that are eroding these rights. The slogan "Free, Safe and Legal" has long been a mantra of the reproductive rights movement. Restrictions on development aid unfairly impact women in developing countries and restrict their ability to access the basic reproductive health care that they most need. We have highlighted both the principled objections to such restrictions and also some of the practical negative outcomes of these policies.

Many are now focused on "Post 2015" global reproductive health goals. Given the improvements in maternal health on a worldwide scale since the ICPD in 1994, it would be a pity if retrograde steps such as restrictions on development aid with regard to family planning services were to become common place. The rhetoric of appeasement such as that evident in the quote from Melinda Gates in this chapter should be challenged. Access to safe abortion cannot be disentangled from access to contraception as part of the protection of women's basic reproductive rights. Attempting to decouple access to safe abortion care goes against accepted development policy since 1994 that has "linked abortion with other key public health and women's health rights issues" (Hessini 2005, 88–100). It is important, therefore, that we ensure that access to *both* contraception and safe abortion care occupies a prominent space in the post-2015 ICPD agenda (Barot 2014).

Notes

1. Other arguments could be made on autonomy grounds. Our claim is not that such arguments cannot be made; we simply wish to focus on the equality argument for this chapter.
2. Attempts to imagine what a similar bodily invasion would amount to for a man are the subject of many philosophical papers, the most famous being Judith Jarvis Thomson's violinist, which is still central to the philosophical debate (Jarvis Thomson 1971).
3. This was first published in 1999 in *Reflections on the Universal Declaration of Human Rights*, but it is reprinted in MacKinnon's 2006 collection of the same title.
4. Furthermore, she continues that "The generational distinctions and their rankings, questionable for men as well, are clearly premised on gendered assumptions, perceptions and priorities" (MacKinnon 2006, 6).
5. Of course, this is one view and many feminists welcome CEDAW as a huge advance in women's rights.
6. http://www.un.org/en/globalissues/briefingpapers/humanrights/quotes.shtml (accessed July 31, 2015).
7. "Reproductive Rights," http://www.un.org/en/development/desa/population/theme/rights/
8. The continuation of forced, or at least coerced, sterilization of Roma in Europe was brought to light in a 2003 report by the Center for Reproductive Rights & Poradña.

The report documents sterilization as a common experience of Roma women. In these instances women go into the hospital when in labor and then, when about to be given a caesarean section, they are told to sign a consent form. This form gives consent not only to a caesarean section but also to tubal ligation.

9. http://www.sexualhealthandrights.ca/wp-content/uploads/2015/07/Global-5_Abortion.pdf

10. http://www.breitbart.com/big-government/2014/06/12/bill-and-melinda-gates-foundation-says-it-will-no-longer-fund-abortion/ (accessed February 21, 2015).

11. http://www.gatesfoundation.org/What-We-Do/Global-Development/Family-Planning

BIBLIOGRAPHY

Amnesty International. 2010. Thousands at risk of forced sterilization in China (Amnesty International. https://www.amnesty.org/en/latest/news/2010/04/thousands-risk-forced-sterilization-china/.

Baird, Karen L. 2004. Globalizing reproductive control: Consequences of the Global Gag Rule. In *Linking visions: Feminist bioethics, human rights, and the developing world*, ed. Rosemarie Tong, 133–145. New York: Rowman & Littlefield.

Barot, Sneha. 2014. Looking back while moving forward: Marking 20 years since The International Conference on Population and Development. *Guttmacher Policy Review* 17: 22–28.

Barot, Sneha. 2013. Abortion restrictions in U.S. foreign aid: The history and harms of the Helms Amendment. *Guttmacher Policy Review* 16: 9–13.

Barot, Sneha. 2011. Unsafe Abortion: The Missing Link in Global Efforts to Improve Maternal Health. *Guttmacher Policy Review* 14: 24–28.

Beijing Platform for Action 1995. http://www.un.org/womenwatch/daw/beijing/platform/.

Berer, Marge. 2014. Down a Garden Path: The Folly of Pitting Contraception against Abortion. *Conscience* 35: 14–21.

Bordo, Susan. 1993. *Unbearable weight: Feminism, Western culture, and the body*. Berkeley and Los Angeles: University of California Press.

Bunch, Charlotte. 1990. Women's rights as human rights: Toward a re-vision of human rights. *Human Rights Quarterly* 12: 486–489.

Center for Reproductive Rights 2010. Whose choice? How the Hyde Amendment hurts poor women. http://www.reproductiverights.org/feature/whose-choice- how-the-hyde-amendment-harms-poor-women.

Center for Reproductive Rights. 2000. The Bush Global Gag Rule: A violation of international human rights (Briefing Paper). http://www.reproductiverights.org/document/the-bush-global-gag-rule-a-violation-of-international-human-rights.

Center for Reproductive Rights & Poradɴa. 2003. Body and soul: Forced sterilization and other assaults on Roma reproductive freedom. http://www.reproductiverights.org/sites/default/files/documents/bo_slov_part1.pdf.

Chesler, Ellen. 2005. Introduction. In *Where human rights begin: Health, sexuality, and women in the new millenium*, ed. Chavkin Wendy, and Ellen Chesler, 1–34. New Brunswick, NJ: Rutgers University Press.

Cohen, Susan A. 2006. The global contraceptive shortfall: U.S. contributions and U.S. hindrances. *Guttmacher Policy Review* 9: 15–18.

Cohen, Susan A. 2012. Access to safe abortion in the developing world: Saving lives while advancing rights. *Guttmacher Policy Review* 15: 2–6.

Colletti, Jennifer. 2013. Harm reduction: An innovative approach to ending unsafe abortion gains momentum. *Because.* http://www.ipas.org/en/Get-Involved/Because/Because-Summer-2013/Harm-Reduction.aspx.

Cook, Rebecca J. 1993. Women's International Human Rights Law: The way forward. *Human Rights Quarterly* 15: 230–261.

Cook, Rebecca J., and Bernard M. Dickens. 2009. From reproductive choice to reproductive justice. *International Journal of Gynecology and Obstetrics* 106: 106–109.

Crane, Barbara B., and Jennifer Dusenberry. 2004. Power and politics in international funding for reproductive health: The US Global Gag Rule. *Reproductive Health Matters* 12: 128–137.

DeGrazia, David. 2012. *Creation ethics: Reproduction, genetics, and quality of life.* New York: Oxford University Press.

Dixon-Mueller, Ruth. 1993. *Population policy and women's rights: Transforming reproductive choice.* Westport, CT and London: Praeger.

de Londras, Fiona. 2015. Constitutionalizing fetal rights: A salutary tale from Ireland. *Michigan Journal of Gender & Law* 22 (2). (Print forthcoming, available online http://papers.ssrn.com/sol3/papers.cfm?abstract_id=2600907).

Erdman, Joanna N. 2014. Procedural abortion rights: Ireland and the European Court of Human Rights. *Reproductive Health Matters* 22: 22–30.

Erdman, Joanna N. 2011. Access to information on safe abortion: A harm reduction and human rights approach. *Harvard Journal of Law & Gender* 34: 413–462.

European Dignity Watch. 2012. The Funding of Abortion through EU Development Aid. http://www.europeandignitywatch.org/fileadmin/user_upload/PDF/Day_to_Day_diverse/Funding_of_Abortion_Through_EU_Development_Aid_full_version.pdf.

George, Robert P., and Christopher Tollefsen. 2008. *Embryo: A defense of human life.* New York: Doubleday.

Hesketh, Therese, and Zhu Wei Xing. 2005. The effect of China's one-child family policy after 25 years. *New England Journal of Medicine* 353: 1171–1176.

Hessini, Leila. 2005. Global progress in abortion advocacy and policy: An assessment of the decade since ICPD. *Reproductive Health Matters* 15: 88–100.

International Conference on Population and Development. 2014. http://www.unfpa.org/icpd.

Jaggar, Alison. 2005. "Saving Amina": Global justice for women and intercultural dialogue. In *Real world justice: Grounds, principles, human rights and social institutions,* ed. Andreas Follesdal and Thomas Pogge, 37–63. Dordrecht, the Netherlands: Springer.

Luna, Zakiya, and Kristin Luker. 2013. Reproductive justice. *Annual Review of Law and Social Science* 9: 327–352.

Luna, Zakiya. 2009. From rights to justice: Women of color changing the face of US reproductive rights organizing. *Societies Without Borders* 4: 343–365.

MacKinnon, Catherine A. 1991. Reflections on sex equality under law. *Yale Law Journal* 100: 1281–1328.

MacKinnon, Catherine A. 2006. *Are women human? And other international dialogues.* Cambridge, MA: Harvard University Press.

One of Us. 2012. http://ec.europa.eu/citizens-initiative/public/initiatives/finalised/details/2012/000005; http://www.oneofus.eu/.

Pateman, Carole. 1983. Feminist critiques of the public/private dichotomy. In *Public and private in social life,* ed. S. I. Benn and G. F. Gaus, 281–303. London: Croom Helm.

Population Action International. 2015. Helms hurts. http://www.helmshurts.com/.

Siegel, Reva B. 2007. Sex equality arguments for reproductive rights: Their critical basis and evolving constitutional expression. *Faculty Scholarship Series*. Paper 1137. http://digitalcommons.law.yale.edu/fss_papers/1137.

Singh, Susheela. 2010. Global consequences of unsafe abortion. *Women's Health* 6: 849–860.

Skuster, Patty. 2004. Advocacy in whispers: The impact of the USAID Global Gag Rule upon free speech and free association in the context of abortion law reform in three east African countries. *Michigan Journal of Gender & Law* 11: 97–126.

Steinbock, Bonnie. 1992. *Life before birth: The moral and legal status of embryos and fetuses.* New York: Oxford University Press.

Thomson, Judith Jarvis. 1971. A defense of abortion. *Philosophy and Public Affairs* 1: 47–66.

Trombley, Stephen. 1988. *Right to reproduce: History of coercive sterilisation.* London: Weidenfeld & Nicholson.

UN Millenium Development Goals. 2000. http://www.un.org/millenniumgoals/.

Vienna Declaration & Programme for Action. 1993. http://www.ohchr.org/EN/ProfessionalInterest/Pages/Vienna.aspx.

Widdows, Heather. 2011. *Global ethics: An introduction.* Durham, NC: Acumen.

World Health Organization. 2014. Eliminating forced, coercive and otherwise involuntary sterilization: An interagency statement OHCHR, UN Women, UNAIDS, UNDP, UNFPA, UNICEF and WHO. http://www.unaids.org/sites/default/files/media_asset/201405_sterilization_en.pdf.

World Health Organization. 2010. Packages of Interventions for Family Planning, Safe Abortion care, Maternal, Newborn and Child Health. http://apps.who.int/iris/bitstream/10665/70428/1/WHO_FCH_10.06_eng.pdf

World Health Organization. 2007. Unsafe abortion: Global and regional estimates of the incidence of unsafe abortion and associated mortality in 2003 (5th ed.). http://www.who.int/reproductivehealth/publications/unsafe_abortion/9789241596121/en/.

CHAPTER 3

··

CONSTRUCTING THE
ABORTION ARGUMENT

··

ROSAMOND RHODES

IN the 1970s and 1980s, the period shortly before and after *Roe v. Wade*, 410 U.S. 113 (1973), the landmark decision by the United States Supreme Court on the permissibility of abortion, a flurry of publications argued the ethical pros and cons of abortion. Although many of the articles from both sides of the debate have been reprinted in anthologies, there have been few contributions to the dialogue since then. At the same time, disagreement over abortion has continued to be one of the most hotly debated and divisive issues in the United States, and there are constant challenges to *Roe v. Wade* on the state and federal levels.

Meanwhile, a few important ethical theories dominate contemporary moral philosophy. In no particular order, the most prominent include utilitarianism, intuitionism, emotivism, and constructivism. Interestingly, however, most of the arguments in the abortion literature rely on none of these theories, but only invoke a crude form of ethical naturalism (Noonan 1970; Warren 1973; Engelhardt 1974; Devine 1978; Sumner 1981; Tooley 1984; Feinberg 1986). Although some subtle versions of ethical naturalism continue to be debated in the metaethics literature, the rudimentary versions employed in the abortion debate attempt to draw ethical conclusions from natural properties in the physical world. Ethical naturalism of this sort has been criticized most prominently by G. E. Moore and R. M. Hare.[1] Moore, who formulated the open-question argument, maintained that saying something has a certain property (e.g., the human genome) does not tell us anything about what ethics requires (Moore 1993). It is still legitimate to ask, for example, "Is it ethically acceptable to do X to that human?" This would be an additional question that is not answered simply by pointing out that the human genome is present. Similarly, Hare explained that words like "right" and "good" are ethical terms that cannot be reduced to descriptive terms (Hare 1952). For example, explaining why killing is wrong cannot be accomplished without employing ethical terms. Regardless of how many descriptive details are added, describing just what George did when he killed Harry cannot provide an account of why what

George did was wrong (i.e., murder). Ethical conclusions can only follow from ethical statements.

In almost all of the arguments over the morality of abortion, the authors have aimed at establishing empirical claims about the human fetus. They have then drawn conclusions about how the fetus may or may not be treated based on those claims. Opponents of abortion typically argue that fetuses have certain physical characteristics and, therefore, have an inviolable right to life. Advocates of the right to abortion typically maintain that fetuses lack some specific psychological qualities, and, therefore, do not have a right to life.

Reflecting on positions that are based on such claims, Don Marquis presents a cogent critical analysis of some of these most celebrated pro-choice and anti-abortion arguments in the rarely reprinted introductory section of his 1989 article, "Why Abortion Is Immoral" (Marquis 1989). According to his crisp analysis, typical versions of both opposing positions have a similar flaw. As he sees it, "[t] he pro-choicer will argue or assert that fetuses are not persons or that fetuses are not rational agents or that fetuses are not social beings" (Marquis 1989, 184). He also notes that the anti-abortionist argues or asserts "that life is present from the moment of conception or that fetuses look like babies or that fetuses possess a characteristic such as a genetic code that is both necessary and sufficient for being human" (Marquis 1989, 188). Marquis points out that both positions suffer from drawing invalid inferences of the same sort or from circularity. The validity problem, which undermines both opponents' arguments, involves inferring a moral conclusion, an "ought," from a factual, nonmoral premise, an "is."[2] The pro-choicers maintain that psychological characteristics (e.g., personal identity, experience of emotions, ability to feel pain, thinking of goals and plans) make a *moral* difference, whereas anti-abortionists take *biological* characteristics to make a *moral* difference.

Proponents of both views are also vulnerable to the pitfall of assuming what they are trying to prove. The pro-choice advocates do this by shifting their discussions from psychological qualities to moral categories and, without argument, introducing moral terms such as "personhood." Anti-abortion advocates make the same sort of mistake when, without argument, they shift their discussions from biological qualities, like "human," to moral categories such as "person" or "innocent." As Marquis points out, such moves have the effect of obliterating the grounds for establishing the "essential premise" in their respective arguments (Marquis 1989, 188); that is, that fetuses lack or have moral standing.

These arguments are typically framed in terms of the right to life. In other words, pro-choice advocates argue that fetuses lack psychological qualities such as an ongoing consciousness of self or the ability to imagine a future or use language, and therefore, have no right to life. Anti-abortion advocates maintain that fetuses have physical characteristics like human DNA or looking human, and therefore, have a right to life. From the inadequacy of these approaches, Marquis concludes that the solution to the abortion question lies in another direction. Perhaps he may have been too hasty in giving up on rights-based ethics and the intuition that the philosophic solution to the abortion question is to be found in the right to life. Just because these discussants employed rights language in their arguments to draw illegitimate conclusions does not imply that a legitimate rights-based argument cannot be developed. Previous discussants may have misused the concept of a right to life, but Marquis may have been too quick to toss out the baby with the bathwater.

He holds instead that the loss of the value of a future like ours is what makes all sorts of killing wrong. Without debating the merits of Marquis's own approach, there are at least two ways of understanding his position. Reading him as making a psychological point about valuing a future like ours is unpersuasive because, on the one hand, fetuses are incapable of valuing anything, and on the other hand, that would make Marquis's approach vulnerable to his own criticism, because the psychological fact that adults value a future cannot explain why ending another's life is wrong. Alternatively, reading him as making the point that valuing a future like ours is the basis for people having a right to life does not adequately explain why we should not kill or why valuing something creates any right, let alone the right to life.

CONSTRUCTIVISM

In what follows, I offer a different sort of approach to the abortion question. I will be presenting a constructivist argument because I find that to be the most reasonable and useful theoretical approach to resolving ethical issues.[3] I shall first present a description of what I take to be key features of constructivist ethics.

Constructivism (and I include its close relations, contextualism and pluralism) is perhaps the most popular ethical theory in contemporary moral and political philosophy. It is the approach presented in the work of today's most influential moral theorists, including John Rawls, T. M. Scanlon, and Christine Korsgaard. These philosophers see morality as a human creation that we construct based on reasons that reflect features of human nature, the world we live in, and the circumstances in which we find ourselves.[4] In political philosophy, where laws are created for governing an entire population, the aim is to identify those principles that would be endorsed by rational and reasonable individuals (following Rawls) or those principles that no one can reasonably reject (following Scanlon). Similarly, in ethics, where the focus is more on individual action and directed at what is the right thing for me or some other individual to do, constructivists aim at identifying the reasons that should govern the actions of any reflective individual who is similarly situated (following Korsgaard).

To generalize, a constructivist position holds that there are no independently existing natural moral obligations and no independently existing natural moral rights (Hobbes 1965). In interpersonal relations, endorsement or assent creates an obligation for oneself, and that undertaking creates a right in another. In that way, all moral rights arise with the creation of obligation, and all moral obligations arise from undertaking commitments. Surprisingly, aside from my writing, as far as I know, no thoroughgoing constructivist approach to the issue of abortion has been offered.

From a constructivist perspective, general obligations can be seen as those duties that every reasonable person could be assumed to have undertaken, typically on conditions of reciprocity. Correlative rights emerge for everyone else, at least so long as reciprocity is observed. For example, each of us can be said to have assumed an obligation to abstain from threatening the survival of every other moral agent, so long as others observe that commitment as well. That assumption of obligation creates a duty for me to everyone else, and for each of them a right with respect to me, and vice versa.

Special obligations would be those duties that only some particular individuals take on. In matters that involve others, they would bring forth rights in the particular individual or group that was the focus of the commitment (e.g., you, as in I will cook you a dinner; a group, as in I will host a dinner party for everyone in our reading group). Both general and special obligations are binding because you assent to them, because you make them laws to yourself for governing your own action.[5]

Identifying the salient reason(s) for a course of action is the first step in constructivist political philosophy and ethics. The second step in constructivism involves the creation of the force that assures compliance with the conclusion of moral deliberation. For a constructivist, when a person takes on an obligation or accepts a duty, a moral force to comply with that commitment is created. In the political domain, laws created by a legitimate political authority require our compliance because we have assured it by a prior contract or an explicit or implicit promise to abide so long as others do as well. That prior commitment to abide by the civil law on the condition of reciprocity is the creation of an obligation to obey the law, the source of the duty of compliance.

In the context of individual action, a commitment to abide by the conclusions of one's own reasoning is, in essence, the creation of a law for oneself. Such commitment is expressed as an endorsement, a promise to oneself, or assent. In interpersonal action, when I commit myself to doing something for another, by that assent I undertake an obligation to another.

For constructivists, undertaking responsibilities creates rights in others. This position is in sharp contrast to the view of ethical naturalists, who see the genesis of moral responsibility as flowing in the opposite direction, and see needs (Gewirth 1978), or valuing (Marquis 1989) or competencies (Sen 2001; Nussbaum 2003) as creating rights. For them, those rights are the source of obligations. One problem with their rights-to-obligations approach is that it cannot explain who has responsibilities, why they have them, and how they got them. For constructivists, at least in the cases of an individual's obligations, the story of how duties are acquired is typically obvious. An individual's duties arise from that person's undertaking the responsibility.

An example of how someone personally creates an obligation in constructivist terms may help to clarify this distinction. There are many in war-torn Africa who are starving. Clearly, those people need food. Philosophers who see moral obligation as running from needs to rights to duties would have to say that every starving person has a right to food, and that all of those who are not responding to their needs are failing to fulfill their obligations. They cannot explain whom I have to feed, how, and why, or how my limited wherewithal affects my obligations.

Those who see the ethics of individual action in constructivist terms will appreciate the same needs of each starving person in Africa and consider their own circumstances and the reasons supporting some response. Upon reflection, and after considering and evaluating the reasons that support doing one thing or another, these individuals may decide to support governmental foreign aid, undertake an individual commitment to a particular child through the U.N.-sponsored Save the Children program, donate to a particular charity that responds to such needs, or do nothing. Any obligation that they undertake is their duty and no other. It is their duty only because of their commitment, not solely because of the others' needs. And if the person who committed to support an individual child through Save the Children fails to provide the promised sum, that person has failed to fulfill that duty.

For constructivists, as John Gray has explained, rights are conclusions (Gray 2000). Rights have no special metaphysical status, but calling something a "principle" or a "right" reflects our thinking that it is a weighty reason that frequently figures in our moral deliberation and that it is a reason that we accept and endorse. Reasons in this sense are prima facie considerations for thinking that some specific action should be done. In this sense, "ethical principles" and "moral rights" are terms used to mark prima facie considerations for doing something, that many people frequently consider important and persuasive, even though they may be overridden in some particular circumstances by more stringent reasons or more pressing obligations.

In interpersonal relationships, when an individual undertakes an obligation, the assent creates a right in the other.[6] For example, the African child who shared her photograph and wrote letters to her sponsor had a right to her ongoing support because her sponsor had committed to providing it. If, however, the sponsor lost his job and could no longer provide for his own children as well as support his sponsored child, it could be morally defensible for the sponsor to fail in his obligation to the sponsored child. Conflicts of duty are part of the fabric of life, and in most cases, the conflicts are resolved by the sacrifice of one duty in order to fulfill another prioritized duty. For a constructivist, a conflict in duties is resolved by providing reasons for why one duty is overriding and then endorsing that decision.

Some reasons for action are commonly accepted because they are tied to features of human nature and our natural world. Thus, when a reason is widely considered to be a very important consideration of the sort that people generally endorse, and one that figures in numerous moral deliberations, we may call it a "right," or even a "human right." We expect that other thoughtful individuals would endorse such a reason and abide by their commitments so long as others do as well. When there are grounds for assuming that reciprocity will be upheld, we consider everyone in the moral community to be obliged to abide by and ethically required to uphold mutually accepted duties, and such obligations may be regarded as duties to respect human rights.

CONSTRUCTIVISM AND THE RIGHT TO LIFE

Although a number of authors have found that framing abortion and other controversial ethical issues in terms of rights is irrelevant or narrow (Raz 1984), others have found that rights are central to explaining morality (Dworkin 1978; Feinberg 1970, 3) In what follows, I side with the latter group and employ a constructivist understanding of rights to account for the right to life and how it figures in an explanation of the ethics of abortion. I go on to show how this concept can be used in an argument for the permissibility of abortion and how it can be used to resolve troubling related questions.

According to most rights theorists, any discussion of rights is also a discussion of duties. Every obligation or duty of A to B implies a right of B against A. Importing this correlativity thesis and applying it to the context of the abortion debate, an argument for an infant, B, having a right to life should explain who has the concomitant duty. Identifying the duty-bound agent also requires an investigation into the origin of the duty.

In her important paper, "A Defense of Abortion," Judith Jarvis Thomson offers a somewhat different approach to the abortion question (Thomson 1971). She begins by granting, for the sake of argument, that the fetus is a person. From there, using her example of the violinist plugged to your body for a nine-month rescue by using your kidneys, she presses her view that even if the fetus were a person and therefore had the right to life, it would not have the right to use your body in order to survive. She is trying to show that granting the fetus the right to life would not prove that abortion is immoral.

Ignoring for a moment the main thrust of her argument, I want to turn instead to a smaller point in her paper and make a big deal of that. In passing, Thomson explains that "nobody has any right to use your kidneys unless you give him such a right" (see note 10, Thomson 1971, at 56). In other words, when you assent to another person's use of your kidneys, that person gets the right to use them, and you get the obligation to allow that person the use.

Because the decision to procreate is primarily the undertaking of an individual or a couple, it should be regarded as a special obligation and seen in the same light as giving someone the right to use your kidney. By this analysis, the right to life should be given a similar account: the right to life must also arise from someone's right-creating act of assuming an obligation. This is the position that I am inclined to accept and the one that seems most fruitful for unraveling the abortion question.

To explain this position further, consider that if the moral right to life does not simply come from some physical quality such as being conceived by a woman or from possession of some particular anatomical characteristics (e.g., blond hair and blue eyes, or 46 chromosomes), then we may consider whether it arises in the way that constructivists regard the origin of other rights. The rights of a dinner guest arise when someone takes on the duties of hosting him. For an immigrant, rights of citizenship come into being by the state accepting the responsibility for him as a citizen. The right of a patient with kidney failure to use your kidneys only arises when you accept the obligation to him. The right of a school administration and students to performance by a teacher comes from the teacher accepting the obligation to be a member of the faculty. In each of these situations the right of B against A comes from A's accepting the obligation to B.

Rights and duties are reciprocal or have corresponding parts. The relation is reciprocal when there is a right to x of A against B and a right to x of B against A. When B accepts the obligation to scratch A's back, A gets the right to have his back scratched by B; if at the same time A also accepts the obligation to scratch B's back, giving B the right to have his back scratched by A, then A and B have reciprocal rights and duties.

The relations of rights and duties have corresponding parts when there is a right to x of A against B and a right to y of B against A. When B accepts the obligation to scratch A's back if A will agree to rub B's feet and if, at the same time, A also accepts the obligation to rub B's feet so long as B agrees to scratch A's back, A gets the right to have his back scratched by B and gives B the right to have his feet rubbed by A. In such a case, A and B have corresponding rights and duties. These should be viewed as cases of simultaneous or conditional assumption of duties.

Some binding acts, however, involve assumption of duties by only one party, oneself (i.e., A = B), thus entailing no reciprocal or corresponding rights in others. For example, someone who resolves to finish her book or to become diligent, thrifty, or thin takes on a duty to herself. And some binding acts create concomitant rights but no reciprocal or corresponding duties. This last arrangement of rights and duties is the one of all gift-givers and their beneficiaries and of woman/parents and child.[7] The woman/parents assume the duty of caring for and nurturing the child,[8] while the child gets the right to be cared for and nurtured.[9]

Following this analysis, the origin of obligation can be pinpointed in time for each parent. Parents who are trying to conceive are bound to constrain their actions in accordance with the requirements for care and nurturing from the time they begin trying. For example, from the moment of their decision they must avoid situations that they believe might endanger the health of their baby. So, because we now know that the health of infants may be adversely affected by a woman's smoking or drinking alcohol during the first days after conception (before the fact of pregnancy could be known), she would be bound not to smoke or drink once she sets herself to try to become pregnant, or at least during any period of time when she was uncertain about her pregnancy status.[10]

ABORTION

When an unplanned pregnancy occurs (e.g., as a result of thoughtlessness, contraceptive failure, rape), there is no obligation on the woman (to the fetus) until she decides to have the child. Because the fetus, at that point, has no right to life, there is no violation of the fetus's right when a woman decides to terminate the pregnancy instead of carrying the pregnancy to term. And whenever a woman takes steps to avoid procreation, she is, in effect, refusing to undertake the responsibility of bearing a child, and in that she does not engender a right to life.

Consequently, when a woman uses an abortifacient for contraception, she undertakes no obligation to the embryos that may develop, so no violation of the right to life is involved in the termination of the pregnancy.[11] The same can be said of a woman who uses postcoital techniques (e.g., morning-after pills, RU-486) to interrupt a pregnancy (Knight and Callahan 1989). She assumes no obligation to the embryo and engenders no right to life. And when a woman plans to undergo a therapeutic abortion if she should become pregnant from unprotected intercourse, she would not be violating the fetus's right to life by terminating the pregnancy because she would not have created any right.[12] Without knowing more about the details of her situation, we might think that she was being imprudent or reckless, but that would not amount to violating the fetus's right to life.

When a pregnant woman decides to bear her child and then place it for adoption, she accepts the duties of acting to preserve her baby's health by arranging for a placement that would provide the baby with adequate care and nurturing.[13] Adopting parents, although not engendering a right to life, acquire the obligation to care for and nurture their baby only because they accept it.

A constructivist approach accepts the abortion of a fetus before the parents invest it with rights. There may, however, be morally relevant reasons in addition to the right to life that should be taken into account in a particular abortion decision. Depending on the circumstances and the relative weight of the additional considerations, the scales could be tipped for or against abortion in a particular case. In some drastic situations, an event that occurs after a fetus is invested with a right to life (e.g., the death of a spouse) could so significantly affect the burdens of other conflicting moral responsibilities that the fetus's right to life could be outweighed.

TOUGH QUESTIONS

In these days of embryonic cell research, assisted reproduction, prenatal diagnosis, and perinatal intensive care, difficult ethical questions arise about the moral status of the embryo, the fetus, and the neonate. The constructivist approach to the genesis of the right to life provides a powerful conceptual tool for navigating many of these complex issues.

Embryos

Although human embryos have human genetic material and have the special potential for developing into a human being, unless and until someone undertakes special responsibility for their care and nurturing, they have no right to life. Consequently, even though we may want to be especially careful and thoughtful about fertilizing human eggs and using them in basic science research or in assisted reproduction, such uses of human embryos would not involve the violation of a right to life. Similarly, discarding unused fertilized human eggs would not violate their right to life, because they have none. Hence, the right to life could not be a reason for concern, and it could not justify a prohibition on creating human embryos for assisted reproduction or basic science research.

Pregnancy Reduction

To improve the chance of achieving a pregnancy, assisted reproduction specialists typically transfer several fertilized eggs into a patient's uterus in a single cycle.[14] It is, therefore, not unusual for a multiple pregnancy to result. A pregnancy of two or more fetuses may put each of the fetuses at greater risk for prematurity or spontaneous abortion than a pregnancy of one fetus. To improve the chance for a healthy live birth, or because some parents want no more than one baby, a procedure to reduce the number of fetuses can be performed.

Because pregnancy is clearly chosen in such cases, we can be concerned about the nature of the commitment to each of the fetuses. If the well-informed parents had intended to have only one baby and planned on pregnancy reduction (i.e., abortion) for any additional resulting fetuses, these situations should be seen as similar to the situation of the woman who plans to use abortion as birth control. Because the parents could foresee that multiple fetuses could be created by having multiple fertilized eggs transferred, they are responsible for them. Nevertheless, they could have specifically withheld a commitment to care for and nurture them all, thereby not investing any of them with a right to life prior to the pregnancy reduction.

Anomalous Fetuses and Neonates

This same approach can also be extended to understanding the situation of anomalous fetuses and neonates. By the time a prenatal diagnosis is made or an infant is born, parents can be presumed to have undertaken a commitment to care for and nurture their child. So when a serious pre- or postnatal diagnosis is made, would a late-term abortion or infanticide violate the right to life?

Perhaps we can analyze the situation this way. When a person undertakes a responsibility of a certain kind, x, he is only bound to accept the duties of that kind. He is not bound to accept, instead, duties of another kind, y, or an additional kind, $x + y$. For example, when I invite you to dinner and you arrive with ten of your relations in tow, all expecting to be fed, I have no obligation to feed your hungry horde. When a teacher accepts a position on a faculty and arrives at his post to discover that the administration expects his service to include providing clothing for the students as well as education, the teacher is not bound to take up the position. The commitment made was to the performance of a certain kind of task that did not include outfitting the students. If I found that you were famished, or if the teacher discovered that his students were less than brilliant and enthusiastic, then unless the teacher and I had been promised otherwise, we would still be obliged to fulfill the obligations we had undertaken. The hostess who extends an invitation and the teacher who accepts a position each accepts the obligation to try to perform the kind of act that she believes she can perform at the level she believes she is expected to perform within a reasonable range of conditions that would count for performance of the task. Variations of these sorts would not change the obligation in kind. A person should anticipate deviations from the ideal conditions in every undertaking.

Similarly, prospective parents accept the obligation to try to perform a certain predictable set of acts, specifically, caring for and nurturing their child until the time when it can be independent and able to assume obligations. When parents are delivered of a severely compromised child that could never be expected to become an independent moral agent, then, the responsibilities entailed, being lifelong, are of a different kind from those obligations that had been undertaken. A responsibility to care for an offspring through its entire life is significantly different from a responsibility to care for one until it can be independent and able to assume obligations as a moral agent. That these responsibilities are different in kind becomes obvious when you notice that it is impossible for the parents of the severely compromised child ever to satisfy the previously assumed obligation for the care and nurturing of their offspring until it can be an independent moral agent, because that time will never come. Because the goal cannot be satisfied, ought implying can, the original resolve is not binding.[15]

Like the host confronted by the hungry horde or the teacher confronted with clothing responsibilities, the prospective parents of a seriously anomalous fetus are not duty bound to continue the pregnancy after the diagnosis is made. Similarly, the parents of a seriously compromised neonate are not obliged to care for the child. Instead, as the host who could choose to welcome all, or the teacher who could, in a new undertaking, assume the obligations of the position that involved clothing the students, the parents of a seriously defective fetus or neonate could, in a new act, choose to accept the responsibility for the care of the child who could never be expected to lead an independent life. Until and unless the prospective parents or parents assume the obligation for the care of their anomalous fetus or seriously compromised neonate, it has no right to life. Having no right to life, aborting the anomalous fetus, or even killing the seriously compromised neonate would not violate its right, and so the actions could not be immoral on that ground.

When health care providers warm, feed, and treat a newborn, and the parents are given no opportunity to refuse, it is not at all clear who has undertaken what responsibility.[16] Insofar as the state will take responsibility for any child that parents refuse, it may be said that the state invests the neonate citizen with the right to life and takes on the concomitant obligations to provide for its lifelong care and nurturing when the parents decline to accept those duties.[17]

The criteria of having the capacity to develop into an individual who is independent and morally responsible for her own actions prevents the possible objection that any less than perfect child may be sacrificed. For a fetus or neonate who had conditionally been granted the right to life, it is the potential for becoming a moral agent, the possibility of achieving the moral status of a member of a moral community, that entitles it to a continued right to life. Although individuals can assume personal responsibilities to entities that are not moral agents (e.g., to pets, farm or research animals, art, natural sites, the environment), only those who are capable of taking on moral responsibility can join the moral community by taking on reciprocal responsibilities. Thus, (1) the capacity to develop into an independent individual and (2) the capacity to develop into one who can be morally responsible for his own actions are each necessary conditions and jointly sufficient conditions for investing a conditionally promised fetus or neonate with a right to life.[18] Perhaps we should just say that potential moral agents are potential (and not actual) rights bearers.

1. Although the set of physical capacities requisite for independence differs in different societies (e.g., a deaf person could be independent in our society but probably not in a jungle society), and although few could be independent of all society, the ability to achieve independence within the society into which an infant is born seems to be a necessary condition for its claim to a right to life. Anyone who cannot be independent will always be dependent on others for his continued existence. If there is no designated person (s) who is obligated to provide needed care, then the dependent individual will have no right to that care, and hence no right to what is necessary for survival. Furthermore, one who will be unable to intentionally act will not become an agent because he will not be able to enact the things a person ought to perform.

2. It is because adult humans can be held liable for their actions that they can form and maintain societies: accountability is what counts in a moral community. Because children and madmen are not accountable for their actions, they are systematically excluded from the rights and duties of citizenship. An infant who, because of its lack of potential, could not become morally responsible for the things he might do could never have all of the rights and obligations of a citizen. No society could tolerate members for whose actions no one was liable. It may not be difficult to imagine a society in which every individual could become independent (think of the government of Bahrain guaranteeing a non-Bahraini body servant to each Bahraini who might need one to achieve independence); still, it is unimaginable that unowned acts of killing or destruction could be allowed. In society, the liability for every human action, and even some omissions, is owned by someone. For every window broken by a thrown baseball, there is someone liable for the repair. Because the members of society are moral agents, they are morally responsible for their own acts and also the acts of those for whom they assume responsibility. When an individual cannot assume responsibility for what he does, and no one who may take up that obligation does so, then he cannot claim the rights of membership in the society.

Invoking these two criteria makes it clear that the minor birth defects of many children would not compromise their right to life. Clearly, a child who is born tongue-tied, with six fingers on one hand, or with crossed toes would be one with birth defects who could be expected to develop into an independent individual. Clearly, a child born with Tay-Sachs disease or trisomy 13 could not.[19] Hence, it follows that the conditional right to life previously granted to fetuses and newborns may be withdrawn when it is determined that the child could not develop into an independent moral agent.

Understanding the acceptance of parental responsibility as the source of a conditional right to life provides a framework for answering questions about the moral permissibility of late-term abortion and the moral parameters for decisions about treatment or euthanasia for defective newborns. Many infants with birth defects die very young if not given special treatment, and withholding treatment from an infant who dies as a result of this denial can be morally equivalent to killing him (Rachels 1975). When withholding treatment from those who will die early prolongs the agony for the infant and parents, and, therein, seems to be unnecessarily cruel. Furthermore, those infants who do not die from this neglect suffer by not having benefited from possible treatment that would have improved the child's condition if it had been administered. When parents accept the obligation for an infant with congenital defects or a serious disease, they become bound to provide it with care and nurturing. Treatment is, therefore, obligatory when it is the means most likely, or indeed, the only possible means of satisfying the infant's need to be free from pain. Treatment is obligatory when it is the most likely means for nurturing whatever development is possible. In contrast, parents who do not assume responsibility for a seriously impaired neonate give it no right to life; therefore, it may be killed. Moreover, if one also accepts the principle of humane alleviation of suffering (infant's, parent's, or both), it ought to be euthanized.

It may seem that this conclusion, which can in some cases tolerate infanticide, could be avoided whenever someone other than the parents was willing to take on the obligation for the lifelong care and nurturing of the seriously defective infant. This, however, is not the case. In bearing the obligation for their actions, parents have the responsibility for the offspring they produce. That obligation gives only them the rights necessary for fulfilling their responsibilities. No benevolent institution or individual has the right to wrest that decision from them.[20] Because the procreative activity only involves the assumption of special responsibilities or potential responsibilities by the parents, only the parents have the right to decide about the fate of their infant who, by having no potential to become an independent moral agent, may not be invested with a right to life.[21]

Violinists, Trespassing Joggers, Shipwrecked Sailors, and Others

Returning to Thomson's argument and the case of the violinist who needs the continued use of your kidneys to survive, recall that she maintained that even though the violinist is a person who had a right to life, it was morally permissible to disconnect the violinist so long as you had never consented to being connected to him. She was confident that this analogy justified abortion.

Let us consider instead another hypothetical example, the common legal situation of a person who wants to be alone on his large estate. His property is posted with unmistakable signs warning trespassers that they will be shot on sight. He awakens one morning to find an apparently unarmed jogger trespassing on his front lawn. Regardless of the fact that he has no right to be there, legal and moral intuition concludes that the property owner has no right to kill him because the jogger has a right to life. This persuasive example suggests the opposite conclusion from Thomson's, that even though the violinist has no right to use your body and the fetus has no right to use the woman's body, you and the woman have no right to kill trespassing others who have a right to life. Thus, the trespassing jogger example suggests that when Thomson grants the fetus personhood or a right to life for the purpose of her thought experiment, the fetus's right to life should take precedence over the woman 's right to determine what happens to her own body for a few months.

To press the point further, consider a variation on the theme. Imagine that you finally have the opportunity to fulfill a lifelong dream to sail solo across the Pacific. You awaken one morning on your amply outfitted but very small boat to find that a shipwrecked sailor has climbed aboard. He displays no threatening intentions and expresses tremendous appreciation for finding your boat because the water is cold and infested with sharks. But you want to be alone, and he smells bad, speaks banalities ungrammatically and very loudly, and, when he is not talking, he sings your least favorite songs off key. And because of the smallness of the boat and the size of the shipwrecked sailor, it is hard to find a position where your bodies are not in contact. Even though he has no right to be on your boat and even though he causes you mental anguish, and even though you suffer an intrusion on your body, the intuition persists that you have no right to push him overboard and that you are duty bound to put up with his company for a few days, weeks, or even months.

Although many people share Thomson's intuitions about abortion, the case of the trespassing jogger and the shipwrecked sailor are also compelling. This disparity of intuitions suggests that there may be a significant dissimilarity in these cases. The constructivist analysis offers an explanation for why these cases should be treated differently.

In the abortion cases discussed earlier, the fetus that is killed has no right to life, so the woman has no obligation not to kill it. The trespassing jogger and the shipwrecked sailor do have the right to life. As a general obligation we can assume that all reasonable people would undertake the duty not to threaten the survival of others so long as others take on a similar obligation to them. Because the property owner and the sailboat owner have no reason to suspect the trespasser or the shipwrecked sailor of reneging on their part of this reciprocal agreement, they have no justification for not respecting their right to life and their duty to not to kill persists.

This distinction also explains why my remarks about infanticide would not extend to a generalized argument for nonvoluntary euthanasia. Once the right to life has been vested, any killing would be a violation of that right. And although some killing in viola-tion of the right to life may be justified, additional arguments would have to be mustered to make the case. Discovering some acts of abortion and infanticide to be permissible when they do not involve a violation of a right to life does not entail judgments about euthanasia in different kinds of situations. Independent arguments based on other con-siderations would be required to show the moral permissibility of euthanasia in other circumstances.

CONCLUSION

According to the constructivist account that I have presented, morality only arises in our freely choosing our responses to the situations that present themselves to us. To the extent that any unintended pregnancy or the conception of a seriously impaired fetus is "chance," "luck," or even an "act of God," no one is morally respon-sible. There is nothing moral or immoral about these events. But treating the continu-ation of fetal and newborn lives as inevitable and therefore not subject to choice is an immoral act of avoiding responsibility. Parents have the obligation to make decisions about their potential offspring. Their moral choices would be either to reject paren-tal duties and accept the responsibility for abortion or infanticide, or to accept and fulfill the standard parental duties or the special duties of being a parent to a severely compromised child.

I would like to draw attention to one further conclusion that follows from this discus-sion. The central feature of this chapter is the account of the generation of the right to life in a fetus or neonate as undertaking a special personal obligation. Viewing the right to life in this light is a drastic departure from the standard approach that presents it as a natural right, in fact, the most fundamental natural right. If my account is at all per-suasive, this constructivist abortion argument presents a dramatic challenge to natural rights theory by undercutting its paradigmatic example.

NOTES

1. H. A. Prichard presents a similar argument in his 1912 paper, "Does Moral Philosophy Rest on a Mistake?"
2. To illustrate, from statements such as, "There are shoes in the middle of the room." and "There is a newspaper on the chair." we cannot conclude either that "John should clean his room." Or that "Mary should make the room look more lived in." Similarly, from state-ments such as "The fetus is genetically human." or "The fetus is incapable of using lan-guage." we cannot conclude anything about how we ought to treat it. Descriptions of the world, by themselves, tell us nothing about what is right or wrong, good or bad, ethically acceptable or prohibited.

3. An earlier and briefer version of this chapter appeared as "Abortion and Assent," in *Cambridge Quarterly of Healthcare Ethics* (1999), 8: 416–427. This paper has benefited from many thoughtful comments by Roger Crisp and Joe Fitschen.

4. This is not intended as a complete account of constructivist ethics. It is offered as a sketch of this type of theory, with the intention of explaining enough to make my approach to the abortion question seem reasonable.

5. H. A. Prichard explains how obligation is created, how binding oneself to fulfill a duty requires a prior general commitment to keep our agreements, and how such a mechanism is necessary for human cooperation. "The Obligation to Keep a Promise," (1949) pp. 169–179.

6. The way that constructivism involves two separate steps has not received much attention. Nevertheless, constructivist authors, such as Rawls, Scanlon, and Korsgaard, distinguish the conclusion of moral evaluation from something like endorsement or commitment. We also find evidence for distinguishing two steps in the process of duty creation in the way Rawls distinguishes the rational from the reasonable as two distinct and essential powers for membership in the moral community. Rationality refers to a thought capability. Reasonableness is the willingness to abide by principles on the condition of reciprocity. We find a similar two-step process in the precursors of constructivism, namely the work of Thomas Hobbes and Immanuel Kant. For Hobbes, the Laws of Nature are the conclusions of our reflection. They become binding action guiding laws when we assent to them. For Kant, first we reflect on the situation before us and formulate a possible action as a categorical imperative. When we then will it to be a law for ourselves, the willing is the commitment to abide by the conclusion.

7. It is often claimed that the child has the corresponding obligation to care for aged parents and that parents have a right to such care. It seems inconceivable that infants so bind themselves. This has already been pointed out by Immanuel Kant in his *De Obligation Activa Et Passiva* (Kant 1963).

8. H. A. Prichard makes a similar point when he notes that deciding to become a parent is like binding oneself or making a promise that "gives rise to the obligation to feed and educate" one's offspring. "The Obligation to Keep a Promise," (1949) p. 170.

9. Paul Gomberg provides an account that resembles mine in some respect. Although he maintains that the duty to nurture one's offspring is gradually acquired as the fetus develops over nine months of gestation (p. 519), he also declares that, "nurturance takes hold when we accept our pregnancy (p. 517).

10. It's not that the woman who is trying to conceive has an obligation to a non-existent entity. Rather, it is more accurate to say that there are periods during which she may be uncertain about whether or not she is pregnant. During that interval, it is prudent for her to behave with caution to avoid failing in her obligation if she should have one.

11. Although I am arguing that a fetus can only have a right to life if its mother/parents create the right to life by undertaking a commitment to provide for its care and nurturance, the decision about whether to invest the fetus with a right to life cannot be put off indefinitely. At a certain point in the pregnancy, it is fair to assume that equivocation is no longer acceptable and that she/they are actually accepting parenting responsibilities and investing the fetus with a right to life. For example, in jurisdictions where abortions are allowed up until 24 weeks of gestation, barring some unusual circumstances, it is fair to assume that a woman who has not terminated the pregnancy by then has undertaken parental

responsibilities and invested the fetus with a right to life. It's fair to make that assumption because the time period is significant enough to allow for due consideration and because it is a legal limitation. Sometimes we may evidence a choice by doing nothing, and sometimes we may take on a responsibility without being fully cognizant of the implications of our action or inaction.

12. This may unfortunately be a prudent approach for a woman who lives in a society where abortion is readily available but birth control is not.

13. Because the biological duties of the birth mother cannot be transferred the way that her social duties for care and nurturing can be, she may have an obligation to leave a blood sample for possible future genetic analysis.

14. Some countries regulate the number of fertilized eggs that can be transferred. In other countries there is no regulatory limitation and the decision is left to the physician and the patient. A variety of considerations can affect the choice (e.g., number of available eggs, age, cost, physician experience, reputation).

15. When a severely handicapped child is born and the kind of care that it will require is significantly different from the standard case, the care can impose a different kind of responsibility. Since the physical, emotional, and financial demands of caring for a severely handicapped child can be beyond the wherewithal of what reasonable parents realistically anticipate, the burden of care may also defeat the original undertaking.

16. Obligation is assumed in any words or actions of a moral agent that are sufficient to mark her intention as assuming that obligation. Any action performed or authorized by a parent that causes her child to continue to live (i.e., prevents it from dying) marks the undertaking of some degree of parental responsibility. For example, feeding an infant may signify the assumption of obligation, although it may only signify the continuation of conditional obligations (e.g., pending the outcome of diagnostic studies). That many people perform such morally significant acts as taking up and caring for their infant without appreciating the significance of those acts does not undercut their importance as moral commitments. (Infants can live unfed without suffering harm for as long as 24 hours after birth.) Some acts are immoral and some agents are morally careless or blind.

17. A society with ample resources could certainly take on the responsibility.

18. It is difficult to lay out the precise parameters of parental reasonable expectations and how much of a deviation makes a situation different in kind from the original undertaking. For the purposes of this discussion, it may be enough to invoke a concept of reasonable expectations and draw broad outlines of the criteria. The resources available within the society and the wherewithal of the parents would also have to be factored into such an assessment. Perhaps ethics can offer no more precision here than a conceptual model.

19. Choosing the moral principle appropriate to the situation and comparing general criteria to particular cases are always matters of moral judgment; these principles and criteria are also used as the tools in making moral judgments. As with other difficult moral dilemmas, a clarification of the issue resolves the question for instances at the extremes. The criterion of having the capacity to develop into an independent, morally responsible individual is useful in deciding most cases. However, solutions to cases falling in the murky middle, e.g., the infant who is blind and deaf or the quadruple amputee, may remain obscurely gray and more subject to considerations of the complex whole of the particular situation.

20. To further illustrate this point, imagine a strong young man wanting to take on the obligation of carrying my heavy packages for me. It seems that I have a right to refuse his assistance, and he has no right to impose that assistance on me. Or, imagine a wealthy dowager who believes that every able child should have ballet lessons since they can be shown to provide the most beneficial form of exercise. If she were willing to take on the obligation of providing ballet classes for all of the children in my community she would not have the right to include my child, and I would I have the right to refuse my child's participation.

21. On this analysis, the time frame for parents deciding whether to assume responsibility for a defective fetus would run up to delivery. The time frame for deciding about taking on responsibility for a defective newborn, however, should be rather brief. Some time should be allowed for an assessment of the infant's condition and prognosis. That window of opportunity cannot, however, remain open indefinitely. Constraints of reasonableness and legality (e.g., vesting of citizenship rights) would limit the period for decision-making.

Bibliography

Devine, P. 1978. *The ethics of homicide*. Ithaca, NY: Cornell University Press.

Dworkin, R. 1978. *Taking rights seriously*. Cambridge, MA: Harvard University Press.

Engelhardt, H. T., Jr. 1974. The ontology of abortion. *Ethics* 94, no. 3: 217–234.

Feinberg, J. 1970. The nature and value of rights. *Journal of Value Inquiry* 4: 243–257.

Feinberg, J. 1986. Abortion. In *Matters of life and death: New introductory essays in moral philosophy*, edited by T. Regan, 256–293. New York: Random House.

Gewirth, A. 1978. *Reason and morality*. Chicago: University of Chicago Press.

Gomberg, P. 1991. Abortion and the morality of nurturance. *Canadian Journal of Philosophy* 1, no. 4: 513–524.

Gray, J. 2000. *Two faces of liberty*. Cambridge, UK: Polity Press.

Hare, R. M. 1952. *The language of morals*. Oxford: Clarendon Press.

Hobbes, T. 1965. *Hobbes's Leviathan*. London: Oxford University Press.

Kant, I. De Obligation Activa Et Passiva. 1963. *Lectures on ethics*. Indianapolis: Hackett.

Knight, J. W., and Callahan, J. C. 1989. *Preventing birth: Contemporary methods and related moral controversies*. Salt Lake City: University of Utah Press.

Marquis, D. 1989. Why abortion is immoral. *Journal of Philosophy* 86, no. 4: 183–202.

Moore, G. E. 1993. *Principia ethica*. Revised edition with preface to the 2d and 3d ed. And other papers. New York: Cambridge University Press.

Noonan, J. T, Jr. 1970. An almost absolute value in history. In *The morality of abortion: Legal and historical perspectives*, edited by J. T. Noonan, Jr., 51–59. Cambridge, MA: Harvard University Press.

Nussbaum, M. 2003. Capabilities as fundamental entitlements: Sen and social justice. *Feminist Economics* 9, no. 2–3: 33–59.

Prichard, H. A. 1949. The obligation to keep a promise. In H. A. Prichard, *Moral Obligation: Essays and Lectures*, W. D. Ross (ed.), 169–179. Oxford: Clarendon Press.

Prichard, H. A. 1912. Does moral philosophy rest on a mistake? *Mind*, 21: 21–37.

Rachels, J. 1975. Active and passive euthanasia. *New England Journal of Medicine* 292: 8–80.

Raz, J. 1984. Against right-based morality. In *Theories of rights*, edited by J. Waldron, 182–200. Oxford: Oxford University Press.

Sen, A. 2001. *Development as freedom*. Oxford: Oxford University Press.

Sumner, L. W. 1981. *Abortion and moral theory*. Princeton, NJ: Princeton University Press.

Thomson, J. J. 1971. A defense of abortion. *Philosophy and Public Affairs* 1, no. 1: 47–66.

Tooley, M. 1984. *Abortion and infanticide*. New York: Oxford University Press.

Warren, M. A. 1973. On the moral and legal status of abortion. *The Monist* 57, no. 1: 43–61.

CHAPTER 4

....

VICTIMS OF TRAFFICKING, REPRODUCTIVE RIGHTS, AND ASYLUM

....

DIANA TIETJENS MEYERS

THE aim of this chapter is to extend and complement the compelling arguments that others have already made for the claim that women who are citizens of economically disadvantaged states and who have been trafficked into sex work in economically advantaged states should be considered candidates for asylum. These arguments cite the sexual violence and forced labor that trafficked women are subjected to along with their well-founded fear of persecution—stigmatization, social ostracism, and retrafficking— if they are repatriated.[1] What has not been considered is that reproductive rights are also at stake. This chapter explains how reproductive rights are implicated in sex trafficking. Moreover, it contends that sex traffickers' abuse of women's reproductive rights is persecutory and that this persecutory abuse obliges destination states to offer asylum to transnational trafficking victims.

I start by tracing the emergence and encoding of reproductive rights doctrine in international human rights instruments. I then examine studies of women who are in post-trafficking recovery programs in order to ascertain the impact of their past experience of forced sex work on their reproductive freedom and health. On the basis of these findings, I maintain that, among other outrages, sex trafficking systematically violates victims' reproductive human rights. In view of this abuse, women trafficked into sex work might seem to be prime candidates for asylum in destination states. Yet economically well-off destination states are not particularly receptive to this idea, and international law provides some justification for their chilliness. Preliminary to challenging them, I explicate four ways in which international antitrafficking law and international refugee law interfere with viewing women trafficked into sex work as refugees and approving their applications for asylum.

The second half of this chapter undertakes to overcome those legal obstacles. In the interest of parsimony and because there are many continuities between US refugee law and antitrafficking law and the policies of similar destination states, I focus mainly on the United States in this part of the chapter. To anchor my argument, I spotlight two precedents in refugee law for taking reproductive human rights seriously and several precedents for treating trafficked women as members of a distinct social group as required by refugee law. I then urge that a law enforcement gestalt has gained undue influence over US legal practices where antitrafficking law intersects with refugee protection law. A human rights gestalt is needed as a counterweight, for otherwise victims of sex trafficking and the reproductive abuse they have suffered are erased. Taking up a human rights perspective and mobilizing precedents, I show that respecting the reproductive human rights of women who have been trafficked into sex work entails that affluent destination states must recognize their right to asylum.

The ethical obligations of destination states that flow from this conclusion are twofold. First, it is incumbent on destination states, especially those that encourage sex trafficking by providing strong markets for paid sex work and little deterrence to sex traffickers, to offer an effective remedy to women victimized by transnational criminal organizations operating in their territory. Because the principal remedies that they have at their disposal are asylum and medical care, there is an ethical imperative to recognize traffickers' violation of the reproductive rights of trafficked sex workers as a form of persecution, to amend antitrafficking legislation to secure the right to asylum for sex trafficking victims, and to link refugee status to appropriate remedial health care. Second, there is an ethical imperative to ensure that immigration judges evaluate asylum claims advanced by trafficked women on their merits. But the conditions in which immigration judges work make them susceptible to being swayed by commonplace implicit biases against undocumented migrants, against poor women of childbearing age, and against sex workers. To curb these subconscious attitudes, I advocate reforming the institutions in which asylum cases are adjudicated in several respects. Without these reforms, equitable statutory remedies for women trafficked into sex work may come to nothing because of the illicit impact of implicit biases against trafficked asylum seekers. Both legislative and procedural reforms are vital to realizing women's reproductive human rights.

A BRIEF HISTORY OF REPRODUCTIVE HUMAN RIGHTS

Reproductive rights have figured in the human rights regime from the beginning. Article 16 of the Universal Declaration of Human Rights states that "men and women of full age . . . have the right to marry and found a family." Subsequent covenants that transformed the aspirations of the Universal Declaration into international law amplify on this theme. Both the International Covenant on Civil and Political Rights and the International Covenant on Economic, Social, and Cultural Rights reaffirm the right to marry and have children. Article 10 of the Covenant on Economic, Social, and Cultural Rights adds that working mothers should receive paid leave from work or leave with social security benefits before and after the birth of a child. Article 12, which recognizes the right to the "highest attainable standard of physical and mental health," also calls for the "reduction of the still-birth rate and of infant mortality." Prenatal care for pregnant women, safe birthing conditions, and adequate pre- and postnatal maternal nutrition are indispensable to achieving these aims. This acknowledgment of gender difference and women's specific role in reproduction is exceptional in the early development of human rights law. Perversely, the only other explicit affirmation of women's reproductive rights in these founding covenants provides for stays of death sentences for pregnant women (ICPR, Art. 6, Sec. 5).

It was not until late in the 1970s that women's reproductive rights gained the attention they deserve in the arena of international law. CEDAW, the Convention on the Elimination of All Forms of Discrimination Against Women, articulates a number of reproductive rights. With respect to employment, CEDAW emphasizes that workplaces should be safe for women in their reproductive years and during workers' pregnancies, that terminating pregnant employees is impermissible, and that provisions must be made for paid maternity leave or comparable social security benefits for working women (Art. 11). For the first time, the topic of family planning is featured prominently in a legally binding human rights document. According to CEDAW, health care services must include provision of family planning methods (Art. 12), and rural women must have access to the same information about and access to family planning techniques as urban women (Art. 14). After reiterating the right to consensual marriage, Article 16 declares women's all-important right "to decide freely and responsibly on the number and spacing of their children and to have access to the information, education, and means to exercise these rights." Whereas previous thinking about reproductive rights had focused on protecting women's reproductive health and function, CEDAW finally affirms women's right to reproductive freedom and self-determination.[2]

The right to found a family together with the right to reproductive health—for most women, this is necessary as a means to exercising the former right—is well established in human rights law. Although controversial in some quarters, the right to reproductive freedom has been steadily upheld in documents issued by international conferences on population and development and women's rights as human rights.[3] Moreover, these consensus documents explicitly urge destination nations to extend full reproductive rights to migrants regardless of their legal status.[4] Although the United States is not a State Party to the International Covenant on Economic, Social, and Cultural Rights, and it is one of the seven nations worldwide that are not States Parties to CEDAW, in practice the United States realizes at least as many of women's reproductive rights as many of the States Parties to all of the treaties that encode these rights. I argue that fully realizing women's reproductive rights and eliminating inconsistencies in US law entail modifications in US refugee law with respect to victims of transnational sex trafficking as well as extending the right to reproductive health to these women.

SEX TRAFFICKING AND
REPRODUCTIVE HEALTH

No one has accurate information about reproductive health outcomes resulting from sex trafficking because all well-designed studies are based on interviews with women who are receiving rehabilitative services and reviews of their medical records. These women represent a tiny minority of trafficked women. However, there is little reason to doubt that complete data would disclose at least as severe a problem. After all, whatever proportion of women who have left forced sex work with previously untreated, fertility-threatening sexually transmitted infections (STIs) and whatever proportion of women who have left forced sex work and report undergoing forced abortions, the proportions are likely to be greatly magnified the longer women are trapped in trafficking schemes.

Two widely cited, Coalition Against Trafficking in Women (CATW)–sponsored studies of the reproductive health consequences of sex trafficking rely on data collected from female sex workers with no attention to possible differences between trafficked and voluntary sex workers or between settings in which sex work is legal and settings in which it is criminalized.[5] Forced sex work is always illegal under international law. The 2000 UN "Protocol to Prevent, Suppress and Punish Trafficking in Persons, Especially Women and Children, Supplementing the United Nations Convention Against Transnational Organized Crime," often called the Palermo Protocol, defines trafficking in persons as:

> the recruitment, transportation, transfer, harbouring or receipt of persons, by means of the threat or use of force or other forms of coercion, of abduction, of fraud, of deception, of the abuse of power or of a position of vulnerability or of the giving or receiving of payments or benefits to achieve the consent of a person having control over another person, for the purpose of exploitation.[6]

The protocol goes on to specifically include sexual exploitation. Thus, trafficked sex workers have been tricked or coerced in the recruitment and relocation process, held in debt bondage or imprisoned in brothels at their destinations, or both. In what follows, I rely on studies that take care to distinguish voluntary sex work from forced sex work and to collect data exclusively from survivors of sex trafficking.

Stolen Smiles, an omnibus study of the health consequences for eastern European women trafficked into sex work in western Europe, reports that the single biggest concern of women in posttrafficking treatment programs is their future fertility.[7] Although the study denies that infertility is an inevitable consequence of forced sex work, it also acknowledges that the women's fears are warranted.[8] Only 38% of the women report consistent use of condoms, but the authors of the study suspect that this percentage is inflated because 29% of the women in this cohort had contracted STIs.[9] Nor did many of them receive medical care befitting the risky nature of their work. Medical care mainly took the form of abortions—a procedure that greatly benefits traffickers and that these trafficked women also value.[10] Unsurprisingly, though, abortions augmented the dangers to these women's reproductive health because they were often performed by unqualified practitioners in unsanitary environments.[11] Likewise, untreated chlamydia, pelvic inflammatory disease, and HIV threaten trafficked women's fertility, as do ectopic pregnancies.[12] Although *Stolen Smiles* is upbeat about some of the benefits of post-trafficking medical intervention, the study's concluding observation is grim: "Infertility and other resulting complications, including cervical cancer, may be the unalterable personal legacies of their nightmare."[13] In violating women's right to reproductive self-determination, sex traffickers violate their right to reproductive health.

A study that documents the reproductive health experiences of Nigerian women trafficked into sex work reports similar but less detailed findings. Sixty-nine percent of the women contracted STIs, and the investigators stress that if left untreated, STIs can lead to pelvic inflammatory disease, ectopic pregnancy, and infertility.[14] Ninety-one percent of the women in the study said they had no access to birth control.[15] In a statistic that is somewhat puzzling in light of the previous one, 80% of the women said their traffickers forced them to have abortions or forced them to use contraceptives.[16] Perhaps this statistic breaks down as follows: The percentage of this cohort that was forced to use contraceptives was very small, and the percentage that was forced to undergo abortions was very large. If so, the seeming tension between the claim that 91% of the women were not provided with contraceptives and the claim that an unspecified percentage of the women in the study were forced to use contraceptives would be resolved. The key point, however, is that regardless of whether women are procured in Eastern Europe or sub-Saharan Africa, sex traffickers trample on their human rights to reproductive self-determination and reproductive health. There is no reason to believe that the reproductive rights of women trafficked from other regions fare better.

WOMEN TRAFFICKED INTO SEX WORK AS CANDIDATES FOR ASYLUM

The purpose of recognizing refugees and granting asylum to them is to protect people from persecution. The 1951 Geneva Convention Relating to the Status of Refugees defines a refugee as a person who "owing to well-founded fear of being persecuted for reasons of race, religion, nationality, membership of a particular social group or political opinion, is outside the country of his [sic] nationality and is unable or, owing to such fear, is unwilling to avail himself [sic] of the protection of that country."[17] The convention never defines persecution. But it is clear that refugees are fleeing a credible and wrongful threat of severe harm in their homeland, a threat that targets them because of their adverse positioning in a stratified social system or their opposition to the state. Moreover, were they to return to their homeland, they would in all likelihood be subjected to renewed persecution.

From one angle, women trafficked into sex work seem like prime candidates for refugee status and asylum. Widely cited legal scholar James Hathaway defines persecution as "a sustained or systemic violation of basic human rights demonstrative of a failure of state protection."[18] By definition, sex trafficking organizations violate their victims' rights to liberty and reproductive self-determination. In colloquial terms, trafficked sex workers are sex slaves—their bodies are under the control of their traffickers and their customers. Moreover, the abusive conditions in which trafficked women are compelled to perform sexual services and the scarcity of medical services provided to them put their reproductive health and thus their right to found a family in jeopardy. These sustained violations of basic human rights notwithstanding, there are major obstacles to classifying trafficked sex workers as refugees.

Call the first obstacle the "smuggled woman" problem. A growing social scientific literature reveals that most adult women trafficked into sex work are also economic migrants—that is, they have knowingly availed themselves of trafficking networks in order to be smuggled into more prosperous nations in the hope of economic betterment. According to Dina Haynes, "Victims of human trafficking are people who [were] determined to improve their lives but had that desire exploited."[19] Likewise, Louisa Waugh points out that women in posttrafficking recovery programs think of themselves as "migrants who'd been brutalized because they'd had to resort to desperate measures."[20] Thus, many trafficking scenarios start with a smuggling scenario. The would-be migrants are neither naïve country girls, nor are they duped about their employment prospects abroad.[21] Rather, they are extremely poor women who have no job opportunities sufficient to meet their needs (often family members' needs as well) in their home countries.[22] Seeking a solution, they allow themselves to be recruited by known traffickers in order to obtain fake travel documents and assistance in crossing otherwise closed borders, all the while hoping to escape from poverty.[23] When they reach their destinations, they are forced into prostitution.

In many host countries, however, their cooperation with transnational criminal gangs in the procurement and transport process earns them the label "smuggled," an epithet that excludes them from the category "trafficked." In the United States, for example, the Trafficking Victims Protection Act of 2000 mandates procedures for handling alleged trafficking cases and for providing benefits to individuals certified as trafficking victims. Under the TVPA, qualifying for benefits comparable to those provided to refugees is contingent on being certified as "severely trafficked." But to obtain certification, a female foreign national working in the US sex industry is for all practical purposes required to prove that she was kidnapped by, sold to, or deceived by a trafficker at her point of origin.[24] If certified as a victim of severe trafficking, the applicant may apply for a T visa, which can but does not automatically lead to permanent residence.[25] Although application numbers and rates of approval for T visas have increased markedly since the inception of the program, government statistics do not differentiate between applications from women trafficked into sex work and individuals trafficked for other types of labor.[26] Moreover, the number of T visas granted is tiny compared to estimates of the number of women trafficked for sex work in the United States.[27] Disappointing as these numbers are, they are unsurprising, for as we have seen, few of the women doing forced sex work are brought to their destinations through force or fraud. Absent certification as a severely trafficked person, trafficked sex workers apprehended by law enforcement officers are relegated to the status of undocumented migrants and processed for deportation despite being forced to perform commercial sexual services in the United States.[28] Consent at any stage of a woman's journey into forced sex work nullifies her claim to be severely trafficked.

Call the second obstacle the "crime stopper" problem. What I have already stated about US policy regarding trafficking victims adumbrates this additional obstacle. As the official title of the UN protocol on trafficking implies, international law views trafficking in persons first and foremost as an issue concerning catching and punishing transnational criminals as opposed to an issue concerning the human rights of trafficking victims. Arresting and prosecuting traffickers are prioritized over rectifying the wrongs done to trafficked victims of human rights abuse. Thus, international law obliges states to pass antitrafficking legislation independent of refugee law. The annual US Trafficking in Persons Report and the favorable treatment accorded countries that score well on prosecuting traffickers reinforce this orientation. One result is that women who claim to have been trafficked into sex work are funneled into the criminal law apparatus—in the United States they must agree to cooperate with prosecutors pursuing cases against traffickers—and into a special system of accreditation for extended residence that need not conform to established criteria for gaining asylum. Indeed, the criteria for obtaining a T visa in the United States are more difficult to satisfy than those that asylum seekers must meet.[29] By splitting antitrafficking law away from human rights law and segregating sex trafficking victims from refugees, the legal system closes off the human rights remedy par excellence—namely, asylum.

Call the third obstacle the "social group" problem. To qualify for refugee status, the Geneva Convention states, you must be persecuted "for reasons of race, religion, nationality, membership of a particular social group or political opinion." Unfortunately, sex traffickers appear to be equal opportunity predators. They do not target women on account of their race, religion, or nationality and certainly not on account of their political views. Nevertheless, there are patterns of vulnerability that are typical of trafficked sex workers. They commonly report a history of domestic violence, alcoholic or absent husbands, children to support, jobs lost and ensuing debt, and/or insufficient income to pay for housing and other essential expenses; they come from regions where women do not enjoy equal rights and that are undergoing economic turmoil coupled with deepening poverty.[30] Still, an asylum claimant must be persecuted because she is a member of a distinct social group, and delineating such a social group for women forced into sex work poses a challenge.

Although persecution on account of gender is a recognized ground for refugee status, the category "women" is too broad to characterize the individuals persecuted by sex traffickers. Yet the social group consisting of women forced into sex work or at risk of being forced into sex work is unacceptable because it is circular—it defines the group targeted for persecution as those who have been persecuted in a particular way or are vulnerable to that type of persecution.[31] If the diverse women trafficked into sex work are to gain access to the refugee system, the group(s) to which they belong must, on the one hand, be demarcated narrowly enough to exclude women who are not targeted by traffickers and must, on the other hand, be demarcated independently of being targeted by traffickers. Under US law and in line with the UNHCR's guidelines, a cognizable social group is one whose members "share a common, immutable characteristic, i.e., a characteristic that either is beyond the power of the individual members of the group to change or is so fundamental to their identities or consciences that it ought not be required to be changed."[32]

Call the last and least of the obstacles the "government role" problem. Recall that the Geneva Convention requires a refugee to be "unable or . . . unwilling to avail himself [sic] of the protection" of the state she has fled, and Hathaway contends that persecutory harms must be "demonstrative of a failure of state protection." Accordingly, paradigmatic cases of persecution are situations in which the state or an agent of the state inflicts or threatens to inflict harm rising to the level of persecution. But transnational trafficking gangs are not government institutions or agents appointed to act on behalf of government institutions. Consequently, it is not obvious that they can count as persecutors, and if they do not count as persecutors, the women whose rights they violate cannot count as refugees and are not eligible for asylum.

Fortunately, recent advances in refugee law render this problem more tractable than the others I have enumerated. In the United States, for example, the persecutor can be "persons or an organization that the government was unable or unwilling to control."[33] Thus, a showing that transnational trafficking organizations operate with impunity or with the complicity of corrupt government officials in a trafficked woman's home country suffices to establish the requisite government role in the persecution. And it is often uncontroversial that sending states have no power or wish to rein in trafficking.

PRECEDENTS FOR ASYLUM FOR WOMEN TRAFFICKED INTO SEX WORK

As I have pointed out, there is an international convention governing the treatment of refugees. For better or worse, implementation of the convention is left to each signatory state. As a result, there is considerable variation in the refugee legislation and judicial history of different States Parties. In the interest of parsimony, but with the caveat that uniformity is not to be found in this evolving and state-relative area of law, I will focus on US refugee law while occasionally noting what I take to be more equitable policies elsewhere.

In 1996, the United States enacted legislation that directly addresses, albeit somewhat obliquely, one aspect of the reproductive rights of migrants. Section 601 of the Illegal

Immigration Reform and Immigrant Responsibility Act makes a special allowance for certain victims of reproductive rights abuse:

> A person who has been forced to abort a pregnancy or to undergo involuntary sterilization, or who has been persecuted for failure or refusal to undergo such a procedure or for other resistance to a coercive population control program, shall be deemed to have been persecuted on account of political opinion, and a person who has a well founded fear that he or she will be forced to undergo such a procedure or subject to persecution for such failure, refusal or resistance shall be deemed to have a well founded fear of persecution on account of political opinion.[34]

Section 601 grants preferential treatment to those victims of reproductive rights abuse whose reproductive rights have been violated in the context of a coercive population control policy. In singling out this subset of victims, the law discounts the primary reason for ensuring access to the right to asylum in cases of persecutory reproductive rights abuse. To wit, coerced abortion and sterilization violate the right to bodily integrity that underwrites the right not to be tortured or subjected to cruel, inhuman, or degrading treatment.

Section 601 seems to have its moral priorities upside down and its psychology muddled. The provision exempts any Chinese person (men are often the beneficiaries of this provision) who has been forced to undergo an abortion or sterilization procedure or fears being forced to do so from proving persecution on account of her political opinion.[35] Yet the proximate wrong would seem to be being subjected to a nonconsensual medical procedure. Ever since the revelations that Nazi doctors performed sadistic experiments on concentration camp inmates, nonconsensual medical procedures have been considered anathema to human rights. Yet Section 601 identifies the principal wrong as a violation of freedom of conscience and the intrusion on bodily integrity as secondary. Unless nonconsensual abortion or sterilization is performed pursuant to a government's population control program, Section 601 provides no remedy. Furthermore, for many Chinese couples, especially in rural, agricultural China, having more than one child is an economic imperative or is dictated by the cultural value placed on begetting a son. It is odd, then, that Congress instructs the Immigration and Naturalization Service (INS) to project dissident political opinions onto people who may have quite different reasons for their resistance. What Section 601 fails to acknowledge is that the right to reproductive self-determination—the entitlement to choose whether and when to have children—is not contingent on people's reasons for exercising it. Even so, US hospitality to these ostensible political dissenters is limited, for Section 601 allows only 1,000 of them to be granted asylum in each fiscal year.[36]

In view of the persistence of uneasy relations between China and the United States, China's one-child policy, and residual opposition to abortion rights in the United States, Section 601 appears to be an extension of US foreign policy and a sop to a US voting bloc that incidentally fulfills international human rights law. Nevertheless, it amounts to a fissure in US defenses against recognizing reproductive human rights for purposes of refugee law that I propose to exploit in the next section.

The groundbreaking US Board of Immigration Appeals (BIA) decision *In Re Fauziya Kasinga* (1996, hereafter *Matter of Kasinga*) furnishes another precedent pertinent to the availability of asylum as a remedy for reproductive rights abuse. *Matter of Kasinga* considers the application of a 19-year-old woman from Togo whose father had protected her from female genital mutilation (FGM) but whose relatives demanded that she undergo the procedure after her father passed away. I will skip over the details of her flight. What is crucial is that she requested asylum upon arrival in the United States. Although initially denied, the BIA granted her request on several grounds:

> FGM is extremely painful and at least temporarily incapacitating. It permanently disfigures the female genitalia. FGM exposes the girl or woman to the risk of serious, potentially life-threatening complications. These include, among others, bleeding, infection, urine retention, stress, shock, psychological trauma, and damage to the urethra and anus. It can result in permanent loss of genital sensation and can adversely affect sexual and erotic functions.[37]

Binaifer Davar, who helped to write the INS guidelines "Considerations for Asylum Officers Adjudicating Asylum Claims From Women" (1995), sums up the *Kasinga* ruling as an "unprecedented recognition and protection of a woman's right to bodily and sexual identity."[38] She then proceeds to argue that *Matter of Kasinga* sets the stage for a full appreciation in US refugee law of the significance of the wrong of sexual violence and its links to violations of reproductive rights as well as the right to bodily and sexual integrity.[39] Davar condemns trafficking as a violation of the right to bodily and sexual integrity. Additionally, she underscores the attention paid in *Matter of Kasinga* to the harmful health consequences of FGM, and she points out that sex trafficking inflicts comparable harms on women.[40] Still, there is a noteworthy oversight in her argument. Although Davar places violations of reproductive rights under the umbrella of sexual violence, she does not make the connection between sex trafficking and violations of reproductive rights. I will make a case for that connection in the next section.

The evidence suggests that granting asylum to sex trafficking victims is by no means a growing trend.[41] Nevertheless, there are US, UK, and Canadian cases in which victims of sex trafficking have been granted asylum.[42] The US case is another slap at China's human rights record. A Chinese woman who was trafficked for sex work within China reached the United States, where she applied for and was granted asylum. The decision in the case notes that she would be vulnerable to retrafficking if repatriated to China. The particular social group to which she belongs and which provides another part of the justification for granting her asylum is "women in China who oppose coerced involvement in government sanctioned prostitution."[43] Again, the case appears to pivot on a political opinion ascribed to the applicant while the harms of forced sex work and the attendant violations of human rights are consigned to the periphery.

The UK case seems less in thrall to ulterior geopolitical posturing and convoluted analysis. It concerns a Ukrainian woman who had been trafficked into Hungary for sex work, who escaped and returned to the Ukraine, but who then fled to the United Kingdom and sought asylum there. This case also recognizes that the woman would be in danger of resumed persecution by criminal gangs that traffic in women if returned to the Ukraine, and it defines the particular social group to which she belongs and on account of which she was initially trafficked as "women in Ukraine who are forced into prostitution against her will."[44] As glad as I am that the United Kingdom provided a safe haven for this woman, I am skeptical that this decision supplies a strong precedent for future asylum cases stemming from sex trafficking. Its definition of the particular social group on account of which the victim was persecuted is vulnerable to the charge of circularity, for it cites gender only in conjunction with persecution by sex trafficking to define the particular social group.

The Canadian case furnishes a potentially far-reaching precedent for granting asylum to trafficked women. This decision grants asylum to another Ukrainian woman who had been trafficked into sex work and cites her membership in the following particular social group as the basis for her persecution: "impoverished young women from the former Soviet Union recruited for exploitation in the international sex trade."[45] In my view, this formulation breaks new ground because it incorporates the gender, age cohort, and economic status of the victim as well as the social and economic upheaval in the victim's homeland into the set of characteristics that define the individuals whom transnational trafficking organizations single out for persecution. Unlike the UK decision, the Canadian decision avoids collapsing into circularity by conjoining gender with multiple attributes that are known to figure in traffickers' targeting tactics.[46] Women are preyed upon because most purchasers of sexual services are heterosexual men; young women are preyed upon because they are perceived as more desirable by the main clientele; poor young women are preyed upon because they are eager to change their economic fortunes; poor, young women in patriarchal societies with foundering economies have no hope of economic betterment in their homelands and thus make ideal targets for traffickers. Like the two preceding decisions, the Canadian decision adds that upon return to the Ukraine there would be a "reasonable possibility that she would be subjected to abuse amounting to persecution at the hands of organized criminals" and that she would not be able to seek protection from Ukrainian authorities in view of the ties between organized crime and the government and the government's inability to combat trafficking.[47]

Summing up, there is plenty of precedent for overcoming the government role problem in asylum cases stemming from sex trafficking. Additionally, these cases make a start at overcoming the social group problem for sex trafficking victims seeking asylum. But whereas reproductive human rights factor into decisions to grant asylum to individuals seeking to escape from state-sponsored forced abortion or sterilization or seeking to escape from customary FGM practices, reproductive rights have yet to become central to understandings of persecution in relation to sex trafficking. I believe that the smuggled woman problem and the crime-stopper problem help to suppress reproductive rights issues in refugee law with respect to sex trafficking victims.

CONSOLIDATING THE REPRODUCTIVE RIGHTS ARGUMENT FOR ASYLUM

A law enforcement gestalt frames both the smuggled woman problem and the crime stopper problem, and both problems privilege sovereign governance over individual human rights. The crime stopper problem fastens attention on incarcerating perpetrators and sidelines victims except in their instrumental role as sources of evidence. The smuggled woman problem compounds this marginalization of victims. In all but a few cases, it denies victimhood in the name of policing borders and exerting state control over the composition of the populace. Once victims of sex trafficking have been classified as malefactors along with traffickers, law enforcement—deporting victims and prosecuting traffickers—becomes the preeminent objective.

In practice, the law enforcement gestalt creates a presumption against refugee status for women trafficked into sex work. We have seen, for example, that US law not only directs women who claim to be sex trafficking victims into the T visa system but also sets more stringent evidential standards for obtaining a T visa than it does for obtaining asylum through regular refugee proceedings. However, this presumption conflicts with US obligations as a signatory and State Party to the Palermo Protocol.[48] Article 14 of the Palermo Protocol states:

> Nothing in this Protocol shall affect the rights, obligations and responsibilities of States and individuals under international law, including international humanitarian law and international human rights law and, in particular, where applicable, the 1951 Convention and the 1967 Protocol relating to the Status of Refugees and the principle of *non-refoulement* as contained therein.

Raising an all but insuperable barrier to asylum for victims of one type of human rights abuse plainly abrogates the obligations of States Parties to the Refugee Convention and violates the rights of victims under the Convention. Similarly, the US distinction between a severely trafficked person and a trafficked person is incompatible with the Palermo Protocol. As Rey Koslowski points out, under the protocol "a smuggled woman becomes a trafficking victim when she arrives at her destination and is forced into prostitution."[49] Coercion in the recruitment and transport process is not a necessary condition for trafficking. I do not doubt the legitimacy of putting legal pressure on the activities of transnational sex trafficking organizations, including their role in smuggling undocumented migrants. However, deporting women who have been forced into sex work at their destinations does not deter traffickers with side businesses in human smuggling. Moreover, implementing the Palermo Protocol requires that a human rights gestalt counterbalance the law enforcement gestalt. In particular, the human rights abuse systematically inflicted on women trafficked into sex work must be brought to the fore and redressed. In addition to bringing US law into alignment with US commitments under international refugee and antitrafficking law, I urge that two glaring inconsistencies regarding reproductive rights in US immigration law be eliminated.

It is altogether arbitrary to confine the remedy of asylum to persons whose human right to reproductive self-determination has been violated pursuant to government-mandated population control policies. Forced contraception (whether temporary or permanent) and forced abortion are no less abhorrent when imposed by sex traffickers than they are when imposed by public officials.

Indeed, the former may well be more deplorable than the latter. Population control, when not an excuse for eugenic population pruning, can be a legitimate state interest. The same cannot be said of the profit motive of gangs of outlaws run amok. As it is acknowledged that traffickers plying their trade in countries with apathetic or complicit governments can be persecutors, the difference between the agents of persecution in the two cases is of no moral significance. If not, the protections of Section 601 of the US Illegal Immigration Reform and Immigrant Responsibility Act should be extended to women trafficked into sex work, for traffickers usurp their right to reproductive self-determination as surely as any government does.

Sex trafficking is also inimical to the right to reproductive health. Although *Matter of Kasinga* does not cite this right as a reason to grant asylum, the decision does cite the adverse effects of FGM on sexual function. Although sexual dysfunction ordinarily refers to problems with sexual desire, arousal, or orgasm and pain during intercourse, *Matter of Kasinga* cites Namib Toubia's research on FGM, which takes a broader view of sexual function. For example, Toubia states that chronic pelvic infection is a common complication of FGM and that chronic pelvic infection heightens the risk of infertility.[50] In the same vein, she points out that many women who have undergone genital mutilation procedures fear becoming infertile because of the condition of their genitals.[51] The similarities between the detriments to reproductive health caused by FGM and those caused by forced sex work are striking. Inasmuch as the BIA has ruled that possessing intact genitals is so fundamental to a woman's identity that she should not be compelled to submit to having them altered, surely an intact capacity to conceive and give birth to a child is also so fundamental to a woman's identity that she should not be compelled to submit to treatment likely to irreparably damage it. It follows that being trafficked into sex work constitutes persecution comparable to being subjected to FGM.

Finally, in many instances, repatriating women who have been trafficked into sex work deprives them of the right to found a family. So valorized is the virginity of brides and so stigmatized is sex work that many sex trafficking survivors are cruelly ostracized when they are returned to their communities of origin. Moreover, once a woman has been trafficked into sex work, her traffickers regard her as their property. Although she may have originally colluded with traffickers in order to migrate, she can expect to be tracked down and retrafficked if she is deported from her destination state.[52] Unable to find work or make a marriage and pursued by transnational trafficking gangs, women trafficked into sex work are highly vulnerable to retrafficking.[53] Thus, repatriation often amounts to *refoulement*—return to persecution—and *nonrefoulement* is a cardinal principle of international refugee law.

All the elements are now in place to justify making asylum available to migrant women forced into sex work. I have argued that the harms resulting from forced sex work rise to the level of persecution. It is indisputable that violations of reproductive human rights can be persecutory. I have identified the persecutory agent. The persecutors are transnational criminal gangs that operate with little or no interference from legal authorities in countries where women are recruited and in destination countries.[54] I have specified the features of the particular social group that is targeted by these transnational gangs. They are poor, young females in states where women are routinely discriminated against in education and employment and/ or where law and order have broken down because of social upheaval, widespread poverty, or recent armed conflict. Although it may be necessary to refine this formulation to reflect changing local conditions in source countries, it provides a legally tenable framework for future asylum claims. Add to all of this the likelihood of *refoulement* if women trafficked into sex work are not granted a safe haven in destination states, and the justification is complete.

THE ETHICAL OBLIGATIONS OF DESTINATION STATES

For the United States (and states with similar trafficking and immigration policies), the overarching obligation that flows from my line of argument in the preceding sections is to modify the laws and practices governing the treatment of women trafficked into sex work in order to secure their right to asylum. Denying this right or constructing elevated requirements for accessing it is inconsistent with the Refugee Convention and the Palermo Protocol. The obligation to reform trafficking and immigration policy in this way is all the more stringent because destination states provide vast markets for commercial sexual services, thereby fostering the high profitability of trafficking sex workers, and also because their enforcement of antitrafficking laws is lax.

But the ethical obligations of destination states do not end with legislative reform, for immigration procedures are organized in ways that allow implicit bias to unfairly shape outcomes and these unreliable procedures must be reformed. Issues concerning stereotyping and bias recur throughout the literature on sex work and migration. Preliminary to suggesting ways in which to counteract implicit bias in immigration hearings, I will comment on three strands of prejudice that distort perception of women trafficked into sex work.

Martha Nussbaum's work on disgust is a good place to start getting a purchase on one relevant type of implicit bias. Nussbaum sums up her understanding of disgust in the following passage:

> Because disgust embodies a shrinking from contamination that is associated with the human desire to be non-animal, it is more likely to be hooked up with various forms of shady social practice, in which the discomfort people feel over the fact of having an animal body is projected outward on vulnerable people and groups.[55]

She goes on to point out that semen is among the types of bodily discharge that are regarded as disgusting, and that this disgust transfers to persons who have frequent contact with it.[56] It is a short step to the observation that "sex itself has something disgusting about it, something furtive and self-contaminating, particularly if it is the body of a female whore (receptacle of countless men's semen) that inspires desire."[57] Along similar lines, Dina Haynes comments that one mechanism through which the victims of sex trafficking are othered hinges on the sexualization of racial/ethnic stereotypes.[58] Because only a disreputable type of person becomes a sex worker, character assassination follows on the heels of victimization.

Another strand of implicit bias concerns poor women of reproductive age. The same attitudes that sparked the wave of resentment against single mothers on welfare that led to the gutting of social benefits for women with dependent children in the United States infect perceptions of women trafficked into sex work. Trafficked women are presumed to be uneducated and unqualified for jobs in today's economy, and an unknown percentage of them fall into trafficking schemes because they are trying to migrate in order to send remittances home to their children. Thus, their immigration cases trigger the stereotype of the lazy, lying, irresponsible, poor young woman. Inasmuch as the statutory grounds for excluding claimants from the United States include the likelihood of becoming a "public charge," this implicit bias can sabotage a trafficked woman's otherwise worthy application for asylum.[59]

A third pair of stereotypes interferes with seeing women trafficked into sex work as refugees and hence as candidates for asylum. On the one hand, we have an image of persecuted individuals as brave opponents of tyranny. On the other hand, we have an image of trafficking victims as helpless, passive pawns of ruthless thugs. Insofar as the latter image frames perception of an applicant for asylum, its irreconcilability with the image of a "proper" candidate for asylum undermines her case. Indeed, because qualifying as a "severe" trafficking victim under US law requires proving that no voluntary action of your own contributed to your plight, the law demands that trafficking victims present themselves as conforming to the helpless, passive stereotype, which in turn undermines their plausibility as asylum seekers.[60]

This pileup of perception problems gives rise to grave epistemic injustice with dire material consequences for many asylum seekers.[61] In asylum hearings, the credibility of the applicant is crucial, but the stereotypes I have sketched, if allowed to prevail, raise doubts about her truthfulness in virtue of her presumptive character as a member of the very sort of group that is apt to be persecuted through sex trafficking. But, as Laurence Kirmayer points out, if the asylum seeker attempts to address probable biases in her sworn testimony, "any trace of this effort will cast doubt on [her] account."[62] In contrast, Fatma Marouf focuses on ways to improve the institutional setting in which US immigration proceedings are conducted rather than on ways asylum seekers or their attorneys can overcome the implicit biases of judges. It seems, therefore, that Marouf's remedies for the problem of implicit bias in asylum proceedings hold most promise.

Marouf exposes a number of institutional arrangements that conduce to the influence of implicit bias in immigration hearings. Immigration judges are Department of Justice civil servants, most of whom previously held positions in the Department of Homeland Security that required regarding prospective immigrants with suspicion.[63] As a result, many judges adopt an "inquisitorial" posture in hearings.[64] To ensure greater impartiality, Marouf recommends separating the appointment of immigration judges from the Department of Justice.[65] She goes on to point out that immigration judges work under appalling conditions. Their calendars of cases are overloaded; they have insufficient support staff to do legal research; and they are expected to deliver oral decisions on the spot.[66] Correcting for implicit bias is possible given familiarity with widespread prejudices, strategies for counteracting them, and time to deliberate carefully. But the highly pressured context in which US immigration judges are currently obliged to work thwarts even the most fair-minded judges. Marouf's solution, of course, is to reduce judges' caseloads and eliminate the rushed schedules they are expected to maintain.[67]

The reforms Marouf advocates would benefit all asylum seekers in the United States, but for my purposes it is key that they would give women seeking asylum in the aftermath of forced sex work a better chance of getting a fair hearing. None of these measures will accomplish much, however, if immigration judges are not sensitized to the prejudicial stereotypes that may mislead them and if they receive no training in how to curb implicit biases. Still, as early as 1995, the INS took the initiative in educating judges about the distinctive issues that persecution on account of gender raises.

"Considerations for Asylum Officers Adjudicating Asylum Claims From Women" acknowledges the distance between salient understandings of persecution and the forms of persecution that primarily impact women, and it instructs judges in how to respond appropriately to gender-based claims.[68] Yet change has come slowly, and the full implications of persecutory abuses of women's reproductive rights remain far from adequately appreciated. For reasons that are easy to fathom, sexual violence and reproductive defilement carry an extraordinarily intense emotional charge that is profoundly unsettling—more so than familiar, though horrifically cruel forms of persecution, such as extrajudicial incarceration, death threats, and torture. As a result, there is strong resistance to extending asylum to women trafficked into sex work based on violations of their reproductive rights.

This resistance is strengthened, perhaps masked, by appeals to the so-called floodgates argument. Floodgates arguments rest on demographic considerations, for they claim that a certain type of persecution is so pervasive that the receiving nation must protect itself from a potentially overwhelming influx of migrants. But by itself this demographic concern is plainly insufficient to justify excluding a particular type of asylum seeker. To be ethically convincing, a floodgates argument must invoke a normative claim that the alleged persecution is so trifling or tractable that the state is justified in barring these victims. Dina Haynes questions the cogency of the demographic worry, for there is no reason to believe that more women would be induced to attempt migration than is presently the case, nor is there reason to believe that women would willingly endure the brutality of forced sex work in order to qualify as refugees in destination states.[69] I have argued that the normative claim is a travesty. On the contrary, acknowledging asylum claims stemming from abuse of trafficked women's reproductive rights is vital both because of the gravity of the reproductive harm inflicted and because equitable application of legal principles demands it.

Still, granting women who have been trafficked into sex work access to the right to asylum is not a sufficient remedy for the human rights violations they have suffered. Asylum in many destination states is an effective guarantee of victims' future reproductive self-determination, but by itself asylum does nothing to restore or limit the damage to their reproductive health. In her capacity as Special Rapporteur on Trafficking in Persons, Joy Ngozi Ezeilo forcefully argues that trafficked persons have a right to an effective remedy and that helping victims to recover from the ordeal of trafficking is an essential component of an effective remedy.[70] Not surprisingly, she emphasizes that furnishing medical and psychological care is often vital to the recovery of trafficking victims.[71] In view of the high incidence of serious harm to the reproductive health of women trafficked into sex work, it follows that providing an effective remedy to them requires, at a minimum, diagnosing and treating STIs.

The reforms that the United States would need to put in place in order to comply with this tenet of international law are somewhat less momentous than the changes in refugee law and implementation that I have advocated so far. Under current trafficking law, persons certified as trafficking victims are eligible for Medicaid, Refugee Medical Assistance, and medical testing and treatment for communicable diseases.[72] If trafficking victims were viewed as asylum seekers, they would receive the same health benefits once their asylum applications were successful. However, in view of the connection between untreated STIs and infertility, the high incidence of STIs among women trafficked into sex work, and the protracted process of applying for asylum, these health care provisions must be extended to victims of sex trafficking during the asylum application process in order to ensure respect for their reproductive human rights. This modest expansion of health care rights would go a long way toward realizing sex trafficking victims' reproductive rights.[73]

Now that covering contraception is mandatory for all US health insurance, sex trafficking victims would be entitled to the means of managing their fertility.[74] However, one recovery scenario poses a serious political problem in the United States. Many states do not pay for abortion through their Medicaid programs, and it remains illegal to use federal funds to pay for abortions. Yet it is altogether possible that some victims of sex trafficking will escape from their traffickers and apply for asylum while pregnant. Studies indicate that many of them will want to terminate their pregnancies, and being able to do so may well be critical to their recovery processes. If so, the United States and other destination states with restrictive abortion policies will need to permit federal funding of abortions for some sex trafficking victims in order to provide an effective remedy for the reproductive abuse these women have endured.[75] In sum, destination states that fail to classify women trafficked into sex work as legitimate asylum seekers or that fail to provide prompt remedial health care to them are flouting ethical obligations of the first magnitude.[76]

Notes

1. Binaifer A. Davar, "Rethinking Gender-Related Persecution, Sexual Violence, and Women's Rights: A New Conceptual Framework for Political Asylum and International Human Rights Law," *Texas Journal of Women and the Law* 6 (1997): 241–256; Tala Hartsough, "Asylum for Trafficked Women: Escape Strategies beyond the T Visa," *Hastings Women's Law Journal* 13 (2002): 77–116; Dina Francesca Haynes, "Used, Abused, Arrested, and Deported: Extending Immigration Benefits to Protect Victims of Trafficking and to Secure Prosecution of Traffickers," in *Women's Rights: A Human Rights Quarterly Reader*, ed. Bert B. Lockwood (Baltimore, MD: Johns Hopkins University Press, 2006); Dina Francesca Haynes, "(Not) Found Chained to a Bed in a Brothel: Conceptual, Legal, and Procedural Failures to Fulfill the Promise of the Trafficking Victims Protection Act," *Georgetown Immigration Law Journal* 21 (2007): 337–381.
2. For a helpful discussion of the links between women's right to reproductive self-determination and the right to life, the right to liberty and security of the person, and the right to found a family, see Rebecca J. Cook, "International Human Rights and Women's Reproductive Health," in *Women's Rights, Human Rights: International Feminist Perspectives*, ed. Julie Peters and Andrea Wolper (New York: Routledge, 1995).
3. Aliya Haider, "Out of the Shadows: Migrant Women's Reproductive Rights Under International Law," *Georgetown Immigration Law Journal* 22 (2008): 429–457, 438.
4. Haider, 438.
5. Elzbieta M. Gozdziak and Elizabeth A. Collett, "Research on Trafficking in North America: A Review of the Literature," *International Migration* 43 (2005): 99–128, 107, 113–114.
6. http://www.unodc.org/unodc/en/human-trafficking/what-is-human-trafficking.html (accessed September 7, 2013).
7. Cathy Zimmerman et al., *Stolen Smiles: The Physical and Psychological Health Consequences of Women and Adolescents Trafficked in Europe*, London School of Hygiene & Tropical Medicine: http://genderviolence.lshtm.ac.uk/files/Stolen-Smiles-Trafficking-and-Health-2006.pdf (2006), 3, 63.
8. Zimmerman et al., 64.
9. Zimmerman et al., 61.
10. Zimmerman et al., 62, 68.
11. Zimmerman et al., 69. A study of the health consequences of sex trafficking in Southeast Asia reports that septic abortions are a major danger faced by trafficked sex workers in Burma and Thailand. Chris Beyrer and Julie Stachowiak, "Health Consequences of Trafficking of Women and Girls in Southeast Asia," *Brown Journal of World Affairs* 10 (2003): 105–117, 106, 111.
12. Zimmerman et al., 64, 65.
13. Zimmerman et al., 69, 70.
14. S. Abdulraheem and A. R. Oladipo, "Trafficking in Women and Children: A Hidden Health and Social Problem in Nigeria," *International Journal of Sociology and Anthropology* 2 (2010): 34–39, 37, 39.
15. Abdulraheem and Oladipo, 37.
16. Abdulraheem and Oladipo, 37.
17. http://www.unhcr.org/3b66c2aa10.html.
18. James C. Hathaway, *The Law of Refugee Status* (Toronto: Butterworths, 1991), 104–105.

19. Haynes 2007, 373; also see Wendy Chapkis, "Trafficking, Migration, and the Law: Protecting Innocents, Punishing Immigrants," *Gender and Society* 17, no. 3 (2003): 923–937, 931–932.

20. Louisa Waugh, *Selling Olga*, xv. Kara notes that in Central and Eastern Europe seduction coupled with promises of lifelong romance in the West is another common ploy to lure women into trafficking schemes. Siddharth Kara, *Sex Trafficking*, 9.

21. Siddharth Kara, *Sex Trafficking: Inside the Business of Modern Slavery* (New York: Columbia University Press, 2009), 7. Louisa Waugh, *Selling Olga: Stories of Human Trafficking and Resistance* (London: Orion Books, 2007), xiv, 63.

22. Suzanne Dayley, "Rescuing Young Women From Trafficker's Hands," *New York Times*, October 15, 2010. Siddharth Kara, *Sex Trafficking*, 7, 23–30, 115, 142. Louisa Waugh, *Selling Olga*, 3, 73

23. Liz Kelly adds a layer of complexity to the economic forces shaping these women's decisions. Many "smuggled" women borrow money from relatives in order to seek their fortunes in foreign sex industries. If they are deported and return empty-handed, they are unable to repay their debts and feel compelled to submit to retrafficking in the hope of making good on their debts if not improving family finances. Thus, the cycle of sexual abuse commonly enters a new iteration. Liz Kelly, "'You Can Find Anything You Want': A Critical Reflection on Research on Trafficking in Persons Within and Into Europe," *International Migration* 43, no. 1/2 (2005): 236–265, 248.

24. Jacqueline Bhabha, "International Gatekeepers? The Tension Between Asylum Advocacy and Human Rights," *Harvard Human Rights Journal* 15 (2002): 155–181, 175–176; April Rieger, "Missing the Mark: Why the Trafficking Victims Protection Act Fails to Protect Sex Trafficking Victims in the United States," *Harvard Journal of Law and Gender* 30 (2007): 231–256, 249; Hartsough, 99.

25. Hartsough, 101.

26. http://www.uscis.gov/USCIS/Resources/Reports%20and%20Studies/Immigration%20 Forms%20Data/Victims/I914t-I918u_visastatistics_2012-dec.pdf

27. As Gozdziak and Collett point out, disputed definitions of sex trafficking, not to mention the underground nature of the enterprise, make accurate counts of victims impossible and estimates highly conjectural (pp. 107–108). Nevertheless, they cite the official US estimate for 2004 of 14,500–517,500 (p. 117).

28. Rieger, 249.

29. Rieger, 252–253.

30. Not surprisingly, some trafficked women tell stories that smack of ambitions to upward mobility and heightened consumerism rather than escape from poverty (Christine M. Jacobsen and May-Len Skilbrei, "Reproachable Victims?" *Ethnos* 75 (2010): 190–212, 199–200). However, because stories of desperate flights from severe poverty and/or domestic abuse and the need to support family back home predominate in the literature, I center my discussion on that background narrative (see Louisa Waugh, 15–16, 31–32; Abdulraheem and Oladipo, 37–38; Hartsough, 80; Natasha Ahmad "Trafficked Persons or Economic Migrants? Bangladeshis in India," in *Trafficking and Prostitution Reconsidered: New Perspectives on Migration, Sex Work, and Human Rights*, ed. Kamala Kempadoo (Boulder, CO: Paradigm Publishers, 2005), 212–213, 224–225; Jan Boontinand, "Feminist Participatory Action Research in the Mekong Region," in *Trafficking and Prostitution Reconsidered: New Perspectives on Migration, Sex Work, and Human Rights*. ed. Kamala Kempadoo (Boulder, CO: Paradigm Publishers, 2005), 186, 192–193; Siddarth Kara, *Sex*

Trafficking: Inside the Business of Modern Slavery (New York City: Columbia University Press, 2009), 25, 114–115, 143, 172.

31. Michelle Foster, *International Refugee Law and Socio-Economic Rights: Refuge From Deprivation* (Cambridge: Cambridge University Press, 2007), 324–325.

32. *Matter of Acosta* (http://www.justice.gov/eoir/vll/intdec/vol19/2986.pdf, accessed September 15, 2013, p. 212.

33. *Matter of Acosta*, p. 222.

34. Quoted by Paula Abrams, "Population Politics: Reproductive Rights and U.S. Asylum Policy," *Georgetown Immigration Law Journal* 14 (2000): 881–905, 882.

35. Canadian law regarding forced abortion or sterilization does not hinge on holding an oppositional political opinion but rather on membership in a particular social group. See *Cheung v. Canada* (http://www.refworld.org/cgi-bin/texis/vtx/rwmain?page=country&category=&publisher=CAN_FCA&type=CASELAW&coi=CHN&rid=&docid=3ae6b70b18&skip=0, accessed September 15, 2013).

36. Abrams, 904.

37. *In Re Fauziya Kasinga* (http://www.justice.gov/eoir/vll/intdec/vol21/3278.pdf, accessed September 14, 2013), p. 361.

38. Davar, 243–244.

39. Davar, 245, 249–250.

40. Davar, 250.

41. Stephen Knight, "Asylum From Trafficking: A Failure of Protection." *Immigration Briefings: Practical Analysis of Immigration and Nationality Issues.* No. 07-07 Thomson/West (July 2007); also see Haynes (2007).

42. Haynes (2007), 476–477.

43. Angelika Kartusch, *Reference Guide for Anti-Trafficking Legislative Review*, (http://www.osce.org/odihr/13986, accessed September 15, 2013), OSCE/ODIHR (2001), 69.

44. Kartusch, 69.

45. Kartusch, 69.

46. The 2006 2nd Circuit Court of Appeals decision in *Gao v. Gonzales* held that "the statutory term 'particular social group' is broad enough to encompass groups whose main shared trait is a common one, such as gender, at least so long as the group shares a further characteristic that is identifiable to would-be persecutors and is immutable or fundamental." *Gao v. Gonzales* 440 F.3d 62 (2d Circuit 2006, p. 3 (http://cgrs.uchastings.edu/documents/legal/gao.pdf, accessed September 21, 2013). Additionally, in the 2012 7th Circuit Court of Appeals decision in *Cece v. Holder*, the majority held that the persecutory harm feared by an asylum seeker could be a component of the definition of the particular social group to which she belongs but could not be the whole of it (http://scholar.google.com/scholar_case?case=17906068323051465130&q=cece+v.+holder&hl=en&as_sdt=2,33&as_vis=1, accessed September 17, 2013).

47. Kartusch, 69.

48. See   https://www.unodc.org/unodc/en/treaties/CTOC/countrylist-traffickingprotocol.html.

49. Rey Koslowski, "Response to 'The New Global Slave Trade' by Harold Honfju Koh," in *Displacement, Asylum, Migration: The Oxford Amnesty Lectures 2004*, ed. Kate E. Tunstall (Oxford: Oxford University Press, 2006), 259–260. Also see UNHCR "Guidelines on International Protection No. 7: The Application of Article 1A(2) of the 1951 Convention and/or 1967 Protocol Relating to the Status of Refugees to Victims of Trafficking and

Persons at Risk of Being Trafficked" 7 April, 2006 http://www.refworld.org/docid/443679fa4.html (accessed February 13, 2014).

50. Namid Toubia, "Female Circumcision as a Public Health Issue," *New England Journal of Medicine* 331, no. 11 (1994): 712–716, 713. (http://www.nejm.org/doi/full/10.1056/NEJM199409153311106, accessed October 15, 2013).

51. Toubia, 714.

52. According to the UNHCR "Guidelines on International Protection Relating to the Status of Refugees to Victims of Trafficking and Persons at Risk of Being Trafficked," a refugee need not have left her country of origin because of persecution or fear of persecution:

> The requirement of being outside one's country does not, however, mean that the individual must have left on account of a well-founded fear of persecution. Where this fear arises after she or he has left the country of origin, she or he would be a refugee *sur place*, providing the other elements in the refugee definition were fulfilled. Thus, while victims of trafficking may not have left their country owing to a well-founded fear of persecution, such a fear may arise after leaving their country of origin. In such cases, it is on this basis that the claim to refugee status should be assessed. (Paragraph 25)

   From the standpoint of international law, then, the smuggled woman problem is a red herring.

53. UNHCR. "Guidelines on International Protection Relating to the Status of Refugees to Victims of Trafficking and Persons at Risk of Being Trafficked." 2006, 7; Haynes (2006), 461–462, 471–472, 476; Waugh, 39.

54. Leslie and John Francis show that lack of enforcement of laws prohibiting sex trafficking is not a problem unique to source countries. It is also a failing of destination states, including the United States. See their "Trafficking in Human Beings: Partial Compliance Theory, Enforcement Failure, and Obligations to Victims," in *Poverty, Agency, and Human Rights*, ed. Diana Tietjens Meyers (New York: Oxford University Press, 2014).

55. Martha C. Nussbaum, "'Secret Sewers of Vice': Disgust, Bodies, and the Law," in *The Passion of the Law*, ed. Susan Bandes (New York: NYU Press, 1999), 22.

56. Nussbaum, 24.

57. Nussbaum, 40.

58. Haynes 2007, 356; also see Haynes (2006), 456. For a recap of the workings of explicit bias in US immigration law, see Fatma E. Marouf, "Implicit Bias and Immigration Courts." *New England Law Review* 45 (2010-2011): 417–434, 422–423.

59. Hartsough, 99; Rieger, 253.

60. Kara Abramson, "Beyond Consent, Toward Safeguarding Human Rights: Implementing the United Nations Trafficking Protocol." *Harvard International Law Journal* 44, no. 2 (2003): 473–502, 495.

61. For a pertinent account of testimonial injustice and hermeneutical injustice that addresses the problem of implicit bias, see Miranda Fricker, *Epistemic Injustice: Power and the Ethics of Knowing* (Oxford: Oxford University Press, 2007).

62. Laurence J. Kirmayer, "Failures of Imagination: The Refugee's Narrative in Psychiatry," *Anthropology and Medicine* 10, no. 2 (2003): 167–185, 174.

63. Marouf, 429.

64. Marouf, 430.

65. Marouf, 430.

66. Marouf, 431–433.

67. Marouf, 434.

68. A 1995 memorandum distributed to the INS Asylum Officer Corps, http://cgrs.uchastings. edu/documents/legal/guidelines_us.pdf (accessed October 21, 2013).

69. Haynes (2006), 479; Haynes (2007), 377.

70. See the 2011 Report to the UN General Assembly of the Special Rapporteur on Trafficking in Persons, Especially Women and Children http://www.ohchr.org/Documents/Issues/ Trafficking/A-66-283.pdf (accessed February 12, 2014).

71. Ibid.

72. See the US Office of Refugee Resettlement's "Fact Sheet: Victim Assistance" http://www. acf.hhs.gov/programs/orr/resource/fact-sheet-victim-assistance-english#Benefits (accessed February 12, 2014).

73. Although the focus of this paper is women from economically disadvantaged, source states who are trafficked into sex work in economically advantaged, destination states, I note that the points I am making about the obligation to provide remedial health care apply equally to native born women who are trafficked into sex work in their home countries.

74. See US Affordable Care Act of 2010 http://www.hrsa.gov/womensguidelines/ (accessed February 12, 2014).

75. The summary of the Justice for Victims of Trafficking Act of 2015, which at this writing has been passed by the US Senate but not the House, states, "The bill prohibits the use of amounts from the Fund for any abortion or for health benefits coverage that includes coverage of abortion, except where the pregnancy is the result of rape or incest or the woman's life is in danger unless an abortion is performed" (https://www.congress.gov/bill/114th-congress/senate-bill/178, accessed April 28, 2015). If the bill is passed and signed into law with this language intact, it is possible that victims of sex trafficking will qualify for funding for abortions. Since sex acts performed by women trafficked into sex work are by definition nonconsensual, any pregnancies resulting from these forced sex acts should count as resulting from rape.

76. I thank Francoise Dussart for helpful discussion of this topic, Jean Connolly Carmalt for valuable suggestions regarding human rights and refugee law, and Leslie Francis for her incisive comments on an earlier draft.

CHAPTER 5

....

THE COMMODIFICATION OF WOMEN'S REPRODUCTIVE TISSUE AND SERVICES

....

DONNA DICKENSON

IT is sometimes alleged that the term "commodification" is vague, overused, or both.[1] This chapter argues the opposite: "Commodification" has quite a nuanced philosophical meaning and can never be used too often in relation to reproductive technologies because the phenomena that it describes are still gaining ground. Commodification is a necessary corrective to the dominance of a much more nebulous and omnipresent term, "choice," because it expands our analysis beyond the individual level and incorporates systemic economic realities of the new reproductive technologies.

However, the terms "commodification" and "objectification" are sometimes used too broadly, or they are run together when they should be distinguished from one another. It is not helpful for our purposes to paint commodification with a very broad brush as "all capitalized economic relations in which human bodies are the token of economic exchanges that are often masked as something else—love, pleasure, altruism, kindness."[2] Nor will we get far in the specific case of reproductive technologies with an all-encompassing definition of objectification as a plurality of denials imposed on human subjects: denials of their agency, autonomy, uniqueness, and dignity.[3]

This chapter will begin by narrowing down and analyzing these key terms, distinguishing commodification from objectification and illustrating how a correct understanding of commodification can be applied to reproductive technologies. The chapter will then go on to illustrate three complicated and compelling instances in which commodification is a genuine and ongoing concern: the sale of eggs for in vitro fertilization (IVF) and research, the banking of umbilical cord blood, and the growth in domestic and international commercial "surrogacy."[4]

COMMODIFICATION IN MORAL
AND POLITICAL PHILOSOPHY

Far from being imprecise jargon of recent vintage,[5] the term "commodification" has a venerable pedigree, even if in these times any analysis that traces back in part, but only in part, to Marx might wrongly be regarded by some as ideological. In Marx's analysis commodification entails assigning *both exchange and use value* to something, whereas objectification *only attributes use value*—the process by which something external to ourselves is made to satisfy human needs and wants.[6] In a pure system of unpaid donation, blood would be objectified but not commodified.[7] The same would be true of genuinely unpaid egg donation, but not of a partially commodified system such as egg "sharing," in which women are given cheaper IVF treatment if they agree to let some of their eggs be used by other patients.[8] Whereas public umbilical cord blood banking began as a system in which cord blood was objectified but not commodified, it is now moving toward a partially commodified state because of the international trade in publicly banked cord blood.[9]

There is nothing inherently wrong with objectification, Marx thinks; indeed, it is necessary to human existence. Even commodification may or may not be inherently unethical in itself, according to some commentators. Carolyn McLeod and Francoise Baylis argue that the act of commodification is permissible or impermissible according to the intrinsic value of the thing commodified, the existence of any moral constraints on alienating the thing from persons, and the favorable or unfavorable consequences of commodifying the object.[10]

Even where the consequences of making an object satisfy our needs and commodifying it are favorable, a Kantian perspective would require us to avoid both objectification and commodification of that which has most intrinsic value in itself: the human subject as a member of the Kingdom of Ends.[11] As subjects in their own right, persons can never be merely the objects of property holding. "Man cannot dispose over himself because he is not a thing; he is not his own property; to say that he is would be self-contradictory; for insofar as he is a person, he is a Subject in whom the ownership of things can be vested, and if he were his own property he would be a thing over which he could have ownership."[12]

Two questions arise. First, does Kant's dictum apply to commodifying individual parts of our bodies as extracted tissue, or only to the contradiction entailed in terms of autonomy by selling one's entire self into slavery?[13] Kant seems to wink at that distinction when he allows the selling of hair, for example, even though he frowns on it as rather disreputable. More seriously, he is willing to allow treating a body part merely as an object when it is necessary to preserve one's life, for example by amputating a diseased limb. Commodification is not involved in this example. however; nor is it entirely clear what the Kantian position would be in terms of saving someone *else's* life by excising an organ, as in living kidney donation or sale. Scholars disagree about that issue,[14] which of course did not arise in Kant's own time because the technology was unavailable.

Different legal jurisdictions have developed radically different responses to this first question—whether it is wrong to commodify individual tissues once taken from the body, or only whole bodies. French law has traditionally taken the strong position that the body and its parts together simply *are* the person, and that any commodification of extracted tissue is therefore unacceptable. However, many French critics regard that equivalence as an insufficiently examined platitude or even as an irrational taboo.[15] Jean-Pierre Baud, for example, argues in favor of overturning the equation of the body and the person with a frank admission that the body is a thing, "but not just any thing: a thing which, by virtue of reality and its sacred nature, is the object of narrowly limited and controlled legal procedures."[16] Although French courts have reiterated the principle that the body is indeed the subject, in practice they have made a series of concessions to medical reality: for example, by allowing blood donation.[17]

In contrast to the French position, an interpretation of the US National Organ and Transplant Act of 1984 has developed whereby in many states, gametes are exempted from the general prohibition on organ sale in the statute. Perhaps this exemption is based on the view that gametes are renewable tissue,[18] but if so, it is mistaken: Eggs, unlike sperm, are not renewable. Commercial sperm banks developed first, however, and that fact may well account for the assumption that egg sale was permissible on the same model.[19]

On a Kantian basis, however, it might well be argued that gametes, both eggs and sperm, should be subject to *stricter* prohibitions against commodification than other tissues. Unlike kidney donation, gamete sale does not save anyone's life; indeed, egg extraction may actually put the seller at risk of ovarian hyperstimulation, with potentially serious or even lethal consequences.[20] In terms of a Kantian concern with selfhood and identity, egg sale could also be suspect because gametes are widely seen to reflect the genetic identity of the donor and to convey that identity to the next generation. Certainly the purchasers think they do have that function: in a highly differentiated market such as California's, commissioning couples are looking for very specific phenotypical identities in egg sellers, which they hope will be reproduced in the resulting babies.[21] While a donated kidney is subject to tissue matching, much more specific profile casting typifies markets in eggs.

Gametes also involve relationships with both future generations and our present partners. In a sense, they are not owned, but rather lent by our ancestors and passed on to our progeny.[22] The French system recognizes this social context, rather than a merely individualistic interpretation, by restricting gamete transfer to the context of a *projet parental* undertaken by a married or long-term cohabiting heterosexual couple.[23,24] This provision was first stated in the bioethics laws of 1994 and reconfirmed in the statutes of 2004 and 2011, although it has occasioned much controversy because of its obviously discriminatory nature. The point here is not to endorse this particular French interpretation of what the social context of gamete transfer ought to be—only to note that at least the French do not consider the provision of eggs and sperm as purely a consumer bargain between seller and buyer.

The second question that arises about the firm Kantian distinction between person as subject and person as object is whether it is increasingly false to the realities of modern biotechnology. Céline Lafontaine argues that while the body has become "a pure object, a malleable material,"[25] underpinning an immense global market, at the same time individual subjects increasingly view their identities as wrapped up with the bodies they choose to manipulate or objectify. Modern biotechnology muddies the distinction between things external to our bodily selves and those intrinsic to us.[26] External objects such as ventilators or pacemakers are incorporated into our bodies, while extracted parts of our bodies such as tissue samples or DNA swabs assume an ongoing existence in stem cell lines or biobanks. As Melinda Cooper and Catherine Waldby write, "The twentieth century brings the production process *inside* the body and puts organs, blood, and cell lines into circulation *outside* the body, scrambling the classical Marxist distinction between the living and the dead."[27] It also confuses the distinction between subject and object.

The essential dilemma underlying both questions—whether it is wrong to commodify individual extracted tissues, and whether we can properly distinguish between person as subject and person as object in modern biomedicine—has been neatly summarized as this: We both *have* and *are* our bodies. As Maria Marzano-Parisoli puts it, "The body is not a simple worldly object, but rather the object which each of us both *has* and *is*; it is a thing, but *sui generis*; it is that over which we dispose, but not in an absolute manner."[28] This tension exists most starkly in the case of the commodification of women's reproductive tissue.[29] Indeed, insofar as commodification has come to dominate international tissue markets, all bodies, even biologically male ones, are effectively rendered open-access and thus feminized.[30] Furthermore, just as women's supposed natural capacity for selfless devotion was used in the nineteenth-century cult of the "True Woman"[31] to camouflage the legal power imbalance then current in marriage, so the language of "gift" is now consciously used to encourage altruism by women in a highly commodified area of reproductive tissue donation, the sale of human ova. It is to this example that the next section will turn.

THE SALE OF HUMAN EGGS FOR IN VITRO FERTILIZATION AND RESEARCH

The language of gift can and does coexist with commodification in the sale of human eggs for IVF and research. Indeed, the process of commodification is eased and abetted by encouraging tissue sellers to view their "gift" as altruistic, even if it is paid for and not really a gift at all. But that process is highly gendered: Although both sexes are encouraged to see their "donation" for IVF as altruistic, women are urged to see it as entirely so, while men are also meant to see it as a job like any other. That complicated reality is well captured by Rene Almeling in her analysis of private and public egg and sperm banks in California as part of the "medical-industrial complex."[32]

The commercial sperm banks that Almeling studied never allow their clients to meet the men from whom they are purchasing sperm, whereas egg "donation" services consciously encourage frequent meetings and a strong sense of relationship between clients and egg providers. The sale of sperm is final, abstract, and contractual, whereas women are paid by brokers to produce eggs for a particular couple, who may reward their "donor" with optional additional gifts beyond the sale price they have agreed with the agency. In short, Almeling concludes, egg sale is structured as gift exchange, whereas sperm sale is set up as paid temporary employment. Men readily use the language of commodification, calling purchasers "customers," agencies "middlemen," and their sperm "assets." Although the price paid for eggs is far higher than that for sperm, women typically deny that the money is earned, even if they admit that much of their original motivation was financial.

That should not be altogether surprising, because women's reproductive labor is simply not regarded *as* labor in either IVF or in the sale of human eggs for research. Indeed, the way in which the monetary value of women's labor is downplayed will be a recurring motif across all three examples in this chapter, showing why it is continually necessary to insist on the term "commodification" in order to emphasize the obvious but widely ignored economic facts of the matter.

In the case of egg sale, although money changes hands in a commodified exchange, agencies have defined women who sell their eggs as donors, not vendors, and the majority of egg sellers studied by Almeling accept that description of themselves.[33] Likewise, most egg vendors do not regard their "donation" as work or labor, although Almeling points out that their acceptance of the altruism narrative actually exposes them to additional emotional labor. Even though it is not part of their contract and has no immediate bearing on the fee they are paid, they worry about whether the recipients of their eggs succeed in becoming pregnant and delivering a healthy child. Perhaps this is partly because they are encouraged to feel almost like part of the commissioning family. As Lisa Okemoto argues, even though the use of contract and the payment of a fee places egg sale in the public sphere, it is still seen as a private, family matter.[34] Calling the sale a "gift" reinforces that illusion and removes it from the public sphere of commodification and exchange.

What is going on here is commodified sale of human reproductive tissue, not gift. If it looks like a duck, walks like a duck, and quacks like a duck, we can be reasonably confident that it is not a swan. But why should it matter whether gift or sale is involved? If gametes can be rightfully given away, why can't they be sold? Clearly the egg brokerage agencies think it does matter, because they go to great lengths to present egg sale as mutual gift.

A more conceptual answer is that property in modern jurisprudence is seen as a bundle of independent, differentiated, and distinct rights.[35] The right to alienate something by gift does not necessarily entail the right to alienate the same object by sale. I may give my vote to my preferred candidate, but I am forbidden to sell it. Guido Calabresi and Douglas Melamed similarly differentiate pure property rules, in which both sale and gift are permitted, from market inalienability or liability rules, which allow gift but not sale, and also from pure inalienability systems, which allow neither gift nor sale.[36] Charlotte Harrison has developed this distinction into an administrative model for tissue collection based on market inalienability, which she views as advantageous because it does not commodify tissue.[37]

Even a moderate interpretation of commodification's ethical status, such as that proposed by McLeod and Baylis, rules it out when unfavorable consequences arise. Unfettered commodification of eggs for IVF in some US states has undeniably produced adverse outcomes, including the apparent unenforceability of professional guidelines on egg pricing, the lack of incentives or mechanisms for clinics to follow up the long-term health of egg providers, and a potential conflict of interests within the role of clinic doctors: the temptation to harvest the maximum number of eggs, against the primary medical duty, *primum non nocere*.[38] As one fertility doctor has put it, "What is certain is that doctors are sworn to 'do no harm.' Donors are as much our patients as the recipients we so willingly serve."[39] Although the comparatively high price paid for eggs should perhaps alert egg sellers to potential risks, there is little indication that it does have that effect.[40] Indeed, one study uncovered widespread economy with the truth about the level of risks actually revealed to egg vendors.[41]

To these harms produced by commodification of eggs for IVF can be added similar qualms about payment for eggs used in research, originally for somatic cell nuclear transfer (SCNT) stem cell research but recently also for "mitochondrial replacement."[42] Although the techniques are not identical,[43] both types of research would require substantial quantities of human eggs. In the most notorious case of SCNT research, the South Korean researcher Hwang Woo Suk used over 2,200 eggs from paid vendors and his own research assistants in his vain attempts to produce personalized stem cell lines.[44] We now know that some 75% of these eggs were purchased for cash, in contravention of South Korean law.[45] But at the time, international reaction to Hwang's fraudulent claim to have succeeded largely ignored the ethical issues surrounding the commodification of human eggs, concentrating almost solely on the status of the embryo and the implications for human cloning. This is the phenomenon I call "The Lady Vanishes"[46]: the women from whom the ova were taken virtually disappeared from view, along with the labor they put into the process of egg extraction and the risks they underwent.[47]

It was nonetheless predictable, as I argued at the time,[48] that ethical issues about harms to egg donors would arise from the similarities between Hwang's technique and that used in producing the cloned sheep Dolly, with its stratospheric levels of sheep ova wastage. It required something like 400 sheep ova to produce one Dolly, implying that very large numbers of human eggs would also be required to produce one stem cell line through SCNT. Because the nuclear genetic content of the eggs is irrelevant in SCNT research, unlike in the highly differentiated IVF markets, there might also be a risk of a race to the bottom in seeking out the vulnerable vendors who will charge the least.[49] Subsequently, some states, including California in 2006, have enacted legislation making it illegal to pay for eggs used in research, but pressure continues to be mounted by researchers who want to see such restrictions overturned.[50] However, women have been reported to be highly reluctant to provide eggs for research for reasons having little to do with financial incentives.[51]

Advocates of paying women for eggs used in research do have one strong argument in their arsenal: at least they present what women do in egg retrieval procedures as genuine labor.[52] Whether donating for IVF or research, women are estimated by the American Society for Reproductive Medicine to put in 56 hours of work in undergoing interviews and procedures when they provide eggs.[53] Recognizing that the labor women undergo in egg procurement actually *is* labor, producing something of exchange value, goes beyond Marx's own analysis. Marx assumed that women's domestic and reproductive labor produced no use values and added no surplus value. It lay outside production and commodification altogether, belonging to the realm of the "merely" natural or repro-duction.[54] Modern assisted reproduction techniques make that premise even more untenable: There is very little "natural" about what women undergo in egg harvesting.

This insight has prompted Melinda Cooper and Catherine Waldby to develop their concept of "clinical labor," linked to the idea of "biocapital" enunciated in the work of Kaushik Sunder Rajan.[55] In this analysis, the life science business and the accumulation of biocapital depend on a property regime that prioritizes and rewards the inventive cog-nitive labor of the scientist. By contrast, this system construes the "clinical labor" of egg donors and research subjects as cheaply and readily available, no matter how risky and potentially harmful the work they perform and the procedures they undergo. This situ-ation has not been sufficiently critiqued or regulated, partly because Anglo-American jurisprudence traditionally viewed tissue taken from the body as no one's property (*res nullius*), available to the first claimant, and partly because neither the Marxist nor the Fordist model of production can accurately describe the 21st-century life science industry.

Although Cooper and Waldby do not explicitly do so, this analysis could be deepened by adding a third reason: the association of women with the merely natural and with the private domestic realm. When a contractual relationship such as egg selling is deliberately treated as gift exchange, outside the economic realm of commodification, we are witness-ing the reduction of women's clinical labor to a private act of love, within the boundar-ies of the relationship that they are encouraged to develop with the contracting couple. Similarly, in the private banking of umbilical cord blood, another new type of clinical labor that creates considerable biovalue for private firms is presented as something any dutiful mother will naturally want to do. It is to this example that the next section will turn.

THE COMMODIFICATION OF UMBILICAL CORD BLOOD

For the past quarter of a century it has been known that umbilical cord blood, taken during or after the final stage of labor,[56] contains hematopoietic (blood-making) cells, similar to although fewer in number than those found in bone marrow. The first use of cord blood cells in clinical medicine was to treat a baby's older sibling who had Fanconi's anemia.[57] As of 2010, the American Academy of Pediatrics estimated that roughly 360,000 cord blood units were stored internationally in public banks, which charge no fee for collection. But in many countries, such as India, that number is far outweighed by units in for-profit private banks, which store the blood on a contractual, paid-for basis. Around the world there are now nearly three units stored privately for everyone in a public bank. (Surprisingly, perhaps, the United States has by far the highest number of public banks in the world, although it also has substantial numbers of private ones charging between $1,500 and $2,000 initially, along with an annual fee of $90 to $200.) A 2013 commercial report, *Capitalizing on Opportunities in Cord Blood Industry Growth*, was decidedly Boosterish about the future, as well it might have been with a price tag of $3,995. The title alone should make it obvious that commercial interests regard cord blood as a commodity like any other, as does the "warning" at the head of the Web page: "Don't read this unless you want to profit from the global cord blood banking market." For anyone left in doubt, the Executive Summary went on to state:

> The cord blood banking industry is one of the fastest growing industries in the world. There were only 23 active cord blood banks as of 2005, and now there are 485 world-wide. Cord blood banks exist in nearly every developed country, as well as within many developing nations. That is a 21-fold increase (2,100%) in the companies involved in the industry, in less than a ten year period. This rapid market growth represents both an opportunity to profit, as well as swarming competition.[58]

Private banks generally store the blood purely for the child's own future use, whereas public banks make it available for others (although they will return the unit to the parents in case of need, assuming the unit is still in their inventory.) Counterintuitively, cord blood banking is most effective if it is *not* performed with the patient's own cord blood, but rather with that taken from other babies and pooled.[59] A comprehensive evidence-based review concluded recently that "the scientific evidence clearly supports public cord blood donation [over private banking] due to the likelihood of clinical need, potential graft vs. leukemia effect, concern over latent disease in the cord blood unit, and quality of autologous [own] cord blood units."[60]

Cord blood is often presented as mere waste that would otherwise be discarded—just as the risks inherent in the provision of ova are sometimes downplayed with the claim that eggs are so plentiful that they can be lost monthly in menstruation. Of course, that is not the means by which eggs are extracted for IVF, and neither is cord blood taken from cords and placentas that have already been discarded. What actually happens in the extraction of cord blood is that the umbilical cord is clamped—a routine although increasingly controversial part of the active management of labor.[61] A portion of the blood is then taken for storage in the hypothetical case of future need (predicted as a 1 in 2,700 chance by American College of Obstetricians and Gynecologists guidelines[62]). It is more common for private banks to take this blood while the placenta is still attached to the uterine wall in order to maximize the volume. Public banks such as the

London Cord Blood Bank more typically harvest cord blood immediately after delivery of the placenta.[63] In public banks there should be less pressure to maximize the donation because cord blood is immunologically naïve: It does not react strongly to tissue from another body, making pooled donations effective, although some tissue matching is still required.[64]

Privately banked cord blood is commodified as part of a service industry: Although no money changes hands for the blood itself, a commercial contract is drawn up between parents and private bank for the provision of the bank's services. Until recently it would have been possible to claim that public banked cord blood was not similarly commodified, but the demarcation lines are no longer drawn so clearly. Some private banks collaborate with not-for-profit agencies—for example, the partnership between Viacord and the National Heart, Lung and Blood Institute—while one private UK bank offers its customers a slightly reduced fee if they offer to donate the greater part of the blood to a public bank.

What most undermines the distinction between uncommodified public banking and commodified private banking, however, is the way in which cord blood units are traded as commodities in the international bioeconomy. Altruistically donated cord blood units in public banks trade internationally at very high prices, between $23,000 and $31,000 per unit.[65] At the end of 2008, this global commerce was already worth over $30 million, with over 40% of all cord blood units being traded across borders. Public cord blood banks in ethnically heterogeneous nations benefit from the comparative rarity value of immunologically typed blood from their minority populations. Very few national banks are diverse enough to meet all domestic demand, except for more ethnically homogeneous nations such as Japan.

This trade engaged in by public cord blood banks does not represent solidarity or altruism, so much as market strategy concerning a crucial commodity.

> The international trade in cord blood is not necessarily a freely given expression of common community. It is instead a form of protection for the trade's participants from the vulnerabilities of being dependent on an import market in premium goods.[66]

In the international cord blood trade, profit is being made—albeit by public banks seeking new means to support their services in a climate of cutbacks and austerity—from women's unpaid and altruistic labor in the labor of childbirth itself. Providing cord blood generally requires women to undergo an additional intervention because they want to do what they believe is best for their baby. (In fact, the medical evidence base suggests that the procedure may actually be harmful, because it lessens the blood flow available to the newborn and may result in adverse sequelae such as jaundice.[67]) Rarely do these women realize that the blood they donate is likely to become a tradeable commodity. Interviews carried out with mothers who donated cord blood to a UK public bank reveal that women were asked to bestow a "double gift": life for their own newborn and also for another child who could be saved by their altruism.[68] The possibility of units being traded was not mentioned in the information they received before giving consent. Furthermore, the fact of an international trade diminishes the likelihood that their child's own unit would be available from the public bank if needed later.

The global bioeconomy of cord blood, in which both private and public banks take part, relies on a substance that is either donated for nothing or that the parents have actually paid to store. It also depends on the mother's willingness to undergo an additional intervention, as well as her "emotional labor" on behalf of her own child and possibly other children as well. If, as Marx thought, productive labor is distinguished by intentionality and control, the mother's decision to allow cord blood to be extracted demonstrates both those qualities. Women must decide in advance that they intend this additional procedure to be performed, possibly extending the process of childbirth and even exposing themselves to some risk if, for example, the attention of delivery room staff is diverted at a crucial moment in the final stage of childbirth.[69] Not only is this form of labor rarely acknowledged *as* labor; most of the literature refers to cord blood as belonging to the child,[70] although physiologically it is the mother's.[71] As well as using the language of "waste" in a manner that disguises the value of the commodity and masks the mother's rights in her own tissue, the cord blood industry also plays on the language of "gift" in a way that ignores the profits made by everyone except the original donor.

The question is not whether women would have wanted a share in those profits: that is not their motivation. It is whether their contribution is being commodified, whether the surplus value of their labor is being transferred to the cord blood banks, and whether their altruism is being exploited. Cooper and Waldby see the cord blood phenomenon as a form of "regenerative labor," typical of a new kind of global bioeconomy that depends crucially on the generative powers of their reproductive tissue and efforts. In commercial gestational surrogacy, they identify a similar phenomenon. It is to surrogacy that this chapter now turns.

SURROGACY: JUST WHAT IS BEING COMMODIFIED?

Eggs sold for cash and cord blood traded on international markets can be clearly identified as commodities, but what constitutes the commodity in commercial surrogacy is far more controversial. Commonly, as in the phrases "renting a womb" or "pregnancy outsourcing," a surrogacy contract is seen to concern the provision of a service, rather than a physical object such as eggs or cord blood. Cooper and Waldby likewise frame commercial surrogacy as a service rather than a good, actually using the popular but incorrect analogy of womb-letting. However, they also classify egg sale as a service, even though a physical object is involved.[72] This apparent anomaly follows from their depiction of reproductive commodification as an instance of the post-Fordist service economy. In their scheme of "clinical labor," both egg sale and commercial surrogacy thus come under the same rubric as the work of research subjects who undertake clinical trials on behalf of contract research organizations: The latter is clearly a service rather than a good.

Although this chapter is entitled "The Commodification of Women's Reproductive Tissue and Services" as an acknowledgment of the widely held presumption that surrogacy involves payment for a service, this section will conclude that the primary object of the contract is neither the service of pregnancy nor the "renting" of a womb, but rather the baby itself. In this respect it harkens back to the argument made by Elizabeth Anderson some 25 years ago. Anderson viewed surrogacy contracts as commodifying both the woman's labor in pregnancy and the purchase of a child, and she condemned both.[73]

Anderson was right to depict surrogacy as baby sale, for reasons that will be detailed later, but academic debate seems to have moved away from her position, at the same time as commercial interests have made surrogacy big business. Instead, the right to enter into a surrogacy contract has often been presented as part and parcel of women's reproductive freedom: "That doctors would be so paternalistic as to deny women the option of using a surrogate if the surrogate were willing to do so is simply outrageous."[74] Yet while a ban on baby selling has been problematized as discriminatory,[75] prohibition remains the position in the majority of legal jurisdictions which take a position on surrogacy.[76] However, France, which continues to maintain that ban, has recently been forced by the European Court of Human Rights to grant citizenship to children born abroad to French nationals who have traveled to countries with a more permissive surrogacy regime.[77]

Even California, one of the US states that allows commercial surrogacy, retains the option of prosecuting what it does term "baby selling" in particular circumstances. More specifically, it prohibits the sale of parental rights to babies and children, while permitting surrogacy arrangements if the "gestational carrier" and the "intending parents" enter into an agreement prior to an embryonic transfer. In 2011 Theresa Erickson was convicted by a California district court for being part of a "baby-selling ring" after she and her conspirators used falsely obtained prebirth adoption declarations to create an inventory of unborn babies who would be sold for $100,000 each.[78] It is indicative that the court did use the term "baby selling," since otherwise the case might seem to fit the contention that what is being commodified is not the child but a limited bundle of parental rights.[79] Another indication that the tide may be turning against commercial surrogacy in the United States is Louisiana State House Bill 187, which would outlaw payment other than medical and travel expenses to a surrogate mother. Any additional payment would incur a penalty of up to 10 years in prison, as sale of a child.[80]

Why is it inappropriate to see surrogacy as womb-letting or pregnancy outsourcing? The recent case of "Baby Gammy" provides a clear example. A 21-year-old Thai surrogate mother, Pattaramon Chanbua, was paid $11,000 by an Australian couple in a commercial arrangement. When Chanbua became pregnant with twins, she was promised an additional $2,000. If surrogacy were indeed womb-letting, that is, if the pregnancy and not the child was the object of the contract, there would be no additional payment for twins: rather a flat rate for the pregnancy. Nor would the Australian couple have withdrawn the offer of the extra $2,000 when one of the twins turned out to have Down syndrome and a congenital heart condition. The Australian couple were widely reported as having refused to accept the "damaged" twin, who was left with the surrogate mother.[81]

Because the Baby Gammy case involved a vulnerable child and an impoverished mother, it occasioned an outcry and provoked Thailand's subsequent decision to criminalize paid surrogacy. But one might also argue that the Baby Gammy case shocked people around the globe because it makes it impossible to avoid the conclusion that babies are indeed being bought and sold in commercial surrogacy. The "damaged" child was effectively being treated as faulty goods.

Viewing the child rather than the pregnancy as the object of the contract also helps to explain another oddity about surrogacy contracts: They enforce specific performance. Other service contracts typically allow the party performing the service to break the agreement by returning any monies paid, perhaps with damages. A housepainter who signs a decorating contract and then reneges on it cannot be physically forced to scale his ladder and get busy with the brushes. Not so with surrogate mothers in jurisdictions such as India, where a draft surrogacy bill includes a provision requiring the mother to surrender the baby on birth—overturning the traditional common-law presumption that the birth mother is the legal mother.

Debra Satz has developed this specific performance argument with precision and clarity. However, she does not view it as entailing the view of surrogacy as baby selling: in fact, she regards that analogy as incorrect. As Satz writes:

> [T]his argument is flawed. Pregnancy contracts do not enable fathers (or prospective mothers, women who are infertile or otherwise unable to conceive) to acquire full ownership rights over children. Even where there has been a financial payment for conceiving a child, the child cannot be viewed as a mere commodity. The father (or prospective mother) cannot, for example, simply destroy or abandon the child.[82]

In the Gammy case, of course, it seems that the commissioning parents did in fact abandon the child. More generally, however, Satz's criticism depends on a view of property as unitary, rather than in terms of the generally acknowledged jurisprudential model of a bundle of rights.[83] We may lack the right to destroy or abandon an object of ownership rights but still maintain other property entitlements in it: for example, physical possession, management, and security against taking by others. These rights are common features of surrogacy contracts, particularly where the birth mother is prevented from "taking" the child back or refusing to surrender the baby in the first place.

The disparity of wealth between the surrogate and the commissioning couple in the Gammy case raises the question of whether the injustice concerns exploitation of the mother as well as commodification of the baby. In some Indian clinics women who miscarry are paid nothing, some critics allege.[84] Far from enhancing women's autonomy and rights, commercial surrogacy undervalues women's reproductive labor, in some instances to the point of ignoring it altogether.[85] This is another reason why use of the phrase "renting a womb" is pernicious: The surrogate mother is not a privileged *rentier* but a worker paid to produce a valuable commodity under conditions of risk and pain. In the *Anna J* case,[86] the judge recognized that the woman was effectively selling her pain and suffering in labor. But that begs the question of why the commissioning parents would want to buy pain and suffering—and in that case the custody judgment went against the surrogate mother.

Conclusion: Commodification, Reproductive Labor, and Exploitation

Labor in childbirth, like women's work in producing eggs or the extra labor that women undergo in banking cord blood, is not widely recognized as the sort of labor that grounds a property right. All three case studies have that phenomenon in common. In each example, the commodification of female reproductive tissue—or, in the case of surrogacy, the commodification of the child—is masked by an assumption that these products of women's reproductive labor are more properly seen as gifts than as commodities. Just as egg donors are encouraged to see their paid dealings with the buyers as a gift relationship, and just as new mothers are encouraged to donate umbilical cord altruistically to banks, which will then go on to trade it as an international commodity, so surrogate mothers, even paid ones, frequently view what they are doing in terms of gift values rather than market ones.[87]

Anderson also asserts that the way in which women are encouraged to adopt a non-economic motivation in providing their reproductive services renders them ripe for exploitation. Whatever the economic imbalance, she discovers exploitation in the mere fact that one party sees the transaction as purely monetary while the other regards what she is doing as mainly altruistic.[88] Yet when everyone else is making a profit from women's tissue, as some commentators assert,[89] isn't it exploitative to expect them to undergo the laborious and risky procedures in egg donation out of pure altruism? One-way altruism is better known as exploitation, even when camouflaged by the language of gift.[90]

This argument from one-way altruism is descended from the Marxist concept of exploitation as disparity of compensation: the imbalance, extracted under conditions of subordination, between the labor value invested in producing an object by the worker and the price the worker is paid for his labor. This external standard of disparity overrides subjective interpretations, including those of the workers themselves. Thus, it is entirely possible for someone to be exploited even if she denies it, as egg sellers and surrogate mothers often do.[91] For example, a UK study of women enrolled in an "egg-sharing" program to obtain IVF at a reduced price found that they typically rejected the language of exploitation, even though they candidly described themselves as "desperate" because the National Health Service would not cover IVF for them.[92]

Although it might seem paternalistic to deny that we must take women at their own word when they deny being exploited—another version of the rather condescending notion of "false consciousness"—their views do not arise in a vacuum. Women are being given a consistent message by commercial egg selling, cord blood, and surrogacy agencies that the object of their reproductive labor should rightfully be seen as a gift. False consciousness is being encouraged for commercial reasons: The language of exploitation cannot arise in the gift relationship. In commercial egg economies, sellers may profess altruism to increase their chances of success in a competitive buyer's market,[93] but are usually motivated in large part by monetary gain, while "the gift of life" has become merely a marketing concept.[94]

Just as early capitalism and its predecessor, the agricultural revolution, were funded by the accumulation of value in labor and land taken from underpaid industrial workers and displaced peasants, so modern commercial biotechnology can be seen as underpinned by systematic and exploitative underpayment of the women who provide the crucial "components" and the labor of artificial reproduction. This systematic transfer of surplus value on a global scale is bolstered by neoliberal governmental policies. In the view of Waldby and Cooper: "What neo-liberalism seeks to make available is not merely a permanent surplus of labor power but also a surplus of reproductivity—a reserve of low-cost suppliers of reproductive services and tissues who perform unacknowledged reproductive labour within the lowest echelon of the bioeconomy."[95]

As Kieran Healy points out, exploitation under capitalism is masked because "Capitalist markets lead people to believe that commodities possess value in their own right, rather than because of the social labor that goes into producing them. This is commodity fetishism."[96] Because under capitalism people are primarily linked through the exchange of goods for money, they lose sight of the original source of value of the goods they purchase. This sets up a major difficulty in establishing a just or fair price for human tissue, which is exacerbated by the rapidity and unpredictability of new developments in reproductive biomedicine. Frequently there is little or no recognition that women's tissue is even involved in biotechnological processes, and even less awareness that women have labored to create the "product."[97]

If human tissue cannot be turned into a commodity without harming people's worth as persons, as a Kantian perspective would suggest, then any form of tissue sale, including but not exclusive to female tissue such as eggs, is in a sense exploitative, whatever price is offered for it. The source of exploitation lies not so much—or not only—in an objective disparity of payment, but in the twin wrongs of commodifying that which should not be commodified and of exploiting another human being. As the French analyst Sylvie Ebelpoin has put it,[98] childlessness is an undeniable source of suffering, but we are not permitted to alleviate one person's suffering by committing a wrong to other persons.

Commodified reproductive technologies such as paid egg donation and commercial surrogacy are often justified on the grounds that they enable new sorts of families and expand reproductive choice. But reproductive choice is not a knockdown argument. We should be particularly wary of it when it also camouflages the interests of increasingly dominant commercial interests.

NOTES

1. Timothy Caulfield and Ubuku Ogbogu, "Stem Cell Research, Scientific Freedom and the Commodification Concern," *European Molecular Biology Organization Reports*, online at doi:10.1038/embor.2011.232, December 2, 2011.

2. Nancy Scheper-Hughes, "Bodies for Sale—Whole or in Parts," *Body and Society* 7 (2002): 1–8, at p. 2.

3. Martha Nussbaum, "Objectification," *Philosophy and Public Affairs* 24, no. 4 (1995): 249–291.

4. The term "surrogacy" wrongly implies that the birth mother is not the real mother, contravening the established common-law presumption, but although "contract motherhood" might be preferable, that term is much less widely recognized.

5. Timothy Caulfield and Ubuku Ogbogu, "Stem Cell Research, Scientific Freedom and the Commodification Concern," *European Molecular Biology Organization Reports*, online at doi:10.1038/embor.2011.232, December 2, 2011.

6. Karl Marx, *Capital*, trans. by Samuel Moore and Edward Aveling, ed. Friedrich Engels (Moscow: Progress, 1954, original edn. 1867), p. 48.

7. Richard Titmuss, *The Gift Relationship: From Human Blood to Social Policy*, eds. Ann Oakley and J. Ashton (London: LSE Books, 1997, 2nd ed.). Titmuss famously thought the United Kingdom was a pure gift system, but it is no longer so except insofar as the donor is not paid, because of the extensive trade in blood products derived from the donation. See Catherine Waldby and Robert Mitchell, *Tissue Economies: Blood, Organs and Cell Lines in Late Capitalism* (Durham, NC: Duke University Press, 2006), ch. 1.

8. For further discussion of the distinction between incomplete or partial commodification and full commodification, see Margaret J. Radin, *Contested Commodities: The Trouble with Trade in Sex, Children, Body Parts and Other Things* (Cambridge, MA: Harvard University Press, 1996).

9. Nik Brown, "Contradictions of Value: Between Use and Exchange in Cord Blood Bioeconomy," *Sociology of Health and Illness* 35, no. 1 (2013): 97–112.

10. Carolyn McLeod and Francoise Baylis, "Feminists on the Inalienability of Human Embryos," *Hypatia* 21(2006): 1–4.

11. Donna Dickenson, *Property in the Body: Feminist Perspectives* (Cambridge: Cambridge University Press, 2007), p. 30.

12. Immanuel Kant, *Lectures on Ethics* (Indianapolis: Bobbs-Merrill, 1963), p. 4.

13. David Resnik, "The Commodification of Human Reproductive Materials," *Journal of Medical Ethics* 24 (1998): 288–293. Resnik takes a strong line that whole bodies which in his view do not contain persons, such as those of anencephalic infants, can legitimately be commodified, as can reproductive materials as mere parts of the body not containing the entire person.

14. Ruth F. Chadwick, "The Market for Bodily Parts: Kant and Duties to Oneself," in Brenda Almond and Don Hill (eds.), *Applied Philosophy: Metaphysics and Morals in Contemporary Debate* (London: Routledge, 1991), pp. 288–298; Nicole Gerrand, "The Misuse of Kant in the Debate about a Market in Human Body Parts," *Journal of Applied Philosophy* 16, no. 1 (1999): 59–67; Jean-Christophe Merle, "A Kantian Argument for a Duty to Donate One's Own Organs: A Reply to Nicole Gerrand," *Journal of Applied Philosophy* 17, no. 1 (2000): 93–101.

15. Dominique Memmi, *Les gardiens du corps: dix ans de magistère bioéthique* (Paris: Editions de l'Ecole des Hautes Etudes en Sciences Sociales, 1996), p. 20.

16. Jean-Pierre Baud, *L'affaire de la main volée* (Paris: Editions du Seuil, 1993), p. 120, translation mine.

17. Maria M. Marzano-Parisoli, *Penser le corps* (Paris: Presses Universitaires de France, 2002), p. 124.

18. Kieran Healy, *Last Best Gifts: Altruism and the Market for Human Blood and Organs* (Chicago: University of Chicago Press, 2006), p. 36.

19. Rene Almeling, *Sex Cells: The Medical Market in Eggs and Sperm* (Berkeley: University of California Press, 2011); Debora L. Spar, *The Baby Business: How Money, Science and Politics Drive the Commerce of Conception* (Cambridge, MA: Harvard Business School Press, 2006).

20. W. Kramer, J. Schneider, and N. Schultz, "US Oocyte Donors: A Retrospective Study of Medical and Psychosocial Issues," *Human Reproduction*, doi: 10.193/humrep/dep309 (September 3, 2009); A. Delavigne and S. Rozenberg, "Epidemiology and Prevention of Ovarian Hyperstimulation Syndrome: A Review," *Human Reproduction Update* 8, no. 6 (2002): 559–577; Allen Jacobs, James Dwyer, and Peter Lee, "Seventy Ova," *Hastings Center Report* 31 (2001): 12–14.

21. Rene Almeling, *Sex Cells: The Medical Market in Eggs and Sperm* (Berkeley: University of California Press, 2011).

22. Donna Dickenson, "Procuring Gametes for Research and Therapy: The Case for Unisex Altruism," *Journal of Medical Ethics* 23 (1997): 93–95.

23. Karène Parizer-Krieff, "La notion de 'projet parental' dans le droit de l'assistance médicale à la procréation (AMP)," *The Tocqueville Review* 34 (2013): 1–39.

24. Code de la santé publique, art. I-152-2.

25. Céline Lafontaine, *Le corps-marché: la marchandisation de le vie humaine a l'ère de la bioéconomie* (Paris: Editions du Seuil, 2014), p. 13, translation mine.

26. Donna Dickenson, *Body Shopping: Converting Body Parts to Profit* (Oxford: Oneworld, 2009), p. 11.

27. Melinda Cooper and Catherine Waldby, *Clinical Labor: Tissue Donors and Research Subjects in the Global Bioeconomy* (Durham, NC: Duke University Press, 2014), p. 12.

28. Maria M. Marzano-Parisoli, *Penser le corps* (Paris: Presses Universitaires de France, 2002), p. 138, translation mine.

29. Donna Dickenson, "Property and Women's Alienation from Their Own Reproductive Labour," *Bioethics* 15, no. 3 (2001): 203–217; "Commodification of Human Tissue: Implications for Feminist and Development Ethics," *Developing World Bioethics* 2, no. 1 (2002): 55–63.

30. Donna Dickenson, *Property in the Body: Feminist Perspectives* (Cambridge: Cambridge University Press, 2007).

31. Donna Dickenson, *Margaret Fuller: Writing a Woman's Life* (Basingstoke: MacMillan, 1994).

32. Rene Almeling, *Sex Cells: The Medical Market in Eggs and Sperm* (Berkeley: University of California Press, 2011). The term "medical-industrial complex" was coined in the 1980s by the then editor of the *New England Journal of Medicine*, Arnold Relman.

33. For a comparable study motivations of donors in Europe, see Guido Pennings, J. de Mouzon, Francoise Shenfield, et al., "Socio-Demographic and Fertility-Related Characteristics and Motivations of Oocyte Donors in Eleven European Countries," *Human Reproduction* (March 13, 2014), doi:10.1093/humrep/deu048. Pennings et al. found

that 47.8% of donors identified their motives as pure altruism, 33.9% altruistic and financial reasons, 10.8% pure financial reasons, 5.9% altruism and own treatment, and 2% own treatment only. The latter two categories comprised egg "sharers."

34. Lisa Okemoto, "Eggs as Capital: Human Egg Procurement in the Fertility Industry and the Stem Cell Research Enterprise," *Signs* 34 (2009): 763–781.

35. Wesley Newcomb Hohfeld, *Fundamental Legal Conceptions* (New Haven, CT: Yale University Press, 1923); A. M. Honore, "Ownership," in *Making Law Bind: Essays Legal and Philosophical* (Oxford: Clarendon Press, 1987), pp. 161–192.

36. Guido Calabresi and A. Douglas Melamed, "Property Rules, Liability Rules and Alienability: One View of the Cathedral," *Harvard Law Review* 85 (1972): 1089.

37. Charlotte H. Harrison, "Neither Moore nor the Market: Alternative Models for Compensating Contributors of Human Tissue," *American Journal of Law and Medicine* 28 (1972): 77–104.

38. In a large literature, see, inter alia: Rene Almeling, *Sex Cells: The Medical Market in Eggs and Sperm* (Berkeley: University of California Press, 2011); Judith F. Daar, "Regulating the Fiction of Informed Consent in ART Medicine," *American Journal of Bioethics* 1, no. 4 (2001): 19–20; Debora L. Spar, "The Egg Trade: Making Sense of the Market for Human Oocytes," *New England Journal of Medicine* 356 (2007): 1289–1291; W. Kramer, J. Schneider, and N. Schultz, "US Oocyte Donors: A Retrospective Study of Medical and Psychosocial Issues," *Human Reproduction*, doi: 10.193/humrep/dep309 (September 3, 2009).

39. Mark V. Sauer, "Egg Donor Solicitation: Problems Exist, But Do Abuses?" *American Journal of Bioethics* 1, no. 4 (2001): 1–2.

40. Jessica Berg, "Risky Business: Evaluating Oocyte Donation," *American Journal of Bioethics* 1, no. 4 (2001): 18–19.

41. Andrea F. Gurmankin, "Risk Information Provided to Potential Oocyte Donors in a Preliminary Phone Call," *American Journal of Bioethics* 1, no. 4 (2001): 3–13.

42. Donna Dickenson and Marcy Darnovsky, "Not So Fast," *New Scientist*, June 14, 2014; Donna Dickenson, "The Commercialization of Human Eggs in Mitochondrial Replacement Research," *The New Bioethics* 19, no. 1 (2013): 18–29.

43. Somatic cell nuclear transfer is a means of producing a stem cell line by inserting a somatic (body) cell from one individual into an enucleated egg from a "donor" in hope of developing a tissue-matched personal "spare parts kit." "Mitochondrial transfer," better termed "nuclear transfer," takes a human egg from a healthy woman and inserts a nucleus from a woman who has mitochondrial disease, before fertilizing the egg with sperm from the second woman's partner.

44. Hwang Woo Suk et al., "Evidence of a Pluripotent Human Embryonic Stem Cell Line Derived from a Cloned Blastocyst," *Science* 303 (2004): 1669–1674; Hwang Woo Suk et al., "Patient-Specific Embryonic Stem Cell Lines Derived from Human SCNT Blastocysts," *Science* 306 (2005): 1777–1783; Francoise Baylis, "For Love or Money? The Saga of the Korean Women Who Provided Eggs for Embryonic Stem Cell Research," *Theoretical Medicine and Bioethics* 30 (2009): 385–396; Azumi Tsuge and Hyunsoo Hong, "Reconsidering Ethics Issues about 'Voluntary Egg Donors' in Hwang's Care in Global Context," *New Genetics and Society* 30 (2011): 241–252.

45. Francoise Baylis, "For Love or Money? The Saga of the Korean Women Who Provided Eggs for Embryonic Stem Cell Research," *Theoretical Medicine and Bioethics* 30 (2009): 385–396.

46. Donna Dickenson, "The Lady Vanishes: What's Missing from the Stem Cell Debate," *Journal of Bioethical Inquiry* 3 (2006): 43–54.

47. One woman was hospitalized twice for ovarian hyperstimulation syndrome, whose overall incidence among the egg providers was abnormally high at 17.7% Francoise Baylis, "For Love or Money? The Saga of the Korean Women Who Provided Eggs for Embryonic Stem Cell Research," *Theoretical Medicine and Bioethics* 30 (2009): 385–396.

48. Donna Dickenson, "The Threatened Trade in Human Ova," *Nature Reviews Genetics* 5, no. 3 (2004): 167.

49. Francoise Baylis and Carolyn McLeod, "The Stem Cell Debate Continues: The Buying and Selling of Eggs for Research," *Journal of Medical Ethics* 33 (2007): 726–731.

50. Dieter Egli, Alice Chen, Genevieve Saphier, et al., "Impracticality of Egg Donor Recruitment in the Absence of Compensation," *Cell Stem Cell* 9 (2011), doi: 10.1016/j.stem.2011.08.002; Charis Thompson, "Why We Should, in Fact, Pay for Egg Donation," *Regenerative Medicine* 2 (2007): 203–209; Erica Haimes, Loane Skene, Angela J. Ballantyne, et al., "Position Statement on the Provision and Procurement of Human Eggs for Stem Cell Research," *Cell Stem Cell* 12 (2013): 285–291. For an opposing position, see Donna Dickenson and Itziar Alkorta Idiakez, "Ova Donation for Stem Cell Research: An International Perspective," *Journal of Feminist Approaches to Bioethics* 1 (2008): 125–144.

51. Catherine Waldby and Katherine Carroll, "Egg Donation for Stem Cell Research: Ideas of Surplus and Deficit in Australian IVF Patients' and Reproductive Donors' Accounts," *Sociology of Health and Illness* 34 (2012): 513–528.

52. For example, Bonnie Steinbock, "Payment for Egg Donation and Surrogacy," *Mt Sinai Journal of Medicine* 71 (2004): 255–265.

53. Ethics Committee of the American Society for Reproductive Medicine, "Financial Incentives in Recruitment of Oocyte Donors," *Fertility and Sterility* 82 (2004): Supplement 1: S240–S244.

54. Modern Marxist feminists, however, particularly Christine Delphy in *Close to Home*, have introduced a new category into conventional Marxism, "domestic relations of production," which includes the products of conception and pregnancy, although not specifically the products of assisted reproductive techniques. See Christine Delphy, *Close to Home: A Materialist Analysis of Women's Oppression* (trans. and ed. Diane Leonard) (London: Hutchinson, 1984); Donna Dickenson, "Property and Women's Alienation from Their Reproductive Labour," *Bioethics* 15 (2001): 205–217; Susan Dodds, "Women, Commodification and Embryonic Stem Cell Research," in James Humber and Robert F. Almeder (eds.), *Biomedical Ethics Review: Stem Cell Research* (Totowa, NJ: Humana Press, 2003), 149–175.

55. Melinda Cooper and Catherine Waldby, *Clinical Labor: Tissue Donors and Research Subjects in the Global Bioeconomy* (Durham, NC: Duke University Press, 2014); Kaushik Sunder Rajan, *Biocapital: The Constitution of Postgenomic Life* (Durham, NC: Duke University Press, 2006).

56. The third or final stage of labor, the expulsion of the placenta, to which the baby is connected by the umbilical cord. Cord blood can either be collected while the placenta remains attached to the uterine wall (in utero) or after the placenta has been delivered (ex utero). Particularly with the in utero method, much of the blood that would naturally flow to the baby will be diverted for storage, resulting in diminished blood flow to the baby with possible risks such as jaundice. This is one reason why professional body guidelines from the American and UK colleges of obstetricians and gynecologists do not recommend routine collection.

57. Eliane Gluckman, H. A. Broxmeyer, A. D. Auerbach, et al., "Hematopoietic Reconstitution in a Patient with Fanconi's Anemia by Means of Umbilical Cord Blood from an HLA-Identical Sibling," *New England Journal of Medicine* 321 (1989): 1174–1178.

58. BioInformant Worldwide, *Capitalizing on Opportunities in Cord Blood Industry Growth*, accessed August 11, 2014, http://www.bioinformant.com/Cord-Blood-Industry-Growth.html

59. V. Rocha, M. Lahaopin, G. Sanz, et al., "Transplants of Umbilical Cord Blood or Bone Marrow from Unrelated Donors in Adults with Acute Leukemia," *New England Journal of Medicine* 351 (2004): 2276–2285.

60. Karen Ballen, "Challenges in Umbilical Cord Blood Stem Cell Banking for Stem Cell Reviews and Reports," *Stem Cell Reviews and Reports* 6 (2010): 8–14.

61. Candice L. Downey and Susan Bewley, "Third Stage Practices and the Neonate," *Fetal and Maternal Medicine Review* 20 (2009): 1–18.

62. American College of Obstetricians and Gynecologists, "Committee Opinion Number 399: On Umbilical Cord Blood Banking," *Obstetrics and Gynecology* 111 (2008): 475–477.

63. Sue Davey, Sue Armitage, Vanderson Rocha, et al., "The London Cord Blood Bank: Analysis of Banking and Transplantation Outcome," *British Journal of Haematology* 125 (2004): 358–365.

64. For a fuller discussion of the evidence base, see Donna Dickenson, *Me Medicine vs. We Medicine: Reclaiming Biotechnology for the Common Good* (New York: Columbia University Press, 2013), chapter 4.

65. Nik Brown, Laura Machin, and Danae McLeod, "The Immunitary Bioeconomy: The Economisation of the International Cord Blood Market," *Social Science and Medicine* 30 (2011): 1–8.

66. Nik Brown, Laura Machin, and Danae McLeod, "The Immunitary Bioeconomy: The Economisation of the International Cord Blood Market," *Social Science and Medicine* 30 (2011): 1–8, at p. 2.

67. H. Rabe, G. Reynolds, and J. Diaz-Rossello, "Early Versus Delayed Clamping in Preterm Infants," *Cochrane Database Systemic Reviews* 4: CD0032248 (2004); E. K. Hutton and E. S. Hassan, "Late vs. Early Clamping of the Umbilical Cord in Full-Term Neonates: Systematic Review and Meta-Analysis of Controlled Trials," *Journal of the American Medical Association* 297 (2007): 1241–1252; Andrew Weeks, "Umbilical Cord Clamping After Birth," *British Medical Journal* 335 (2007): 312–313.

68. Helen Busby, "The Meanings of Consent to the Donation of Cord Blood Stem Cells: Perspectives from an Interview-Based Study of a Public Cord Blood Bank in England," *Clinical Ethics* 5 (2010): 22–27.

69. This concern is strongly expressed in the professional bodies' recommendations against routine banking; see Royal College of Obstetricians and Gynaecologists (UK), *Opinion Paper 2: Cord Blood Banking* (London: RCOG, 2002) and the equivalent report in 2006.

70. For example, Stephen Munzer, "The Special Case of Property Rights in Umbilical Cord Blood for Transplantation and Research," *Rutgers Law Review* 51 (1999): 493–568.

71. Royal College of Obstetricians and Gynaecologists (UK), *Opinion Paper 2: Cord Blood Banking* (London: RCOG, 2002); Emily Ann Meyer, Kathi Hanna, and Christine Gebbie (eds.), *Cord Blood: Establishing a National Hematopoietic Cell Bank Program* (Washington, DC: Institute of Medicine of the National Academies, 2004).

72. Melinda Cooper and Catherine Waldby, *Clinical Labor: Tissue Donors and Research Subjects in the Global Bioeconomy* (Durham, NC: Duke University Press, 2014), p. 20.

73. Elizabeth Anderson, "Is Women's Labor a Commodity?," *Philosophy and Public Affairs* 19 (1990): 71–92.

74. Summer Johnson, "Ethics of Reproductive Tourism Questioned," *Blog Bioethics Net*, May 20, 2010.

75. See, for example, Ruth Macklin, "Is There Anything Wrong with Surrogate Motherhood?," in Larry Gostin (ed.), *Surrogate Motherhood: Politics and Privacy* (Bloomington, IN: Indiana University Press, 1990), pp. 136–150; Kimberly D. Krawiec, "Price and Pretense in the Baby Market," in Michele Bratcher Goodwin (ed.), *Baby Markets: Money and the New Politics of Creating Families* (New York: Cambridge University Press, 2010), pp. 41–55; Mary Anne Case, "Bringing Fundamentalist Feminism to US Baby Markets," in Michele Bratcher Goodwin (ed.), *Baby Markets: Money and the New Politics of Creating Families* (Cambridge: Cambridge University Press, 2010), pp. 56–68.

76. Sonia Allan, "Surrogate Mother Cares for Baby Abandoned Because of Down Syndrome," *Biopolitical Times*, August 4, 2014, accessed August 13, 2014.

77. RFI English, "European Human Rights Court Orders France to Recognise Surrogate-Mother Children," June 26, 2014, accessed August 13, 2014, http://www.english.rfi.fr.

78. Federal Bureau of Investigation, "Baby-Selling Ring Busted," based on statement by US Attorney's Office, Southern District of California, August 9, 2011, accessed August 13, 2014, http://www.fbi.gov/sandiego/press-releases/2011/baby-selling-ring-busted.

79. Richard Arneson, "Commodification and Commercial Surrogacy," *Philosophy and Public Affairs* 21 (1992): 131–164, at p. 149.

80. Michelle Millhollon, "Surrogacy Bill Sails Through House Committee," *The Advocate (Louisiana)*, March 27, 2014, accessed August 21, 2014, http://www.geneticsandsociety.org/article.php?id=7634.

81. Sonia Allan, "Surrogate Mother Cares for Baby Abandoned Because of Down Syndrome," *Biopolitical Times*, August 4, 2014, accessed August 21, 2014, http://www.biopolitical-times.rsvp1.com/article.php?id=7953&mgh=http%3A%2F%2Fwww.biopoliticaltimes.org&mgf=1.

82. Debra Satz, *Why Some Things Should Not Be For Sale: The Moral Limits of Markets* (New York: Oxford University Press, 2011), p. 124.

83. Wesley Newcomb Hohfeld, *Fundamental Legal Conceptions* (New Haven, CT: Yale University Press, 1923); A. M. Honore, "Ownership," in *Making Law Bind: Essays Legal and Philosophical* (Oxford: Clarendon Press, 1987), pp. 161–192.

84. Ranjana Kumari of the New Delhi-based Centre for Social Research, quoted in Grant Peck and Kriten Gellneau, "Thai Case Casts Spotlight on Business of Surrogacy," *Biopolitical Times*, August 7, 2014, accessed August 21, 2014, http://www.geneticsandsociety.org/article.php?id=7977.

85. For further discussion of this point, see Donna Dickenson, *Property, Women and Politics: Subjects or Objects?* (Cambridge: Polity Press, 1997), especially pp. 161–165.

86. *Anna J. v. Mark C.*, 286 Cal. Rptr. 369 (1991).

87. Philip Parker, "Motivation of Surrogate Mothers: Initial Findings," *American Journal of Psychiatry* 140 (1983): 117–118; Carol A. Rose, "Women and Property: Gaining and Losing Ground," chapter 8 in *Property and Persuasion: Essays on the History, Theory and Rhetoric of Ownership* (Boulder, CO: Westview Press, 1994); Helena Ragone, *Surrogate Motherhood: Conception in the Heart* (Boulder, CO: Westview Press, 1994).

88. Elizabeth Anderson, "Is Women's Labor a Commodity?," *Philosophy and Public Affairs* 19 (1990): 71–92.

89. Debora L. Spar, *The Baby Business: How Money, Science and Politics Drive the Commerce of Conception* (Cambridge, MA: Harvard Business School Press, 2006); Bonnie Steinbock, "Payment for Egg Donation and Surrogacy," *Mt Sinai Journal of Medicine* 71, no. 4 (2004): 55–65.
90. Donna Dickenson, "Commodification of Human Tissue: Implications for Feminist and Development Ethics" *Developing World Bioethics*, 2 (2002): 55–63; *Body Shopping: Converting Body Parts to Profit* (Oxford: Oneworld, 2009), p. 161.
91. See, for example, the comment by an Indian surrogate mother denying that contract motherhood is exploitation, compared to her usual work of crushing glass, in Donna Dickenson, *Bioethics: All That Matters* (London: Hodder Education, 2012), p. 29.
92. Erica Haimes and Ken Taylor, "An Investigation of Women's Experiences of an IVF Egg-Sharing Scheme for Somatic Cell Nuclear Transfer Research," paper presented at the PEALS 12th annual symposium on "The Uses of Human Reproductive Tissue in Research and Treatment: Principles and Practice," Newcastle, UK, February 23, 2011.
93. Laura Crimaldi, "Stalled Economy Fertile Ground for Baby Business," *Boston Herald*, January 25, 2009.
94. Financial motivations were found to be paramount for egg providers in Andrea M. Braverman, "Exploring Ovum Donors' Motivations and Needs," *American Journal of Bioethics* 1, no. 4 (2001): 16–17. Karla Momberger, in "Breeder at Law" *Columbia Journal of Gender and Law* 11 (2002): 127–174, describes the way she negotiated with several egg brokerage agencies to obtain the highest price. For the idea that the gift of life has become a marketing concept, see Michele Bratcher Goodwin, *Black Markets: The Supply and Demand of Body Parts* (New York: Cambridge University Press, 2006), p. 25 ff.
95. Catherine Waldby and Melinda Cooper, "The Biopolitics of Reproduction: Post-Fordist Biotechnology and Women's Clinical Labor," *Australian Feminist Studies* 23, no. 55 (2008): 57–73.
96. Kieran Healy, *Last Best Gifts: Altruism and the Market for Human Blood and Organs* (Chicago: University of Chicago Press, 2006), p. 4. For Marx's own analysis, see *Capital*, volume 1, section 4, "The Fetishism of Commodities and the Secret Thereof."
97. For further development of my arguments about exploitation and women's reproductive labor, see Donna Dickenson, "Exploitation and Choice in the Global Egg Trade: Emotive Terminology or Necessary Critique?" in Michele Goodwin (ed.), *The Global Body Market: Altruism's Limits* (New York: Cambridge University Press, 2013), pp. 21–43.
98. Sylvie Ebelpoin, "Gestation pour autrui: une assistance médicale a la procréation comme les autres?" *L'Information psychiatrique* 27 (2011): 7.

BIBLIOGRAPHY

Almeling, Rene. 2011. *Sex cells: The medical market in eggs and sperm.* Berkeley: University of California Press.
Anderson, Elizabeth. "Is Women's Labor a Commodity?" *Philosophy and Public Affairs* 19 (1990): 71–92.
Baylis, Francoise. 2009. For love or money? The saga of the Korean women who provided eggs for embryonic stem cell research. *Theoretical Medicine and Bioethics* 30: 385–396.
Baylis, Francoise, and McLeod, Carolyn. 2007. The stem cell debate continues: The buying and selling of eggs for research. *Journal of Medical Ethics* 33: 726–731.

Brown, Nik. 2013. Contradictions of value: Between use and exchange in cord blood bioeconomy. *Sociology of Health and Illness* 35: 97–112.

Brown, Nik, Machin, Laura, and McLeod, Danae. 2011. The immunitary bioeconomy: The economisation of the international cord blood market. *Social Science and Medicine* 30: 1–8.

Busby, Helen. 2010. The meanings of consent to the donation of cord blood stem cells: Perspectives from an interview-based study of a Public Cord Blood Bank in England. *Clinical Ethics* 5: 22–27.

Calabresi, Guido, and Melamed, A. Douglas. 1972. Property rules, liability rules and alienability: One view of the cathedral. *Harvard Law Review* 85: 1089–1128.

Cooper, Melinda, and Waldby, Catherine. 2014. *Clinical labor: Tissue donors and research subjects in the global bioeconomy*. Durham, NC: Duke University Press.

Daar, Judith F. 2001. Regulating the fiction of informed consent in ART medicine. *American Journal of Bioethics* 1: 19–20.

Dickenson, Donna. 2009. *Body Shopping: Converting Body Parts to Profit*. Oxford: Oneworld.

Dickenson, Donna. 2002. Commodification of human tissue: Implications for feminist and development ethics. *Developing World Bioethics* 2: 55–63.

Dickenson, Donna. 2001. Property and women's alienation from their own reproductive labour. *Bioethics* 15: 203–217.

Dickenson, Donna. 2007. *Property in the body: Feminist perspectives*. Cambridge: Cambridge University Press), second edition forthcoming.

Dickenson, Donna. 2013. The commercialization of human eggs in mitochondrial replacement research. *The New Bioethics* 19: 18–29.

Dickenson, Donna. 2006. The lady vanishes: What's missing from the stem cell debate. *Journal of Bioethical Inquiry* 3: 43–54.

Gurmankin, Andrea F. 2001. Risk information provided to potential oocyte donors in a preliminary phone call. *American Journal of Bioethics* 1: 3–13.

Harrison, Charlotte H. 1972. Neither Moore nor the market: Alternative models for compensating contributors of human tissue. *American Journal of Law and Medicine* 28: 77–104.

Healy, Kieran. 2006. *Last best gifts: Altruism and the market for human blood and organs*. Chicago: University of Chicago Press,.

Hohfeld, Wesley Newcomb. 1923. *Fundamental legal conceptions*. New Haven, CT: Yale University Press.

Honore, A. M. 1987. Ownership. In *Making Law Bind: Essays Legal and Philosophical*, pp. 161–192. Oxford: Clarendon Press.

Jacobs, Allen, Dwyer, James, and Lee, Peter. 2001. Seventy ova. *Hastings Center Report* 31: 12–14.

Kramer, W., Schneider, J., and Schultz, N. September 3, 2009. US oocyte donors: A retrospective study of medical and psychosocial issues. *Human Reproduction*, doi:10.193/humrep/dep309.

Lafontaine, Céline. 2014. *Le corps-marché: la marchandisation de le vie humaine a l'ère de la bioéconomie*. Paris: Editions du Seuil.

McLeod, Carolyn, and Baylis, Francoise. 2006. Feminists on the inalienability of human embryos. *Hypatia* 21: 1–4.

Marzano-Parisoli, Maria M. 2002. *Penser le corps*. Paris: Presses Universitaires de France.

Marx, Karl. 1954. *Capital*, trans. by Samuel Moore and Edward Aveling, ed. Friedrich Engels. Moscow: Progress, original edn. 1867.

Munzer, Stephen. 1999. The special case of property rights in umbilical cord blood for transplantation and research. *Rutgers Law Review* 51: 493–568.

Okemoto, Lisa. 2009. Eggs as capital: Human egg procurement in the fertility industry and the stem cell research enterprise. *Signs* 34: 763–781.

Pennings, Guido, de Mouzon, J., Shenfield, Francoise, et al. Socio-demographic and fertility-related characteristics and motivations of oocyte donors in eleven European countries. *Human Reproduction* (March 13, 2014), doi:10.1093/humrep/deu048.

Radin, Margaret J. 1996. *Contested commodities: The trouble with trade in sex, children, body parts and other things.* Cambridge, MA: Harvard University Press.

Resnik, David. 1998. The commodification of human reproductive materials. *Journal of Medical Ethics* 24: 288–293.

Royal College of Obstetricians and Gynaecologists (UK). 2002. *Opinion Paper 2: Cord Blood Banking.* London: RCOG.

Satz, Debra. 2011. *Why some things should not be for sale: The moral limits of markets.* New York: Oxford University Press.

Scheper-Hughes, Nancy. 2002. Bodies for sale—whole or in parts. *Body and Society* 7: 1–8.

Spar, Debora L. 2006. *The baby business: How money, science and politics drive the commerce of conception.* Cambridge, MA: Harvard Business School Press.

Titmuss, Richard. 1997. *The gift relationship: From human blood to social policy,* 2nd ed, ed. Ann Oakley and J. Ashton. London: LSE Books.

Waldby, Catherine, and Mitchell, Robert. 2006. *Tissue economies: Blood, organs and cell lines in late capitalism.* Durham, NC: Duke University Press.

CHAPTER 6

TWENTY-FIRST-CENTURY EUGENICS

CHRISTOPHER GYNGELL
AND MICHAEL J. SELGELID

THE term "eugenics" is commonly employed in debates about the development and use of reproductive technologies. For example, when discussing the impact of preimplantation genetic diagnosis, Jeanne Freeman (1996) claims that these technologies represent a "disturbing tendency toward eugenics."[1] In justifying their call for a ban on gene editing, a recent United Nations Educational, Scientific and Cultural Organization (UNESCO) panel claimed that such technologies could "renew eugenics."[2] Marcy Darnovsky, the executive director of the nonprofit organization The Centre for Genetics and Society, believes that gamete selection technologies "could encourage the dangerous idea that science should be used to breed 'better' people, breathing new life into the specter of eugenics that has long hung over the field of genetics."[3]

Though appeals to "eugenics" play a significant role in debate surrounding the ethics of reproductive genetic technologies, exactly what it means for a practice to be "eugenics," and why this is ethically relevant, is (all-too-often) not made clear. Although many use the term "eugenics" in a pejorative sense, several scholars have argued that, on certain interpretations of "eugenics," it is not necessarily a bad thing.[4]

In this chapter we provide a conceptual analysis of eugenics and discuss its relevance to ethical debates about twenty-first-century reproductive technologies. We begin by providing an overview of existing and developing technologies that enable greater control over the heredity of future generations. Next, we explore the origins of the term "eugenics" and the history of the eugenics movement. Then, we discuss whether the use of reproductive genetic technologies (RGTs) should be considered eugenics. Finally, we outline the moral significance of eugenics, and we discuss the difference between the recent liberal eugenics movement and the view we call moderate eugenics, and argue in favor of the latter.

REPRODUCTIVE GENETIC TECHNOLOGIES

Prenatal Testing and Selective Abortion

In a seminal article in the journal *Nature* in 1956, Fuchs and Riis[5] described a technique for using extractions of amniotic fluid to determine whether embryos possessed specific genetic factors. This formed the basis of the first prenatal test. By the mid-1970s prenatal tests were regularly used to test embryos for a range of conditions, including Down syndrome (trisomy 21) and muscular dystrophy. In addition to identifying chromosomal abnormalities, contemporary prenatal tests can detect the presence of single gene mutations associated with conditions such as cystic fibrosis, and also genetic predispositions to complex diseases such as breast and ovarian cancer.[6]

The invention of prenatal tests marked an important milestone in human reproduction. When used in combination with abortion, prenatal tests enable parents to avoid having children with particular genes and chromosomes. Women who do not wish to have a child with Down syndrome can utilize prenatal tests to check for the extra chromosome associated with this condition and abort the fetus if it is detected. Prenatal tests were the first reproductive technology to give parents some control of the genetic makeup of their children.[7]

However, prenatal diagnosis and selective abortion only give parents very limited control over their children's genetic constitution. Although it is an effective method of selecting against undesirable genetic diseases or predispositions (in cases where causal links between genes and disease have been established), its usefulness as a method to *select for* positively desired traits is more limited. Selective abortion involves destroying a fetus with no guarantee that it will be possible to conceive another one with (or without, for that matter) the positively desired genetic characteristics in question. Given the physical, psychological, and (arguably[8]) moral costs involved, selective abortion is, and will likely continue to be, primarily used to select against serious diseases and disabilities.[9]

In Vitro Fertilization and PreImplantation Genetic Diagnosis

The advent of in vitro fertilisation (IVF) in the 1970s marked another important milestone in human reproduction. For the first time in history, human embryos could be created entirely outside the body of the mother.[10] This innovation was followed in the early 1990s by preimplantation genetic diagnosis (PGD), in which the embryos created in vitro were tested for the presence or absence of particular genes.[11]

PGD was initially developed as an alternative to prenatal testing and selective abortion. It allowed parents to avoid having children with serious disabilities without the costs associated with abortion. However, the potential for IVF and PGD to be used for nonmedical purposes soon became apparent. IVF enables creation of multiple embryos,[12] all of which can be tested before implantation. It is thus technologically possible for parents to choose between embryos based on the presence of genetic sequences associated with nonmedical traits such as height or intelligence. Choosing an embryo that is likely to be taller, for example, comes at little extra cost to the mother and does not raise concerns about the morality of abortion.

Many human traits have a strong genetic component and could thus potentially be targeted though PGD. Geneticists have already identified genetic sequences associated with height,[13] intelligence,[14] and musical ability.[15] As our knowledge of genetics increases, it will likely become possible to perform quite sophisticated genetic analyses on embryos before implantation. Hence, IVF and PGD could (depending upon the purposes for which use of such technologies is allowed/offered) potentially provide parents with a mechanism to influence a wide variety of traits in their children.

In Vitro Gamogenesis

Technologies are currently being developed which promise to greatly increase the selective power of IVF and PGD. In vitro gamogenesis (IVG) involves artificial production of germ cells (oocytes and sperm). Since 2004, methods have been available that allow embryonic murine and adult murine[16] stem cells to be turned into sperm or egg cells in a petri dish. These cells are functional and have resulted in the birth of fertile offspring.[17] This technology potentially allows any adult to generate thousands of germ cells from the stem cells contained in their bone marrow.

Importantly, it has also been reported that fertile offspring have been produced with oocytes derived from induced pluripotent murine stem cells (IPS cells).[18] IPS cells are somatic cells that have been specially treated, so that they act like stem cells. The fact that these somatic cells can be turned into germ cells is significant because it means individuals can potentially generate thousands of germ cells from any cells in their body.

Although most IVG research to date has been carried out in mice, there are several interesting possibilities for reproductive medicine in humans. The technique could one day allow people with no functional germ cells to produce children using standard IVF techniques. The technique could therefore have significant therapeutic benefits for those who are infertile.

In addition, the technique could greatly increase the selective power of IVF and PGD.[19] The power of IVF is currently limited by the number of viable embryos a couple can produce. In an average IVF cycle, nine oocytes are gathered, meaning that the maximum number of embryos that can be created is nine.[20] Using IVG, any woman could potentially make hundreds or thousands of oocytes from her somatic cells. These could be used to make hundreds of embryos, all of which could undergo PGD. This would greatly increase the ability of IVF and PGD to be used to target polygenic traits[21]—or multiple genetic traits at the same time. For example, imagine that 20 different genes contribute to a particular trait. If a couple aims to use PGD to select for 20 different alleles[22] in an embryo, they may need to create around 10,000 embryos to produce one that will have the desired combination at all 20 loci.[23] This is impossible through IVF and PGD today, but it could become possible in the future through IVG.

Genetic Engineering

In addition to being able to select embryos based on their genetic makeup, parents may soon have the ability to modify embryos directly, using genetic engineering technologies. Genetic engineering technologies could potentially allow (absent) desired genetic sequences to be inserted into embryonic DNA; and they could allow existing genetic sequences to be modified or deleted. These technologies, if perfected, could (like IVG[24]) potentially be used to create much more significant changes to the traits of children than is currently possible via IVF and PGD.

Genetic engineering technologies have been successfully used on other species to alter their physical, cognitive, and social characteristics. For example, in 2007 scientists at Case Western Reserve University used genetic engineering technologies to alter a gene called "PEPCK-A" in mice. The resulting transgenic mice could run for 6 kilometers without a break—30 times longer than the normal mouse limit of 200 meters. They also had extended lifespans compared to their unaltered counterparts, and they retained the ability to breed well into old age.[25] In 1999, scientists engineered mice to overexpress the gene NR2B, which codes for a nerve cell receptor. This was shown to lead to dramatic improvements in memory, with transgenic mice being able to remember objects and experiences for many days longer than unaltered mice.[26] The social characteristics of some animals have also been altered using genetic engineering technologies. Polygamous voles can be turned monogamous by modifying genes associated with the vassopressin V1a receptor.[27]

Recent advances in genetics have increased the probability of genetic engineering technologies being used in human reproduction. The early genetic engineering methods used to create transgenic animals used modified viruses to to insert and delete genetic sequences. Using viruses to alter DNA often only changes one out of two copies of a target gene, meaning heterozygote animals (who only have one copy of the target gene) have to be bred together to make the modifications effective. Furthermore, this method is very imprecise, and it commonly makes random changes to large segments of the genome. As a result, only a small proportion of the animals subjected to these technologies have not suffered serious side effects. Hence, early genetic engineering methods have not been suitable for human use.[28]

Gene Editing

A revolution in genetic engineering started in 2010 with the development of techniques that used engineered enzymes, rather than viruses, to alter DNA. These techniques were given the collective moniker "gene editing" to reflect their increased efficiency and precision in comparison with older methods. The CRISPR technique uses customizable snippets of RNA to guide a DNA cutting mechanism, Cas9, to precise locations in the genome. It then triggers DNA repair mechanisms that can alter a gene by inserting an alternative DNA sequence from another template. It has already been used to make precise genetic modifications to primate embryos that have been subsequently expressed in adult organisms.[29] In 2015, the technique was used for the first time in human embryos, with mixed success.[30]

Gene-editing techniques are improving very rapidly. Whereas the rate of "off- target" mutations was originally considered a major barrier to the technique ever being used as a reproductive technology, more precise methods have been developed and off-target mutations are now virtually undetectable in some applications.[31] It may be only a matter of time before gene-editing techniques will be considered sufficiently safe to meet common research and clinical safety standards.

Selective Fertilization and Gamete Modification

Recent advances in genomics have given parents yet another way to influence the genetic makeup of their children. Rather than selecting between embryos, or modifying existing embryos, parents may soon be able to *create* embryos with desirable genetic characteristics. This possibility first received widespread attention when personal genomics company 23andMe patented a technology called "gamete donor selection based on genetic calculations."[32] This technology would allow individuals accessing assisted reproductive services to choose between sperm or egg donors based on the statistical likelihood of the resulting child having a certain phenotype. Using 23andMe's technology, a woman wanting a blue-eyed child could select sperm donors to maximize this probability.

Similar techniques could provide an alternative to PGD for couples accessing IVF. Rather than performing genetic tests on embryos and then choosing which to implant based on the results of those genetic tests, testing could be done directly on primordial germ cells. Particular sperm could then be combined with particular eggs based on the likelihood of the resulting embryos having certain genes.

Importantly, these selective fertilization techniques could be used in combination with the genetic modification technologies described earlier. The CRISPR technique could be used to modify the DNA of sperm. Modified sperm could then be combined with particular eggs—perhaps produced via IVG and/or with edited genomes—to create embryos with specific genetic characteristics.

EUGENICS

The ethical implications of reproductive genetic technologies (RGTs) have been at the center of numerous debates within bioethics for the past two decades.[33] One constant theme of these debates has been the relationship between RGTs and eugenics. As discussed in the introduction, nearly all of the aforementioned RGTs have been labeled as eugenics at some point. To better understand the relevance of eugenics to RGTs, it is important to understand the term's historical context.

A Brief History of Eugenics

The term "eugenics" was first introduced by Francis Galton to denote "science of improving stock, which is by no means confined to questions of judicious mating, but which, especially in the case of man, takes cognisance of all influences that tend in however remote a degree to give to the more suitable races or strains of blood a better chance of prevailing speedily over the less suitable than they otherwise would have had]."[34] Galton later also defined "eugenics" as "the study of all agencies under human control which can improve or impair the racial quality of future generations."[35]

Galton was inspired by studying the family histories of eminent men and finding that exceptional talent and genius ran in their families.[36] He thought this showed that there was an innate, heritable component to exceptional ability. If gifted men and women were encouraged to breed more, according to Galton, then this would lead to more people having exceptional ability and other desirable traits such as health. In addition to benefiting individuals, he argued, this would be better for society as a whole.[37]

Eugenics spread quickly and was widely embraced. Although Galton described eugenics as a "science"—it quickly became a social movement, guiding policy as much as inspiring empirical research. The idea of eugenics appealed to politicians across the political spectrum.[38] Eugenic-inspired policies were passed in countries as diverse as Sweden, Italy, Brazil, France, Peru, Australia, Japan, and the United Kingdom.[39]

Eugenics practices and policies took different forms in different countries. The eugenics movements in France and Latin America, for example, were motivated by concern that heredity was being degraded by environmental factors, and so they emphasized improved neonatal care, public health, and sexual hygiene.[40] Eugenics programs in most of Europe and the United States, by contrast, were primarily focused on controlling reproduction. In the United States, many believed the good of society was threatened by "degenerate" persons who were biologically predisposed to lives of immorality, criminality, and sickness generally.[41] In response to this perceived threat, many states enacted legislation aimed to limit reproduction of those considered genetically inferior. This included marriage restrictions, immigration restrictions (from countries deemed to have a high number of "degenerates"), and compulsory sterilization laws. Sterilization efforts initially focused on the disabled, but later expanded to include repeat criminals. Over 60,000 people were involuntary sterilized for eugenic reasons in the United States between 1907 and 1964.[42]

The most heinous eugenics polices were enacted by Nazi Germany. The eugenically motivated Nazi program of "Racial Hygiene" called for compulsory sterilization of all those with "congenital mental defect, schizophrenia, manic-depressive psychosis, hereditary epilepsy, hereditary chorea, hereditary blindness, hereditary deafness, severe physical deformity, and severe alcoholism."[43] The culmination of the eugenics movement under the Nazis was the Holocaust, involving the murder of over 5 million Jews. The Nazis characterized their victims as "worthless eaters" or those with "lives unworthy of life."[44]

Eugenics fell into disrepute after World War II. Eugenic thinking was closely associated with Nazi ideology and the Holocaust. There was thus strong impetus for governments and institutions to distance themselves from eugenics, as a way of distancing themselves from the horrible actions of the Nazis. Another contributing factor to the demise of eugenics was the realization that (though eugenicists included some of the very best scientists of the time period in question) much of the science behind eugenics was deeply flawed. Inter alia, eugenic "science" reflected bias and prejudice, and its practitioners drew premature and oversimplified conclusions about heredity without properly considering environmental influences upon human characteristics. The "old eugenics" of the early twentieth century was thus ultimately abandoned for both political and scientific reasons.[45]

EUGENICS AND REPRODUCTIVE
GENETIC TECHNOLOGIES

Though the early eugenics movement was abandoned decades ago by governments and institutions, many believe eugenics is still relevant to modern bioethics. As seen in the introduction, many claim that the use of RGTs involves eugenics—and this label is most commonly used in a pejorative sense. Saying that a technology, or a particular use of a technology, involves eugenics is (for many) supposed to show that it is immoral, or at least that there are moral reasons against it. This raises two distinct questions:

- Does the use of RGTs involve eugenics?
- Is eugenics necessarily a bad thing?

Do Reproductive Genetic Technologies Involve Eugenics?

The broadest way to interpret eugenics is as an attempt to improve heredity. The concept of heredity—that there are innate biological components to character that are passed from parents to children—began to get widespread attention in the nineteenth century.[46] The idea that heredity was contributing to social problems, and indeed could be altered by social practices, was a key driver of twentieth-century eugenics practices and policies.

However, during the nineteenth century there were very different theories regarding the nature of heredity. This resulted in a considerable diversity of goals, beliefs, and policies in the eugenics movements around the globe.[47] As alluded to earlier, the eugenics movements in France and Latin America were influenced by Lamarckian views about heritable transmission of acquired characteristics.[48] Improving heredity under a Lamarckian view involves improving environmental conditions that influence transmissible (acquired) traits.

Galton himself and many other European and American eugenicists believed in a "germ plasm" theory of heredity, whereby heritable material is passed directly from the germ cells of parents to the next generations.[49] On this view, acquired characteristics have either no or very little influence on the heredity of the next generation. Many who adhered to this theory saw hereditable traits as being mostly immune to environmental influences.[50]

Three other views about the nature of heredity shaped the eugenics movement in Europe and the United States.[51] The first was that complex behavioral traits were heritable in a relatively simple way. Early eugenicists thought that traits like "pauperism" and "thallasophilia" (the latter meaning "love of the sea") were directly passed from parent to child. Likewise, it was believed that intelligence was governed by a single heritable factor. The view that complex behavioral traits were straightforwardly heritable strengthened the belief that social problems like crime and poverty were caused by poor heredity. The second common view about heredity that influenced the early eugenics movement was that the quality of heritable material in populations was declining rapidly. Fears of degeneration plagued nineteenth and early-twentieth-century European social thought.[52] Many thought that the lower classes were outbreeding higher classes and thereby spreading poor hereditable material throughout the population. In addition, many were concerned that advances in medicine, and poverty relief, were thwarting natural selection by allowing people with bad heredity to continue breeding. A third common view about heredity that influenced eugenics, particularly in Germany, was that there were significant differences in heredity between different races. Many thought that some races had objectively better heritable material than others. This led to the belief that, in order to improve society's genetic stock, a greater proportion of society should be of the superior race—a population must become more racially homogenous.[53]

Contemporary views of heredity, informed by modern genetics, reject all three of the aforementioned views. Complex behavioral traits are not thought to be heritable in a straightforward manner, but rather to be the result of complex interactions of many genes and environmental influences. Rather than being governed by a single gene, the heritability of intelligence is thought to be highly complex and is still largely unknown.[54] Although there is a theoretical concern that the accumulation of germline mutations as a result of modern medicine may one day harm future generations,[55] there is no evidence to suggest that this process is having any significant effect on the current population.

The idea that some racial groups have genes which are objectively better than others is inconsistent with modern genetics. For one, it is known that there is only a minor genetic difference between different races. Approximately 85%–90% of genetic variation is found within racial groups, and only an additional 10%–15% of variation is found between them.[56] Furthermore, the very notion that some races have genotypes that are objectively better than others is problematic. Genotypes only have effects within particular environmental contexts. Genotypes that are advantageous in one environment may be detrimental in another. For example, a variant of the DARC gene which codes for an antigen found on red blood cells provides protection against malaria. For individuals who are likely to encounter malaria, this genotype is likely to be beneficial. However, this genotype also makes individuals more susceptible to HIV.[57] For individuals who live in regions where HIV, but not malaria, is prevalent, this genotype will likely be harmful.[58] Whether any particular genotype is beneficial or harmful depends on the environment with which it interacts.

Given contemporary views about heredity, how should eugenics be understood? When eugenics is discussed today, it is often defined in the parlance of modern genetics. For example, eugenics is often defined as *the attempt to improve the human gene pool*,[59] or *the positive selection of "good" versions of the human genome and the weeding out of "bad" versions.*[60] We believe, however, that we should resist the view that eugenics should be defined solely in terms of *genetic inheritance* improvement. Much recent work in biology has highlighted the importance of epigenetic inheritance—the transmittance of information from one generation to the next, without changes in DNA sequences. For example, severe stress can change patterns of gene expression in cells, which can then be passed on to children in the next generation.[61] Epigenetic inherence involves transmission of acquired characteristics, and thus represents a type of Lamarckian inheritance.

Any attempts to improve epigenetic heredity (for example, by trying to reduce severe stress in parents to be) should be considered as a type of eugenics. Indeed, such a program could be seen as a direct successor to the French and Latin American eugenics programs discussed earlier. If we define eugenics solely in terms of improving gene pools and genomes, this unnecessarily narrows eugenics to being solely about genetic inherence. Though some interpret "eugenics" in this narrow fashion, a broader interpretation of eugenics, which understands it as an attempt to improve heredity—genetic or otherwise—is both plausible and consistent with (some) early use of the term.[62]

Regardless, it is clear that both attempts to improve gene pools and genomes fall under this broad conception of eugenics. They are *forms* of eugenics (broadly conceived), rather than what eugenics (broadly conceived) reduces to. Because the modern use of RGTs targets improvement in heredity, it is clear they are eugenic in this broad sense.

Is Eugenics Bad?

When eugenics is understood in this way, as an attempt to improve heredity, it is clear it is not necessarily a bad thing. The term "improve" implies making changes for the better. When eugenics is defined in terms of making beneficial changes, it is difficult to see how it could necessarily be bad. Few would argue that the Lamarckian-inspired eugenic initiatives in Latin America, such as improved neonatal care, were wrong. Conversely, it is clear that many of the acts carried out in the name of eugenics in Europe and the United States were horrendous. Whether eugenic practices are good or bad clearly depends on the specifics of how they are implemented.

What about the modern use of RGTs? Consider the case of prenatal screening. Prenatal genetic diagnosis is routinely performed for mothers at risk of giving birth to offspring with genetic diseases. When these tests reveal that the child-to-be would be at risk of severe genetic disorder, then abortion is often sought, followed by re-attempt of conception (of offspring without the disorder in question). This is clearly eugenic in a broad sense as it reflects the aim to improve heredity. Specifically it aims at ensuring that people with better genomes (which are not predisposed to disease) are born rather than people with genomes predisposed to disease. For those not absolutely opposed to abortion, prenatal diagnosis and selective abortion of fetuses that test positive for the most severe kinds of genetic disease is usually considered to be morally acceptable. Similarly imagine a future case where gene editing is used at the embryonic stage to correct the mutation that causes cystic fibrosis. The only result of this edit is that a future child develops who does not develop cystic fibrosis. Again this clearly involves eugenics (broadly conceived) in the sense that it is an attempt to improve heredity. However, such a case seems morally acceptable. Indeed, such a case seems morally equivalent to curing a child's cystic fibrosis soon after birth.

What about the use of RGTs to *enhance* individuals rather than avoid disease? The ethics of human enhancement is complex and has been discussed at length elsewhere. For reasons of space, we will not delve into these issues here. However, it is clear that insofar as enhancement is an attempt to improve heredity, it involves eugenics (broadly conceived). Our claim is that the mere fact human enhancement involves eugenics (broadly conceived) does not generate moral reasons against it.

Moving away from the use of RGTs to target individuals, what about the use of RGTS to improve the gene pool—a practice commonly equated with eugenics?[63] Though improving the gene pool is not (as far as we know) the explicit/admitted aim of any current practices, we can conceive of cases in the future where it would be a legitimate goal. Imagine a program that encouraged gene-editing technologies to be used to edit out the cystic fibrosis gene in carriers, rather than just those who would suffer from the disease. The motivation of this program would be to remove the cystic fibrosis gene from the gene pool, rather than reduce the number of people who suffer from cystic fibrosis in the next generation (although this would be a clearly good side effect). This would be a clear case of improving gene pools and would clearly involve eugenics (even according to more narrow definitions of eugenics than we have been operating with). However, assuming such a program (was fully safe and) respected the reproductive freedoms of individual parents and there was informed consent to editing, it is hard to see how such a program would be intrinsically morally problematic. Because future generations would likely benefit from the removal of the cystic fibrosis gene from the gene pool, there may be good moral reasons in favor of such a program. (We here, of course, take that is safe to assume that there are not currently, and not likely to be in the future, envirnonments where having cystic fibrosis or being a carrier would be advantageous.)

Similarly imagine an initiative that aimed to reduce the number of mutations that accumulate in the human germline as a result of modern medicine and delayed paternity. Under such a program parents are offered the opportunity (and perhaps even incentives) to use gene-editing technologies to reverse any naturally occurring deleterious mutations that occur in their children's DNA. The aim of such program would be to protect the gene pool—so that future generations are not negatively affected by the accumulation of mutations. Provided such a program was (fully safe and effective and) conducted in ways which did not comprise the reproductively liberty of parents, it is not clear why such a program would be unethical. Indeed, insofar as we have obligations to benefit future generations, there would be moral reasons in favor of such a program.

In sum, the modern use of RGTs to pursue eugenic aims (even narrowly conceived[64]) is not clearly immoral. There are moral reasons to improve the lives of individuals, including by altering their heredity. Similarly, there are moral reasons to try to benefit future generations, including by improving the gene pool. It appears that there are often pro tanto moral reasons in favor of improving gene pools and genomes. We will look at the implications of such reasons in the next section.

Old, Liberal, and Moderate Eugenics

Let's assume that there are moral reasons to pursue eugenic aims. What actions and practices might this justify?

In the old eugenics movement, the pursuit of eugenic aims was often thought to justify highly coercive, state-enforced practices. States sought to improve heredity through the control of reproduction. This was pursued in two different ways: encouraging those with (or thought to have) good heredity to breed more (often known as "positive eugenics") and discouraging—and/or brutally preventing—those with (or thought to have) bad heredity from breeding (known as "negative eugenics"). Because not many individuals will voluntarily choose to stop having children at the request of the state, negative eugenics was implemented by highly coercive and deceptive means, especially in the United States and Germany. Many victims of the US sterilization program were not even aware that they were being sterilized.[65] The eugenic policies carried out in Nazi Germany were highly coercive and involved gross violation of the most basic human rights (including the right to life).

In the aftermath of the old eugenics movement, many identified the coercive, state-based nature of eugenic practices as a central reason for their moral failings.[66] In response, many advocate a "liberal eugenics," which emphasizes state neutrality.[67] Individuals, on this view, should be free to pursue eugenics using RGTs. The state should remain neutral with regard to heredity and simply allow free choice with regard to use of RGTs.

Liberal eugenics can draw on certain moral principles that seem to justify individual eugenic acts, but not state-level acts. Take Julian Savulescu's principle of procreative

beneficence (PB). PB holds that "couples who decide to have a child have a significant moral reason to select the child who, given his or her genetic endowment, can be
expected to enjoy the most well-being."[68] PB aims at improvements in heredity, with
improvement understood as increases in expected well-being. Whereas PB is clearly
a eugenics principle (broadly conceived), it only applies in certain contexts—that is,
when couples have decided to have a child, and selection is possible. PB thus justifies
individuals acting eugenically, but it does not justify any state-based eugenic practices.
Similarly, Douglas and Devolder's "principle of procreative altruism" (PA) holds that
"parents have significant moral reason to select a child whose existence can be expected
to contribute more to (or detract less from) the well-being of others than any alternative
child they could have."[69] PA is also a eugenic principle that only generates moral reasons
in the context of parental reproductive decisions. One could use such principles to show
that parents have pro tanto moral obligations to act eugenically. As these principles do
not apply to states, they cannot be used to justify state-based eugenic practices.

   However, allowing individuals to freely pursue eugenics has clear risks. Take the case
of collective action problems.[70] If RGTs are widely available to parents, and parents use
them in ways that are expectedly best for their children, it could inadvertently have
an overall harmful effect on society and future generations. The collective effects of all
parents rationally pursuing eugenic aims could make everyone worse off. For example,
say RGTs are available that allow parents to target the height of their future children.
Research suggests that height is correlated with a range of measures thought relevant
to well-being. If RGTs that target height were available, we might expect rational parents to use these RGTs to attempt to have taller children. However, if every parent
used RGTs to have taller children, this would negate any positive effect on well-being.
This is because everyone's relative height would stay more or less the same, and it is
relative height rather than absolute height that is associated with subjective well-being.
Furthermore, there are ways in which the widespread provision of height enhancements would make everyone worse off. Increasing the average height of a population
could lead to economic as well as environmental costs relating to increased resource
use.[71] It has also been speculated that collective action problems could arise for genes
related to innate immunity and for certain cognitive traits.[72]

   Cases like collective action problems reveal serious reasons for worrying about leaving eugenics in the hands of individuals. Each parent (freely) acting in his or her child's
own self-interest could end up making everyone worse off. This shows that the state
might be justified in restricting access to RGTs.

   More extremely (though we assumed voluntary informed consent to use of RGTs in
much of the earlier discussion), it might even be permissible for the state to coercively
enforce certain uses of RGTs. Suppose that safe, precise, gene-editing technologies that
can make individuals immune to a number of infectious diseases become available in
the future. Given state's (arguably legitimate) use of coercive measures to ensure people get vaccines, they might also be justified to coerce people into getting these types of
preventative gene edits—particularly if this was safer and more effective than vaccine-
based prevention.

Rather than embrace a fully *liberal* eugenics, we should instead endorse a *moderate* eugenics.[73] On this view both individuals and states have reason to attempt to improve heredity. However, these reasons are not overriding, and they must be balanced against other values, such as procreative liberty and social equality (neither of which is itself overriding). The right to reproduce without interference from third parties is recognized by international law and moral theories from a host of ethical traditions.[74] Given the strong moral reasons against interfering with reproductive liberty, eugenic considerations would only exceptionally rarely—if ever—justify stringent state control over who reproduces. However, less restrictive state interference in the name of eugenics (broadly conceived) might often be justified. For example, restricting access to particular usages of RGTs, or coercing parents to use RGTs in ways that protect populations against disease, may be legitimate.

CONCLUSION—LESSONS FROM EUGENICS

As we proceed into the twenty-first century, reproductive technologies will provide humankind with powerful means through which to influence the heredity of future generations. It is vital that society makes good decisions about how to use such technologies. When the term "eugenics" is used in debates regarding the regulation of RGTs, it is important to clarify exactly what conception of eugenics is being referred to. When eugenics is understood in its broadest sense, as an attempt to improve heredity, it is not necessarily a bad thing. We have likewise shown that eugenics is not necessarily ethically unacceptable even on more narrow conceptions (e.g., according to which it is thought that the aim to improve genetic inheritance and/or the use of state coercion are essential to eugenics). There are often moral reasons in favor of altering heredity (genetic or otherwise)—either to benefit individuals or future generations. These reasons may justify not only eugenic acts by parents but also state-based programs. The term "eugenics" thus need not be used pejoratively.

We should not abandon eugenics as a concept, and indeed we should be encouraging discussions about how we can improve heredity. These discussions should not be limited to improving genetic inheritance. One important lesson from the old eugenics movement is the risk of aiming to improve heredity when one has a poor understanding of it. If we do not understand something properly, it is difficult to improve it. Today we still know very little about the inheritance of complex traits. This is illustrated by the phenomenon of missing heritability.[75] For many complex diseases and traits (for example, intelligence, cardiovascular disease, diabetes) twin and family studies indicate they are strongly heritable. However, individual genetic differences only account for a small portion of the observed heritability. One hypothesis to explain missing heritability is that epigenetic inheritance is playing a much larger role in the heritability of these traits than has been traditionally thought.[76] Events in an individual's life can make cellular changes that affect gene expression and be passed down multiple generations. This may explain why closely related individuals resemble each other in these traits. If we do not approach the improvement of these complex traits by looking at both genetic and non-genetic forms of inheritance, we risk repeating the mistakes of the old eugenics movement. Our efforts to improve these features of our character by focusing on particular genes may be ineffective and inadvertently do more harm than good.

However, there are some aspects of our heredity we understand very well. The inheritance of many Mendelian disorders has been understood for decades. Because we understand the heredity of these conditions, and the effects of the genes involved, we can make better decisions regarding their alteration. In many cases it is likely we would gain much and lose little from removing these genes from the human genome.

These considerations show the need for a moderate approach to eugenics. We should recognize that there are clear reasons in favor of eugenics, broadly conceived. However, these reasons must be balanced against the risk of altering our heredity without a proper understanding of it. Furthermore, we need to balance the goods of eugenics against other ethical values like individual liberty and social equality.

NOTES

1. Jeanne Salmon Freeman, "Arguing Along the Slippery Slope of Human Embryo Research." *Journal of Medicine and Philosophy* 21, no. 1 (1996): 61–81.
2. The United Nations Educational, Scientific and Cultural Organization. UNESCO panel of experts calls for ban on "editing" of human DNA to avoid unethical tampering with hereditary traits. Available at http://en.unesco.org/news/unesco-panel-experts-calls-ban-editing-human-dna-avoid-unethical-tampering-hereditary-traits (accessed November 11, 2015).
3. The Center for Genetics and Society (CGS). (2013). "Center for Genetics and Society Calls on 23andMe to Disavow Designer Babies": Controversial New Patent Raises Critical Questions. Available at http://www.geneticsandsociety.org/article.php?id=7193 (accessed November 11, 2015).
4. Philip Kitcher, *The Lives to Come* (New York: Simon & Schuster, 1996). Allen Buchanan, Dan Brock, Norman Daniels, and Daniel Wikler; *From Chance to Choice: Genetics and Justice* (Cambridge: Cambridge University Press, 2007); Michael J. Selgelid, "Neugenics," *Monash Bioethics Review* 1, no. 4 (2000): 9–33; Nicholas Agar, *Liberal Eugenics: In Defence of Human Enhancement* (Malden, MA: Wiley-Blackwell, 2004).
5. Fritz Fuchs and Povl Riis, "Antenatal Sex Determination." *Nature* 177 (1956): 330–330.
6. Nancie Petrucelli, Mary B. Daly, and Gerald L. Feldman, "Hereditary Breast and Ovarian Cancer due to Mutations in BRCA1 and BRCA2." *Genetics in Medicine* 12 (2010): 245–259.
7. Of course, individuals have long had nontechnological means of influencing the genetic makeup of their children through partner choice.
8. Michael J. Selgelid, "Eugenic Abortion, Moral Uncertainty, and Social Consequences," *Monash Bioethics Review* 20 (2001): 26–42.
9. The major exception to this is sex—which is a significant nondisease trait that can easily be selected for through the use of prenatal tests and selective abortion. However, there are more readily available technologies that enable sex selection, like ultrasonography. Imaging techniques like ultrasonography have been a much more significant driver of sex selection than prenatal tests in countries where social sex selection is common. For

example, see Jing-Bao Nie, "Non-medical Sex-selective Abortion in China: Ethical and Public Policy Issues in the Context of 40 million missing females," *British Medical Bulletin* 98 (2011): 7–20.

10. In vitro means "in glass."

11. Anastasia A. Theodosiou and Martin H. Johnson, "The Politics of Human Embryo Research and the Motivation to Achieve PGD." *Reproductive Biomedicine Online* 22 (2011): 457–471.

12. It is standard IVF practice to produce more embryos than will actually be implanted.

13. Sonja I. Berndt et al., "Genome-wide Meta-analysis Identifies 11 New Loci for Anthropometric Traits and Provides Insights Into Genetic Architecture," *Nature Genetics* 45 (2013): 501–512.

14. S. Desrivieres et al., "Single Nucleotide Polymorphism in the Neuroplastin Locus Associates With Cortical Thickness and Intellectual Ability in Adolescents." *Molecular Psychiatry* (2015). doi: 10.1038/mp.2013.197

15. J. Oikkonen et al., "A Genome-Wide Linkage and Association Study of Musical Aptitude Identifies Loci Containing Genes Related to Inner Ear Development and Neurocognitive Functions." *Molecular Psychiatry* 20 (2015): 275–282.

16. Murine means from the rodent family—for example, mice, rats, and so on.

17. Erna Magnusdottir and M. Azim Surani, "How to Make a Primordial Germ Cell." *Development* 141 (2013): 245–252.

18. Erna Magnusdottir and M. Azim Surani, "How to Make a Primordial Germ Cell." *Development* 141 (2013): 245–252.

19. Douglas Bourne and Julian Savulescu, "Procreative Beneficence and In Vitro Gametogenesis." *Monash Bioethics Review* 30 (2012): 29–48.

20. Sesh Kamal Sunkara et al., "Association Between the Number of Eggs and Live Birth in IVF Treatment: An Analysis of 400 135 treatment cycles," *Human Reproduction* 26 (2011): 1768–1774.

21. Polygenic traits result from the expression of multiple genes.

22. Alleles refer to the different forms that any given gene may take.

23. Douglas Bourne and Julian Savulescu, "Procreative Beneficence and In Vitro Gametogenesis," *Monash Bioethics Review* 30 (2012): 29–48.

24. Depending on how well these technologies are developed/perfected, they could potentially enable even more control than IVG.

25. Parvin Hakimi et al., "Overexpression of the Cytosolic Form of Phosphoenolpyruvate Carboxykinase (GTP) in Skeletal Muscle Repatterns Energy Metabolism in the Mouse." *The Journal of Biological Chemistry* 282 (2007): 32844–32855.

26. Ya-Ping Tang et al., "Genetic Enhancement of Learning and Memory in Mice." *Nature* 401 (1999): 63–69.

27. Miranda M. Lim et al., "Enhanced Partner Preference in a Promiscuous Species by Manipulating the Expression of a Single Gene," *Nature* 429 (2004): 754–757.

28. Helen Shen, "First Monkeys With Customized Mutations Born." *Nature* (2014). doi: 10.1038/nature.2014.14611

29. Y. Niu et al., "Generation of Gene-Modified Cynomolgus Monkey via Cas9/RNA-Mediated Gene Targeting in One-Cell Embryos," *Cell* 156 (2014): 836–843.

30. Puping Liang, Yanwen Xu, Xiya Zhang, Chenhui Ding, Rui Huang, et al. "CRISPR/Cas9-Mediated Gene Editing in Human Tripronuclear Zygotes." *Protein & Cell* 6, no. 5 (2015): 363–372.

31. Iyer, Vivek, Bin Shen, Wensheng Zhang, Alex Hodgkins, Thomas Keane, Xingxu Huang, and William C Skarnes, "Off-Target Mutations Are Rare in Cas9-Modified Mice." *Nature Methods* 12, no. 6 (2015): 479–479.

32. US patent: US 8,543,339.

33. For an overview of the ethical issues raised by RGTs, see Allen Buchanan and Dan Brock, eds., *From Chance to Choice: Genetics and Justice* (Cambridge: Cambridge University Press, 2007); Jonathan Glover, *Choosing Children: Genes, Disability, and Design* (Oxford: Oxford Clarendon Press, 2006); John Harris, *Enhancing Evolution: The Ethical Case for Making Better People* (Princeton, NJ: Princeton University Press, 2007); President's Council on Bioethics, *Beyond Therapy: Biotechnology and the Pursuit of Happiness* (New York: Harper Collins, 2003).

34. Francis Galton, *Inquiries Into Human Faculty and Its Development* (London: Macmillan, 1883).

35. Francis Galton, "Eugenics: Its Definition, Scope, And Aims," *American Journal of Sociology* 10, no.1 (1904): 1–25.

36. Francis Galton, *Hereditary Genius* (Bristol, U.K.: Thoemmes Press, 1998).

37. Op. cit note 35.

38. Daniel J. Kevles, *In the Name of Eugenics* (Los Angeles, CA: University of California Press, 1985).

39. Nancy Leys Stepan, *"The Hour of Eugenics": Race, Gender, and Nation in Latin America* (Ithaca, NY: Cornell University Press, 2015).

40. This will be discussed in further detail later.

41. Teryn Bouche and Laura Rivard, *America's Hidden History: The Eugenics Movement.* Available at http://www.nature.com/scitable/forums/genetics-generation/america-s-hidden-history-the-eugenics-movement-123919444 (accessed October 19, 2015).

42. Daylanne K. English, *Unnatural Selections: Eugenics in American Modernism and the Harlem Renaissance* (Chapel Hill, NC: University of North Carolina Press, 2004).

43. Benno Muller-Hill, *Murderous Science: Elimination by Scientific Selection of Jews, Gypsies, and Others in Germany 1933–1945* (New York: Cold Spring Harbor Press, 1988).

44. Benno Muller-Hill, *Murderous Science: Elimination by Scientific Selection of Jews, Gypsies, and Others in Germany, 1933–1945* (New York: Cold Spring Harbor Press, 1988).

45. Daniel J. Kevles, *In the Name of Eugenics* (Los Angeles, CA: University of California Press, 1985).

46. J. Waller, "Parents and Children: Ideas of Heredity in the 19th Century," *Endeavour* 27, no. 2 (2003): 51–56.

47. Allen Buchanan, Dan Brock, Norman Daniels, and Daniel Wikler, *From Chance to Choice: Genetics and Justice* (Cambridge: Cambridge University Press, 2007).

48. Allen Buchanan, Dan Brock, Norman Daniels, and Daniel Wikler, *From Chance to Choice: Genetics and Justice* (Cambridge: Cambridge University Press, 2007).

49. Michael Bulmer, *Francis Galton: Pioneer of Heredity and Biometry* (Baltimore, MD: Johns Hopkins University Press, 2003).

50. John C. Waller, "Parents and Children: Ideas of Heredity in the 19th Century." *Endeavour* 27, no. 2 (2003): 51–56.

51. Allen Buchanan, Dan Brock, Norman Daniels, and Daniel Wikler, *From Chance to Choice: Genetics and Justice* (Cambridge: Cambridge University Press, 2007).

52. Allen Buchanan, Dan Brock, Norman Daniels, and Daniel Wikler, *From Chance to Choice: Genetics and Justice* (Cambridge: Cambridge University Press, 2007).

53. François Haas, "German Science and Black Racism—Roots of the Nazi Holocaust." *The FASEB Journal* 22 (2007): 332–337.
54. Christopher F. Chabris et al., "Most Reported Genetic Associations With General Intelligence Are Probably False Positives." *Psychological Science* 23, no. 11 (2012): 1314–1323.
55. Russell Powell, "In Genes We Trust: Germline Engineering, Eugenics, and the Future of the Human Genome." *Journal of Medicine and Philosophy* 40, no. 6 (2015): 669–695.
56. Lynn B. Jorde and Stephen P. Wooding, "Genetic Variation, Classification and 'Race.'" *Nature Genetics* 36 (2004): S28–S33.
57. Weijing He, Stuart Neil, Hemant Kulkarni, Edward Wright, and Brian K. Agan, "Duffy Antigen Receptor for Chemokines Mediates Transinfection of HIV-1 From Red Blood Cells to Target Cells and Affects HIV/AIDS Susceptibility." *Cell Host Microbe* 4 (2008): 52–62.
58. See Chris Gyngell and Thomas Douglas, "Stocking the Genetic Supermarket: Reproductive Genetic Technologies and Collective Action Problems." *Bioethics* 29 (2015): 241–250.
59. Stephen Wilkinson and Eve Garrard, *Eugenics and the Ethics of Selective Reproduction* (Keele, UK: Keele University, 2013).
60. Robert Pollack, "Eugenics Lurk in the Shadow of CRISPR." *Science* 348 (2015): 871–871.
61. Rachel Yehuda, Nikolaos P. Daskalakis, Amy Lehrner, and Michael J. Meaney, "Influences of Maternal and Paternal PTSD on Epigenetic Regulation of the Glucocorticoid Receptor Gene in Holocaust Survivor Offspring." *American Journal of Psychiatry* 171 (2014): 872–880.
62. It should also be noted that some use a narrower interpretation of eugenics on which "only procedures enforced by the state, using authoritarian coercive methods, can really be classed as eugenics." For discussion, see Stephen Wilkinson and Eve Garrard, *Eugenics and the Ethics of Selective Reproduction* (Keele, UK: Keele University, 2013).
63. Improving gene pools is more complex than the idea of improving a genome. Gene pools do not have interests or experiences. Hence, it is not immediately obvious what the idea of improving the gene pool consists of. One approach has been to specify that we improve the human gene pool by increasing the long-term persistence of the human species. For an in-depth discussion, see Chris Gyngell, "Enhancing the Species: Genetic Engineering Technologies and Human Persistence," *Philosophy & Technology* 25, no. 4 (2012): 495–512.
64. Expect if eugenics is narrowly conceived of as requiring authoritarian coercive methods. See note 62.
65. Alexandra Minna Stern, "Sterilized in the Name of Public Health: Race, Immigration, and Reproductive Control in Modern California," *American Journal of Public Health* 95 (2005): 1128–1138.
66. Arthur Caplan, Glenn McGee, and David Magnus, "What Is Immoral About Eugenics?" *Western Journal of Medicine* 171 (1999): 335–337.
67. Nicholas Agar, "Liberal Eugenics." *Public Affairs Quarterly* 12 (1998): 137–155.
68. Julian Savulescu, "Procreative Beneficence: Why We Should Select the Best Children." *Bioethics* 15 (2001): 413–426; Julian Savulescu and Guy Kahane, "The Moral Obligation to Create Children With the Best Chance of the Best Life." *Bioethics* 23 (2009): 274–290.
69. Thomas Douglas and Katrien Devolder, "Procreative Altruism: Beyond Individualism in Reproductive Selection." *Journal of Medicine and Philosophy* 38, no. 4 (2013): 400–419.
70. Michael J. Selgelid, "Ethics and Eugenic Enhancement." *Poiesis and Praxis: International Journal of Ethics of Science and Technology Assessment* 1(3) (2003): 239–261. Allen Buchanan, Dan Brock, Norman Daniels, and Daniel Wikler, *From Chance to*

Choice: Genetics and Justice (Cambridge: Cambridge University Press, 2007; Peter Singer, "Parental Choice and Human Improvement." In *Human Enhancement*, Julian Savulescu and Nicholas Bostrom, eds. (Oxford: Oxford University Press, 2009), pp. 277–290; Chris Gyngell and Thomas Douglas, "Stocking the Genetic Supermarket: Reproductive Genetic Technologies and Collective Action Problems." *Bioethics* 29 (2015): 241–250.

71. Allen Buchanan, Dan Brock, Norman Daniels, and Daniel Wikler, *From Chance to Choice: Genetics and Justice* (Cambridge: Cambridge University Press, 2007).

72. See Chris Gyngell and Thomas Douglas, "Stocking the Genetic Supermarket: Reproductive Genetic Technologies and Collective Action Problems." *Bioethics* 29 (2015): 241–250.

73. Michael J. Selgelid, "Moderate Eugenics and Human Enhancement." *Medicine, Health Care and Philosophy* 17 (2014): 3–12.

74. Arthur Caplan, Glenn McGee, and David Magnus, "What Is Immoral About Eugenics?" *Western Journal of Medicine* 171 (1999): 335–337.

75. Evan E. Eichler et al., "Missing Heritability and Strategies for Finding the Underlying Causes of Complex Disease." *Nature Reviews Genetics* 11, no. 6 (2010): 446–450.

76. Marco Trerotola, Valeria Relli, Pasquale Simeone, and Saverio Alberti, "Epigenetic Inheritance and the Missing Heritability." *Human Genomics* 9 (2015). doi: 10.1186/s40246-015-0041-3.

CHAPTER 7

··

PROCREATIVE RIGHTS IN A POSTCOITAL WORLD

··

KIMBERLY M. MUTCHERSON

Just as the absence of fitting and effective regulation is ethically problematic, so too is overly burdensome or unjustifiable regulation of practices that alleviate human suffering and bring great joy. The possible costs and drawbacks of potential regulation must themselves be counted among the concerns that drive our interest in this field.[1]

FAMILY structures reflect a society's organization and how individuals understand their place in the social order. Thus, families, no matter their form, are foundational in any civilization. In many countries during the past decades, there has been a profound shift in societal understanding of what constitutes a family and who is worthy of making families, especially families with children. In the United States, the rise of single-parent families, families headed by same-sex couples, multiracial families, and families created by unmarried opposite-sex couples speaks to the ability and willingness to expand the societal and legal understanding of family.

These shifts in family life, however, have not emerged without controversy. At the same time that the law and ethics have grappled with new family structures, they have also continued to value traditional beliefs about what families are for, and to describe the optimal relationships among family members, and between families and the law. All of this while dealing with significant technological advances that expand the manner in which children can be conceived. This chapter focuses on how the rise of assisted reproduction has ushered in a postcoital world in which the law simultaneously embraces change and reinforces existing hierarchies of reproduction. These reproductive hierarchies rest on the state's decision to value procreation and family formation by some while actively or passively suppressing procreation and family creation by others frequently based on discrimination rooted in identity categories, including sexual orientation.

Even as change happened, barriers to broadening the legal and social understanding of family remain. One of the greatest of these is convincing governmental actors to embrace and encourage pluralistic families and procreative pluralism. "Pluralistic families" as used here refers not only to families that fit a traditional nuclear model but also the wide range of families that eschew tradition, such as those headed by same-sex couples, single parents, or those that are multiracial. Procreative pluralism refers to the variety of ways in which people create offspring, including with the assistance of reproductive technology.[2] The relationship between pluralistic families and procreative pluralism and the law matters because while people can make families outside of the law, the law provides significant benefits to the families that it recognizes. And, in doling out those benefits, ample evidence suggests that the law privileges certain types of familiar familial structures, which works to the detriment of other families.

The vision of family life and human freedom at the center of this chapter narrowly focuses on childbearing and childrearing familial units. This focus does not mean that families do not exist without children or that people who opt not to procreate are inferior to those who do procreate. This chapter is about families with children and responds to the reality that many people desire adding children to their families and that there are various ways to make that happen, including through adoption, coital reproduction, and assisted reproductive technology (ART).[3] While this is not the life path chosen by all, it is a life path chosen by many and therefore warrants attention, especially to the extent that the state opts to regulate access to the tools of reproduction in discriminatory ways.

First, the chapter briefly discusses the revolutionary nature of assisted reproduction and ART and the ways in which new forms of procreation create or enhance ethical and moral quandaries about procreation and families. Second, the chapter describes how reproductive hierarchies have long existed in the world of coital reproduction. This means that structures of inequality, sometimes reinforced by law, serve to demarcate worthy and state-supported procreative decisions and acts from those which the state denigrates or does not sanction. This section argues that similar hierarchies exist in the context of noncoital reproduction and that the law should work to dismantle rather than reinforce them. Finally, in order to support a claim for legal protection of a right to procreate noncoitally, this section argues about the importance of procreation, coital or noncoital, and the ways in which assisted reproduction demands the recognition of a more elastic notion of what it means to procreate. In its third section, the chapter lays out noncoital procreation as a constitutional and human right and argues that it is unjust to deny access to such a right on the basis of nonrelevant categories. The fourth section urges protection of the right to noncoital reproduction by first acknowledging its importance in law and policy and refusing to base access to assisted reproduction on discredited reproductive hierarchies. Without taking a position on what kinds of procreative regulation might be appropriate and sound, this chapter seeks to set a foundational standard for how the law should understand the fundamental importance of noncoital reproduction.

NONCOITAL REPRODUCTION IN
THE MODERN WORLD

In prior writing, this author has argued for the significance of distinguishing procreation from parenting.[4] No doubt, the two are often interlocking, but they are not incontrovertibly bound to each other. Thus, it is important to be analytically precise about what is at stake in the context of assisted reproduction. One part of what is at stake is the ability to procreate in the sense of participating in a process by which one's genes are propagated and a child comes into being. This is in line with the most basic definition of *procreation*, which is to "produce children or offspring."[5] Another equally if not more important element at stake is the ability to parent a child irrespective of whether there is a genetic or biological link between parent and child. One need not procreate in order to parent and one need not parent as a consequence of procreation. Adoption is an example of how both of these things can be true. Through the adoptive process, people who have not participated in a process of producing children can become legal and social parents. Adoption also allows people who have produced children to free themselves from the legal rights and responsibilities of parenthood.

This chapter centers on those who enter the thicket of assisted reproduction with the intention of participating in a procreative process in some way and following that procreative process with parenting.[6] Positioning the discussion in this way allows this author to draw parallels to coital reproduction while acknowledging that regulation surrounding coital reproduction is also complicated and flawed. This chapter seeks to avoid the trap of assuming that coital reproduction has been treated equally across different categories of people who reproduce coitally. The arguments in this chapter begin by considering the experiences of those for whom procreation has been and continues to be contested territory, thus making legal protection more vital for them in their quest to procreate and become parents.

It is uncontested that the ability to conquer infertility through the use of medical techniques like in vitro fertilization (IVF) is one of the most significant advances in medicine in the last century.[7] Long before IVF became possible, artificial or alternative insemination (AI), in which sperm is introduced into a woman's body without intercourse in order to produce a pregnancy,[8] made it possible for women whose husbands were incapable of creating pregnancies to become pregnant.[9] More recent advances in reproductive medicine raise a host of ethical conundrums even as they shift the landscape of reproductive possibilities for thousands of people around the globe. For instance, intracytoplasmic sperm injection (ICSI), a technique that allows men with very low sperm counts to become genetic fathers,[10] may also lead to the birth of boys who will share their father's infertility, thus creating the next generation of fertility patients.[11] Preimplantation genetic diagnosis (PGD), which involves the testing of embryos to determine characteristics, generally related to disease or disability, in order to assist would-be parents and their health care providers in deciding which of several embryos to use in IVF,[12] raises issues about how a society and would-be parents decide which lives are worth being brought to fruition and which are not. The buying and selling of gametes is a stark reminder that the fertility industry is a business that traffics in the creation of human beings and the sale of precious body products.

The list of ethical concerns about the fertility industry, both intrinsic and as practiced, is extensive. Other chapters in this volume carefully explore a range of these concerns in exacting detail. This chapter's goal is to articulate positively the case for a right to procreate using assisted reproduction as a matter of law, policy, and ethics and leaves the necessary critique to be launched by others. Thus, even with appropriate ethical caveats, assisted reproduction opens the world of procreation to people who seek a very common and often welcome human experience. But it also allows people to exercise a degree of choice over that procreative process that many find jarring at best and unethical at worst. That ART is both liberating and confining creates dilemmas for the law.

Hierarchies of Reproduction and the Reproduction of Hierarchy

Assisted reproduction might create some new ethical dilemmas related to the manipulation of embryos, but, for the most part, it simply recreates or reinforces historically entrenched hierarchies of reproduction. The state has long exercised or at least attempted to exercise some manner of control over who can procreate and with whom. Restraints on reproduction are a common tool of reproductive oppression, and the United States, like many nations, has used various tools, including law, to constrain and deny procreative choices and to elevate some choices and some procreative actors over others.

Historical antecedents for present-day reproductive oppression include decades of sterilization abuse of poor women and women of color in state-run facilities, which has been well documented, if not sufficiently recompensed.[13] States proudly and unabashedly created and defended eugenics-based programs that allowed for the coerced or wholly unconsented sterilization of people, especially women, living with developmental disabilities.[14] Antimiscegenation laws that made it a crime for White people to marry non-Whites were not just about who could marry, but very much about the creation of biracial or multiracial children and the fear of diluting the purity of the White race.[15]

Lest one think that the days of state-sponsored reproductive control are over, in the more modern era, so-called welfare caps that deny public benefits to beneficiaries who exceed a state-determined acceptable number of children also place barriers in the way of people with low incomes who wish to procreate. It remains true that poorer women and women with developmental disabilities are at greater risk for sterilization abuse in part based on beliefs about their ability to procreate and parent responsibly.[16] Prisons are an ongoing site for such abuse and in 2014 the California legislature passed a bill that bars its state prison system from sterilizing prisoners,[17] in response to an investigative report that revealed that in a 5-year period ending in 2010, health care providers performed at least 148 unapproved tubal ligations on female inmates.[18]

Criminal courts and state legislatures in the United States have used their powers to make procreation an excuse for punishment for certain parents or would-be parents. Courts can use their judicial power to encourage or require sterilization or refraining from procreation for women and men whose criminal conduct marks them as unfit for parenthood. For instance, judges have imposed nonprocreation as a condition of parole for men who are delinquent on their child support.[19] Women who use illegal drugs while pregnant have faced prosecution for their pregnancy-related behavior, which may deter the drug-using behavior of the pregnant woman but can also lead her to terminate her pregnancy in order to avoid prosecution.[20] These prosecutions can deter other women from pursuing pregnancy for fear that they will also be punished for their pregnancy-related behavior. Additionally, the denial of conjugal visits for prisoners prevents female prisoners from becoming pregnant and keeps male prisoners from impregnating wives or girlfriends during the pendency of their prison terms.[21] The denigration of procreation by some can even be seen in prison policies that allow for the shackling of pregnant prisoners while they are in labor.[22] Again, not only do these policies act as barriers to procreation; they send a message about the state's desire that these bodies not participate in any procreative process because they are not worthy.

As the reproductive justice movement has shown,[23] reproductive oppression is not limited to withholding access to procreation. It also extends to systems that disestablish relationships between children and parents deemed unfit for the task of raising children. Data reveal that child welfare agencies disproportionately target poor families and families of color, especially African American families, for disruption and rupture.[24] The overrepresentation of Black families in the child welfare system speaks not to an abundance of abuse and neglect in this community but to heightened levels of surveillance, biased notions of proper family life, and a porous social safety net, which make it difficult for many families to sustain themselves adequately.[25] Similarly, the widespread history of removing Native American children from their homes so that they could be raised away from their cultural origins ultimately led to the passage of the Indian Child Welfare Act to protect tribes from decimation.[26] These examples and more define a landscape in which the state consents to efforts to thwart procreation and parenting by some. That these hierarchy-sustaining acts continue to happen even in the face of fundamental rights to parent and procreate speaks to the precariousness of those rights for those who are different and whose desires for children and family exist at the margins of acceptability.

As both history and present-day reality attest, it has long been the case that socioeconomic markers such as race, income, sexual orientation, marital status, and disability status have been relevant to how the law and society value or devalue certain people who procreate and certain family structures within which reproduction takes place. Laws and policies of this type have a negative impact on the procreative experiences of those whose lives they touch, but they also have a larger expressive value in signaling that procreation is a privilege to be granted to those who are worthy by virtue of not being poor, disabled, or otherwise less desirable.

As assisted reproduction has become an available option for those living with medical infertility[27] and, increasingly for some living with social infertility, existing hierarchies of reproduction are instantiated within the realm of noncoital reproduction. Unsurprisingly, the history of assisted reproduction shows that it was first used and intended for opposite-sex married couples who were contending with medical infertility.[28] In the early days, in fact, married couples often kept their use of ART secret to avoid sharing the knowledge of their own infertility or that one or both social parents were not genetically related to their child. Thus, the early goal in the use of ART was to mimic coital reproduction, which translated into the presence of a two-parent dyad, a father and a mother, in a committed, monogamous, legally sanctioned union. As other populations have begun to seek out greater access to ART to build nontraditional families, the law has sometimes acted as a barrier to these new technologically enabled families.

The reinforcement of hierarchy can be seen in fertility providers who will not provide services to those who are socially, but not medically infertile.[29] This means that single women and same-sex couples are turned away from some providers, a form of discrimination for which the law may, but does not always, provide a remedy.[30] Similarly, people living with a range of disabilities,[31] including transmissible diseases like HIV, might be turned away from accessing assisted reproduction services even if the use of those services is the best way to avoid disease transmission while trying to get pregnant.[32] Insurance can also act as a barrier to procreation with assisted reproduction. In the United States, public insurance programs do not typically cover the cost of assisted reproduction, which can be very expensive, depending upon the type of service being accessed.[33] Private insurance might cover those services, but only for certain populations of people, and it is sometimes restricted based on age or a required diagnosis of medical infertility.[34]

On a global scale, the regulation of procreation via rules that limit access to or uses of assisted reproduction are plentiful and stark. Rules include banning access to assisted reproduction for people in same-sex relationships or who are single.[35] Some countries make it illegal to use gametes other than those that come from the couple who plan to parent.[36] Still other countries engage in significant screening in order to evaluate parental worth before an individual or couple can avail themselves of assisted reproduction. In the United Kingdom, where the fertility industry is subject to dense legal regulation, fertility providers must evaluate the parental potential of would-be parents before they can provide them with fertility services, which includes passing judgment on their planned family structures.[37] For many years, the Human Fertilisation and Embryology Authority (HFEA), which regulates access to assisted reproduction in the United Kingdom, made access to assisted reproduction difficult for single women or women in same-sex relationships because part of the review of their attempt to use assisted reproduction required them to show that they would provide an adequate father figure for any child brought into their home.[38]

Some countries have instituted adoption rules that make it impossible for both partners in a same-sex couple to be parents of a child who is brought into their relationship with the use of assisted reproduction.[39] India, which has otherwise proven to be a popular nation for surrogacy services, has barred same-sex couples from hiring surrogates there.[40] To signal broader disdain for the use of surrogacy services, for many years France did not allow children born abroad via surrogate to be awarded French citizenship even if those children were being raised in France by French parents.[41] Many governments around the world have banned surrogacy, especially commercial surrogacy, because of concerns about exploitation of the women hired to participate in the practice and the concern that this practice is akin to baby selling.[42] General bans on surrogacy make procreation difficult if not impossible for some opposite-sex couples and same-sex male couples. This message reinforces the primacy of coital reproduction and the second-class status of other means of creating children.

Several countries ban the purchase or sale of gametes on an anonymous basis based on concerns about the children born of these arrangements who do not have access to information about their genetic progenitors.[43] This can result in substantially weakening the market for gametes in these countries. Where gamete markets become weak, those who need to purchase gametes as part of their use of assisted reproduction must do so in a foreign country, adding expense and, perhaps, legal complications to their attempts to have a family with children.[44]

Countries also regulate the use of techniques like preimplantation genetic diagnosis (PGD) because it is a tool used to reject certain embryos, which will then be discarded.[45] Without access to PGD, some couples and individuals run the risk of having children with life-threatening or significantly life-altering conditions, which could be avoided through technology. Italy's law regulating assisted reproductive technology does not allow would-be parents to refuse to transfer embryos based on information discovered using PGD.[46] Governments may also, more specifically, ban practices like sex selection, especially when it is disconnected from concerns about disease.[47] The denial of access both impairs the procreative interests of would-be parents but also creates the paradoxical situation in which these would-be parents might instead end up seeking abortions if prenatal diagnosis shows a future child who will be impaired. These rules, in addition to other impacts, imply that true procreation, state-valued procreation, demands that would-be parents be unable to pursue preferences related to the children they will parent until after pregnancy has begun or, in some cases, after a child is born. Restrictions of this type also support a norm of pregnancy as a status best achieved with minimal or no technological intervention. In this vision of procreation, would-be parents, especially would-be mothers, should be grateful for any pregnancy and should not act as consumers who pick and choose the kind of child they would like to give birth to or parent.

A belief that coital reproduction is an improper space for legal intervention protects some, but not all, from attempts to alter or extinguish access to procreation. As a result of law and policy, the ideal of family, even families created through assisted reproduction, continues to center around an opposite-sex parental dyad. Legal rules, therefore, can deny access to procreation or can leave children in precarious forms of legal limbo when their parents cannot legally legitimate their relationship to each other or to their children.

In the end, these disparate rules about who can use technology and how it can be used serve a range of purposes, and one such purpose is to elevate some who procreate above others. Just as welfare caps and procreation affecting probation conditions signal ideas about procreation by those who have low incomes, so, too, do bars on single or same-sex couples using assisted reproduction or refusals to work with people living with disabilities help to reinforce restrictive norms of acceptable procreation and adequate parents.

THE PLASTICITY OF REPRODUCTION

In fascinating and challenging ways for the law, assisted reproduction highlights the plasticity of procreation in that what it means to procreate is not static. Focusing simply on technology, the elastic nature of procreation is revealed in the inherent fact that procreation refers not to a single act, but to a series of events taking place over an extended period of time and potentially involving multiple parties, some of whom may be strangers to each other. The procreative act can begin not with two people having sexual intercourse, but with those two people perusing Web sites to find a source of sperm and/or eggs to use to create embryos. The next step is purchasing those gametes and having them sent to a fertility doctor's office, where they will be combined in a petri dish in the hope of creating viable pre-embryos. Those pre-embryos may sit in cryopreservation for months or years or might be transferred to a woman's uterus, not necessarily the uterus of the woman who plans to parent any children born of this procreative process. Once inside a woman's body, the fertilized eggs may implant and morph from embryos to fetuses and eventually into babies, at which point one could ask who exactly has procreated.

The people who provided the genetic material have procreated because they contributed the necessary genetic building blocks that created the baby. The woman who gestated the fetus, now child, has procreated because, for now, gestation inside a female body is an indispensable and valuable, if not always valued, part of the procreative process. As a general matter, people tend to be content to limit procreation to those who have genetic or biological ties to a child, but much can be said of the other parties involved in this process. The people whose desire to parent led them to initiate the process culminating in the child's birth have also procreated in some sense. Unlike the gamete providers, they do not have a genetic link to the child and unlike the gestational carrier they do not have a biological link to the child born of the intimate physical intertwining and dependence created by pregnancy. But, at the most granular level, the people who initiate the process that leads to the child's creation are the most important part of the entire procreative process. Without them, none of the other pieces of the procreative puzzle would have become connected in such a way so as to create this child at this moment in time.[48] Thus, the foundational creators of a child conceived through assisted reproduction are the people who, for whatever social or physical reasons, set in motion the procreative process. It is proper, then, to see the interest in initiating the procreative process, make some decisions related to that process, and parent a child born of that process as being worthy of significant concern and legal protection. And, of course, when genetics and gestation overlap with intention to parent, the interest of would-be parents are even clearer, though not necessarily more important.

Assisted reproduction, which can decouple parenting from genetic connection and sex from procreation, requires those who participate in these arrangements to define their connection to children in ways that can be discomfiting to individuals for whom genetic and biological connections are paramount. Worries about shifting relationships between parents and children are fundamentally concerns about shifts in family form. For those who believe that children are best served by being raised in two-parent households with married parents of opposite genders,[49] the opportunities that assisted reproduction creates to upend that traditional dyad are disquieting. Single parents, male or female; unmarried parents; same-sex parents; older parents; parents living with significant disabilities; and other *outsider* parents challenge the idea that there is one best way to procreate and parent or that there is one best way to be a family. For those who believe in procreative and familial pluralism, these new family formations are a boon, but that is not a feeling shared by all, as evidenced by varying attempts to exclude some families from the protection of the law and some individuals from access to procreation.

The litany of anxieties attendant to assisted reproduction related to family destruction, exploitation, and rights violations are not simply discussions that happen in scholarly literature about technologically enhanced procreation. They are very much the foundation of law and policymaking that aims to limit and regulate access to assisted reproduction often based on the characteristics of the individuals or families that seek the service. Even where laws are meant to be neutral or focus on protecting children or sellers in the market, their impact is felt most acutely by those for whom access to assisted reproduction is a necessary precursor to creating the families of their choice. Therefore, it is necessary to view laws about assisted reproduction with a critical and discerning eye.

ACCESS TO PROCREATION AS A CONSTITUTIONAL AND HUMAN RIGHT

Procreation, the ability to propagate one's genes, matters greatly to many people and in many cultures. It is equally true that the right to parent, either one's own progeny or children with whom one creates a parental relationship legally or otherwise, is a right considered fundamental to existence in a legal and ethical sense.[50] That procreation, with or without parenting, matters so deeply on an individual and societal level explains why state-sanctioned denial of access to procreation has a painful history of being used as a tool to demarcate worthy citizens from those who are not worthy. As already articulated earlier in this chapter, the well-documented past and present of state control over who can procreate and with whom includes targeted forced sterilization laws, anti-miscegenation laws, and disproportionate use of the child welfare system in some communities. Justice in reproduction continues to be denied to many individuals and communities as a means of delimiting procreative worth.

The bald discrimination in access to reproductive justice is especially stark given that the US Constitutional scheme has long protected a right to procreate. Beginning with *Skinner v. Oklahoma* in 1942,[51] a case involving a forced sterilization law for habitual criminal offenders, the US Supreme Court has continually explicitly held that marriage and procreation are fundamental rights. This, of course, does not mean that the state has no power to regulate in this realm, but only that such regulation must be narrowly tailored to meet a compelling interest of the state. Over the years, courts have found sufficient state interests to allow for intrusion into the otherwise private realm of family formation and procreation across an array of contexts. As suggested earlier in this chapter, the space in which the courts seem to find state intrusion into the realm of procreation most acceptable is when that intrusion ostensibly seeks to protect children. So, for instance, state child welfare agencies have significant powers that allow them to remove children from the custody of their parents or terminate parental rights altogether when a parent fails to provide a minimally adequate level of care to a child. Controversially, states have even been allowed to exercise power over pregnant women in the interest of protecting a fetus either through criminal or civil systems.[52] While there is state power here, that power is limited and is too often wielded against those whose procreative choices fail to conform to a narrow standard of normal or, in the case of assisted reproduction, natural.

Despite the uneven hand of regulation in the context of coital reproduction, critics have expressed disdain at the comparative lack of regulation of the fertility industry in the United States.[53] The critique is that the lack of regulation places actors in the industry at risk for ill treatment or harm, including people who sell gametes, women who act as surrogates, and children born to parents who are not screened for parental fitness.[54] It may be true that the lack of specific regulation has negative consequences for some, but, given the nature of restrictions seen in other countries, this lack of regulation is also protective of the interests of others because when countries regulate they do not always do so justly. Some nations ban access to commercial surrogacy altogether.[55] In other cases, the use of surrogates is limited to those who have a medical need for such services— a diagnosis that is not always available to same-sex couples or single women.[56] Some states that require insurance coverage for IVF also limit the circumstances under which insurance must cover the use of the technology, including creating age caps.[57] Thus, while more regulation in the United States will perhaps create greater protections for some, it will, justly or unjustly, erect greater barriers for others.

By placing limits on who may procreate using assisted reproduction and what technologies can be accessed and for what reasons, the state uses its regulatory power to shape family life within its borders. Of course, those with means can leave their homes of origin to seek services elsewhere, but this does not guarantee a smooth journey to parenthood as law can still negatively impact the recognition of the family upon return to the home country.[58] And as referenced earlier, other countries continue to exercise procreative and parental control over their citizens through citizenship and adoption rules that make it difficult or impossible for intended parents to create legal ties to children born through assisted reproduction abroad who are brought back to the parental home country to live.[59]

None of this is to say that shaping family life is beyond the scope of rights, and perhaps even duties, accorded to the state. In the United States, courts have long held that states have significant interests in families and can regulate family life within certain limits.[60] Despite the fundamental nature of the rights at stake, the state parens patriae interest in children gives it wide latitude to regulate in order to protect those who cannot protect themselves.[61] The state can and should act to protect children, but what that means for the power to regulate procreation is a matter worthy of debate. As Professor I. Glenn Cohen has eloquently argued, the regulation of procreation to meet the best interests of future children will often have the impact of ensuring that certain children never come to exist in the first instance, which is difficult to count as a benefit to those children.[62] Even so, while Cohen's argument may resonate for some, it is undoubtedly the case that the state often blurs the distinction between regulating procreative actors and protecting future children. It is naïve to think that this line would ever be anything but diaphanous given the range of interests the state has asserted under the rubric of parens patriae, but as a matter of law and policy states should be called to offer some justification for an interest in and right to engage in regulation that protects children by denying would-be parents the ability to procreate.

And even to the extent that ART implicates the state's parens patriae interest in children, it is not clear how that interest should be weighed in the context of procreation versus parenting. When a child exists in the world and is no longer in the womb of a pregnant woman, a developed body of child welfare law provides direction to the state and policymakers in thinking about how to effectuate the state interest in children.[63] Given these interests and concerns, it is right that parenting choices are subject to some level of state surveillance and perhaps control, though the extent to which the state's eye trains itself on some families disproportionately warrants significant oversight of this system.[64] But it is not clear how an interest in parenting choices translates into an interest in procreative or preparenting choices. In light of conflicts about the nature of a fetus as a person or potential person, the latter interest demands independent justification from the former.[65] States may act in the interest of live children, and in some instances they may also act so as to protect those who have not yet been born, but the state's ability to protect those not yet conceived stands on shaky ground. Denying access to the tools of procreation is not only a way of policing who will parent; it is a way of policing who will be born at a time when there is no child to protect and, in fact, when *protection* means preventing a child from coming in to being.[66]

Some scholars have long taken the position that the overlap between coital and noncoital reproduction is so significant that there is no valid claim to make that one should be left unprotected while the other receives the protection of being considered a fundamental right, thus demanding the most exacting level of constitutional scrutiny by courts when states seek to alter or extinguish the right involved.[67] Others are reluctant to extend the same level of protection to noncoital reproduction as is afforded to those who procreate coitally.[68] Using human rights jurisprudence as intellectual precedent and building on a long-existing constitutional right to procreate, for the law to exclude noncoital reproduction from the purview of legal protection declares that procreation truly matters only to those who procreate through sexual intercourse. Drawing lines of exclusion in this way serves only to reinforce hierarchies and discount the deep desire for procreation and parenting that animates those for whom procreation happens noncoitally.

In the United States, the European Union, and many other countries, state power to deny procreation is cabined. For decades, the U.S. Supreme Court has reiterated that the rights to marry, procreate, and parent are fundamental and, for the most part, state laws that interfere with those rights must be subjected to the most exacting level of constitutional scrutiny when they are challenged.[69] Therefore, as a matter of law, the claim here is not that the state has no role to play in the regulation of family life, including access to assisted reproduction. Rather, the concern is the ways in which the state chooses to interfere and the threshold of acceptability to which the courts will subject those laws and regulations when and if they are challenged. As a matter of constitutional rights, the state should tread lightly and without pernicious bias when it regulates noncoital reproduction.

The Constitution is just one source of limitation on state power over procreation because freedom from unwarranted governmental interference in procreation is also a human right. Foundational human rights documents such as the Universal Declaration of Human Rights articulate a human right to procreate.[70] As described by the International Conference on Population and Development Programme of Action:

> [R]eproductive rights embrace certain human rights that are already recognized in national laws, international human rights documents and other consensus document. These rights rest on recognition of the basic right of all couples and individuals to decide freely and responsibly the number, spacing, and timing of their children and to have the information and means to do so, and the right to attain the highest standard of sexual and reproductive health. It also includes the right to make decisions concerning reproduction free of discrimination, coercion, and violence as expressed in human rights documents.[71]

The availability of assisted reproduction has created the necessity of deciding whether the human and constitutional right to procreation extends beyond coital reproduction to those individuals who must or choose to build their families using technology. Though the US Supreme Court has not had an occasion to describe the relationship between noncoital reproduction and the fundamental right to procreate, human rights courts dealing with the issue of postcoital procreation have reinforced that access to the right to procreate can include access to the technology of procreation. For instance, in a 2012 case called *Murillo et al. v. Costa Rica*, the Inter-American Court of Human Rights ruled that the Costa Rican ban on IVF violated the right to privacy, the right to a family, and the right to personal integrity.[72] The *Murillo* Court wrote in part, "the Court considers that the decision of whether or not to become a parent is part of the right to private life and includes, in this case, the decision of whether or not to become a mother or father in the genetic or biological sense."[73]

Beyond a rights-based regime, the ethical principle of justice also countenances significant respect for and protection of a right to noncoital reproduction. Whether by an accident of birth or an act of will, that some individuals cannot or do not procreate coitally should not have a bearing on whether their desire to procreate warrants acknowledgment and protection by the government that serves them. If procreation is an experience of significant human value and worth, then the terms upon which that experience is denied to some should be clear and justifiable. And, in the context of assisted reproduction where many rights denials are based on indefensible reproductive hierarchies, this basic standard of fairness cannot be met.

PROTECTING THE RIGHT TO NONCOITAL REPRODUCTION

There are a variety of tools that governments use to create tiered access to procreation and to reinforce hierarchies of reproduction. Around the globe, governments use their regulatory powers to make clear that access to assisted reproduction is, first and foremost, warranted for those whose desire to reproduce and whose families, if they are successfully created, will most closely mimic traditional family structures. This accounts for rules that exclude single people from accessing assisted reproduction or that reserve access to assisted reproduction for people who are in opposite-sex couples. Though the regulation of the fertility industry in the United States is relatively slight as compared to many other countries, regulation does still exist and where it does exist in can often act to the detriment of people whose desire to procreate is considered fringe or unwelcome. It is known that fertility providers play a gatekeeping role in deciding who should have access to assisted reproduction and that role can be used to exclude a range of potential parents, including those who are single, those who are in same-sex relationships, or people living with various disabilities.[74]

As a matter of justice and equality, when society and the law accord procreation different value based on invidious categories of discrimination, the deleterious impact of those decisions is felt most acutely by those who the states deems unworthy to procreate. As indicated earlier in this chapter, denying people access to the tools of procreation does more than simply keep them from being the parents that they would like to be; these access rules have an expressive outcome even if not an expressive intent. And what they express is that procreation is a thing worthy of protection for some and worthy of derision and denial for others.

One of the most basic ways to justify restricting access to assisted reproduction is by first carving out noncoital reproduction as not just physically but also intellectually and philosophically different in kind and character from coital reproduction. But marking these territories as so distinct is ultimately an unsuccessful task. There is no evidence to suggest that would-be parents who use coital reproduction are, as a class, more unfit than parents who coitally reproduce. There is no evidence to suggest that children born of assisted reproduction are less well-adjusted or lead less productive lives than their coitally created counterparts. In fact, what evidence there is indicates that these children are as happy, healthy, and well-adjusted as their coitally conceived counterparts.[75] And there is no evidence to suggest that the desires for parenthood that animate those who reproduce noncoitally are disturbing or suspect when compared to the desires of those who reproduce coitally. In fact, one could argue that noncoital reproduction, as considered from the point of view of future parents and future children, has distinct benefits over coital reproduction. It requires a specific intent to create a pregnancy— something that is often sorely lacking in the context of coital reproduction, where approximately 50% of all pregnancies in a given year are unintended.[76] It requires planning and forethought, which is also lacking in many coital pregnancies, given the number of such pregnancies that are unplanned. It subjects participants to outside review of their choice to become parents, for better or for worse, which is not present at the start of most coitally created pregnancies. None of this is to say that coital or noncoital reproduction is preferable to the other. Rather, the core interests that are valued when people coitally reproduce are also present for those who reproduce noncoitally: namely, a desire for propagating one's genes; a desire to create interdependence with a child; and an interest in creating a family unit with dependents. If the only thing that differentiates coital reproduction from noncoital reproduction when it comes to those seeking parenthood is that one route involves sex and the other does not, it seems difficult to justify differing treatment under the law on anything other than the law's beliefs about sex, rather than larger principles about parenthood and family.

Restrictive regulation of assisted reproduction strikes some as intuitive while others see it as anathema. For others, the possibility of regulation presents a difficult conundrum for "supporters and providers of reproductive health services have good reasons to be skeptical of government regulation in the area of reproduction"[77] because "too often, laws and regulation have been designed to restrict access to reproductive health services ... especially for the most vulnerable groups of women."[78] However, with the caveat of proceeding with caution, others assert that "we need to step up and begin designing public policies that responsibly regulate the application of reproductive technologies and the industry that develops and depends on them."[79] But before we can decide if and how to regulate, we are bound to make a determination about how to conceive of a right to procreate in the absence of coital reproduction, and there the right answer seems to be that a right to procreate that does not embrace noncoital reproduction is anemic and unnecessarily discriminatory.

Given the intimate nature of regulating procreation, the default position that emerges from this chapter's claim about the primacy of the right to procreate, both coitally and noncoitally, is that there should be no or little restrictive regulation of ART. In a constitutional sense, the party seeking to shift away from the default position of no regulation bears the burden of making the strongest claim possible for a state exercise of control over noncoital reproduction. As a matter of policy, a society that prides itself on inclusion and nondiscrimination should avoid reproductive regulation premised on nonrelevant categories of identity. And, as a matter of ethics, justice requires that the benefits of access to the tools of reproduction be made widely available.

Translating this position into positive law requires nuance and care. The position that access to noncoital reproduction is a fundamental right does not assume that it is an unassailable right. States may, given the appropriate confluence of interests, enact laws that restrict access to fundamental rights. For instance, in the case of marriage, states have long created constitutional restrictions on those under the age of 18 who want to marry or those who wish to marry close relatives.[80] So, too, legal marriage has been restricted only to two individuals and plural marriages have not traditionally been able to acquire the imprimatur of legality.[81] But, where marriage restrictions have served to support bigotry and express disdain for certain groups of people, as courts have found to be true in the context of bans on same-sex marriage, those restrictions have fallen.[82] The point, then, of arguing for recognizing noncoital reproduction as part and parcel of a fundamental right to procreate is to ensure that the laws that seek to restrict the right are subjected to an appropriate level of scrutiny. The hope, too, is that those who would legislate in this arena will, by dint of the looming threat of legal challenge, feel inspired to tread lightly and with an eye toward equality and justice rather than pernicious discrimination. Thus, legislative acts might well survive constitutional challenge where legislation legitimately sought to protect important constituencies. Examples might include laws that protect women or men who are selling their gametes by ensuring that consent to participate in sales of this sort comes only with proper information about potential physical consequences. Similarly, a law meant to protect children born through third-party reproduction by ensuring that those responsible for their creation are required to take on the legal rights and responsibilities of parenting when a child is born could also survive a constitutional challenge.

As the Supreme Court wrote in *Planned Parenthood v. Casey*, "matters, involving the most intimate and personal choices a person may make in a lifetime, choices central to personal dignity and autonomy, are central to the liberty protected by the [Fourteenth] Amendment."[83] As it slowly chips away at a woman's right to make choices related to terminating a pregnancy, the Court has not lived up to the promise of this expansive language. But the message conveyed in this passage from *Casey* is instructive in its call to set a high bar for governmental interference in access to reproductive health services, including fertility treatment for purposes of this chapter, that are important and worthy of constitutional protection. Making sure to classify properly the right is even more important in a world in which even coital reproduction has not, in practice, been accorded the same level of deference across hierarchies of reproduction. Excluding those who procreate noncoitally from the highest levels of legal protection only makes it that much easier for biases related to family formation and parenting to become enshrined in law.

CONCLUSION

There are broad interests at stake in the regulation of assisted reproduction that reach to the heart of procreation as a right of individuals to entangle themselves in the lives of others and form units of dependence. Families come to be because of the ways that people choose to organize their lives. Choice, as always, must be tempered by the reality that all choices are exercised within contexts that can be confining and determinative. As such, in a society that believes in justice, individual decisions about procreating, becoming a parent, and building a family that includes children, if so desired, are decisions worthy of societal protection. Therefore, it behooves a society that cares about equality and justice to reduce or eliminate unwarranted discrimination in doling out the benefits attendant to being a legally recognized family.

The landscape of procreation and the power that the state has wielded over it is complex. Procreation has long been and will continue to be a site of oppression and dominance as well as a site for assertions of power by outsiders and others living on the fringe of acceptability. Given its place of prominence as a locus of political struggle, procreation is an activity that matters. Any belief that restrictive regulation of access to assisted reproduction is constitutionally possible leaves many unanswered questions about what should be regulated, how it should be regulated, and what checks there should be on state interference into this private realm. This chapter has focused on the ways in which the state might restrict or support access to assisted reproduction and, more broadly, the state's relationship to individuals' desires and attempts to conceive. Ultimately, the assertion of state powers over assisted reproduction should be subject to significant checks. Even within the world of coital reproduction, the state does not always act with equal reverence for the rich history of fundamental rights protection. The ability to treat the reproduction of some as suspect and second-tier is even greater where we mark technologically assisted reproduction as fundamentally less worthy than coital reproduction. To regulate appropriately, we must first begin with the belief that the thing being regulated, noncoital reproduction, is worthy of a high level of respect and that level of respect is one that recognizes that though the ways that people come to procreation may be different, the reasons that they come to procreation are often identical.

ACKNOWLEDGMENTS

Many thanks to Leslie Francis, Judy Daar, and Katie Eyer for their helpful editing and critique of this chapter.

NOTES

1. The President's Council on Bioethics, *Reproduction and Responsibility* (March 2004).
2. For a broader account of the overall good of procreative pluralism, see Kimberly M. Mutcherson, "Procreative Pluralism," *Berkeley Journal of Gender, Law & Justice* 30 (Winter 2015): 22.
3. The Centers for Disease Control defines assisted reproductive technology as "includ(ing) all fertility treatments in which both eggs and sperm are handled. In general, ART procedures involve surgically removing eggs from a woman's ovaries, combining them with sperm in the laboratory, and returning them to the woman's body or donating them to another woman. They do NOT include treatments in which only sperm are handled (i.e., intrauterine—or artificial—insemination) or procedures in which a woman takes medicine only to stimulate egg production without the intention of having eggs retrieved." Centers for Disease Control and Prevention, "What Is Assisted Reproductive Technology?," accessed February 20, 2015. http://www.cdc.gov/ART/. To signal a broader focus, this chapter will use the term "assisted reproduction" to refer to multiple forms of technologically assisted procreation, including IVF, with or without a surrogate and with or without purchased gametes, as well as alternative or artificial insemination.
4. Mutcherson, "Procreative Pluralism."
5. Merriam-Webster Dictionary (online).
6. The limitation that this author places on this discussion does not imply that there are no important arguments about parenting that need to be made in favor of those, for instance, who are discriminated against in the adoption market. It also does not deny the need to think about and create policy around the needs of those who participate in the market for fertility services not as possible parents but as vendors, specifically gamete providers and gestational carriers. These are things that matter and the exclusion of those issues from this text is not meant to elevate the concerns discussed herein but only to illuminate them.
7. In 2010, Dr. Robert Edwards received the Nobel Prize for Physiology or Medicine for his work developing in vitro fertilization (IVF). Nicholas Wade, "Pioneer of In Vitro Fertilization Wins Nobel Prize," *New York Times*, October 4, 2010. IVF is a process by which eggs and sperm are joined outside of the body in order to create fertilized eggs that can then be returned to a woman's uterus in the hope that they will grow and become healthy babies. MedlinePlus, "In Vitro Fertilization (IVF)," Accessed February 10, 2015. http://www.nlm.nih.gov/medlineplus/ency/article/007279.htm.
8. Artificial or alternative insemination is a process, which involves the collection of sperm from a man and the transfer of that sperm to a woman's body in the hope that the sperm will fertilize an egg and a pregnancy will commence. American Society of Reproductive Medicine, "Third-Party Reproduction: A Guide for Patients," 9–11 (2012).
9. As Kara Swanson describes in her history of banking body products, in its early incantations, donor insemination was used primarily for married women whose husbands were unable to create a pregnancy because of problems related to their sperm. Kara W. Swanson, *Banking on the Body: The Market in Blood, Milk, and Sperm in Modern America* (Cambridge, MA: Harvard University Press, 2014), 227–229. This model, in which physicians acted as gatekeepers, largely left single women and lesbians without access to a basic fertility service if they desired to have children. Ibid.
10. Intracytoplasmic sperm injection (ICSI) is a technique that allows men with very low sperm counts to become genetic fathers as it requires only that a single sperm be

injected directly into the cytoplasm of a woman's egg as part of IVF. "Fact Sheet: What Is Intracytoplasmic Sperm Injection (ICSI)?, American Society for Reproductive Medicine, accessed February 10, 2015. http://www.reproductivefacts.org/uploadedFiles/ASRM_Content/Resources/Patient_Resources/Fact_Sheets_and_Info_Booklets/ICSI-Fact.pdf.

11. Ibid. ("Some of the problems that cause infertility may be genetic. For example, male children conceived with the use of ICSI may have the same infertility issues as their fathers.")

12. See, e.g., Ethics Committee of the American Society for Reproductive Medicine, "Use of Preimplantation Genetic Diagnosis for Serious Adult Onset Conditions: A Committee Opinion," *Fertility and Sterility* 100 (July 2013): 54–57 (discussing the ethics of using PGD for detecting nonchildhood diseases).

13. See, e.g., Alexandra Minna Stern, "Sterilized in the Name of Public Health," *American Journal of Public Health* 95 (2005): 1128–1138.

14. Paul Lombardo, *Three Generations, No Imbeciles* (Baltimore: Johns Hopkins University Press, 2008), 8–19.

15. See, e.g., Kevin Noble Maillard and Rose Cuison Villazor, eds., *Loving v. Virginia in a Post-Racial World—Rethinking Race, Sex, and Marriage* (Cambridge: Cambridge University Press, 2012) (essays exploring the history of laws regulating interracial intimacy and the legacy of those laws in present day America).

16. See generally, e.g., Jessica Arons, *More Than a Choice: A Progressive Vision for Reproductive Health and Rights* (Center for American Progress, September 2006), 8; Jael Silliman et al., *Undivided Rights: Women of Color Organize for Reproductive Justice* (Boston: South End Press, 2004); Dorothy Roberts, *Killing the Black Body* (New York: Vintage Books, 1997); Paul A. Lombardo, ed., *A Century of Eugenics in America: From the Indiana Experiment to the Human Genome Era* (Bloomington: Indiana University Press, 2011).

17. Cal. Pen. Code §3440 (2014) (prohibiting the sterilization of prisoners for the purpose of birth control).

18. Patrick McGreevy and Phil Willon, "Female Inmate Surgery Broke Law," *L.A. Times*, July 14, 2013.

19. See, e.g., *State v. Oakley*, 629 N.W.2d 200 (2001) (upholding probation conditions that required probationer to refrain from procreation until he demonstrated that he could monetarily support his existing children as well as any new children). In 2012, a Wisconsin judge ordered Corey Curtis, a man who owed $90,000 in back child support for nine children, to avoid procreating as part of his probation. "Judge's Unusual Order to Man With Nine Kids: Stop Procreating," NBC News, December 5, 2012. Accessed February 10, 2015. http://usnews.nbcnews.com/_news/2012/12/05/15700788-judges-unusual-order-to-man-with-nine-kids-stop-procreating?lite.

20. Lynn M. Paltrow and Jeanne Flavin, "Arrests and Forced Interventions on Pregnant Women in the United States, 1973–2005: Implications for Women's Legal Status and Public Health," *Journal of Health Politics, Policy and Law* 38 (2013): 299–343.

21. See, e.g., *McCray v. Sullivan*, 509 F.2d 1332(1975) (finding that denying conjugal visits to prisoners does not deny them federal constitutional rights).

22. *CAT Shadow Report: The Shackling of Incarcerated Pregnant Women* (September 2014). Accessed February 10, 2015. https://ihrclinic.uchicago.edu/sites/ihrclinic.uchicago.edu/files/uploads/Report%20-%20Shackling%20of%20Pregnant%20Prisoners%20in%20the%20US%20%28Final%201.8.14%29.pdf.

23. Reproductive Justice is a movement begun by women of color activists that focuses equally on the right to have a child, the right to avoid having a child, and the right to

parent one's children and raise them in safe and clean communities. Loretta Ross, "What Is Reproductive Justice?" in *Reproductive Justice Briefing Book: A Primer on Reproductive Justice and Social Change*. Accessed February 10, 2015. https://files.zotero.net/4338391260/Reproductive%20Justice%20Briefing%20Book.pdf.

24. Dorothy Roberts, *Shattered Bonds: The Color of Child Welfare* (New York: Basic Civitas Books, 2001) (describing significant racial disparities in the child welfare system in the United States).

25. Ibid.

26. Congress passed the Indian Child Welfare Act in 1978 to "protect the best interests of Indian children and to promote the stability and security of Indian tribes and families." Indian Child Welfare Act, 25 U.S.C. § 1902.

27. Medical infertility is defined as a failure to become pregnant after one year of unprotected heterosexual intercourse. MedlinePlus, *Infertility*. This medical diagnosis can be contrasted with social infertility, which is a term that is generally associated with those who use assisted reproduction for reasons other than a documented medical condition such as single women and same-sex couples. For a discussion of lesbians and access to infertility services, see Laura Mamo, *Queering Reproduction: Achieving Pregnancy in the Age of Technoscience* (Durham, NC: Duke University Press, 2007). Reproductive technology can also be used by would be parents who wish to avoid the transmission of disease or disability but who are not otherwise medically infertile.

28. Margaret Marsh and Wanda Ronner, *The Empty Cradle* (Baltimore: The Johns Hopkins University Press, 1996): 171–209.

29. The Ethics Committee of the American Society for Reproductive Medicine, "Access to Fertility Treatment by Gays, Lesbians, and Unmarried Persons: A Committee Opinion," *Fertility & Sterility* 100 (December 2013): 1524–1527.

30. Susan Donaldson James, "Doctors Deny Lesbian Artificial Insemination," ABC News, May 28, 2008.

31. National Council of Disabilities, *Rocking the Cradle: Ensuring the Rights of Parents with Disabilities and Their Children*. Accessed February 10, 2015. http://www.ncd.gov/publications/2012/Sep272012/Ch11 (describing case of a blind woman who was denied AI until she could get an assessment of her home to prove that it was safe for a baby).

32. Julie Stanitis, et al., "Fertility Services for Human Immunodeficiency Virus-Positive Patients: Provider Policy, Practice and Perspectives," *Fertility and Sterility* 89 (May 2008): 1154, 1156–1158.

33. Jessica Arons and Elizabeth Chen, *Future Choices II—An Update on the Legal, Statutory, and Policy Landscape of Assisted Reproductive Technologies* (March 2013), 7. ("While insurance coverage of fertility treatments has expanded over time, states continue to deny coverage for such treatments to recipients of public medical assistance.")

34. Ibid. at 4–6.

35. See, I. Glenn Cohen, "Circumvention Tourism," *Cornell Law Review* 97 (2012): 1309, 1323 (listing numerous restrictive ART laws from around the globe).

36. Andrea Boggio, "Italy Enacts New Law on Medically Assisted Reproduction," *Human Reproduction* 20 (2005): 1153, 1153.

37. "A woman shall not be provided with treatment services unless account has been taken of the welfare of any child who may be born as a result of the treatment (including the need of that child for supportive parenting), and of any other child who may be affected by the birth." Human Fertilisation and Embrylogy Act of 1990 (as amended), Section 13 (5). In its

previous incantation, this section's language read "including the need of that child for a
father."

38. Dr. Evan Harris, November 7, 2005, "The HFEA's Silence on the Need for a Father," *Bionews*
(noting how the language about the need for father's adversely impacted lesbians and single women).

39. Babies may be stateless, parentless, or both when born to surrogates to parents who originate from countries that ban the practice. Emma Batha, "International Surrogacy Traps
Babies in Stateless Limbo," *Reuters* (U.S.), September 18, 2014 (citing cases involving parents from Norway and Belgium who hired surrogates abroad who gave birth to stateless
children). France's ban on French citizenship for children born by surrogate to French
intended parents was ruled a human rights violation by the European Court of Human
Rights in 2014. *Mennesson v. France*, European Court of Human Rights, September 26,
2014. A decision from the high court overturned the part of Germany's surrogacy ban
that made it impossible for parents, including same-sex parents, to become legal parents
of a child born to a surrogate abroad no matter whether the foreign country recognized
the parental status of the German parents. "Limited win for surrogacy, gay parenthood
in Germany," *Deutsche Well*, December 19, 2014, accessed February 10, 2015. http://www.
dw.de/limited-win-for-surrogacy-gay-parenthood-in-germany/a-18142883.

40. Trudy Ring, "India Bars Gay Couples From Surrogacy Services," Advocate.com, January
18, 2013, accessed February 10, 2015. http://www.advocate.com/health/health-news/2013/
01/18/india-bars-gay-couples-surrogacy-services.

41. In 2014, the European Court of Human Rights found that France's refusal to register children born in the United States to French parents as the legal children of those French parents, and thus entitled to French citizenship, violated the children's human right to respect
for their family and private life. *Mennesson v. France*, European Court of Human Rights,
September 26, 2014.

42. According to the *Mennesson* Court, "A comparative-law survey conducted by the Court
shows that surrogacy is expressly prohibited in fourteen of the thirty-five member States
of the Council of Europe—other than France—studied." Ibid.

43. The brisk commercial market in gametes that exists in the United States is not a
global phenomenon. Several countries limit or forbid compensation for those who
sell their gametes. See, e.g., Human Fertilisation and Embryology (HFE) Act 1990
(as amended) § 12(1)(e) (restricting compensation to egg and sperm donors) and the
Assisted Human Reproduction Act (Canada) (forbidding compensation for selling
eggs or sperm).

44. See, e.g., Gaia Bernstein, "Unintended Consequences: Prohibitions on Gamete Donor
Anonymity and the Fragile Practice of Surrogacy," *Indiana Health Law Review* 10
(2013): 291.

45. Boggio, "Italy Enacts New Law on Medically Assisted Reproduction."

46. In 2012, the European Court of Human Rights decided that Italy's Assisted Reproduction
law, which mandated the use of embryos created for IVF and limited access to preimplantation screen of those embryos, was a violation of human rights. *Costa and Pavan v. Italy*,
August 28, 2012.

47. As of 2009, research indicated that 31 countries that had policies on sex selection prohibited its use for nonmedical reasons. Marcy Darnovsky, "Countries With Laws or Policies
on Sex Selection," Center for Genetics and Society (April 2009). Accessed February 10,
2015. http://geneticsandsociety.org/downloads/200904_sex_selection_memo.pdf.

48. As the court concluded in the *Buzzanca* case, "Even though neither [of the intended parents] are biologically related to Jaycee, they are still her lawful parents given their initiating role as the intended parents in her conception and birth." *In re Marriage of Buzzanca*, 61 Cal. App. 4th 1410, 1428(1998).

49. See, e.g., Brief of Amici Curiae United States Conference of Catholic Bishops; National Association of Evangelicals; The Church of Jesus Christ of Latter-Day Saints; The Ethics & Religious Liberty Commission of the Southern Baptist Convention; and Lutheran Church—Missouri Synod in Support of Defendants-Appellants and Supporting Reversal in *Bishop and Barton v. Smith* (10th Circuit Court of Appeals) (arguing that stable marriages between men and women are the ideal childrearing unit).

50. European Charter of Fundamental Rights and Freedoms, Right to Private and Family Life, Art. 7.

51. *Skinner v. Oklahoma*, 316 U.S. 535 (1942) (holding that marriage and procreation are fundamental rights protected by the Constitution).

52. Paltrow and Flavin, "Arrests and Forced Interventions on Pregnant Women in the United States, 1973–2005: Implications for Women's Legal Status and Public Health."

53. The American Society for Reproductive Medicine argues that "ART is already one of most highly regulated of all medical practices in the United States." American Society for Reproductive Medicine, *Oversight of Assisted Reproductive Technology* (2010), 11.

54. Debora L. Spar, *The Baby Business: How Money, Science, and Politics Drive the Commerce of Conception* (Boston: Harvard Business School Press, 2006), xviii; Naomi Cahn, *Test Tube Families: Why the Fertility Market Needs Legal Regulation* (New York: New York University Press, 2009).

55. States banning commercial surrogacy include New York, Michigan, Washington, and the District of Columbia. See D.C. CODE §§ 16-401 to 16-402 (LexisNexis, 2001) (punishing both commercial and altruistic surrogacy); MICH. COMP. LAWS ANN. § 722.859 (West, 2002); N.Y. DOM. REL. LAW § 123(1) (McKinney, 1999); WASH. REV. CODE ANN. §§ 26.26.210–.260 (West, 2005).

56. See, e.g., Gestational Surrogacy Act, 750 ILCS 47/25 § 20(b)(2).

57. See, e.g., Hawaii Rev. State § 431:10A-116.5 and § 432.1-604 (1989, 2003) (to qualify for IVF, a couple must have a history of infertility for at least 5 years or prove that the infertility is the result of a specified medical condition); R. I. Gen. Laws § 27-18-30 (limiting insurance requirement to IVF to women between the ages of 25 and 42 years).

58. For instance, a child born abroad to a foreign surrogate who is not biologically related to a US citizen parent may experience difficulty returning to the United States and establishing citizenship. US Department of State, Bureau of Consular Affairs, "Important Information for U.S. Citizens Considering the Use of Assisted Reproductive Technology (ART) Abroad." Accessed February 10, 2015. http://travel.state.gov/content/travel/english/legal-considerations/us-citizenship-laws-policies/assisted-reproductive-technology.html.

59. See, e.g., "Avoid International Surrogacy, Says Expert in Wake of B.C. Couple's Fight for Twins," *CBC News*, January 28, 2015 (describing Canadian couple who had twins by surrogate in Mexico who faced legal barriers to bringing the children home); "Legal Wrangle Continues Over Surrogate Child," *Journal of Turkish Weekly*, September 26, 2014 (describing case of male couple from Switzerland who had a child via surrogate in California who were being thwarted in their attempt to both be recognized as the child's parents in their home country); *Fact File: How Easy Is It to Bring Overseas-Born Surrogate Babies Back to Australia and What Are Their Parents' Rights?*, ABC Premium News, August 19, 2014

(describing the sometimes difficult and onerous process of establishing Australian parent-age and citizenship for children born to surrogates overseas).

60. As the U.S. Supreme Court wrote in *Prince v. Massachusetts*, "But the family itself is not beyond regulation in the public interest, as against a claim of religious liberty.... And neither rights of religion nor rights of parenthood are beyond limitation. 321 U.S. 158, 166 (1944) (internal citation omitted).

61. Ibid. at 167. ("[T] the state has a wide range of power for limiting parental freedom and authority in things affecting the child's welfare ....").

62. I. Glenn Cohen, "Sperm Donor Anonymity," this volume; I. Glenn Cohen, "Regulating Reproduction: The Problem With Best Interests," *Minnesota Law Review* 96 (2011): 423.

63. For a comprehensive discussion of state child abuse and neglect statutes, see Child Welfare Information Gateway, "Definitions of Child Abuse and Neglect: Summary of State Laws," Accessed February 10, 2015. http://www.childwelfare.gov/systemwide/laws_policies/state/index.cfm?event=stateStatutes.processSearch.

64. Roberts, *Shattered Bonds: The Color of Child Welfare*; Nina Bernstein, *The Lost Children of Wilder* (New York: Pantheon Books, 2001).

65. I. Glenn Cohen, "Beyond Best Interests," *Minnesota Law Review* 96 (2012): 1187 (rejecting the idea of regulating procreative choices based on the rationale of the best interest of the resulting child).

66. See generally, Cohen, "Regulating Reproduction: The Problem With Best Interests."

67. See, e.g., John Robertson, "Assisting Reproduction, Choosing Genes, and the Scope of Reproductive Freedom," *George Washington Law Review* 76 (2008): 1490, 1491–1495. See also Mutcherson, "Procreative Pluralism."

68. See, e.g., Radhika Rao, "Equal Liberty: Assisted Reproductive Technology and Reproductive Equality," *George Washington Law Review* 76 (2008): 1457.

69. *Loving v. Virginia*, 388 U.S. 1 (1967); *Meyer v. Nebraska*, 262 U.S. 390 (1923); *Skinner v. Oklahoma*, 316 U.S. 535 (1942).

70. "Men and women of full age, without any limitation due to race, nationality or religion, have the right to marry and to found a family." Universal Declaration of Human Rights (1948).

71. International Conference on Population and Development Programme of Action, para. 7.3, October 18, 1994.

72. *Murillo et al v. Costa Rica*, Inter-American Court of Human Rights, November 28, 2012.

73. Ibid. In a similar case decided by the European Court of Human Rights known as *Evans v. United Kingdom*, and decided in 2007, the Court held that "private life [...] incorporates the right to respect for both the decisions to become and not to become a parent." *Evans* at paras. 71 and 72. Specifically in reference to the regulation of IVF, that Court wrote, "the right to respect for the decision to become a parent in the genetic sense, also falls within the scope of Article 8." *Id.* The same year, in *Dickson v. United Kingdom*, also discussing assisted reproduction, the Court held that "Article 8 is applicable to the applicants' complaints in that the refusal of artificial insemination facilities concerned their private and family lives which notions incorporate the right to respect for their decision to become genetic parents." *Dickson* at para. 66. Finally, in *S.H. and Others v. Austria*, the Court wrote, "the right of a couple to conceive a child and to make use of medically assisted procreation for that purpose is also protected by Article 8, as such a choice is an expression of private and family life." *S.H.* at para. 82.

74. As the American Society for Reproductive Medicine notes, "Fertility programs often receive requests for treatment from single persons, unmarried heterosexual couples, and lesbian and gay couples, but programs vary in their willingness to accept such parents." The Ethics Committee of the American Society for Reproductive Medicine, "Access to Fertility Treatment by Gays, Lesbians, and Unmarried Persons: A Committee Opinion," *Fertility and Sterility* 100 (December 2013): 1524, 1524. The law can even facilitate discrimination through insurance mandates for assisted reproduction that implicitly or explicitly exclude single people or those who are LGBT. Jessica Arons, *Future Choices: Assisted Reproductive Technologies and the Law* (December 2007): 8.

75. See, e.g., S. Golombok et al., "The European Study of Assisted Reproduction Families: Family Functioning and Child Development," *Human Reproduction* 11 (1996): 2324–2331; G. T. Kovacs, et al., "Functioning of Families With Primary School–Age Children Conceived Using Anonymous Donor Sperm," *Human Reproduction* 28 (2013): 375–384. See also ASRM, "Access to Fertility Treatment by Gays, Lesbians, and Unmarried Persons: A Committee Opinion," 1525–1526.

76. According to the Guttmacher Institute, about 51% of the 6.6 million pregnancies in the United States each year are unintended. Guttmacher Institute, *Fact Sheet: Unintended Pregnancy in the United States* (December 2013).

77. Editorial, "Assisted Reproduction and Choice in the Biotech Age: Recommendations for a Way Forward," *Contraception* 83 (2011): 1–4, 1.

78. Ibid.

79. Ibid.

80. See, e.g., N.J.S.A. §37:1-1 (prohibiting incestuous marriages); N.J.S.A. § 37:1-6 (requiring special consent for marriages involving parties under the age of 18).

81. See, e.g., *Reynolds v. United States*, 98 U.S. 145 (1878) (statute punishing bigamy did not violate the Free Exercise Clause of the Constitution); *State v. Holm*, 137 p.3d 726 (Sup. Ct. Utah 2006) (upholding conviction for bigamy).

82. See, e.g., *United States v. Windsor*, 133 S.Ct 2675 (2013) (striking down portion of the Defense of Marriage Act that defined marriage as being between one man and one woman).

83. *Planned Parenthood of Southeastern Pa. v. Casey*, 505 U.S. 833 (1992).

CHAPTER 8

....

REPRODUCTION AS
A CIVIL RIGHT

....

ANITA SILVERS AND LESLIE FRANCIS

In calling for access to the health care people need to make their reproductive goals achievable, defenders of reproductive freedom typically appeal to rights. But what kinds of rights are these? Are they human rights or civil rights? Are they rights to protection from interference or undue impediment, such as rights to due process, equal treatment, liberty, or privacy? Or may the requisite rights include substantively more? May they, for instance, underwrite the distribution of resources to individuals who for one or another reason are undeservedly hampered in regard to reproduction but whose disadvantage is susceptible to a health care cure?

In analyzing rights and their implications, a crucial initial distinction lies between ideal justice and the requirements of justice under conditions of injustice (e.g., Stemplowska 2008, 2009; Valentini 2012). What rights there are, and how these rights are to be understood, may be very different as seen from these two theoretical stances. As a matter of ideal justice, for example, freedom of speech or freedom to choose what will be done with one's body may be prevailing rights. In contexts where injustice pervades, however, the practice of freedom of speech may become problematic: consider protests outside of abortion clinics, physicians expressing opinions to patients that abortions cause breast cancer, or states requiring women seeking abortions to view videos of fetal development or barring pediatricians from asking parents whether there are firearms in the home. There are similar problems with freedom to choose what will be done to or with one's body, as practices of female genital alteration (to use a neutral term) or child sexploitation aptly illustrate. And because resource distribution is always affected by the availability of resources, rights to resources for health care, including reproductive health care, call for theorizing about justice under conditions of wealth disparity, not for ideal justice theory.

To set out the scope of our inquiry into reproductive rights, we note that in regard to reproduction many different kinds of disadvantage can occur. And at least some initially may seem antithetical to each other. For example, low sperm count and poor ovarian reserve (oopause) impose reproductive disadvantage on people who desire offspring, but being fully fertile can be reproductively disadvantageous in case people instead desire to be free of the imposition of a parental role. Thus, depending on individual circumstance, fertility and infertility each may occasion harm, or at least conceivably be contrary to someone's interests.

Reproduction plainly is a natural biological process that enables continuation of the species for every kind of living thing. So it also may seem plain that when humans invoke a right to reproduction, we are simply expressing our claims to what our human nature means for us to do. To the contrary, however, an examination of twentieth-century legal history where the capacity to reproduce is defended as a right exposes flaws in taking a human rights approach to equitable access to reproduction. To illustrate, reproduction of, or by, individuals identified as disabled remains a contentious topic, first because there have been, and still are, practices of preventing the birth of people with disabilities but not far behind because there have been and still are practices of preventing parenting by people with disabilities. Construing reproductive rights as civil rather than human rights illuminates these controversies and helps resolve them, or so we argue here.

The rapid advent of more and more applications of biotechnology now enables previously unimaginable control over reproduction: prenatal or even preimplantation identification of biological anomalies, interventions to select among embryos, in vitro initiation of pregnancies, perimortem and postmortem extraction of sperm for insemination, successful outcomes of high-risk preterm births, and a replete repertoire of interventions for contravening fertility. Nor have natural boundaries, or other looming limitations standing in the way of still further technological advances, appeared.

With the advent of powerful techniques to facilitate or discourage reproduction, the need to consider alternative approaches to reproductive access, such as the civil rights view we explore here, becomes more imperative. In this chapter we contrast human rights and civil rights approaches to reproduction-related health care. We argue that it is too easy for a human rights view to assume that it is species-typical individuals who are bearers of reproductive rights. So we examine instead the plausibility, power, and more capacious inclusiveness of a civil rights point of view.

ATYPICAL HUMANS
AND REPRODUCTIVE RIGHTS

Consider the contrast between *Buck v. Bell* and *Skinner v. Oklahoma*, rulings on mandatory sterilization handed down by the US Supreme Court. *Buck v. Bell*[1]—to this day not overruled—remains one of the most notorious decisions in the history of the US Supreme Court, holding that mandated sterilization of persons believed to be intellectually deficient is constitutionally permissible because "three generations of imbeciles are enough." The premise is that the state may call upon its citizens—explicitly here its presumptively biologically deficient citizens—to sacrifice the natural inclination to become parents for society's overall greater good.

The declaration in *Skinner*, only 15 years later, that Oklahoma's Habitual Criminal Sterilization Act was unconstitutional is celebrated as a watershed decision that a state has overstepped its power with respect to reproductive rights.[2] But Justice Douglas's opinion for the Court rejecting sterilization of an habitual thief, along with Chief Justice Stone's concurrence, take care to refer with unequivocal approval to the sterilization of Carrie Buck, the 18-year-old rape victim institutionalized in the Virginia State Colony for Epileptics and Feebleminded. With the exception of a concurrence by Justice Jackson, none of the Justices of the Supreme Court seem troubled by their rejecting sterilization for the supposedly biologically criminal Skinner while reaffirming endorsement of sterilization of the supposedly biologically cognitively impaired Buck.

Oklahoma's statute at issue in *Skinner* defined a habitual criminal as a person convicted two or more times for a felony involving moral turpitude and thereafter convicted in Oklahoma of a third such felony and sentenced to prison. Oklahoma's attorney general could then start a sterilization proceeding after giving the defendant notice and an opportunity to be heard on whether he or she (most likely he) was a habitual criminal and whether sterilization would be detrimental to his health—but notably not on the heritability of his condition.

Justice Douglas, in writing the opinion for the Court, began thus with an invocation of human rights: "This case touches a sensitive and important area of human rights . . . a right which is basic to the perpetuation of a race—the right to have offspring."[3] It is the presence of such human rights that brings equal protection into play. Relying explicitly on *Buck v. Bell*, Justice Douglas observes that equal protection is a last resort of constitutional argument: states are free to classify people differently for even minimally plausible reasons, but not when fundamental rights like reproduction are transgressed.

Habitual felons have these rights, like other human beings, and Oklahoma did not advance any reasoned account of why the particular group of habitual felons it singled out was any different from other accused felons not subject to the sterilization provision. That is, Oklahoma stripped out people who happened to have committed certain felonies from protections against sterilization, but without any explanation of why other kinds of criminals retained their reproductive rights. Justice Douglas distinguished this reasoning from the sterilization in *Buck v. Bell* not because Buck had been given a hearing but because he thought her sterilization potentially improved equality for her as it would allow her to leave the institution for life in the community. And, he thought that even with strict scrutiny, "'the law does all that is needed when it does all that it can, indicates a policy, applies it to all within the lines, and seeks to bring within the lines all similarly situated so far and so fast as its means allow'" (at 540, quoting *Buck v. Bell*).

Chief Justice Stone criticized this equal protection reasoning as insufficiently robust. Oklahoma would equally lack empirical support for the lines it drew among groups if it classified different crimes as felonies involving moral turpitude and hence warranting sterilization for supposedly heritable traits, or even all criminals as having similarly heritable deleterious traits. Without such empirical support, the state must acknowledge individuals' right to be heard by granting them a hearing about their individual circumstances, Chief Justice Stone argued. Thus, the state must accord due process rights to individuals who are subject to a sterilization decision and must prove the heritability of socially injurious tendencies in their particular case. This it had not done for Skinner.

In their analyses, both Justice Douglas and Chief Justice Stone referred approvingly to *Buck v. Bell*. Justice Douglas, in the passage just quoted, assumes the reasonableness of the state's decision to sterilize people whom it determines to be mentally deficient. Chief Justice Stone, in his opinion, cited *Buck v. Bell* for what he judged to be the "undoubtedly" correct proposition that "a state may, after appropriate inquiry constitutionally interfere with the personal liberty of the individual to prevent the transmission by inheritance of his socially injurious tendencies."[4] His only point was that it requires a hearing to make this determination. Neither Justice Douglas nor Chief Justice Stone seems to have noticed the incongruity of their apparent readiness to countenance the sterilization of members of one disfavored group while roundly condemning the sterilization of some, or all, members of another such group.

A natural explanation of their oversight is that without reflection they presume Buck's kind of defect disqualifies her as a full human rights bearer while Skinner's kind of defect does not debilitate his human rights (cf. Silvers 2012). Nor do they seem concerned that the due process right they do allow to her affords only scant security, if any at all. The deprivation of individuals who fail to function normally may feel natural to them and thereby inoffensive to the ideal of fairness under the law.

By contrast, Justice Jackson's concurrence deploys several elements of what we regard as a civil rights approach. He was insistent that scientific evidence be assembled before claims about certain kinds of individuals being unfit for society or injurious to it are advanced. Expressing general skepticism about the state of scientific support for the heritability of intelligence, he asked whether similar doubts might be directed to legislative assumptions about the heritability of stealing chickens (the transgression that introduced Skinner to his life of crime). With these considerations, Justice Jackson underlined the importance of marshaling systematic evidence rather than mere suppositions to scrutinize legislative justifications that are susceptible to scientific evaluation. This is emphatically the case for legislation that introduces categorizations that disadvantage some kinds of individuals in comparison to others.

Moreover, Justice Jackson insisted that even when categorizations are justifiable, there must also be what anti-discrimination law now calls an individualized assessment rather than the application of stereotypes to individuals within these categories. That is, a judgment such as that thieves can be subject to sterilization because they are likely to beget further thieves is insufficient to show that a particular thief is likely to be reproductively dangerous to society in this way.

Furthermore, Justice Jackson appears to be considering whether societal practices thought to serve the overall good can be justified in light of minority differences, although he does not say so explicitly. He emphasized that, even if there were scientific support for believing that intellectual disability was heritable, "[t]here are limits to the extent to which a legislatively represented majority may conduct biological experiments at the expense of the dignity and personality and natural powers of a minority—even those who have been guilty of what the majority define as crimes."[5] These limits are set for multiple reasons, including equality and due process of law. And they may be set differently in different circumstances: When the boundaries of categories are very narrowly drawn, due process might only require a hearing to determine whether the individual is a member of the category; when categories are more loosely drawn, individualized hearings will be critical because of the likely differences among individuals within the category.

Although not saying so explicitly, Justice Jackson appears to be assuming the possibility of contexts in which differing types of injustice might be operative and thus different types of critical legal scrutiny employed. This, too, is a core feature of a civil rights approach. To summarize, Justice Jackson's opinion emphasizes the importance of types of careful scrutiny, sensitive to the social circumstances and even to the impermissibility of applying some types of categorization to individuals, especially when the result is to treat those individuals disadvantageously differently with respect to certain basic interests.

In the spirit of Justice Jackson's observations, this chapter explores what it means to view reproductive rights as civil rights rather than human rights. From a civil rights perspective, rights are seen as tools that both emerge from and enable the kinds of human interactions that shape social environments, and not as ontological entailments of the kinds of creatures humans are constructed to be. In what follows, we address the impact of such a strategic progressive stance on opportunities for different kinds of atypical people to acquire access to medical technology in order to reproduce, or not—that is, so as to bring their reproduction under their own control. Of course, decisions about whether and how to form families are central to intimate interactions in the lives of many—hence, the importance of reproduction, as Justice Douglas affirmed. But it does not follow from the centrality of these interests to human well-being that they must be conceptualized in human rights terms.

Rights: Human and Civil

Familiarly, "human" rights are invoked in grand fashion to counter abuses across the globe. "Civil" rights may appear, by contrast, to offer a slighter—indeed a substandard—version because they are socially, politically, and legally formed, informed, and propelled, and consequently are relativized to cultural contexts. Yet as a matter of political history, the sweeping symbolic force of human rights may have mainly ephemeral efficacy, while the trajectory of civil rights movements, over the past century especially, seems to have established a record of continuing progress.

Human Rights

Human rights theory is premised on the conviction that all humans share some critically important feature in virtue of which they are owed the fundamental protections that rights bring. As such, human rights are inclusive of all members of the human species—or so they are supposed to be. Thus, the Universal Declaration of Human Rights begins: "Whereas recognition of the inherent dignity and of the equal and inalienable rights of all members of the human family is the foundation of freedom, justice and peace in the world . . . " (United Nations 1948) And the US Declaration of Independence proclaims: "We hold these truths to be self-evident, that all men are created equal, that they are endowed by their Creator with certain unalienable Rights, that among these are Life, Liberty and the pursuit of Happiness" (US Congress 1776).

This account of human rights is an expression of "human exceptionalism": the belief that rights belong only to humans uniquely in virtue of some defining characteristic of humanity, whether that characteristic be viewed as natural, god given, or simply postulated (Silvers 2012). For such human exceptionalism not to be merely arbitrary, humans must be distinguishable from other animals in some way that can be articulated and defended. *Contra* defenders of ascribing rights to nonhuman animals, human exceptionalism restricts rights bearing to humans only and consequently has been condemned as "speciesist," a fault analogous to racism in the view of its critics (Singer 1975, 2009).

Rights claims pertaining to biological individuals who might resemble humans in some—indeed, in many or even most—respects are open to being dismissed on ontological grounds based on the absence of a purportedly essential human-making property (Silvers 2012).

If this view is to be defended, all humans—or at least all humans who are bearers of what are thought to be human rights—must have the common property. Thus, John Finnis, attributing the concept of human rights to St. Thomas Aquinas: "[t]hough he never uses a term translatable as 'human rights,' Aquinas clearly has the concept. He articulates it when he sums up the 'precepts of justice' by saying that justice centrally . . . concerns what is owed to 'everyone in common' or 'to everyone alike . . . ' rather than to determinate persons for reasons particular to them . . ." (Finnis 1998, 136).

Indeed, depending on what property is in question, entities that do not yet have the property but that may in time—as fetuses are characterized by some—cannot be said to have rights either, although they may be entitled to protection in virtue of the likelihood that they will come to have these rights (Marquis 1989). Conversely, humans who do not have the property at all and who will not predictably come to have the property will not be the bearers of rights. And so, based on their supposed deficits in essential human capacities, people with disabilities often are excluded from legal recognition as full persons and thereby denied the status of rights bearers.

Human rights are supposed to be universal, but standardly adduced essential human-making properties such as the capacity for reason are not coextensive with the class of individuals who are biologically human. Thus, contrary to any mandate of equality in human rights, this strategy divides individuals whose heritage is human into classes of higher and lower status, with the former but not the latter group enjoying protection through having rights. That affirmation of their full legal standing (UN CRPD 2006, Art. 12), including enjoyment of rights, has been hard for disabled people to attain suggests the hazards of invoking species-definitive physical, psychological, or mental capacities in validating human rights. These problems are nowhere more apparent than in regard to reproduction, as will be seen shortly.

We have argued elsewhere that two different components of human nature have been cited as the proper basis for recognizing human rights. One kind of property is a broadly construed psychological, intellectual, or mental property. The other is a broadly construed biological or material property (Silvers 2012; Silvers and Francis 2013).

The argument for human rights based on distinctively human psychological or mental properties typically cites a crucial cognitive or other kind of mental capacity to differentiate humans from other species. For example, Tooley (1972, 44) argued that "An organism possesses a serious right to life only if it possesses the concept of a self as a continuing subject of experiences and other mental states, and believes that it is itself such a continuing entity." A further step equates distinctively human psychological capacity with the capacity for self-governed rational conduct, and especially for formulating aims for action through self-reflection (Wasserman et al. 2013). Each person therefore should respect the capacity of adult humans to execute the requisite kind of rational action and to accept self-reflective responsibility for what they have done. But exercising these exceptional human capacities, it is contended, requires being sufficiently self-directing and free from social and political subordination to self-determine the good for one's self (Silvers and Francis 2010).

Placing rights on this basis, however, precludes the possibility that human rights can attach to all human beings. People with cognitive disabilities commonly have been judged as failing to meet the standard of capacity for self-reflective, self-governing (and thereby responsible) action (Francis 2009). And, indeed, even people whose deficits are solely corporeal rather than cognitive not unusually are treated as so dependent as to suffer from a similarly attenuated capacity for self-direction. In sum, individuals who are biologically human but are perceived as lacking some human capacity to a crucial degree have been denied the usual moral and legal protections that human rights are expected to bestow.

These judgments reflect a practice—rising almost to a disposition—of underestimating the capacities of individuals owing to their disabilities (Amundson and Tresky 2007). For centuries, intellectually disabled people, as well as people with other kinds of disabilities such as hearing impairments, were denied schooling and then condemned as being unable to learn because they lacked reading and writing skills. This illustrates the effect of bias on accurate assessment of disabled people's capacity (Murdick, Gartin, and Crabtree 2006). Such underestimations have been especially apparent in reproduction, where people with disabilities have been assumed to be asexual, kept from developing sexually[6] (O'Reilly 2007), sterilized when they behave in sexual ways,[7] denied access to reproductive assistance (Orentlicher, this volume, Chapter 16), or deprived of custody of the children they do have (Oeullette 2011, Ch. 5). Such treatment of reproduction and persons with disabilities underscores the importance of Justice Jackson's insistence on the corrective force of scientific evidence and individualized assessments.

If humankind's exceptional capacities are not the hallmark of rights bearers, perhaps the universality of human rights lies in the other familiar articulation of human exceptionalism, that humans are all equally products of a special and singularly successful biological evolutionary process. In its nonrelational contemporary version, this view equates bearing rights with the presence of a human genome. In reply to the apparent arbitrariness of drawing such a critical ethical line between humans and nonhumans on the basis of genetic difference (e.g., McMahan 2005; Singer 2009), Kittay (2005) has developed a relational view of the import of the biological evolutionary process.

The basic idea here is that humans are naturally constructed to be concerned about ourselves, and for those we believe to be our close biological kin as well. We biologically bond with kin to care for our offspring, and we naturally also ally with the smaller and larger circles of humans on whom our own welfare and our family's welfare depend. This is especially the case for parents and their children, according to Kittay (2012; see also Vehmas 1999).

This relational version of human exceptionalism also lends itself to privileging some humans and marginalizing or excluding others, however. If kinship is supposed to be the basis of each human's duty to acknowledge human rights of others, individuals with stronger and deeper familial bonds will enjoy a more secure status than others, depending on the strength and breadth of their familial bonds (Silvers 2012). Adrienne Asch and Erik Parens (2000), among others, have developed powerful criticisms of the disability discrimination implicit in these views, especially when relational bonds encircle the nondisabled but leave out the disabled, as is the case for those opponents of abortion who nevertheless countenance the procedure to prevent potentially disabled children from being born (see also Lawson 2006).

A reply is that we are all bound together by our common humanity; this is the broad relational categorization that steps into the gap when familial or other special relationship ties are not apparent. No one will be left out, for then everyone will have someone to care for them in virtue of the ties that bind human beings together. But it is difficult to see how this position differs from a nonrelational biological approach. The observation of common humanity does not construct special relationships; it simply postulates biological humanness as relational, thus assuming what needs to be argued.

Virginia Held has argued that care ethics can be deployed globally with the development of wider, admittedly weaker, care relationships:

> Weaker but still *caring* relations can be seen and should be far more developed in the wider contexts of political and social life and global relations. The connections of civil society, much more appreciated in recent years than in the past, are understood as necessary for political and legal systems to function, or function well. They may be thought of as weak but caring relations. For the rights of fellow citizens to be respected or their interests promoted, we have to care sufficiently about our fellow citizens. This caring should gradually be extended to our fellow inhabitants of the globe, so that we can live in peace with one another, and so that the moral outrage of still widespread poverty is overcome. (Held 2014, 113)

However, it is an empirical question whether the expansion of such ties actually does develop so as to expand their influence across the globe, for the predictability of achieving such universal social evolution is neither simply presumable nor assured.

Civil Rights

The alternative approach sketched here, a civil rights approach, rejects metaphysical contentions about essential human-making properties upon which rights-bearing turns. Instead, it bases rights claims on expanding possibilities for inclusion in the acceptability or attraction of particular configurations of social institutions and arrangements. Individually as well as collectively, we humans are both creators of our own political and cultural values and yet we also are creatures of the constricting or liberating political and cultural conditions we construct for ourselves or inherit from our predecessors.

It follows that we humans possess individual and collective powers to narrow or expand who are recognized as the parties included in such tacit cooperative agreements. And we can, also collectively and cooperatively, regulate the repertoire of roles available to offer access to social participation and thereby to facilitate different kinds of individuals' inclusion. (For a further discussion of constructivist accounts of rights, see Rhodes, this volume, Chapter 3.)

Thus understood, civil rights underwrite claims that are pressed within the relationships established by social arrangements. Humans live and interact in communities, developing, shaping, testing, and reshaping norms by which to live together. The requirements of political morality are context dependent and ever evolving. As Ruth Anna Putnam (2000, 177) points out, "Unlike other social animals, we are able to reflect on the ways in which we cooperate and on the effects of the manner of our association on ourselves and others."

As we have argued elsewhere (Silvers and Francis 2005), justice is constructed through building trust relationships that are inclusive of outliers and should be understood always as a work in progress. Despite the attractions of prescribing ideally and fully realized fair outcomes as the only goal of the search for justice, we should not expect that fully inclusive and therefore universal justice can be a fait accompli—or even a fully articulated goal. Instead, justice in practice calls for ongoing examination and reexamination of social arrangements that are barriers to flourishing for disregarded kinds of individuals. Civil rights claims, in short, are asserted as particularly important commitments for breaking down these barriers.

As such fundamental commitments, civil rights claims mandate consideration of equality among those in civil society. Civil rights operate less like the tools of formal equality and more like instruments for infusing practical equality into the lives people are able to live. Secured within, rather than transcending, social communities (Carreira da Silva 2013), their function is to press political institutions to recognize what is necessary for all members to lead flourishing lives within them, hence their acknowledgment of universal aspiration.

Understood pragmatically, civil rights are instruments for expanding pragmatic equality among different kinds of individuals who happen to be interacting with one another. In the spirit of Justice Jackson, their expression thus resists schemes that appoint some individuals as more deserving of flourishing or relegate them to lesser forms of flourishing than others. As such, civil rights claims both reflect and challenge extant social arrangements along with the resource commitments and constraints that both shape and sustain these arrangements. In so doing, they build on what exists in the continuing effort to create social conditions under which all have the opportunity to flourish.

From a practical political organizing perspective, calls for civil rights engagement are familiar inspiration for progressive pragmatic efforts. They are not claims for the elimination of differences or a guarantee of equal outcomes. Rather, civil rights propel the mediating effects of social institutions: how these institutions construct barriers to inclusion by making unsubstantiated assumptions about certain types of people, structure resource support that enables some but is inaccessible to others, or underwrite apparently neutral practices that fit the capacities of some but handicap other individuals in effective enjoyment of opportunities.

Within this context, in the first instance civil rights are claims on social attention to remove disparately deployed barriers that disadvantage disregarded kinds of people but not favored kinds. Such barriers include not only laws that prohibit members of disfavored groups from using public accommodations, consign them to separate schools, or mandate their sterilization, but also include architectural designs that block access to health care clinics for individuals who cannot climb stairs or equipment designs such as medical examining tables that some kinds of individuals cannot mount (Pendo 2008). Civil rights claims also can be calls for attention to how unfairly resources continue to be distributed despite awareness of human differences. A familiar example is educational materials that can be read by those who are sighted and manually unimpaired, but are not reproduced in digitized format to make them usable to print-disabled people as well. Other examples might also be providing parental education only in formats designed for nondisabled parents, and health care facilities that are located conveniently to affluent communities but are more difficult for other groups—especially nondrivers—to reach.

Civil rights claims also can critique accepted practices that foster flourishing for some but may impede others from developing or exercising capacities central to well-being. Examples include rules that insist upon typical or popular ways of performing tasks without considering effective alternatives. Consider differences in ways of parenting described by Adam Cureton in Chapter 18 in this volume. Civil rights claims may be bolstered by demonstrating benefits beyond their target group. A familiar example is how installation of curb cuts enables transit both for people with mobility impairments who use wheelchairs to ambulate and unimpaired people who are pushing baby carriages.

Negative and Positive Rights

When they are invoked to remedy injustices arising from imposition of majority preferences on everybody alike, civil rights claims have often been cast predominantly as what some call "negative rights"—rights to protection from interference. A primary source of injustice against which progress is sought is the use of state power by social majorities to regulate or suppress social minorities—as Jim Crow laws did and as mandatory sterilization laws did as well. This is why, as Justice Jackson noted, we may need to insist on both equal protection and due process working together: We need scrutiny of the correctness of categorizations along with scrutiny of their applicability in particular cases. But this is not invocation of purely abstract or formal equal protection or due process. The state must not only refrain from treating powerless, vulnerable minorities disadvantageously—it should also scrutinize whether institutionalized social practices embed bias that disadvantages minorities.

Whether there is a distinction between rights to protection from interference and rights to resources is a central dispute within the rights literature. Civil rights approaches question this division, noting that the types of protections or resources required for inclusion may vary with the social context. Instead, the gravamen of civil rights claims is to address categorical allocations that fail to take differences into account in addressing the needs of each.

An example is questioning whether there are important differences between security against unsanitary or adulterated food products and support in purchasing and preparing meals for the minority too impaired to do so themselves. How to address these different needs under conditions of resource constraints is a matter of constant adjustment and reconsideration of how more can be achieved without compromising other critical needs. Civil rights approaches do not demand specified minimum levels of resources. But they do call for developing and deploying resources to further more equitable flourishing of disregarded groups.

Our contention in this chapter is that implementation and exercise of these rights should be understood within a pragmatic rather than a metaphysical framework. Rights must be grounded explicitly in acknowledgment of people's differences rather than rooted in claims about how humans essentially are the same. Moreover, rights instantiation takes place in given social contexts rather than as theoretical idealization: how rights are put in place specifically in a given social context is affected by the normative understandings at that time and the resources that are reasonably available in that place.

These tacit understandings are not static, of course. They are continually being pressed to make progress for comparatively disadvantaged groups by expanding avenues for flourishing. When rights to health care are understood as civil rights rather than human rights, for example, they can be seen to be always in transition as medicine develops new techniques that expand the dimensions of well-being that cutting-edge health care can improve, as well as new awareness of who should be facilitated in benefitting from these techniques.

Existing assumptions and resources are only the start, however. Their inclusiveness is subject to ongoing challenge in terms of whether they allow everyone equally to lead flourishing lives in accord with their own conceptions of their good.[8] The idea here is that the right to health care should not be understood in terms of a fixed set of services provided to all; rather, what the right requires should be developed through testing and challenging the extent to which allocations can and should be arranged to permit each to flourish.

REPRODUCTIVE RIGHTS AS CIVIL RIGHTS

In this section, we explore how reproductive rights may be helpfully understood as civil rights. So as to address issues of access to fertility treatment and to consider the need for social support in parenting, we argue that a civil rights approach may help to counter the view that reproductive rights can do no more than offer protection from interference with reproductive choices. In contrast, human rights approaches, by idealizing the species-typical human agent, may encourage problematic assumptions about the kinds of protections these agents need and about reproduction as only for those who can do so in the species-typical way.

Civil Rights and Reproductive Liberty

In the liberal tradition, it is common to privilege the liberty rights that free individuals from interference over rights to resources such as food or shelter. Assumptions about features shared by typical human beings can make this distinction seem plausible and maintainable. From Hobbes and Locke on, liberal theorists have recognized that human beings cannot rely on themselves for protection of their physical security from invasion by others and have predicated the authority of the state on this need for protection from others. On this picture, the primary role of social institutions with the power of coercion is to protect individuals from one another rather than to assure access to resources.

Once protections of the state are in place, a familiar version of this liberal picture assumes, ordinary humans are capable of providing for their needs in other respects. Children and the elderly aside, human beings may appear able for the most part to do this, perhaps by purchasing insurance to guard against unanticipated costs. In the background, however, the role of supportive social institutions—the family, social institutions in the private sector, or economic institutions—in fulfilling these needs may go unrecognized. Such oversimplified versions of liberalism thus miss the myriad ways in which social institutions may affect abilities to flourish within civil society.

Also on this picture, when others who do not meet assumed norms in some way need help in fulfilling their needs—even for basic food or shelter—these may be seen as welfarist demands. Such nonidealized protection may be characterized as conferring "benefits" or "welfare" or "special privileges" rather than civil rights, and they may be subjected to criticism as such. Such objection leaves behind those who cannot benefit from the standard protections—rather as individuals with mobility impairments might be left behind by emergency evacuation procedures suited just to the needs of individuals with the ability to walk or even to run. The established protective framework will not seem burdensome to those meeting the standard for whom it was designed. Concomitantly, alterations in it to accommodate more kinds of individuals may be seen as inappropriately burdensome impositions on those for whom opportunity is not expanded due to the changes.

In regard to reproduction, this account may play out as protecting reproductive choices from coercive interferences on the part of others, whether those choices are the right to avoid or to engage in reproduction. That is, it may be seen as a right to reproductive liberty rather than as a right to effective implementation of reproductive choices. Thus, libertarian views about reproductive rights emphasize removing legal barriers to contraception or abortion but not rights to low-cost contraception or to funding for abortions. Such views also condemn coercive state policies limiting family size such as China's one-child policy—but not policies that as a practical matter make the process of reproduction especially difficult, whether to initiate or to halt. *Harris v. McRae*, for example, is a US Supreme Court decision concluding that the right to choose an abortion does not extend to the right to funding for that procedure.[9]

Any claimed rights to resources needed for effective implementation of reproductive choice may be criticized as ill defined and excessively demanding. So proposals for rights to health care have been criticized as boundless when they are conceptualized to include all care that might be beneficial to anyone. To respond requires a plausible account of how limits may be drawn in particular contexts. One such response has been to invoke the normal, for example as Norman Daniels (1985) did at one point by delineating justice in health care in terms of the care required for normal species-typical functioning over an ordinary life span. But even this narrow approach may be criticized as representing an uneasy compromise between placing great demands on social resources to the extent that it is achievable at all (Buchanan 1984; Barlow 1999) and leaving out those who are incapable of normal species-typical functioning (Silvers, Wasserman, and Mahowald 1998, 156).

Leaving abstinence aside (which may not even be a possibility for those who cannot protect themselves against nonconsensual sex), contraception (including the limiting case of sterilization) and abortion are the medical means to prevent reproduction. Both legalization of contraception and abortion, and their funding and availability, can be seen as civil rights questions. A civil rights perspective examines the significance of the practical unavailability of these procedures to those who do not fit paradigms of normalcy, in comparison to those who do fit this standard.

Consider, first, rights to contraception. When contraception is seen as a right to noninterference with its acquisition and use, the focus is on legal barriers to its availability. Such barriers in US law were addressed in the Supreme Court's decision in *Griswold v. Connecticut*,[10] the case declaring that Connecticut's prohibition on the use of contraceptives was an unconstitutional limit on the right to privacy. But there also should be focus on coerced requirements for its use, as there have been with mandatory sterilization of disfavored groups in the United States or with liberal objections to China's imposition of the one-child policy.

If the paradigm of the contraceptive user is the typical patient who is motivated by personal preferences, acting on noncoerced choices, and competently acting on independent decisions about personal preferences, there may seem to be no justification for social resources to provide contraception. This portrayal of the so-called average agent disregards how social arrangements might deter or facilitate the ready availability of contraception (McGuinness and Widdows, this volume, Chapter 2). And those who are discouraged by social arrangements from contraceptive use may face very unattractive choices if they are fertile but do not wish to reproduce. Like Carrie Buck, poor women too often are unjustifiably blamed for having the sex that resulted in an unplanned pregnancy (Whitaker 2014). The cheapest option may be sterilization that disproportionally denies them the opportunity for reproduction should they so choose at a later point in time. And those who cannot use contraception in the normal manner—for example, those with physical conditions that make them unable to administer or use currently available forms of contraception or those with intellectual disabilities that make them unreliable contraceptive users—may face coerced contraception in the form of sterilization, made more palatable if they are not seen as bearers of reproductive rights at all (Pfeiffer 1994).

Indeed, any practice of sterilization imposed on or recommended for individuals due to disability evokes suspicion about a discriminatory normalcy standard because the history of sterilization is a history of abuse of people with disabilities. Sterilization is, after all, a comparatively inexpensive and permanently effective method to insure that someone will not reproduce. *Buck v. Bell*[11]—never overruled and hence potentially more than a symbol of abuse long past (Eisenberg 2013)—legitimizes sterilization on the basis of the burdens people with disabilities supposedly place on society. The words of Justice Holmes—"three generations of imbeciles are enough"—echo today in some permitted sterilization practices.

Although US courts now generally view compelled sterilization as a clear interference with constitutional liberty rights,[12] and thus subject to due process guarantees (Eisenberg 2013, 220–221), such rights can be overcome in what is supposed to be the narrowly tailored pursuit of a compelling state interest but may in fact may be allowed much wider scope. The most recent return of the sterilization issue to the US Supreme Court, albeit nearly 40 years ago, gave full immunity to a trial court judge who clearly violated due process in a sterilization decision.[13] There is also evidence that states vary in the extent to which they accord the protections of the law to people with disabilities faced with compulsory sterilization, particularly when the disability is intellectual or psychiatric (Volz 2006, 209–211; Kundnani 2013).

As with contraception, abortion, even though legal, may be practically unavailable for many. As a practical matter, factors such as cost or availability of providers may make it far more difficult for some kinds of people than for others to obtain abortions: those who cannot travel or those who lack resources to pay for the procedure. Even if such categorizations are de facto rather than de jure, they raise civil rights questions of equal treatment if they continue unexamined and unabated.

Furthermore, the normality standard may resurface in judgments about who should be protected from pressures to abort. Abortion may too readily be judged to be "therapeutic" when the pregnant woman is a person with a disability, even when the pregnancy is intended and desired by her (e.g., Hoglund and Larsson 2013). Civil rights analysis can serve as a reminder of the need for evidence about pregnancy management and outcomes so that women with disabilities are not stereotyped as reproductive risks and unjustly pressured to avoid pregnancies or to terminate them (Lebel et al. 2012, concluding that pregnancy outcomes are not worse for women with documented scoliosis; NCD 2012, Ch. 13).

With abortion, the normality of the fetus is also in play. Many who would oppose abortion generally are more willing to accept it for fetuses that are predicted to develop into children with disabilities, as well as for women who are perceived as being too disabled to care for the fetus should it be carried to term (Asch and Parens 2000). Leslie Reagan (2010) documents how rhetoric of the horror of fetal anomalies and disabled children historically has spurred efforts to legalize abortion. Both the German measles epidemic of 1963–1965 and the thalidomide "tragedy" of the early 1960s brought widespread publicity about "damaged" fetuses and the burdens these children might impose on families and the larger society. Popular magazines such as *Time* published stark, medicalized photographs and exaggerated and unsubstantiated reports of actual disabilities (Reagan 2010, Ch. 2). Parents were encouraged to institutionalize children in light of their supposed inabilities to function, especially when the children had intellectual impairments (Reagan 2010, 66). A hostess for a local version of the television show "Romper Room," Sherri Finkbine, mother of four who had taken thalidomide early in her fifth pregnancy, made a highly publicized trip for an abortion to Sweden, where the procedure was legal; her plight drew widespread sympathy for legalization of abortion in the United States (Planned Parenthood Advocates of Arizona 2012).

This advocacy omitted the dismal levels of social support for children with disabilities to enable them to live in the community—indeed, much was based on the presumed need for institutionalization of these children. Even today, lack of social supports together with exaggerated prognoses of incapacities may significantly influence parents' unwillingness to carry through with pregnancy and parenting by themselves or others (Dresser 2009; Le Dref et al. 2013).

Achieving Reproduction? Civil Rights and Infertility

Technological advances have made pregnancy possible for many who could not achieve it on their own. Such inability may be physiological as with early menopause or social as with same-sex couples. Although under the Americans with Disabilities Act fertility clinics are public accommodations subject to a nondiscrimination requirement, evidence persists that reproductive clinics are unwilling to provide fertility care to women with disabilities (Mutcherson, this volume, Chapter 7). In one court case, for example, Kijuana Chambers, blind since birth, sought in vitro fertilization and was refused services by fertility physicians who were concerned that she would be unable to care for the child. The jury decided in favor of the physicians in Chambers's suit for damage.[14] Chambers found another clinic to do the procedure and gave birth to a daughter in 2001.[15]

Judgments of normality also surface as the view that infertility is a matter of shared concern when it results from disease but not when it occurs naturally. For example, in his seminal discussion of justice in health care, Norman Daniels struggles to determine whether infertility is the kind of deviation from normal functioning that requires attention in a just health care system (Daniels 1985, 32; compare Daniels 2008, 145; Ram-Tiktin 2012). If infertility results from disease such as treatment for cancer, Daniels originally argued, health care systems should address it, but not if it is a species-typical variation such as earlier menopause.

When reproductive rights are seen only as rights to protection from interference, claims for support of individuals who cannot reproduce without specialized fertility care or people for whom reproduction requires other forms of support are left aside (see Mutcherson, Chapter 7; Darr, Chapter 10; Orentlicher, Chapter 16). The Affordable Care Act (ACA) requirement about what health insurance plans must cover as essential health benefits illustrates (ASRM 2015). These essential benefits include items and services within 10 broad categories; one of the categories is maternity and newborn care. But the category extends only to treatment for pregnancy, birth, and pediatric care, not to achievement of pregnancy.

In the few states mandating coverage of infertility care, state benchmark plans based on insurance plans already in existence within the state will cover infertility care. But in other states, they will not. Moreover, although the US government has postponed implementation of this part of ACA, eventually federal subsidies for insurance will not cover any part of premiums attributable to state mandates that go beyond federally mandated essential health benefits.

Civil rights approaches can question this limitation as unjust treatment of people who cannot achieve reproduction unassisted. The problem is equality in achieving what may be important life goals for many—to have children. Health insurance as presently structured in the United States, for example, may bear extensive costs for pregnancy and newborn care; recent estimates put the cost of the 4 million births annually in the United States at over $50 billion (Rosenthal 2013) and the cost for the 10% of babies needing care in a newborn intensive care unit at over $3,000 per day (Kornhauser and Schneiderman 2010). But support for reproductive technology is far less generous.

Attempts to draw lines for access in practice to reproductive technology in terms of normalcy may inappropriately disadvantage or damage individuals who do not fit the norm while privileging other people just because they are typical. In contrast, a civil rights approach does not depend on viewing some capacities as crucial to being human and therefore can be more responsive to human differences. A civil rights view also can offer a different perspective on drawing limits by considering what may be achieved to mitigate, within existing resources, disparate impact due to biological or other differences.

For example, while the biological identity of members of female same-sex couples and single celibate women may permit each to reproduce heterosexually, their interpersonal identity does not. Consequently, they require reproductive medical intervention to conceive. Some propose that it is unjust for medical insurance to refuse to underwrite such treatment while doing so, for example, for women who were diagnosed with endometriosis. One advocate argues that it is discriminatory on the part of health care insurers to pay for treatment for a heterosexual couple where neither partner has an adequate sperm count but not for a female same-sex couple for whom the same absence obtains (Fairyington 2015).

Support for Parents as a Civil Right

What matters most obviously for civil rights is state interference with parental liberty, termination of parental rights but also including parents' choices about how their children will be raised, educated, or treated medically. As Adam Cureton (Chapter 18, this volume) shows, parenting can be as importantly central an interest for people with disabilities as for nondisabled people.

Pregnancy itself provides an initial illustration of these concerns. Recent evidence indicates that although women with intellectual disabilities are carrying pregnancies more frequently than in the past, attention has not been directed toward studying these pregnancies and how they can go well. Evidence indicates that women with intellectual disabilities reach prenatal care later, may not receive care that attends to their needs, and have significantly worse pregnancy outcomes (Mitra et al. 2015).

According to the National Council on Disability (NCD), reproductive health care professionals have not developed sufficient knowledge about caring for this community (NCD 2012, Ch. 13; Weiner and Hammond 2009). For instance, many women with disabilities are encouraged to have a cesarean section "simply because of anxiety on the provider's part" (NCD 2012 at n. 1095). In the same vein as the assumptions regarding the need to rely on cesarean delivery, many women with disabilities are unnecessarily referred to high-risk pregnancy specialists. According to one expectant mother with a disability, when she visited the specialist her physician had referred her to, she was told that her pregnancy was not high risk but that many providers make that assumption if the mother has a disability. The specialist said, "You're probably the least high-risk woman to come into my practice, but you make providers nervous because you're not in their textbooks" (Andrews 2011).

A further civil rights point is that for individuals with disabilities, parenting may be achievable only if there are social supports. The NCD points out that the legislative history of the Americans with Disabilities Act supports a mandate to eliminate disability-based discrimination in the child welfare system and dependency courts. The NCD takes alteration of practice and allocation of resources to be accommodations required for the equitable accommodation of parents with disabilities. For example, currently in the United States, state-provided personal assistance services do not extend to accommodating parents with disabilities in executing parenting tasks (NCD 2012, Ch. 13). Absent the availability of family members or friends willing to fill in as assistants, lack of such childrearing resources can restrict the freedom of individuals with disabilities to fulfill parenting functions even when they can do so in unconventional ways (Cureton, this volume, Chapter 18). Furthermore, the very small inventory of accessible housing usually is not designed with room for families of children. The NCD concludes that "A significant increase in affordable, accessible, and integrated housing is required for parents with disabilities and their families, as well as increased funding for home modifications" (NCD 2012, Ch. 13).

Even when they have become parents, all too frequently thereafter parents with disabilities lose custody of or even contact with their children because they parent differently or require different forms of support in comparison to parents without significant disabilities. People with disabilities, especially intellectual disabilities or mental illness, have historically been subject not only to sterilization efforts but to termination of parental rights over children they bear. One recent study reported that as many as 70%–80% of parents with severe mental illness no longer have custody of their children (Mason, Subeti, and Davis 2007). A Minnesota study found that parents who had a disability label in their school records are more than three times more likely to have parental rights terminated than parents without a disability label (NCD 2012, Ch. 5; LaLiberte et al. 2015). According to the National Council on Disability, "Parents with disabilities and their families are frequently, and often unnecessarily, referred to the child welfare system." (NCD 2012, 71)

In fact, nearly all the parents with whom NCD spoke reported living in constant fear that they would eventually be reported because of their disability. For example, a study of blind mothers found that they felt vulnerable about their parental rights because the custodial rights of parents with disabilities are frequently questioned solely on the basis of the parents' disabilities (Conley-Jung and Olkin 2001). Here again, presumptions of normalcy infect social policies in ways a civil rights perspective might correct.

Like sterilization, termination of parental rights requires clear and convincing evidence of unfitness (Smith 2014–2015). Unlike sterilization, however, the interests of existing children lie in the balance; keeping children safe must be paramount. Yet courts have frequently found these interests overriding, without further consideration of whether it might be possible to support the interests of both parents and children. A civil rights perspective is once again that of Justice Jackson: Judgments about fitness require careful, individualized scrutiny of the evidence and cannot be based on stereotypes about the ability of different groups to parent. Cureton (this volume, Chapter 18) discusses the pervasiveness of stereotyping in assessing parenting by people with disabilities.

In recent years, US courts have engaged in more careful scrutiny of efforts to terminate parental rights based on disability. For example, a 2015 decision by the Georgia Court of Appeals held that the state lacked clear and convincing evidence to terminate the parental rights of a mother with physical disabilities that included multiple sclerosis and lupus.[16] An interracial Missouri couple who both were blind suffered removal of their newborn, an action initiated by a report that the mother had trouble breastfeeding. Their infant eventually was returned—but only after the newborn was held in protective custody for 57 days (Schultz 2010). And there still are cases in which parental rights are terminated when parents have intellectual disabilities and lack apparent support for raising their children; these cases take place in contexts without state resource support for such parents and in which the only possible legal choices are complete termination of parental rights or independent placement of the child with the parent who cannot fully raise the child on his or her own.[17]

One recent investigation by the Civil Rights Division of the US Department of Justice brings multiple aspects of the civil rights approach into play together: evidence rather than stereotyping or assumptions, even-handed treatment, and supports and modifications that are reasonable under the circumstances (US Department of Justice 2015). The facts of the situation were these. Ms. Gordon, a woman with intellectual disabilities, gave birth to her first child. While she was still in the hospital, when her child was 2 days old, the Massachusetts Department of Children and Families (DCF) removed her child from her. The hospital had contacted DCF after observing difficulties Ms. Gordon had with feeding the child: Ms. Gordon's inability to read a digital clock led her to miss a feeding and hospital policy precluded relatives other than a spouse or father from remaining with the mother in the hospital after visiting hours, so her parents were not available to help her with the repetition she required to learn to feed her daughter.

In removing the child, DCF ignored the facts that Ms. Gordon's mother had quit her job to help her daughter care for her child and would assume guardianship of the child and that Ms. Gordon and her child would live with her parents. Instead, DCF placed the child in foster care, gave Ms. Gordon limited opportunities to visit with her, ignored her successful efforts to improve her parenting skills with education, did not give her adequate parent aide services, and ultimately changed the care plan from family reunification to adoption. In insisting on adoption, DCF also ignored the evidence of community-based service providers, experts, and a Foster Care Review panel that a family-supported parenting plan would be appropriate.

In reviewing the case, the US Department of Justice determined that DCF had committed "extensive, ongoing" violations of both the Americans with Disabilities Act and the Rehabilitation Act by discriminating against Ms. Gordon. DCF's discrimination included the failure to make the required individualized assessment of Ms. Gordon's parenting abilities in her situation—a failure of evidence. The discrimination also included a failure of equal treatment: at the same time as it was criticizing Ms. Gordon's parenting, DCF "repeatedly overlooked numerous concerns" in the child's foster care placement, including physical injuries such as a black eye and burnt hands. Moreover, DCF's own regulations required parent aide and homemaker services be provided to parents to enable them to maintain their family units; although these services were routinely made available to parents without disabilities and Ms. Gordon requested them, they were not made available to her. And DCF even separated her from her own supports by evaluating her in the absence of her parental supports. The frequency with which DCF supports and services were made available to others, the US Department of Justice concluded, meant that providing them to Ms. Gordon would not be a fundamental alteration of DCF programs—in other words, so great a change as to disrupt services made reasonably available to others. And DCF had no evidence—other than unsubstantiated stereotypes—that Ms. Gordon's plans for supported parenting posed threats to the safety of her child. Following up on cases like Ms. Gordon's, the US Department of Justice and the Department of Health and Human Services Office of Civil Rights issued technical assistance for state and local child welfare agencies to help them comply with nondiscrimination laws (Department of Health and Human Services 2015).

Conclusion

Reproductive rights—both rights to prevent and rights to achieve reproduction—spark recurring social controversy. Human rights approaches, tracking norms of humanity, may prove too little and too much. They may prove too little to the extent that they track protections for those who can reproduce in the species-typical way and fail to address how social institutions entrench disadvantages of difference. They may prove too much by insisting on absolute rights for some but failing to accommodate difference when it would be reasonable to do so.

In contrast, a civil rights approach, as illustrated by Justice Jackson in *Skinner*, insists on careful scrutiny of justifications for differential treatment, whether these be differences in protections from interference or in the distribution of social services. With reproduction, as with other important human interests, the application of civil rights approaches suggests ways to accommodate differences so that all kinds of people may, increasingly, be socially enabled to lead lives that are meaningful for them.

In this chapter, we have explored how a civil rights approach might provide a way forward in regard to some of these controversies. As people with disabilities infamously have suffered from various forms of socially imposed bias against their becoming parents, and continue to do so to this day, both the history and the current state of their treatment in this regard illustrate various ways in which reproductive liberty has been and still is compromised. Additionally, the slow but steady strengthening of disabled people's civil rights shows the way to achieve heightened social protection and facilitation for family making for all.

Author Note

Some of the material in this chapter is drawn from our earlier work on human rights, civil rights, and health care, especially Silvers and Francis (2013, 2015) and Silvers (2012).

Notes

1. 274 U.S. 200 (1927).
2. *Skinner v. State of Oklahoma ex rel. Williamson*, 316 U.S. 535 (1942).
3. 316 U.S. at 536.
4. 316 U.S. at 544.
5. 316 U.S. at 546.
6. The so-called Ashley treatment involved suppressing puberty, removing breast tissue, and removing sexual organs from a girl with significant intellectual disabilities. A primary goal of the treatment was to ensure that she never attained the size, physical characteristics, and fertility of a grown woman (Liao, Savulescu, and Sheehan 2007).
7. As *Buck v. Bell*, 274 U.S. 200 (1927), illustrates.
8. We have argued elsewhere that people who are not articulate nevertheless may be able to formulate conceptions of their good that require respect from others (Francis and Silvers 2007; Silvers and Francis 2010).
9. 448 U.S. 297 (1980).
10. 381 U.S. 479 (1965).
11. 274 U.S. 200 (1927).
12. *Skinner v. Oklahoma*, 316 U.S. 535, 535-36 (1942).
13. *Stump v. Sparkman*, 435 U.S. 349 (1978).
14. *Kijuana Chambers v. Rocky Mountain Women's Health Care Center* (D. Colo. 2003), http://www.morelaw.com/verdicts/case.asp?n=00-CV-1794&s=CO&d=26278.
15. Chambers testified that she had always wanted a child, but it seemed unlikely because she is a lesbian. http://usatoday30.usatoday.com/news/nation/2003-11-21-fertility-lawsuit_x.htm.
16. *In re S.R.R.*, 330 Ga. App. 817, 769 S.E.2d 562 (2015).
17. For example, In re T.G., 318 G. App. 191, 733 S.E. 2d 777 (Ga. App. 2012).

Bibliography

American Society for Reproductive Medicine (ASRM). 2015. Disparities in access to effective treatment for infertility in the United States: An Ethics Committee opinion. *Fertility and Sterility*. Epub ahead of print, http://dx.doi.org/10.1016/j.fertnstert.2015.07.1139.

Amundson, R., and S. Tresky. 2007. On a bioethical challenge to disability rights. *Journal of Medicine and Philosophy* 32: 541–561.

Andrews, E. E. 2011. Pregnancy with a physical disability: One psychologist's journey. American Psychological Association, *Spotlight on Disability Newsletter* [online] (December), http://www.apa.org/pi/disability/resources/publications/newsletter/2011/12/pregnancy-disability.aspx.

Asch, A., and E. Parens. 2000. *Prenatal testing and disability rights*. Washington, D.C.: Georgetown University Press.

Barlow, P. 1999. Letter: Health care is not a human right. *British Medical Journal* 319: 321.

Buchanan, A. E. 1984. The right to a decent minimum of health care. *Philosophy and Public Affairs* 13, no. 1: 55–78.

Carreira da Silva, F. 2013. Outline of a social theory of rights. A neo-pragmatist approach. *European Journal of Social Theory* 16, no. 4: 457–475.

Conley-Jung, C., and R. Olkin. 2001. Mothers with visual impairments who are raising young children. *Journal of Visual Impairment and Blindness* 91, no. 1: 15.

Daniels, N. 1985. *Just health care*. New York: Cambridge University Press.

Daniels, N. 2008. *Just health: Meeting health needs fairly*. New York: Cambridge University Press.

Department of Health and Human Services. 2015. HHS and DOJ issue technical assistance for child welfare systems under the Americans with Disabilities Act and section 504 of the Rehabilitation Act, http://www.hhs.gov/news/press/2015pres/08/20150810a.html.

Dresser, R. 2009. Prenatal testing and disability: A truce in the culture wars? *Hastings Center Report* 39, no. 3: 7–8.

Eisenberg, H. 2013. The impact of dicta in *Buck v. Bell. Journal of Contemporary Health Law and Policy* 30: 184–221.

Fairyington, S. 2015. Should same-sex couples receive fertility benefits? *The New York Times* [online] (November 2), http://well.blogs.nytimes.com/?module=BlogMainandaction=Clic kandregion=Headerandpgtype=Blogsandversion=Blog%20PostandcontentCollection=He alth.

Finnis, J. 1998. *Aquinas: Moral, political, and legal theory*. Oxford: Oxford University Press.

Francis, L. P. 2009. Understanding autonomy in light of intellectual disability. In *Disability and disadvantage*, ed. Kimberley Brownlee and Adam Cureton, pp. 200–215. Oxford, UK: Oxford University Press.

Francis, L. P. and A. Silvers. 2007. Liberalism and independently scripted accounts of the good: Meeting the challenge of dependent agency. *Social Theory and Practice* (Spring 2007): 311-334.

Held, V. 2014. The ethics of care as normative guidance: Comment on Gilligan. *Journal of Social Philosophy* 45, no. 1: 107–115.

Hoglund, B., and M. Larsson. 2013. Struggling for motherhood with an intellectual disability— A qualitative study of women's experiences in Sweden. *Midwifery* 29, no. 6: 698–704.

Kittay, E. F. 2005. At the margins of moral personhood. *Ethics* 116: 100–131.

Kittay, E. F. 2012. Getting from here to there: Claiming justice for the severely cognitively disabled. In *Medicine and social justice: Essays on the distribution of health care*, 2nd ed. R. Rhodes, M. Battin, and A. Silvers, eds., 313-324. New York: Oxford University Press.

Kornhauser, M., and R. Schneiderman. 2010. How plans can improve outcomes and cut costs for preterm infant care. *Managed Care* [online] (January), http://www.managedcaremag. com/archives/1001/1001.preterm.html.

Kundnani, R. 2013. Protecting the right to procreate for mentally ill women. *Southern California Review of Law and Social Justice* 23: 59–89.

LaLiberte, T., E. Lightfoot, S. Mishra, and K. Piescher. 2015. Parental disability and ter- mination of parental rights in Chile protection (ML #12revised), http://cascw.umn. edu/portfolio-items/parental-disability-and-termination-of-parental-rights-in-child- protection-ml-12revised/.

Lawson, K. L. 2006. Perceptions of deservedness of social aid as a function of prenatal diagnos- tic testing. *Journal of Applied Social Psychology* 33, no. 1: 76–90.

Le Dref, G., B. Grollemund, A. Danion-Grilliat, and J.-C. Weber. 2013. Towards a new pro- creation ethic: The exemplary instance of cleft lip and palate. *Medicine, Health Care and Philosophy* 16, no. 3: 365–375.

Lebel, David E., R. Sergienko, A. Wiznitzer, G. J. Velan, and E. Sheiver. 2012. Mode of delivery and other pregnancy outcomes of patients with documented scoliosis. *Journal of Maternal and Neonatal Medicine* 25, no. 6: 639–641.

Liao, S. M., J. Savulescu, and M. Sheehan. 2007. The Ashley treatment: Best interests, convenience, and parental decision-making. *Hastings Center Report* 37, no. 2: 16–20.

Marquis, D. 1989. Why abortion is immoral. *Journal of Philosophy* 86: 183–202.

Mason, C., S. Subeti, and R. B. Davis. 2007. Clients with mental illness and their children: Implications for clinical practice. *Issues in Mental Health Nursing* 28, no. 10: 1105–1123.

McMahan, J. 2005. Causing disabled people to exist and causing people to be disabled. *Ethics* 116: 77–99.

Mitra, M., S. L. Parish, K. M. Clements, X. Cui, and H. Diop. 2015. Pregnancy outcomes among women with intellectual and developmental disabilities. *American Journal of Preventive Medicine* 48, no. 3: 300–308.

Murdick, N. L., B. Gartin, and T. L. Crabtree. 2006. *Special education law*, 2nd ed. Englewood Cliffs, NJ: Prentice Hall.

National Council on Disability. 2012. *Rocking the cradle: Ensuring the rights of parents with disabilities and their children*, https://www.ncd.gov/publications/2012/Sep272012.

Oeullette, A. 2011. *Bioethics and disability: Toward a disability-conscious bioethics*. New York: Cambridge University Press.

O'Reilly, K. B. 2007. Physician-ethicist explains "Ashley treatment decision." *American Medical News* [online], http://www.amednews.com/article/20070312/profession/303129960/7/.

Parens, E., and A. Asch. 2000. The disability rights critique of prenatal genetic testing: Reflections and recommendations. In *Prenatal testing and disability rights*, E. Parens and A. Asch, eds., 3–43. Washington, D.C.: Georgetown University Press.

Pendo, E. 2008. Disability, equipment barriers, and women's health: Using the ADA to provide meaningful access. *St. Louis University Journal of Health Law and Policy* 2: 5–56.

Pfeiffer, D. 1994. Eugenics and disability discrimination. *Disability and Society* 9, no. 4: 481–499.

Planned Parenthood Advocates of Arizona. 2012. Sherri Finkbine's Abortion: Its Meaning 50 Years Later (August 15), http://advocatesaz.org/2012/08/15/sherri-finkbines-abortion-its-meaning-50-years-later/.

Putnam, R. A. 2000. Neither a beast nor a god. *Social Theory and Practice* 26, no. 2: 177-200.

Ram-Tiktin, E. 2012. The right to health care as a right to basic human functional capabilities. *Ethics Theory and Moral Practice* 15: 337–351.

Reagan, L. J. 2010. *Dangerous pregnancies: Mothers, disabilities, and abortion in modern America*. Berkeley, CA: University of California Press.

Rosenthal, E. 2013. American way of birth, costliest in the nation. *The New York Times* [online] (June 30), http://www.nytimes.com/2013/07/01/health/american-way-of-birth-costliest-in-the-world.html.

Schultz, E. 2010. Blind Independence couple gets newborn back after 57 days. KSBH Kansas City [online] (July 22), https://web.archive.org/web/20150716062716/http://www.kshb.com/news/local-news/blind-kansas-city-couple-gets-newborn-back-after-57-days.

Silvers, A. 2012. Moral status: What a bad idea! Why discard it? What replaces it? *The Journal of Intellectual Disability Research* 56, no. 11: 1014–1025.

Silvers, A., and L. P. Francis. 2005. Justice through trust: Disability and the "outlier problem" in social contract theory. *Ethics* 116, no. 1: 40-77.

Silvers, A. and Francis, L. P. 2010. Thinking about the good: reconfiguring metaphysics (or not) for people with cognitive disabilities. In *Cognitive disability and its challenge to moral philosophy*, E. Feder Kittay, and L. Carlson, eds. Hoboken, NJ: Wiley-Blackwell.

Silvers, A., and L. P. Francis. 2013. Human rights, civil rights: Prescribing disability discrimina-
    tion prevention in packaging essential health benefits. *Journal of Law, Medicine and Ethics*
    41, no. 4: 781–791.
Silvers, A., and L. P. Francis. 2015. Human and civil models of rights: Healthy and ill disabled
    and access to healthcare. In *Human rights and disability*, ed. J.-S. Gordon.
Silvers, A., D. Wasserman, and M. Mahowald. 1998. *Disability, difference, discrimination:
    Perspectives on justice in bioethics*. Lanham, MD: Rowman and Littlefield.
Singer, P. 1975. *Animal liberation: A new ethics for our treatment of animals*. New York:
    Harper-Collins.
Singer, P. 2009. Speciesism and moral status. *Metaphilosophy* 40, no. 3–4: 567–581.
Smith, C. 2014–2015. Finding solutions to the termination of parental rights in parents with
    mental challenges. *Law and Psychology Review* 39: 205–238.
Stemplowska, Z. 2008. What's ideal about ideal theory? *Social Theory and Practice* 34: 319–340.
Stemplowska, Z. 2009. On the real world duties imposed on us by human rights. *Journal of
    Social Philosophy* 40: 466–487.
Tooley, Michael. 1972. Abortion and Infanticide. *Philosophy & Public Affairs* 2, no. 1: 37–65.
United Nations. 1948. Universal Declaration of Human Rights. http://www.un.org/en/docu-
    ments/udhr/.
United Nations. 2006. Convention on the Rights of Persons with Disabilities [UN CRPD],
    http://www.un.org/disabilities/convention/conventionfull.shtml.
US Congress. 1776. Declaration of Independence. http://www.archives.gov/exhibits/charters/
    declaration_transcript.html.
US Department of Justice. 2015. Re: Investigation of the Massachusetts Department of Children
    and Families by the United States Departments of Justice and Health and Human Services
    Pursuant to the Americans with Disabilities Act and the Rehabilitation Act (DJ No. 204-36-
    216 and HHS No. 14-182176), ma.docf_lof.doc.
Valentini, L. 2012. Ideal vs. non-ideal theory: A conceptual map. *Philosophy Compass* 7, no.
    9: 654–664.
Vehmas, S. 1999. Newborn infants and the moral significance of intellectual disabilities. *Journal
    of the Association for Persons with Severe Handicaps* 24, no. 2: 111–121.
Volz, V. 2006. A matter of choice: Women with disabilities, sterilization, and reproductive
    autonomy in the twenty-first century. *Women's Rights Law Reporter* 27: 203–216.
Weiner, S. L., and C. Hammond. 2009. Gynecologic and obstetric issues confronting women
    with disabilities. *Global Library of Women's Medicine* [online], https://web.archive.org/web/
    20150716062404/http://www.glowm.com/section_view/item/76.
Wasserman, D., A. Asch, J. Blustein, and D. Putnam. 2013. Disability: Definitions, models,
    experience. In *The Stanford Encyclopedia of Philosophy* (Summer 2016 Edition, ed. E. N.
    Zalta. <http://plato.stanford.edu/archives/sum2016/entries/disability/>.
Whitaker, M. 2014. Family decay, single moms get blame for poverty from GOP. MSNBC [online]
    (January 9), http://www.msnbc.com/politicsnation/gop-single-moms-still-blame-poverty.

PART II

PROVIDERS

CHAPTER 9

CONSCIENTIOUS OBJECTION IN REPRODUCTIVE HEALTH

ARMAND H. MATHENY ANTOMMARIA

THE conflict regarding conscientious objection in health care is primarily between health care providers who assert their authority not to provide particular goods or services and patients who seek these goods or services. In the domain of reproductive health, the conflict has centered on induced abortion, contraception including emergency contraception, sterilization, and assisted reproductive technology. The conflict is exacerbated by objectors' refusal not only to perform the actions they consider immoral but also to cooperate with others performing these actions. Conscientious objections have the potential to restrict patients' access to goods and services and to cause significant harm.

Equitable resolution of this conflict depends, in part, on the role responsibilities of health care providers. Some commentators have argued that anyone who is not willing to offer all legally available treatments should not enter the field. Although this assertion is overstated, providers nonetheless have fiduciary obligations to their patients. Their objections should at least not make patients substantially worse off than they would be otherwise. Systems should be developed to try to protect both providers' and patients' interests. Controversy persists over whether there is an absolute duty to refer and whether providers can legitimately object to providing a good or a service to a particular category of patients. Similar arguments regarding duties and accommodations apply to claims made by organizations.

CONSCIENCE AND COOPERATION

Some health care providers object to providing goods or services that they consider immoral. (These arguments apply to the members of all medical professions, including physicians, nurses, and pharmacists, and are not substantially modified by the provider's specific or relative role in the health care delivery team. I will, therefore, generally use the term "provider.") For example, a Roman Catholic obstetrician may object to performing abortions or sterilizations or an evangelical Protestant perioperative nurse may object to assisting in abortions. These refusals are frequently framed as conscientious objections. This topic generated substantial public attention in the mid-2000s around physicians' refusals to prescribe and particularly pharmacists' refusals to dispense emergency contraception (Cantor and Baum 2004). (Emergency contraception is the use of a drug or device after unprotected or inadequately protected intercourse to prevent an unintended pregnancy. This term is preferable to the morning-after pill because the latter may mislead individuals about the duration of time the drugs are effective—up to 72 or 120 hours.)

In analyzing this issue, it is important to clarify what the conscience is and what it is not. Conscience is neither an inner sense that distinguishes right from wrong nor the internalization of external, parental or societal norms. Viewing conscience as an inner sense of right and wrong makes it difficult to account for individuals with conflicting understandings of what is morally right or individuals who act conscientiously but immorally. Conceiving conscience as the internalization of external norms leaves open the question whether these norms are valid (Benjamin 1990).

Conscience is better understood as a sense of moral integrity—the congruence between one's fundamental moral beliefs, words, and actions (Benjamin 1990). Fundamental or core moral beliefs are integral to one's identity. Individuals also have more peripheral moral beliefs, but objections based on them do not constitute conscientious objections (Wicclair 2011). Objections based on unpleasantness, potential criticism, or physical risks are not based on core moral beliefs and should not be considered conscientious objections (American College of Obstetricians and Gynecologists 2007). In the context of military service, for example, conscientious objections are differentiated from objections centered on self-preservation.

Although one may retrospectively judge one's prior action to have been wrong, one has an obligation to act according to what one currently believes is right. Acting inconsistently with one's fundamental beliefs can result in guilt, shame, or remorse (Benjamin 1990). It may also cause others to perceive an individual to be unreliable or to lose trust in him or her (Wicclair 2011).

Claims regarding one's own conscience are not binding on others. It would be incoherent to assert, "It would violate *my* conscience if *you* did X." Individuals may, however, object to cooperating with others who perform an action they consider immoral. To take a nonmedical example, we evaluate a bank manager who involuntarily provided robbers access to the safe because they took his or her family hostage differently from a manager who accepted a bribe to provide access to the safe.

The analysis of which forms of cooperation are immoral is complex. The Roman Catholic moral tradition draws a fundamental distinction between formal and material cooperation. In formal cooperation, the cooperator and the wrongdoer share the same immoral intention and this is always morally wrong. In material cooperation, the wrongdoer and the cooperator do not share the same intention. The tradition makes a subsequent distinction between immediate and mediate material cooperation. In immediate material cooperation, the cooperator shares in the act itself, and this is also always immoral. The reason for cooperating must be separate and proportionately serious. The analysis of mediate material cooperation depends on a number of factors, including how proximate or remote the cooperation is, whether the cooperation is necessary for the act to be performed, whether the cooperator is under duress, and whether observers are likely to believe that the cooperator agrees with the immoral act. Mediate material cooperation may be moral, but there are no bright dividing lines (Griese 1987). Whether a particular type of cooperation is immoral can itself become a matter of conscience.

Although many claims of conscience involve the refusal to perform or participate in an action, individuals may also assert positive claims of conscience—the assertion that failing to perform an action would violate an individual's conscience. A provider could, for example, assert the obligation to perform an abortion. Mark Wicclair (2011) argues that, from the perspective of respecting moral integrity, there is no basis for preferentially protecting negative, as opposed to positive, appeals to conscience. Negative and positive appeals may, however, differ significantly in practice. Some positive claims of conscience are illegal, for example, violating restrictions on abortions that one considers unduly burdensome or unethical. Such assertions should be analyzed under the category of civil disobedience rather than conscientious objection (Childress 1985). Other positive claims of conscience would require the cooperation of those morally opposed to the action, for example, an attending physician at a Roman Catholic hospital performing a tubal ligation following a caesarean section. These practical implications may make it difficult to protect positive claims of conscience.

Conscientious Objection in Health Care

Conscientious objection in health care has become a more frequent and divisive issue as morally controversial treatments and practices have been incorporated into medicine. Roman Catholic providers have historically objected to contraception, sterilization, and abortion. Evangelical Protestants have objected to contraception by unmarried individuals and abortion. The legalization of abortion and contraception created initial conflicts resulting in legislation to protect individual and corporate claims of conscience in 1973 (Lynch 2008).

Emergency contraception has been a subsequent nidus of conflict. One of the concerns is whether providers make patients aware of its availability and, if providers do not, whether patients know enough to ask for it. A second concern is whether women, especially in underserved or rural communities or with limited economic means, are able to access emergency contraception in time for it to be effective. For example, a woman reported in an editorial in *The Washington Post* in 2006, before Plan B was available over the counter, that she became pregnant and subsequently had an abortion after she was unable to obtain emergency contraception from her obstetrician/gynecologist and her internist (Dana 2006).

Outside of reproductive health, conflicts have arisen regarding withholding or withdrawing life-sustaining treatment, physician-assisted suicide, and donation after circulatory death.

Although this discussion will focus on the debate in the United States, it should be noted that conscientious objection in reproductive health is an international issue (Casas 2009; Diniz, Madeiro, and Rosas 2014).

As citizens, individuals have limited obligations to assist others. Conscientious objection in health care should, however, be analyzed in terms of professional obligations. Professions are groups of individuals with specialized knowledge and expertise that have been granted social prerogatives, including a degree of self-regulation, in exchange for corresponding obligations (Lynch 2008; Wicclair 2011).

There are a number of ways to conceptualize the basis of this commitment (Wicclair 2011). Some view it as intrinsic to the practice of medicine or the provider–patient relationship. Edmund Pellegrino and David Thomasma (1993), for example, emphasize patients' illness and vulnerability and physicians' promise to help and heal. Others may conceptualize it as a social or a special contract. In the social contract model, the public grants the medical profession certain privileges, such as control over knowledge and skills, in exchange for certain obligations. This contract may be renegotiated over time. One might also see the obligations as a minimal set of commitments that professionals consent to by entering the profession. These different conceptual bases have similar practical implications.

Professions entail both privileges and obligations. There is a knowledge and power differential between professionals and their clients. Given this differential, professionals may constrain access to services by failing to inform clients of their availability. Professional self-regulation also limits client access by preventing others from offering the services (Lynch 2008). In the medical domain, for example, certain pharmaceuticals must be prescribed by a physician, physician assistant, or nurse practitioner and dispensed by a pharmacist. To protect clients and promote their interests, professionals accept certain fiduciary obligations to their clients (Lynch 2008). For example, providers are expected to respect patients' confidentiality—not disclose patients' private information without their permission.

Some have argued that professionals are obligated to provide patients with all legally available goods and services within the scope of their competency and that if one is unwilling to do so, he or she should not enter the profession. Julian Savulescu (2006, 294; see also Rhodes 2006; Schuklenk 2015), for example, famously asserted, "If people are not prepared to offer legally permitted, efficient, and beneficial care to a patient because it conflicts with their values, they should not be doctors." (Savulescu later conceded that objections should be accommodated if they do not compromise the quality, efficiency, or equitability of health care.) There are a number of rejoinders to this argument:

- This position may have negative effects on the profession and on patients. Not accommodating conscientious objections may dissuade individuals who value moral integrity from entering the profession. Requiring individuals to act contrary to their consciences may also result in a decline in individuals' moral character and in less commitment to professional values (Wicclair 2011). A lack of integrity may harm patients. Conscientious objection may also be a basis for refusing constraints inappropriately placed on practice such as "gag rules" or reporting undocumented patients (American College of Obstetricians sand Gynecologists 2007; see also Lynch 2008). Maintaining diversity and protecting providers' consciences may promote debate among various viewpoints and improve decisions. It may also permit patients who desire to be to be cared for by providers with similar values (Lynch 2008).
- Being a professional is not necessarily one's sole or dominant identity. A professional may have other roles or identities such as spouse, child, and/or parent. A professional is not generally expected to place his or her professional duties before all these other role responsibilities. For example, if one is both a gynecologist and a parent and one's child is injured on the playground at school and taken to the emergency department, it would be reasonable to reschedule routine appointments in order to be with one's child if another immediate family member is unavailable. It is not unreasonable to suggest that some duties entailed by being a member of a religious tradition might, on some occasions, have similar priority (Lynch 2008). Expecting individuals to compartmentalize the different aspects of their identity might also be psychologically damaging (Lynch 2008).
- Critics of conscientious objection would need to be able to clearly distinguish personal and professional values. It has been, however, difficult to define terms such as "health" and "disease" in a value-neutral way. Many medical conceptions involve ethical claims and are sufficiently general as to involve personal interpretation (Wicclair 2011). For example, the boundaries between personal, social, and professional in the debate about nonmedical sex selection are indistinct (see Ethics Committee of the American Society for Reproductive Medicine 2015).
- The assertion also erroneously assumes that professional and personal values are static. Medicine changes over time and some of the controversies involve new technologies such as emergency contraception and assisted reproductive technology. Personal values may also change over time. The most dramatic example would be a religious conversion. It would be difficult to track what treatments or interventions one voluntarily committed to when one entered the profession. It would also be expecting a great deal for one to leave his or her profession and train for a new career as a result of a significant change in personal values or beliefs.
- The objection ignores processes of specialization. Individual providers cannot offer all medical services—specialists and subspecialists only offer a range of services. Individual providers' practices may be further specialized apart from specific recognition by board certification (Wicclair 2011). Individuals may never have achieved competency in the provision of particular goods or services or may no longer be competent in goods or services they were initially trained in. It is not clear that they

have an affirmative obligation to attain or maintain competency in the provision of these goods or services (Lynch 2008). This argument may, however, be less applicable in obstetrics and gynecology, where interventions, such as performing dilatation and curettage or prescribing emergency contraception, have a relatively low threshold for competency that is generally crossed in routine clinical practice.

- The threshold "legally permitted" is too low. The number of procedures that are illegal is small. "Female genital mutilation," defined as circumcising, excising, or infibulating the whole or any part of the labia major, labia minora, or clitoris of a minor, is an exception. Performing female genital mutilation or transporting a minor outside the United States to obtain it is illegal under federal law (18 C.F.R. § 116). (Exceptions include procedures performed by licensed practitioners necessary for the health of the individual or in connection with labor or birth.) Twenty-three states also have laws against "female genital mutilation" (Equality Now 2015).

In contrast, although many surgeons would object to amputating a patient with body integrity identity disorder's healthy limb, it is not illegal. Individuals with body integrity identity disorder perceive a mismatch between their sense of self and their anatomy. They believe that amputation of a major limb or paralysis will make them complete or whole. They do not believe that the limb is defective nor do they feel embarrassed or ashamed by it. For most patients with this condition, the primary motivation is not sexual arousal. Individuals may injure a limb to justify its amputation, attempt to amputate it themselves, or seek a surgical amputation (First 2005). There is debate about whether individuals with body integrity identity disorder are capable of giving informed consent (compare Muller 2009 with White 2014). Although amputating a healthy limb is not illegal, many surgeons would nonetheless object.

- Finally, it is not clear that a patient is harmed if another provider provides the service (Lynch 2008). Imagine, for example, an emergency department with a large staff of physicians and nurse practitioners where at least two are scheduled at any one time. One of the physicians has a moral objection to prescribing emergency contraception. Her colleagues evaluate all patients for whom such a prescription might be relevant, including all victims of sexual assault. Triage and preliminary evaluation by other providers makes unexpected requests very unlikely. It is not clear that implementing such a system would be intrinsically unethical.

Balancing Patients' and Providers' Interests

Rather than refuting claims to conscientious objection, these arguments make clear that the primary issues are how both providers' integrity and patients' access can be protected and which takes precedence in exceptional circumstances when the conflict cannot be resolved. The dominant approach to this issue is to identify systems to accommodate both parties' interests (Antommaria 2008; Lynch 2008; Wicclair 2011). Accommodations may be implemented at different levels of the health care system, including the clinic, pharmacy, hospital, insurance company, state licensing board, or legislature.

Before proceeding, it should also be noted that an alternative mechanism to avoid conflicts is to remove the good or service from professional oversight. Some have argued for expanding the range of providers who can offer a good or service and/or removing some services from professional oversight altogether (Potts and Denny 1995). For example, some women's health advocates have argued that hormonal contraceptives should be available over the counter and, after a protracted conflict, emergency contraception is currently available over the counter.

In 2006, the US Food and Drug Administration (FDA) granted approval for Plan B (Levonorgestrel, Teva Pharmaceutical Industries Ltd) to be available without prescription to women 18 years old and older. Because pharmacists were required to verify women's ages, this was referred to as under or behind, rather than over, the counter. A court later lowered the minimum age to 17 years. The manufacturer petitioned to move the product to full over-the-counter status. In 2011 the FDA's Center for Drug Evaluation and Research determined that adolescents were able to use Plan B without their physician's supervision, but Secretary of Health and Human Services Kathleen Sebelius overruled this decision. The courts overturned Sebelius's action and in 2013 the one-dose form of Plan B and its generic forms became available in pharmacies without prescription or age restriction (Sifferlin 2013). Ella (ulipristal acetate, Laboratoire HRA Pharma) is only available by prescription (Afaxys 2014).

Although eliminating or loosening professional oversight is an option for some goods and services, it is not feasible for all goods and services. Surgical abortion may be an example. Although some of the morbidity and mortality of "unsafe abortions" may be the result of legal prohibitions or stigma, these outcomes suggest that lay providers are not competent (Grimes et al. 2006). Studies have demonstrated that midlevel providers are competent to perform vacuum aspiration (Warriner et al. 2006). This technique is, however, only recommended up to 12 to 14 weeks of gestation. Physicians are required to perform dilatation and evacuation after this time. (Some additional restrictions on providers or facilities, such as admitting privileges or transfer agreements, may nonetheless be unnecessary to ensure patients' safety [Gold and Nash 2013].)

It is also important to note that provider behavior that clearly contravenes professional norms should not be accommodated. Some women report being lectured or berated by objecting providers (Cantor and Baum 2004). Others report having their prescriptions destroyed so that they cannot be filled elsewhere. Such disrespectful or obstructionist behavior is clearly ethically inappropriate.

Providers with potential objections have an obligation to notify potential patients as well as employers and/or facilities. Prospective patients should be aware of objections so they do not invest time or money in establishing a relationship with a provider unwilling to provide goods or services that they desire. Notification of employers and/or facilities provides opportunities to arrange staffing or other accommodations to avoid potential conflicts (Lynch 2008; Wicclair 2011).

There are, however, limits as to what accommodations are reasonable. The precise limits, however, may be difficult to establish. The expectation that the process should be invisible to patients so that they do not perceive any criticism of their moral views or experience any delay or inconvenience is excessive. The threshold of a substantial burden may nonetheless be difficult to determine. This is particularly the case because what constitutes a burden is dependent on the patient, the condition, the treatment, and the context. Patients have different levels of health literacy and economic resources, conditions have different degrees of severity, treatments have different urgencies, and the context may vary considerably in terms of alternatives.

The analysis of access in underserved areas is particularly complex. A new local provider who has a conscientious objection to particular goods or services may be preferable to the current distant providers who do not have any objections. It may not, however, be clear whether the presence of a provider with an objection impedes others without objections from entering the market.

At the system level, there are some accommodations that are clearly unreasonable. It is unreasonable to require an abortion provider to hire a clinician who is conscientiously opposed to performing abortions. Providing a particular good or service may be a bona fide requirement of certain positions. Employers should also not be expected to make accommodations that result in excessive burdens similar to the requirements for accommodating religious practices or disabilities (Lynch 2008). This also entails not unduly burdening colleagues or coworkers. A court, for example, considered a pharmacist's demand that colleagues prescreen all telephone calls and onsite customers unreasonable (Wicclair 2011).

Some protections may occur at the legislative level. Legislatures may provide protections for objecting providers referred to as conscience clauses. At the federal level, providers are protected from having to perform abortions or sterilizations (Lynch 2008). There was substantial controversy following the American College of Obstetricians and Gynecologists' publication of an opinion on conscientious objection (Rovner 2008). The opinion recommended that "physicians and other health care professionals have the duty to refer patients in a timely manner to other providers if they do not feel that they can in conscience provide the standard reproductive services that their patients request" (American College of Obstetricians and Gynecologists 2007, 1207). The Secretary of Health and Human Services Michael Leavitt (2008) expressed concern to the American Board of Obstetrics and Gynecology that physicians could be denied or lose board certification for refusing to refer. In the waning days of the Bush administration, the Department of Health and Human Services (2008) issued a final rule prohibiting discrimination against health care professionals for conscientiously refusing to perform or assist in the performance of a lawful sterilization procedure or abortion. Some groups argued that the definition of "assist in the performance," which included counseling, referral, training, and other arrangements, was too vague or broad. The

Obama administration revised or rescinded these regulations (Department of Health and Human Services 2011; see also Stein 2011).

States vary in whether they provide protection for claims of conscience and, if they do, in terms of what types of providers are protected and for what types of interventions (Guttmacher Institute 2015). Protection may be included in general statutes or specific legislation authorizing particular practices. (Executive branch agencies have also become involved, especially state pharmacy licensing boards.) Legislatures should seek to balance provider protections with patient access.

In the end, choices regarding the burdens placed on providers and patients are a matter of judgment and general rules will be necessary. Analogous debate occurs over whether restrictions on women's access to abortion are unduly restrictive. The countervailing risk, that providers will not enter or exit the profession, potentially making patients worse off, should be considered.

The most difficult cases are life-threatening emergencies in which an alternative provider is not available. One can imagine a situation in which an abortion is necessary to save a pregnant woman's life or a woman is seeking emergency contraception after a sexual assault. In underserved communities, qualified alternative providers may be unavailable within the necessary time frame. In such cases, the providers would have a professional obligation, based on the power differential and access constraints, to provide the good or service (Lynch 2008; Wicclair 2011). If they failed to do so, they could legitimately face sanctions such as the loss of their licenses. In some cases this threat may be sufficient to defeat the provider's objection. In others, the provider may continue to feel obligated to withhold the good or service. This reinforces the obligation to try to prevent such situations from arising.

INFORMED CONSENT, REFERRAL, AND DISCRIMINATION

Within these broad outlines, several specific issues should be addressed in greater detail: informed consent, referral, and discrimination (Antommaria 2010).

Informed Consent

One of the fundamental obligations of providers is to seek to obtain informed consent. Patients may not have sufficient knowledge of the potential benefits, risks, and alternatives to make an informed decision. Problematically, they may not even know what they do not know and that they should seek additional information elsewhere.

Inadequate informed consent has been a substantial issue in cases regarding emergency contraception and preterm premature rupture of membranes. Preterm premature rupture of membranes may substantially decrease the likelihood of a successful pregnancy and increase the risk of morbidity and mortality to the pregnant woman. Termination of the pregnancy is a treatment option. Women have asserted that Catholic hospitals did not inform them of this option and they suffered harm as a result (Uttley et al. 2013).

Although providing adequate informed consent should not generally be considered immoral, even if it were, it is a professional obligation. Providing informed consent should not generally be understood as formal cooperation because the provider's intention is to communicate relevant information about the patient's condition and treatment options rather than promote or condone the morally prohibited option. It is also generally not immediate material cooperation because neither the provider nor patient is, at that time, performing the morally prohibited treatment. Disclosing treatment options may at most be remote material cooperation because intervening steps are required to bring about the prohibited option such as obtaining and filling a prescription (Panicola and Hamel 2006). The discussion may provide the opportunity for objecting providers to explain respectfully why they consider certain treatment options immoral. Even if providing informed consent constituted immoral cooperation, informed consent should nonetheless be considered a professional duty (Lynch 2008; Wicclair 2011). Not providing patients with adequate informed consent may have severe negative effects on patient access. It may be sufficiently intrinsic to and frequent within the patient–provider relationship that it would be very difficult to develop satisfactory accommodations.

There is some debate about the scope of the obligation to obtain informed consent and the terminology that should be used in the process. American College of Obstetricians and Gynecologists (2007, 5) states, "Health care providers must impart accurate and unbiased information so that patients can make informed decisions about their health care. They must disclose scientifically accurate and professionally accepted characterizations of reproductive health services."

There is a debate, for example, over emergency contraception's mechanism of action and the definition of abortion. The major methods of emergency contraception are pills containing synthetic hormones and copper intrauterine devices. A levonorgestrel-containing pill (Plan-B) was approved by the FDA in 1999 and an ulipristal acetate–containing pill (ella) in 2010. (Although mifepristone can also be used as emergency contraception, it is not approved for this indication in the US.) Although copper intrauterine devices are the most effective form of emergency contraception, pills are generally considered more convenient (Gemzell-Danielsson, Berger, and Lalitkumar 2013).

Lovonorgestrel and ulipristal acetate's primary mechanism of action is preventing or delaying ovulation. (Delaying ovulation can prevent pregnancy because sperm are only viable for 4–5 days.) Lovonorgestrel inhibits, delays, or blunts the leuteinizing hormone peak and, therefore, delays or arrests follicular development. Ulipristal acetate also directly inhibits follicular rupture and, therefore, has a longer duration of action (Gemzell-Danielsson, Berger, and Lalitkumar 2013). There is debate about the existence and frequency of alternative mechanisms of action, specifically whether lovonorgestrel and ulipristal acetate also effect endometrial receptivity and embryo implantation, due to lovonorgestrel and ulipristal acetate's effectiveness even if follicular rupture occurs

(Noe et al. 2011; Kahlenborn, Peck, and Severs 2015). Copper intrauterine devices, in contrast, affect sperm function preventing fertilization, fallopian tube activity resulting in destruction of fertilized oocytes, and may also affect endometrial receptivity preventing embryo implantation (Gemzell-Danielsson, Berger, and Lalitkumar 2013). Mifepristone is capable of interrupting established pregnancies.

Physicians generally define abortion as the interruption of an established pregnancy; that is, the interruption of a pregnancy after the early embryo has implanted in the uterine wall. Using this definition, it would be inaccurate to refer to hormonal emergency contraceptives as abortifacient (Barot 2010). Some individuals and traditions, however, believe that individuals have moral standing from the time of fertilization and include actions that destroy embryos or prevent them from implanting within the term "abortion" (United States Conference of Catholic Bishops 2009). Depending on how morally scrupulous they are, how important it is to them to not perform an immoral act, the possibility that hormonal emergency contraction may act through postovulatory mechanisms may be relevant to some patients' decision making.

The goal of informed consent is to provide patients adequate information to make decisions based on their values and beliefs. There are several potential standards for informed consent: professional practice, rational person, and subjective. The professional practice standard requires a provider to disclose the information that his or her peers would disclose; the rational person standard, the information relevant to a hypothetical rational person; and the subjective standard, the information relevant to the individual patient (Beauchamp and Childress 2009). For example, a professional athlete or musician with a hand injury may have different information needs about the benefits and risks of the available treatments than the hypothetical rational person because of the higher level of function required by his or her profession.

The professional practice standard is inadequate for a number of reasons, including the fact that a customary standard may not exist and, even if one does, it may nonetheless be inadequate. The subjective standard is preferable, but not sufficient, because patients may not know what information is relevant to them and it is unreasonable to expect providers to analyze thoroughly patients' background and character to determine what information is relevant to them. The rational person standard is the most commonly used legal standard (Beauchamp and Childress 2009).

Even if stating that emergency contraception is not abortifacent were consistent with the rational person standard, it should be acknowledged that this would not provide all patients the information that is relevant to their decision making. Given the controversy regarding emergency contraception, it may be reasonable to expect providers to define how they use the term "abortion" or to ask patients how they define this term.

Referral

Referral is also an unresolved issue (Lynch 2008; Wicclair 2011). Part of the issue centers on different definitions of the term. For the sake of argument, I will define "referral" as providing the patient with contact information for a provider or organization the referring provider knows is willing to offer the service or perform the procedure that the referring provider considers immoral. Some individuals consider referral to be an unethical form of cooperation, while others consider it a necessary professional duty. Patrick C. Beeman (2012), for example, argues that referral is implicit formal cooperation because obtaining the immoral good or service is integral to the actions involved in the referral process; the goal of completing a referral form is obtaining the good or service for which the referral is being made.

This analysis has focused on patient access and, in some cases, referral may not be necessary to assure access. Other individuals or organizations may provide referral services. For example, a health care system or an insurance company may provide referral services. In reproductive health, pharmaceutical companies and private organizations may also provide referral services. For example, the manufacturers of emergency contraceptives (Afaxys 2014; Teva Women's Health, Inc. 2014) as well as the Office of Population Research and the Association of Reproductive Health Professionals (2014) provide Web-based tools to help women obtain emergency contraception. When such information is readily available, referral by the objecting provider should not be required. It should only be required when the information is not readily available, the patient lacks the skills or abilities necessary to locate the information, or the intervention is emergent.

A patient seeking goods or services from another provider is not necessarily a sufficient reason for the original provider to terminate the relationship. If the patient does choose to transfer all of his or her care, the initial provider should continue to provide other goods and services until the new provider assumes responsibility. The former provider should also transfer the patient's records to the new provider in a timely manner. Failing to do so would constitute an attempt to obstruct the patient's access to treatment and be unethical.

Discrimination

An additional topic is whether refusal to provide treatment based on an individual's characteristics constitutes unethical or invidious discrimination. Refusing to provide all medical care to an individual because of his or her race, sexual orientation, or marital status would clearly be unethical. It would, for example, be unethical to refuse to accept a patient because she is a lesbian (see American College of Obstetricians and Gynecologists 2012).

Some individuals have also argued that objecting to provide treatments related to women's reproductive health, such as contraception, also constitutes invidious discrimination because only women can become pregnant (Blackman 2007). It is not, however, clear that this is the case if one refused to prescribe or dispense all forms, or only particular forms, of contraception. For example, a pharmacy owner might object to all forms of contraception and refuse to stock condoms. Alternatively, a nurse practitioner might only object to forms of contraception that inhibit the implantation of the early embryo and be willing to prescribe other forms of contraception. Such decisions affect both men and women or only some women.

The third variation is a provider who refuses to offer particular goods or services to particular categories of patients. For example, in *North Coast Women's Care Medical Group, Inc. v. San Diego County Superior Court* (189 P. 3d 959 [Cal. 2008]), a provider did not refuse all treatment for an unmarried lesbian patient, only certain assisted reproductive technology. (There was dispute at trial whether the refusal was due to the patient's sexual orientation or marital status because California law at the time only prohibited sexual orientation discrimination.) The objection, however, may not be based on animosity to the individual's identity or class per se but on a moral objection to the particular choice he or she is making, for example, the decision to become pregnant outside of a heterosexual marriage. It, however, should be acknowledged that patients might experience the refusal as a dignitary harm.

Permitting objections based on individual patient characteristics also creates the possibility that the provider may violate the patient's privacy to inquire about factors the provider considers morally relevant. Hormonal contraception, for example, is also indicated for the control of dysmenorrhea, metrorrhagia, endometriosis, and acne. It would be inappropriate for a pharmacist to ask an unmarried client why she is filling a prescription for oral contraceptive pills in order to satisfy his or her own curiosity.

It may, therefore, be preferable to only permit categorical objections. For example, in the military context, individuals must be morally opposed to war in any form, not just particular wars, to be granted conscientious objector status (Greenawalt 1971). A potential negative consequence of this position is that some providers may not offer some goods and services that they would otherwise offer.

ORGANIZATIONS

Similar issues arise at the organizational level. Health care facilities owned by a Roman Catholic entity, such as a religious order or diocese, are expected to follow the US Conference of Catholic Bishops' *Ethical and Religious Directives for Catholic Health Care Services* (2009). These directives prohibit abortion, sterilization, and contraception. The local bishop oversees their implementation. Health care institutions that enter into business agreements with Roman Catholic–sponsored facilities are generally expected to adhere to some or all of these restrictions. These restrictions may continue to be binding even if the sponsored facility is sold or the affiliation is dissolved.

Roman Catholic–sponsored or Roman Catholic–affiliated facilities are a significant sector of the US health care system. Between 2001 and 2011, the number of Roman Catholic–sponsored or Roman Catholic–affiliated acute care hospitals grew by 16% and these facilities accounted for 10% of all acute care hospitals. They accounted for over 20% of all acute care hospitals in some states, and 30 were designated "sole community providers" by the federal government (Uttley et al. 2013).

Although the concept of conscience does not apply univocally to organizations, it can apply analogically (Wildes 1997; Sulmasy 2008). Health care institutions are not simply aggregates of people. They may have an identity and purpose, act intentionally, and make decisions that are worthy of praise or blame. Because they have a core identity and actions, they can be said to have consciences that attempt to maintain consistency between the two.

Certain obligations incumbent on providers should also be incumbent on these institutions and systems such as notice and informed consent. The Centers for Medicare and Medicaid Services may have mechanisms through reimbursement eligibility requirements to support the fulfillment of these obligations. Efforts may also be made to assure that consolidation does not unduly limit patient access. Potential mechanisms include state oversight through the granting of licenses or certificates of need. Effective use of these mechanisms may require legal authorization of regulators or expansion of the types of transactions reviewed. Mergers may also be challenged based on antitrust and charitable trust laws. Antitrust laws attempt to protect consumers from decreased competition or monopolies, and charitable trust laws prevent groups from significantly altering the mission of charitable institutions subject to the law. Conscience clauses may also apply to institutions and should be appropriately framed (Sloboda 2001).

Other types of organizations also have recently begun to assert claims of conscientious objection related to reproductive health. In an effort to expand health care coverage, the Obama administration proposed, and the Senate and Congress approved, the Affordable Care Act. Rather than establishing a single-payer health care system, the Act requires all employers meeting certain qualifications to provide health insurance to their employees. The coverage is required to meet certain minimum standards, including the provision of preventive care and contraceptives. Places of worship and their "integrated auxiliaries" are exempt from the so-called contraceptive mandate. Other employers, such a closely held private companies and religious non-profits, have objected that this requirement violates their consciences. Litigation has focused on what types of organizations are entitled to claim an exemption and what constitutes complicity or an undue burden. In *Burwell v. Hobby Lobby Stores, Inc.* (573 U.S. ___, 134 S.Ct. 2751 [2014]), the United States Supreme Court ruled that the contraceptive mandate violated the rights of closely held corporations under the Religious Freedom Restoration Act. The administration subsequently proposed regulations to shift the burden of paying for contraceptive coverage from the employer to the insurance company. Several organizations, including the Little Sisters for the Poor Home for the Aged, have argued that the requirement that they notify the Department of Health and Human Services of their objection nonetheless makes them complicit in the provision of contraceptives and therefore creates a substantial burden on their religious exercise. They argue that this violates the Relgious Freedom Restoration Act's requirments that the government have a compelling interest and utilize the least restrictive means. The Supreme Court heard oral arguments on these issues on March 23, 2016. Reaching a decision may be complicated by the current vacancy on the Supreme Court following Justice Antonin Scalia's death.

CONCLUSIONS

Conscientious objection should be understood as an effort to maintain an individual's or institution's moral integrity. Although integrity should be valued, objection by health care providers or institutions entails the risk of limiting patients' access to goods and services. This is particularly problematic because of the power and knowledge differential between health care professionals and patients and the restrictions on patients obtaining goods and services through other means. Although professional obligations entail clear duties such as notification, informed consent, and emergency treatment, efforts should be made to respect objections while maintaining access. Referral to a willing provider, for example, may not be necessary to assure access. Whether refusal to provide services to particular categories of individuals constitutes invidious discrimination remains an unresolved issue within this emerging consensus on systemic approaches to these conflicts.

BIBLIOGRAPHY

Afaxys. 2014. ella. http://www.ellanow.com/.

American College of Obstetricians and Gynecologists. 2007. ACOG Committee Opinion No. 385 November 2007: The limits of conscientious refusal in reproductive medicine. *Obstetrics and Gynecology* 110: 1203–1208.

American College of Obstetricians and Gynecologists. 2012. ACOG Committee Opinion No. 525: Health care for lesbians and bisexual women. *Obstetrics and Gynecology* 119: 1077–1080.

Antommaria, A. H. 2008. Defending positions or identifying interests: The uses of ethical argumentation in the debate over conscience in clinical practice. *Theoretical Medicine and Bioethics* 29: 201–212.

Antommaria, A. H. 2010. Conscientious objection in clinical practice: Notice, informed consent, referral, and emergency treatment. *Ave Maria Law Review* 9: 81–99.

Barot, S. 2010. Past due: Emergency contraception in U.S. reproductive health programs overseas. *Guttmacher Policy Review* 13: 8–11.

Beeman, P. C. 2012. Catholicism, cooperation, and contraception. *National Catholic Bioethics Quarterly* 12: 283–309.

Beauchamp, T. L., and J. F. Childress. 2009. *Principles of biomedical ethics* (6th ed.). New York: Oxford University Press.

Benjamin, M. 1990. *Splitting the difference: Compromise and integrity in ethics and politics.* Lawrence: University Press of Kansas.

Blackman, D. E. 2007. Refusal to dispense emergency contraception in Washington State: An act of conscience or unlawful sex discrimination? *Michigan Journal of Gender & Law* 14: 59–97.

Cantor, J., and K. Baum. 2004. The limits of conscientious objection—May pharmacists refuse to fill prescriptions for emergency contraception? *The New England Journal of Medicine* 351: 2008–2012.

Casas, L. 2009. Invoking conscientious objection in reproductive health care: Evolving issues in Peru, Mexico and Chile. *Reproductive Health Matters* 17: 78–87.

Childress, J. F. 1985. Civil disobedience, conscientious objection, and evasive noncompliance: A framework for the analysis and assessment of illegal actions in health care. *The Journal of Medicine and Philosophy* 10: 63–83.

Dana, L. 2006. What happens when there is no Plan B? *The Washington Post.* June 4. http://www.washingtonpost.com/wp-dyn/content/article/2006/06/02/AR2006060201405_2.html.

Department of Health and Human Services. 2008. Ensuring that Department of Health and Human Services funds do not support coercive or discriminatory policies or practices in violation of federal law. *Federal Register* 73: 78072–78101. (Amending 45 CFR Part 88). http://www.gpo.gov/fdsys/pkg/FR-2008-12-19/pdf/E8-30134.pdf.

Department of Health and Human Services. 2011. Regulation for the enforcement of federal health care provider conscience protection laws. *Federal Register* 76: 9968–9977. (Amending 45 CFR Part 88). http://www.gpo.gov/fdsys/pkg/FR-2011-02-23/pdf/2011-3993.pdf.

Diniz, D., A. Madeiro, and C. Rosas. 2014. Conscientious objection, barriers, and abortion in the case of rape: A study among physicians in Brazil. *Reproductive Health Matters* 22: 141–148.

Equality Now. 2015. Female genital mutilation (FGM) in the United States. http://www.equalitynow.org/sites/default/files/EN_FAQ_FGM_in_US.pdf.

Ethics Committee of the American Society for Reproductive Medicine. 2015. Use of reproductive technology for sex selection for nonmedical reasons. *Fertility and Sterility* 103: 1418–1422.

First, M. B. 2005. Desire for amputation of a limb: Paraphilia, psychosis, or a new type of identity disorder. *Psychological Medicine* 35: 919–928.

Gemzell-Danielsson, K., C. Berger, and P. G. L. Lalitkumar. 2013. Emergency contraception—Mechanisms of action. *Contraception* 87: 300–308.

Gold, R. B., and E. Nash. 2013. TRAP laws gain political traction while abortion clinics—and the women they serve—pay the price. *Guttmacher Policy Review* 16: 7–12.

Goldman, M. B., J. S. Occhiuto, L. E. Peterson, J. G. Zapka, and R. H. Palmer. 2004. Physician assistants as providers of surgically induced abortion services. *American Journal of Public Health* 94: 1352–1357.

Greenawalt, K. 1971. All or nothing at all: The defeat of selective conscientious objection. *The Supreme Court Review* 1971: 31–94.

Griese, O. N. 1987. *Catholic identity in health care: Principles and practice.* Braintree, Mass.: The Pope John Center.

Grimes, D. A., J. Benson, S. Singh, M. Romero, B. Ganatra, F. E. Okonofua, and I. H. Shah. 2006. Unsafe abortion: The preventable pandemic. *Lancet* 368, no. 9550: 1908–1919.

Guttmacher Institute. 2015. State policies in brief: Refusing to provide health services. http://www.guttmacher.org/statecenter/spibs/spib_RPHS.pdf.

Kahlenborn, C., R. Peck, and W. B. Severs. 2015. Mechanism of action of levonorgestrel emergency contraception. *The Linacre Quarterly* 82: 18–33.

Leavitt, M. O. 2008. Letter to Norman F. Gant. March 14. https://wayback.archive-it.org/3926/20131018161929/http://www.hhs.gov/news/press/2008pres/03/20080314a.html.

Lynch, H. F. 2008. *Conflicts of conscience in health care: An institutional compromise.* Cambridge, MA: The MIT Press.

Muller, S. 2009. Body integrity identity disorder (BIID)—Is the amputation of healthy limbs ethically justified? *The American Journal of Bioethics* 9: 36–43.

Noe, G., H. B. Croxatto, A. M. Salvatierra, V. Reyes, C. Villarroel, C. Munoz, G. Morales, and A. Retamales. 2011. Contraceptive efficacy of emergency contraception with levonorgestrel given before or after ovulation. *Contraception* 84: 486–492.

Office of Population Research and Association of Reproductive Health Professionals. 2014. The emergency contraception website: Get emergency contraception NOW. http://ec.princeton.edu/get-EC-now.html.

Panicola, M. R., and R. P. Hamel. 2006. Conscience, cooperation, and full disclosure. Can Catholic health care providers disclose 'prohibited options' to patients following genetic testing? *Health Progress* 87: 52–59.

Pellegrino, E. D., and D. C. Thomasma. 1993. *The virtues in medical practice.* New York: Oxford University Press.

Potts, M., and C. Denny. 1995. Safety implications of transferring the oral contraceptive from prescription-only to over-the-counter status. *Drug Safety* 13: 333–337.

Rhodes, R. 2006. The ethical standard of care. *American Journal of Bioethics* 6: 76–78.

Rovner, J. 2008. New ob/gyn guidelines stir ethics, legal debate. *NPR.* March 19. http://www.npr.org/templates/story/story.php?storyId=88552296.

Savulescu, J. 2006. Conscientious objection in medicine. *BMJ* 332: 294–297.

Schuklenk, U. 2015. Conscientious objection in medicine: Private ideological convictions must not supersede public service obligations. *Bioethics* 29: ii–iii.

Sifferlin, A. 2013. Timeline: The battle for Plan B. *Time.* June 11. http://healthland.time.com/2013/06/11/timeline-the-battle-for-plan-b/.

Sloboda, M. 2001. The high cost of merging with a religiously-controlled hospital. *Berkeley Women's Law Journal* 16: 140–156.

Stein, R. 2011. Obama administration replaces controversial "conscience" regulation for healthcare workers. *The Washington Post.* February 18. http://www.washingtonpost.com/wp-dyn/content/article/2011/02/18/AR2011021803251.html.

Sulmasy, D. P. 2008. What is conscience and why is respect for it so important? *Theoretical Medicine and Bioethics* 29: 135–149.

Teva Women's Health, Inc. 2014. Plan B one-step: Store locator. http://www.planbonestep.com/toolkit.aspx?id=store.

United States Conference of Catholic Bishops. 2009. Ethical and religious directives for Catholic health care services: Fifth edition. http://www.usccb.org/issues-and-action/human-life-and-dignity/health-care/upload/Ethical-Religious-Directives-Catholic-Health-Care-Services-fifth-edition-2009.pdf.

Uttley, L., S. Reynertson, L. Kenny, and L. Melling. 2013. Miscarriage of medicine: The growth of Catholic hospitals and the threat to reproductive health care. https://www.aclu.org/sites/default/files/field_document/growth-of-catholic-hospitals-2013.pdf.

Warriner, I. K., O. Meirik, M. Hoffman, C. Morroni, J. Harries, N. T. My Huong, N. D. Vy, and A. H. Seuc. 2006. Rates of complication in first-trimester manual vacuum aspiration abortion done by doctors and mid-level providers in South Africa and Vietnam: A randomised controlled equivalence trial. *Lancet* 368, no. 9551: 1965–1972.

White, A. 2014. Body integrity identity disorder beyond amputation: Consent and liberty. *HEC Forum* 26: 225–236.

Wicclair, M. R. 2011. *Conscientious objection in health care: An ethical analysis.* Cambridge: Cambridge University Press.

Wildes, K. W. 1997. Institutional identity, integrity, and conscience. *Kennedy Institute of Ethics Journal* 7: 413–419.

CHAPTER 10

THE ROLE OF PROVIDERS IN ASSISTED REPRODUCTION

Potential Conflicts, Professional Conscience, and Personal Choice

JUDITH DAAR

THE blessings and curses of assisted reproductive technology (ART) are well known to the millions of families formed over the past three-plus decades, thanks to this specialized field of medicine.[1] Given a choice, one suspects virtually every parent whose procreation is attributable to this marvel of modern science would have preferred to reproduce the old-fashioned way: in private, for free, and in intimate association with just one other person. Instead, ART transforms a prospective parent into a patient whose physical, financial, and psychological compartments are thrust open for medical inspection, a process that many describe as humiliating, stressful, and depressing.[2] Infertility, whether medical (the inability to conceive and maintain a pregnancy after 12 months of unprotected heterosexual intercourse) or social (the inability to conceive and maintain a pregnancy within a particular social structure without medical assistance), expands the traditional two-party, male–female dyad into a multiparty process in which nonintimate collaborators are entrusted to assist in fulfilling another's reproductive desires. Not only are the intended parents transformed but so too are physicians, who often face moral and professional dilemmas unique to the provision of fertility treatment.

Provider challenges in reproductive medicine arise from two factors that distinguish natural from assisted reproduction. First, in a medically assisted pregnancy the physician steps into a role historically occupied only by nature. In a natural cycle, whether or not a woman conceives is essentially a determination outside the scope of human manipulation. True enough, the course of a naturally occurring pregnancy can be assured and enhanced by medical interventions, but whether a sperm and egg successfully unite in a fallopian tube is a matter entirely devoid of human judgment. The infertile cannot avail themselves of this natural process but instead must look to physicians to provide the necessary treatment that will eventually place them on equal footing with naturally conceiving parents. Second, a unique feature of assisted conception, particularly in vitro fertilization (IVF), is that it creates a window of opportunity for investigating and choosing among developing embryos based on their perceived suitability for continuation or discard. Deciding which embryos should become born humans and which should not converts providers from those who merely usher in new life to those imbued with the capacity to make decisions heretofore reserved to nature. Thus, assisted reproduction necessarily injects human judgment into the procreative equation, giving ART physicians the power to decide whether a particular person is worthy of parenthood and whether a particular embryo is worthy of birth.

This chapter explores the panoply of physician challenges in reproductive medicine, focusing on specific conflicts that routinely arise in the provision of ART services. The first section explores conflicts that plague first-party reproduction, assisted conception treatment in which the patient is both the intended parent and the gamete provider. Herein called "intimate reproduction," the quest for ART services by intended parents is not always obliged by those skilled to provide such treatment. The formation of a doctor–patient relationship is a matter entrusted primarily to the physician, thus admitting an element of provider discretion. Both law and ethics reject a "vending machine" model in which patients can successfully demand any desired service of a licensed professional. That said, physicians must balance their professional autonomy and personal choice against legal regimes designed to combat unlawful conduct, including illegal discrimination. Survey and other data reveal that prospective ART patients have been turned away for a variety of stated reasons. In this section, treatment denials based on physician assessment of child welfare and parental entitlement are interrogated from legal, ethical, and clinical perspectives.

The second section moves the imposition of physician discretion along the biologic timeline to decisions about which embryos should be transferred for possible implantation and birth. Sophisticated technologies permit prospective parents to peek into their potential child's genetic makeup, enabling selection on the basis of sex and genetic health. The provider's dilemma in the face of these technologies is deciding whether to offer these selection opportunities to patients at all or, if so, under what circumstances. Such decision making pits patient reproductive liberty against physician professional autonomy, two values that are vital to the stability of the ART world. Thematic throughout this chapter is the tension between the individual's quest for biologic parenthood and the provider's exercise of professional conscience.

CONFLICTS IN INTIMATE ASSISTED REPRODUCTION

The vast majority of ART cycles performed in the United States are intimate, meaning the intended parents are able to reproduce without recruiting third parties as gamete donors or surrogates to participate in the treatment plan. Often called first-party assisted reproduction, intimate ART gives rise to at least one, and possibly two doctor–patient relationships. First and invariably, intimate ART creates a doctor–patient relationship between the provider and the treatment-seeking woman; she is the intended mother as well as the egg and womb supplier (no egg donor or gestational carriers will be involved).[3] Whether a second doctor–patient relationship arises between the sperm supplier and the treating physician depends upon the interactions between these two parties.

The male component of intimate ART is either the spouse or partner of the female patient who supplies his sperm and intends to parent any resulting child, or an anonymous sperm donor whose specimen is provided through a commercial sperm bank. As discussed herein, the use of donor sperm remains an act of intimate ART because only the specimen—and not the individual—is brought into the reproductive plan. The distinguishing feature of intimate ART in the context of provider relations is that the treating physician will typically enter into a doctor–patient relationship only with the intended parent (in the case of a single woman using donor sperm) or intended parents (in the case of a male–female couple using the partner's sperm, or a female couple using donor sperm). As these configurations suggest, establishment of doctor–patient relationships in ART is both complex and essential to the flow of professional duties in a medical setting. The existence of a doctor–patient relationship imposes several duties on the provider, including the duty of informed consent, the duty to meet clinical standards of care, and the duty not to abandon a patient.[4]

Commonsense analysis reveals that when a woman receives ART treatment for medical or social infertility via IVF or sperm insemination, she is regarded as a patient of the treating physician for all intents and purposes. Legal analysis supports this view. Under common law, "a patient-physician relationship is generally formed when a physician affirmatively acts in a patient's case by examining, diagnosing, treating or agreeing to do so."[5] Women receiving ART care are clearly subjected to the types of physical interactions with physicians that are at the heart of the common law definition of a doctor–patient relationship. In an ART setting, a less clear-cut scenario is the legal relationship, if any, between the male sperm provider/intended father and the treating physician. As an aside, it should be noted that no patient–physician relationship arises between the provider and an anonymous sperm donor who, upon donation, waives any rights to the sperm or to any future offspring, and who is unknown to all but the bank supplying the specimen.[6] But when a sperm provider is both known to the treating physician and invested in becoming a parent via the requested treatment, is the man a patient of the ART provider? Application of common law principles suggests the answer is yes.

When a man provides sperm for use in ART, a medical process ensues. The sperm must be processed by trained technicians to maximize its effectiveness in the treatment process.[7] While the sperm retrieval process may not require medical assistance in most cases, the specimen is subsequently examined and treated—the very activities that give rise to a doctor–patient relationship. The fact that the activity is applied to an excised part of the "patient's" body should not detract from the legal duty of care that attaches when a person entrusts the direct manipulation of a body part to a medical professional.

Lawsuits in which sperm is wrongfully thawed or destroyed are treated as claims of medical malpractice, which arise only in the context of a patient–physician relationship.[8] On the other hand, it would seem to follow that no doctor–patient relationship arises between a provider and the non-gamete-providing intended parent presenting in an ART scenario. A female or male partner of the treatment-seeking woman (who uses donor sperm) has no "medical" interaction with the physician, absenting any basis on which a relationship could arise.[9] The lack of a physician–patient relationship does not mean categorically that a provider owes no duties to such a third person, rather that any such duties would be founded outside of this specific relationship.[10]

Knowing that a doctor–patient relationship exists presupposes the parties have voluntarily entered into this relationship, an event that has its own legal parameters. A major tenet of American health law is that "the physician-patient relationship is . . . a voluntary and personal relationship which the physician may choose to enter or not for a variety of reasons."[11] While negotiated provider contracts and civil rights laws do limit a doctor's ability to refuse treatment, in the main the principle of physician autonomy allows providers to pick and choose among prospective patients with impunity. In the ART context, refusing to accept a person as a patient means depriving that individual of the opportunity for parenthood. The ability to provide or decline fertility treatment vests the provider with tremendous power over the procreative future of another. As such, it provokes accusations that ART doctors are "playing god," co-opting the randomness of nature. In practice, provider judgment factors into the reproductive narratives of prospective parents at two key moments, empowering physicians to decide whether a person will become a parent and, if so, to what kind of child? A discussion of these two opportunities for provider discretion in ART follows.

Treatment Denied, Parenthood Deprived

People who reproduce naturally face no institutional barriers to parenthood; they need not explain or justify their desire to anyone. In fact, the right to reproduce has been enshrined by the US Supreme Court as a "basic civil right[] of man . . . fundamental to the very existence and survival of the race."[12] Whether reproduction with medical assistance occupies this same lofty constitutional space remains debated, but resolution does not change the fact that ART inserts a physician into another's reproductive decision-making process. If we accept the argument that physicians are not to be regarded as vending machines, at the ready to deliver whatever treatment requests are made of them, then we must understand that providers will have a valued point of view on treatment seekers and their reproductive goals. In most instances, a physician's values will be compatible with the provision of treatment; in rare but important instances, a values clash will result in treatment denial.

ART providers' decisions to decline fertility treatment dwell in the interlocking worlds of physician autonomy, paternalism, contractual obligations, and antidiscrimination legal regimes.[13] Assuming that a physician is under no contractual duty to provide care (such as in an HMO or managed care arrangement) and that the authentic, nonpretextual reason for treatment refusal does not trigger liability under prevailing federal or state antidiscrimination laws, the likely foundation for such a refusal is the physician's belief either that (1) any child born to the inquiring individual(s) will be harmed by their conception or thereafter by their rearing, or (2) the prospective parents are not suitable for parenthood and should not be assisted in bringing a child into the world. Both rationales sound in protectionism, with the former professing concern for the health and safety of a child born to particular parents, and the latter expressing concern for society's well-being should a child of these particular parents be born. Child welfare and parental entitlement justifications for ART treatment denials are equally problematic, yet research suggests both are prevalent in contemporary practice.

Child Welfare Concerns: Harms From Conception

ART treatment denials grounded in child welfare concerns highlight potential harms to a future child's health and/or safety. In the health arena, a provider might be concerned that if a particular person or couple reproduces, the resulting child will be born unhealthy.[14] Two examples may be instructive. Case 1 involves a married couple in which the wife has blocked fallopian tubes, necessitating IVF. She reveals to the provider that she carries the genetic mutation for Huntington's disease, a devastating neurodegenerative genetic disorder that typically becomes symptomatic in mid-adult life. There is no known cure for Huntington's and those affected have a 50% likelihood of passing the mutation to their genetic offspring.[15] While preimplantation genetic diagnosis (PGD) to detect the presence or absence of the Huntington gene in early embryos can be done, suppose the patient refuses such an intervention. Could a physician refuse to provide IVF on the grounds that the resulting child faces a high likelihood of acquiring a devastating illness, albeit one that would permit the child decades of healthy living?

Case 2 imagines an unmarried heterosexual couple in which the male is HIV infected. While the couple could try to reproduce naturally, they want to reduce the risk of transmitting HIV to the uninfected female, and then possibly to the resulting child. Ample research conducted over decades suggests that ART clinics can significantly reduce—and even eliminate—the risk of HIV transmission by a sperm-washing technique.[16] Once the sperm has been processed, it can be used in either intrauterine insemination (IUI) or IVF. Still, the provider is concerned that introducing HIV-infected sperm into the uninfected female could pose a risk to her and her fetus and declines to accept the couple into the practice. Are the physician's actions in Case 1 and Case 2 legal? Are they ethical?

The probable controlling law in these scenarios in the United States is the federal Americans With Disabilities Act (ADA) that prohibits discrimination in the provision of public accommodations, including health care, on the basis of disability.[17] Disability is defined under the ADA as "a physical or mental impairment that substantially limits one or more of the major life activities of an individual." Turning first to Case 2 (the HIV-infected treatment seeker), in 1998 the Supreme Court held that HIV infection constitutes a disability because, at the time the case was decided, reproduction was considered high risk and thus impaired the ability of infected persons to engage in the major life activity of reproduction.[18] Scholars have recently rethought the applicability of the ADA to HIV-infected individuals seeking ART care in light of scientific evidence that with today's antiretroviral treatment protocols, HIV does not impair a person's reproductive capacity. Still, those steeped in the field continue to warn that ART treatment denials based on a person's HIV status alone would violate the ADA.[19]

Despite this straightforward analysis that denying infertility care to HIV-infected individuals violates federal law,[20] nearly every ART clinic in the country declines treatment requests from this population. Fewer than 3% of all US fertility clinics registered with the Society for Assisted Reproductive Technologies (SART) report accepting patients in which either one or both partners are HIV infected.[21] This access barrier persists, in large measure, because it is supported by both the federal government and the ART industry. The federal government's position on HIV and infertility care is contained in a 1990 recommendation by the Centers for Disease Control (CDC) that counseled "against insemination with semen from HIV-infected men" based on a single case of transmission to the uninfected female following suboptimal sperm-washing techniques.[22] Despite pleas for this outdated report to be withdrawn, the CDC has taken no formal steps to revise its longstanding recommendation.[23] As a result, clinics are reticent to defy federal recommendations that sperm from infected males not be used in assisted reproduction. Strategically, physicians seem more concerned about legal action by the federal government than individual lawsuits by HIV-infected patients.

As for the industry perspective, the American Society for Reproductive Medicine (ASRM) has issued guidelines on the provision of ART services to HIV-infected patients. In its most recent Practice Guideline addressing HIV and ART, ASRM does not counsel against treatment but "highly recommend[s] that samples from viral carriers be processed in a separate laboratory or designated space within the main laboratory, utilizing a dedicated storage tank, to minimize the risk of cross contamination."[24] Since most ART providers are not specifically trained in delivering fertility care to HIV-infected individuals and most clinics do not have the financial resources or laboratory space to support the recommended separate facilities to process gametes from HIV-infected patients, treatment refusals are accepted as nondiscriminatory and based on legitimate clinical and business rationales. The ASRM Ethics Committee approaches the issue from the premise that clinics *ought to* provide care because current techniques are highly effective in reducing the risk of transmission, but qualifies its admonition by concluding, "[f]ertility clinics, to the extent it is economically and technically feasible, should offer services to HIV-infected individuals and couples who are willing to use risk-reducing therapies."[25] This final provision—that infected individuals use risk-reducing therapies—figures prominently in our analysis of Case 1 (the female carrier of Huntington's disease).

Physician concern about conceptive harm to offspring of HIV-infected individuals seems almost irrational in light of abundant data showing horizontal transmission (partner to partner) can be virtually eliminated and vertical transmission rates (from mother to baby) hover at less than 2% when the mother is treated with antiretroviral therapy.[26] In contrast, concerns about the well-being of a child conceived by a genetic parent with the mutation for Huntington's disease is understandable and rational given the high likelihood (50%) of inheritance. Could a physician with sincere and profound moral and ethical objections to assisting in the conception of a child under these circumstances be permitted to do so?

At law, the woman patient would likely be captured by the ADA even if she has not yet manifested symptoms of the disease. Interestingly the text of the law, including recently issued regulations, does not specifically name Huntington's disease as a qualified disability but does include "HIV (whether symptomatic or asymptomatic)" as a physical or mental impairment under the ADA.[27] Arguably, the similarities between asymptomatic HIV and presymptomatic Huntington's counsel in favor of ADA coverage of the latter disease.[28] Assuming that the woman is covered by the ADA, could a physician refuse treatment on the grounds of lack of expertise or adequate facility—as is done routinely with HIV infection? No. There is no special skill or clinical component required to assist an otherwise healthy female conceive with IVF. Objecting physicians, however, are not without legal recourse.

A key exception embedded in the ADA excuses withholding of public accommodations if "to permit an individual to participate in or benefit from the goods, services, facilities, privileges, advantages and accommodations . . . poses a direct threat to the health or safety of others."[29] As Professor Kimberly Mutcherson explains, "the evaluation of a direct-threat-to-others claim is a four-part test. First, is the harm posed by the patient in question serious in nature or severity? Second, is the risk temporary and fleeting, or could it endure for a significant period of time? Third, how great is the likelihood that the threatened harm will occur? . . . Fourth, . . . is the harm imminent; in other words, how suddenly might it occur?"[30] Professor Mutcherson applies these factors to a scenario in which an HIV-infected woman seeks ART, concluding that "[o]nly where a woman . . . assert[s] no interest in taking steps to reduce the risk of transmission would a physician be justified in refusing care, and then only if such care would be denied to any person who posed a similar threshold of risk to a child."[31] Based on this analysis, a similar conclusion would obtain in the case of a Huntington's carrier seeking IVF who refuses PGD; the harm to the resulting child is serious, enduring, and highly likely if a genetic parent is a carrier. The only questionable factor is the imminence of the harm, but likely the affliction's severity would overshadow the adult-onset nature of the disease.

Analysis of Cases 1 and 2 suggests that the acceptability of treatment denials based on the threat of conceptive harm is extremely limited and might apply only in instances of serious and certain harm wherein patients refuse to adopt proven risk-reduction modalities. In these cases, providers balance the certainty of diminished child health against the reproductive desires of prospective parents who decline to maximize the health status of their future children. The balancing of child welfare against parental behavior yields less certainty when the perceived harm is predicted to occur post birth. Can and should providers refuse fertility care when they harbor sincerely held beliefs that the prospective parents lack the ability to safely rear a resulting child?

Child Welfare Concerns: Harms From Rearing

Outside the parameters of disability discrimination, there is a larger, arguably more pressing issue that arises when physicians refuse to assist ART seekers based on child welfare concerns. If the individuals or couple *could* reproduce naturally, would it be acceptable for the government to prohibit such couplings out of concern for the welfare of the child? Most would find it unthinkable for the government to prohibit the couples in Cases 1 and 2 from having children via natural conception. A law outlawing reproduction by HIV-infected or Huntington's afflicted individuals would constitute a substantial infringement on procreative liberty and would not withstand constitutional challenge. Why, then, does the government essentially permit physicians to impose such prohibitions in cases of assisted reproduction? Should the fortuity of infertility bestow upon state-licensed providers a power the government lacks in natural reproduction scenarios?

Consider Case 3 in which an unmarried opposite-sex couple has two existing children, both of whom have been placed in foster care as a result of the parents' persistent abuse and neglect. The mother has long struggled with substance abuse and the father has served jail time for child abuse. Imagine this couple presents to a fertility clinic, remorseful and unable to conceive the old-fashioned way. Would it be acceptable for a provider to refuse service to this couple? Whatever the appropriate legal or ethical response, the clinical reality is that a vast majority of ART providers asked about this hypothetical scenario responded they would be "very or extremely likely to turn away" this pair.[32] While the survey did not plumb the responders' rationales, likely the providers would assert some degree of confidence that the couple would continue to mistreat any future children in the same horrendous manner. On balance, depriving these parents another bite at the procreative apple imposes far less harm than facilitating the birth of future abuse and neglect victims. The problem with this analysis is that it assumes a high degree of predictive capacity on the part of the providers.

Even if we agree that no provider possesses an ability to predict how parents will act in the future, should this lack of complete certainty prevent physicians from denying service to those the government has deemed unworthy of parenting? If a physician can take predicted postbirth welfare into account, how serious and certain must the harm be? The ASRM Ethics Committee has considered this question, concluding that "[f]ertility programs may withhold services from prospective patients on the basis of well-substantiated judgments that those patients will be unable to provide minimally adequate or safe care for offspring."[33] The Ethics Committee acknowledges the "ethical paradox" in respecting the interests of children in the context of infertility—as a decision to deny treatment deprives the child the opportunity to be born (to some, the ultimate harm). Balancing the relevant interests, the Committee supports consideration of future harm to offspring in treatment assessments. Such harm includes direct maltreatment of children as well as the significant costs and burden imposed on the larger society by parental unfitness.[34]

The ASRM recommendation can be described as positioning itself midway between natural conception and adoption. As asserted earlier, governmental restrictions on natural reproduction face longstanding and revered constitutional barriers that make a showing of "compelling state interest" difficult to amass.[35] On the other end of the spectrum, adoption regulation is robust; laws protecting existing children derive from the doctrine of parens patriae, which imbues the state with inherent authority to protect persons who are legally unable to act on their own behalf. The state's role in adoption requires assessment of parental fitness that is gleaned from a host of measures, including psychological testing, home visits, and reference checks. While the ASRM position is carefully distinguished from the adoption model (for example, making clear that fertility practices need not conduct a home study), decisions to deny treatment are urged to be grounded in facts. To aid providers, the ASRM policy suggests scenarios in which the empirics would support a finding that "significant harm to future children is likely."[36] These include uncontrolled or untreated psychiatric illness, substance abuse, ongoing physical or emotional abuse, or a history of perpetrating physical or emotional abuse. Our couple in Case 3 falls squarely within these parameters.

What about cases in which providers are less certain, but nevertheless concerned, about a patient's rearing ability? For example, imagine patients with sensory or mobility deficits such as blindness, deafness, or quadriplegia. Would these deficits/disabilities rise to the level of evidence that a person is likely to be unable to provide minimally adequate or safe care for offspring? Perhaps an obvious point, but it is worth highlighting that disability alone is not a sufficient basis upon which to deny fertility treatment. In addition to protections under the federal ADA, state laws offer additional protections against discrimination in health care on the basis of disability.[37] Scholars warn that deprivation of infertility care on the basis of predicted (and often stereotypic and inaccurate) assessments of disabled persons' parenting capacities is highly problematic, and almost invariably illegal.[38]

The real concern surrounding ART treatment for people with disabilities is not child-rearing ability but lack of access to services. According to Professor Alicia Ouellette, "[u]nfortunately, disability-based discrimination is common in the fertility industry." Citing a recent report by the National Council on Disability, Professor Ouellette highlights, "Many prospective parents with disabilities encounter significant, and sometimes insurmountable, barriers to receiving assisted reproductive technologies . . . Access to ART is often impeded by discriminatory practices against people with disabilities, as well as the growing costs of treatment combined with limited coverage by health insurance."[39] This quote reminds us that barriers to ART extend well beyond provider discretion. Even if a physician agrees to provide treatment, an infertile person may lack the necessary resources to avail herself of those family formation services. While the impact of cost on access to ART is beyond the scope of this chapter, no discussion of infertility treatment should proceed without mention of this huge obstacle to assisted reproduction.

In sum, treatment denials in first-party reproduction on the basis of child welfare concerns present in a variety of clinical scenarios, including concerns about conceptive harm, concerns about adult-onset health harms, and concerns about harms arising from a parent's perceived lack of rearing ability. In each case, clinical practice proceeds in the face of questionable assumptions about the certainty and extent of harms, and in defiance of longstanding legal regimes prohibiting the very discrimination at the heart of these treatment denials. Reproductive suppression in the ART world stands in contrast to unfettered access to procreative liberty through natural conception. This contrast highlights the impact of provider discretion in the lives of those who depend upon assisted conception to achieve their parental goals.

Treatment Denied, Parenthood Despised

In addition to concerns over offspring welfare, the second area in which physician discretion plays a role in ART access is the realm of parental entitlement. Judgments about parental entitlement are distinct from judgments about parental fitness, discussed earlier, in that the former involve assessment of a prospective patient's worthiness to parent based on demographic features. A person's race, ethnicity, socioeconomic status, sexual orientation, and marital status can and do figure into his or her ability to access fertility treatment. Provider concern is shifted from concern for child welfare to concern for societal welfare should individuals within certain demographic categories birth children. While stereotyping and outright prejudice do play a role in constructing demographic access barriers, history and law have sadly added substance to the claim that selective infertiles are denied access to ART based on who they are and whom they love.

Provider Views of Parental Demographics: On Stereotyping and Deprivation by Proxy

Disparities in health and health care along racial and ethnic lines in the United States are well known and amply documented.[40] In 2002, the prestigious Institute of Medicine (IOM) released a comprehensive study documenting difference in health status, available treatment, and clinical outcomes according to patient race and ethnicity.[41] The IOM report summarized data from over 100 studies addressing racial differences in health care, concluding that racial and ethnic disparities are consistent and extensive across a range of medical conditions and health care services. As health law scholar Dayna Matthew laments, even after controlling for differences in socioeconomic status, health insurance, and geographic differences, "Blacks and Latinos receive fewer and inferior clinical services than whites."[42] Unfortunately but unsurprisingly, research reveals that similar disparities plague the provision of ART care in the United States, with racial and ethnic minorities experiencing a greater incidence of infertility, a lower rate of treatment seeking, and overall worse assisted reproductive health outcomes.[43]

The reasons for this "stratified reproduction" in ART are multiple and complex, ranging from physiological (for example, minority women experience greater incidents of fertility-threatening uterine fibroids) to cultural (minority women who experience infertility are more likely to wait longer before seeking medical care, worsening outcomes) to historical (history of racism in health care delivery and mistreatment of racial minorities contributes to aura of suspicion among minority patients) to financial (minority patients tend to have lower incomes and lower rates of health insurance).[44] For purposes of this chapter, stratification of assisted reproduction will be explored in the context of the patient–physician relationship. Specifically, what, if any, gatekeeping roles do ART providers play that contribute to unequal racial and ethnic access to and opting for fertility services in the United States? Researchers, scholars, and patients argue that ART providers engage in both direct discrimination as well as discrimination by proxy against patients of color.

Direct discrimination against racial and ethnic minorities in the provision of fertility care has been documented as arising from stereotyping about the reproductive lives of these groups. According to Dr. Marcia Inhorn, caricatures of minority men as hypersexual and minority women as hyperfertile "can lead to the convenient denial of their legitimate reproductive health needs."[45] The clinical impact of racial stereotyping is, at times, a circular loop that melds patient and physician attitudes and actions. On the one hand, according to Professor Dorothy Roberts, "[t]here is evidence that some physicians and fertility clinics may deliberately steer Black patients away from reproductive technologies."[46] She cites the tendency of physicians to diagnose White professional women with infertility problems such as endometriosis that can be treated with IVF. Black patients who fail to conceive are more likely to be diagnosed as having pelvic inflammatory disease (PID), often treated with sterilization.[47]

Lower referral rates of minority patients to infertility specialists from primary care physicians serve to increase suspicion amongst prospective patients about their health care providers' ability to deal with their reproductive complaints effectively and without prejudice.[48] If women of color anticipate a physician will respond to their infertility by either subtly or explicitly suggesting that they do not "need" to birth any (more) children, one can understand why these women shy away from seeking treatment. On the other hand, physicians report that minority women with signs of infertility, particularly Black women, seek out treatment less than White women. Writing on the blog for infertile women of color, one patient noted, "my own doctor has told me how hard it is to not only get women of color to admit to the issue, but also to follow-through with just the preliminary testing."[49]

Indirect discrimination or discrimination by proxy in the ART world takes shape in several ways, including geography, advertising, and financial means testing. As to geography, a list of all ART clinics in the United States coupled with a map showing population by race reveals that few if any fertility clinics are located in minority neighborhoods. For example, a website tracking fertility practices in Los Angeles County lists eight ART programs with clinics in 13 locations.[50] Those clinics are clustered in the west Los Angeles and south San Fernando Valley areas (Beverly Hills, Santa Monica, Encino, Tarzana), which are inhabited by a majority White population (85%). In contrast, there are no fertility clinics located in South Los Angeles (57% Latino and 38% Black) or Southeast Los Angeles (70% Latino, 7% Black, and 14% White).[51] Given that engaging in fertility treatment involves numerous trips to a medical facility for tests, treatments, and follow-ups, geography matters to patients. The point can be comfortably made—clinic location likely contributes to lower access to ART care for minority patients.

Discrimination by proxy along racial and ethnic lines can also be detected in ART clinic online advertising. Since at least the dawn of the twenty-first century, the majority of patients and potential patients from all socioeconomic levels have used the Internet to research their infertility issues.[52] Knowing this, Professor Jim Hawkins conducted an empirical assessment of the advertising found on fertility clinics' websites. One of his queries centered on the racial and ethnic diversity, or lack thereof, of images shown on the home page of clinic websites. Professor Hawkins viewed nearly 300 ART clinic websites, finding 63% presented pictures of only White babies on the home page, while 1% presented images of only Black babies, or only Asian babies or only Latino babies.[53] Looking for pictures with babies of different races, 97% of all websites contained an image of at least one White baby in the group.

What does this mean? As a preliminary response, Hawkins discusses the possibility that the image disparities help explain usage disparities because "pictures of white babies give social proof to white individuals considering fertility care but not to people who are of other races, driving up the number of white patients and driving down the number of patients from other races."[54] Thereafter, Hawkins suggests a deeper, darker theory; clinics are purposefully using the race of babies to draw in White patients, "confirming the charge of some academics who argue that fertility treatments entrench racist norms."[55] Relying on the social psychology theory that people are inclined to like people who are similar to them, Hawkins surmises that clinics' tendencies to advertise with a high percentage of White-only baby images is designed to create a "halo effect" for the clinic in the minds of White patients. Correspondingly, minority patients find it harder to imagine themselves patronizing a "Whites-only" clinic, even sensing an abjectly dismissive attitude toward their infertility. Other researchers who have noted the "Whiteness" of fertility clinic advertising and the homogeneity of infertility depiction in general as a Caucasian-only issue, charge that such behavior imposes an invisibility and marginalization of infertile minority couples. The lack of pictorial representation of people of color in the infertility narrative makes them invisible, unimportant, and shunned, sending a message that their childbearing is unwelcome in the ART world.[56]

The final example of discrimination by proxy draws in the behemoth barrier to ART access: affordability. ART is expensive (averaging $12,000 for one cycle of IVF) and largely excluded by the vast majority of private health insurance plans.[57] As a result, those who can afford treatment pay out of pocket. Thus, access to fertility treatment is highly correlated to a person's wealth status. One would think that the source of one's wealth would not be relevant to one's ability to access treatment, but survey data suggest otherwise. In a study looking at provider attitudes on access to ART care, physicians were queried about a host of hypothetical scenarios and asked whether they would be likely to treat or deny treatment in each case. When asked about a patient's payment source, nearly half of all physician respondents said they would refuse to treat a couple whose income source is some form of public assistance.[58]

Can public assistance serve as a proxy to race and ethnicity such that physicians and clinic policies that refuse service on the basis of income source are in effect turning away patients on the basis of race or ethnicity? Interestingly, the survey did query physicians about whether they would turn away a biracial couple, and 100% responded they were "not at all or slightly likely to turn away" this couple. So is there any racial bias in the treatment of low-resource patients? Statistically, minorities represent a larger percentage of Americans receiving public assistance than their overall representation in the population.[59] These numbers suggest that public assistance could be a pretext for discrimination on the basis of minority status. Thus, whether individual, institutional, direct or indirect, discrimination on the basis of race and ethnicity does play a role in access to fertility care. The hope herein is that highlighting these obvious and subtle barriers to ART access will spark a dialogue about much-needed reform.

Provider Views of Parental Entitlement: On Marital Status and Sexual Orientation

Today it is estimated that over 40% of US births are to unmarried women.[60] Most of those births will be achieved through natural conception but some will be ART induced. Despite the prevalence of marriageless parenthood, a subset of ART providers express discomfort in aiding an unmarried woman, man, or couple to achieve their parental dreams. In the same attitudinal survey referenced earlier, one in five respondents said they would be "very or extremely likely to turn away" a woman who does not have a husband or partner.[61] Seventeen percent said they would not treat a lesbian couple who wanted to use donor insemination, and 48% answered they would decline service to a gay couple wanting to use a surrogate, with one of the men serving as the sperm source. These survey findings are consistent with reported instances of treatment denials on the basis of marital status or sexual orientation, some of which have been litigated in American courts.[62] Granted, this survey is now nearly a decade old and might look very different today, but in all likelihood some portion of the respondents would remain steadfast in their beliefs.

Why would a physician deny service to a gay or straight single person or unmarried couple, or even a married same-sex couple? The answer lies in some combination of personal objection to so-called nontraditional families and reputed concern for the welfare of the resulting children. This latter rationale is of dissipating value and persuasiveness, as numerous studies continue to reveal that unmarried individuals and same-sex couples produce the same parenting outcomes as their married counterparts, and that children of these "nontraditional" parents fare equally well (and equally badly) as children of married heterosexual parents.[63] Despite the swell of empiric data assuring the equal well-being of children born to opposite sex married couples, single individuals, and same-sex couples, unequal access to assisted conception remains a clinical reality. An additional factor may be the law itself, which is oddly and regrettably structured to support treatment denials on the basis of marital status and sexual orientation.

As noted earlier, physicians are free to treat or turn away prospective patients as an exercise of their professional autonomy so long as their conduct does not violate prevailing antidiscrimination laws. US laws against discrimination in the provision of medical services (which include treatment for infertility) are contained in federal and state statutory schemes that delineate protected demographic categories. At the federal level, Title VI of the Civil Rights Act of 1964 prohibits physicians and hospitals receiving federal funding from discriminating in the provision of health care on the basis of race, color, or national origin.[64] Glaringly, several categories are excluded from this federal civil rights protection, including sex, marital status, and sexual orientation. While portions of other federal laws provide categorically broader protection against discrimination in other areas of daily life,[65] many Americans remain vulnerable to physician bias under the 50-year-old national civil rights law. This void has been acknowledged and addressed by a number of states with far more robust protections against discrimination in access to public accommodations, including health care facilities.

Today about half of all state civil rights laws prohibit discrimination in the delivery of health care services on the basis of marital status, and another third include sexual orientation as a protected category.[66] The fertility industry has publicly renounced provider discrimination on the basis of marital status or sexual orientation, urging ART physicians to "treat all requests for assisted reproduction equally without regard to marital/partner status or sexual orientation."[67] These formal and informal protections are promising, but the law still leaves many prospective patients without recourse should they be turned away based on their social structure, that is, whether they are married, partnered, or in a same-sex relationship. In fact, some lawmakers have worked to institutionalize discrimination on the basis of marital status, with elected officials in two states introducing bills that would have prohibited physicians from providing ART services to unmarried individuals.[68] While the bills failed to pass, they remind "nontraditional" patients of their vulnerability to physician bias and embolden providers who hold the power to judge another's worthiness for parenthood.

Internationally, physician discretion over the provision of ART services is sometimes embedded in formal law. In the United Kingdom, for example, the provision of all ART services is regulated under the Human Fertilisation and Embryology Act (HFEA), which empowers a centralized agency to license and oversee every clinic that offers assisted conception. In addition to establishing a system of licensure, the HFEA authorizes limits on the provision of services to all UK patients. One such limit that has been the subject of particular controversy involves the social structure of the treatment-seeking patient. As originally drafted in 1990, the UK law provided, "A woman shall not be provided with treatment services unless account has been taken of the welfare of any child who may be born as a result of the treatment (including the need of that child for a father), and of any other child who may be affected by the birth."[69] This provision linking the welfare of a child to the need for a father was controversial in England, especially among supporters of single and same-sex (female) parenting. The British law was amended in 2008, removing this language and replacing it with "the need for supportive parenting."[70] The concept of supportive parenting, as outlined in the HFEA Code of Practice, instructs providers to consider "a commitment to the health, well being and development of the child ... Where centres have concern as to whether this commitment exists, they may wish to take account of wider family and social networks within which the child will be raised."[71] Outside the United States, providers may expressly consider a prospective parent's social, as well as medical, qualifications for assisted conception services.

In the United States, treatment denials on the basis of marital status and sexual orientation are impliedly authorized in a number of state laws that condition their requirements for the provision of insurance coverage for fertility treatment on the marital status of the covered patient. At least five states limit coverage for infertility treatment to married individuals, and another four require that coverage be limited to "medically necessary" treatment, thus excluding treatment for single and same-sex couples who may be medically fertile but socially unable to procreate without medical assistance.[72] If state lawmakers sanction discrimination against unmarried and LGBT patients, survey data and case law reporting physician discomfort with providing treatment to these individuals should come as no surprise. Clearly the road ahead needs to include advocacy and action to broaden insurance coverage to include anyone who needs medical assistance to become a parent. Changing provider hearts and minds might well begin at ground zero of the American health care system: the insurance industry.

CONFLICTS IN EMBRYO SELECTION

Conflicts between ART physicians and patients do not necessarily end once treatment begins. Ideally, both the doctor and the patient(s) share a mutual interest and desire for the birth of a healthy child, but the science of baby making presents several opportunities for the parties to disagree over how treatment should proceed. In the main, these disagreements arise in the context of embryo selection—deciding which and how many embryos should be transferred to a female uterus for implantation, gestation, and birth. The fact that such decisions can be made by a physician or prospective parent is a display of the enormity of reproductive medicine. Both philosophically and medically complex, the assertion of human discretion into embryo selection and deselection ought to be seriously regarded for the impact that it has on individuals and society. Current technology permits human selection in three areas: selection based on genetic sex, selection based on genetic health, and selection of the number of embryos to be transferred in any given IVF cycle.

Selection Based on Genetic Sex

A quarter century ago scientists developed a technique allowing the genetic makeup of an early embryo to be investigated prior to implantation, giving parents (and possibly providers) an opportunity to choose or discard embryos on the basis of some genetic feature.[73] Styled preimplantation genetic diagnosis (PGD), the procedure begins with the biopsy of one or more cells from the in vitro embryo.[74] Once removed, the cells can be analyzed using one of several techniques with the goal of visualizing the genetic material of the would-be person. A basic analysis of the organism's genetic composition begins with a chromosome count. The normal human genome has 46 individual chromosomes in 23 pairs, with the final pair containing the sex chromosomes. PGD can reveal if the embryo is an XX (girl) or XY (boy) or even some other anomalous configuration such as XO (girl with Turner syndrome) or XXY (boy with Klinefelter syndrome). Selection on the basis of a Pair 46 anomaly is considered within the ambit of medical selection, while selection for purely social, personal, or cultural reasons is considered nonmedical sex selection.

The ethics of nonmedical sex selection using PGD have been much debated, with most air time going toward the benefits and harms arising from parental manipulation of this genetic characteristic in their future children. For purposes of this chapter, the topic shifts to the provider's role in this realm. The provider's role in nonmedical sex selection is paramount because there are few, if any, legal barriers surrounding its use in the United States.[75] Other than compliance with general antidiscrimination laws, physicians are under no legal duty to either provide or refuse to provide the means for selecting embryos on the basis of sex.[76] Thus, the principle of physician autonomy permits providers to calibrate their practices according to their own values and beliefs about the merits of the technology. How have physicians exercised this autonomy?

In a study published in 2008, researchers surveyed ART practices to learn their parameters on the use of PGD. While nearly all PGD-providing clinics offered the technique to detect aneuploidy (a missing or extra chromosome associated with a particular disease), only 42% offered PGD for nonmedical sex selection.[77] Of these clinics, 47% were willing to provide screening under all circumstances, including selecting the sex of a first child. Forty-one percent of those offering nonmedical sex selection limited prospective parents to choosing the sex of a second or subsequent child, presumably to balance their existing family. The survey also revealed that the use of nonmedical sex selection is fairly low as a percentage of genetic screening overall, with only 9% of all PGD cycles involving sex selection for nonmedical reasons.[78]

A more recent study investigated physician attitudes toward PGD for nonmedical sex selection, querying primary care physicians and ART specialists about their views toward the technology. Interestingly, the two groups of doctors had decidedly different perspectives on the ethics of assisting parents in the selection of their children's sex. Primary care physicians (who are not trained and do not offer PGD) generally disfavored the practice, citing concerns about whether women could truly express free choice under family and community pressure. They questioned the value of family balancing and worried that sex selection technologies involved invasive medical interventions in the absence of therapeutic indications, contributed to gender stereotypes that could result in neglect of children of the lesser desired sex, and were not a solution to domestic violence.[79] In contrast, ART providers (who are trained and do offer PGD) viewed sex selection as an expression of women's reproductive rights and a sign of female empowerment that allowed couples to make well-informed family planning decisions. This group believed the availability of nonmedical sex selection prevented unwanted pregnancies and abortions, and minimized the abuse of wives and/or neglect of children.[80]

In addition to the threshold decision of whether to offer nonmedical sex selection as part of their practice, ART providers are free to make further, nondiscriminatory choices about the particular circumstances under which the technique will be made available. For example, as noted earlier, some providers will only offer PGD for family balancing, requiring that a patient have an existing child and, presumably, wish to birth a child of the other sex. Imagine Case 4 in which a fertile married couple with three sons presents to a "family-balancing-only" ART clinic for IVF and PGD. The couple tells the physician that they relish the homogeneity of their offspring and wish to ensure that their fourth child is another boy. Is this family balancing? The parents might argue that they are balancing their family in a way that fulfills their reproductive desires. The physician might worry that the couple is discriminating against girls or is requesting a medical procedure that is wholly unnecessary and needlessly exposes the woman and potential child to IVF-related risks. Could a clinic that provides PGD for family balancing decline to treat this couple?

At the outset, we might search for preexisting written policies that spell out the clinic's definition of family balancing. If the policy expressly limits PGD to selection for an opposite-sex child, then treatment denial seems to be on solid ground. But if the policy is less clear, or the clinic does not limit PGD to family balancing, declining treatment may be more problematic. Imagine further in Case 4 that the couple are immigrants from India, where preferences for sons are well documented.[81] Could a physician decline to treat this couple but agree to provide PGD to a White couple with the same request? Would such action be a violation of Title VI that prohibits discrimination in the provision of health care on the basis of national origin? How about the possible violation of a state law prohibiting discrimination on the basis of sex? Is refusing to help this couple birth another boy discrimination against boys? These and myriad other questions we could pose display the complex nature of physician autonomy in the ART world. Even when obvious barriers to autonomous decision making are removed—whether self-imposed or required by law—physicians will continue to grapple with how best to exercise their power over another's reproductive choices.

Selection Based on Genetic Disease

PGD was originally developed to detect the presence of genetic mutations associated with serious diseases, and its success in so doing is remarkable. Today, the technique can detect over 100 genetic conditions, including Down syndrome, Tay Sachs, cystic fibrosis, thalassemia, sickle cell anemia, Gaucher disease, and hemophilia. In addition to these diseases that impact a child's health at birth and throughout his or her life, PGD can detect other genetic disorders that pose minimal risk to a child's health or arise later in a person's life, often in the third or fourth decade and thus are called adult-onset diseases. The wide spectrum, penetrance, and symptomology of genetic disorders raise questions about the appropriate use of a technology that is so blunt in its application. Because medical science has yet to truly crack the code of repairing genetic anomalies, today's parental choices in the face of PGD results are threefold: implant, discard, or freeze.

Ethical debate over the use of PGD to detect genetic disease, like the debate over elective sex selection, has witnessed many voices expressing a wide range of opinion. Some argue that parental selection against embryos with a disease-related genetic anomaly—no matter how mild, how likely to present, or how late in life to appear—is a protected expression of reproductive autonomy over which neither the state nor the physician should exercise control. Others argue that unfettered selection will result in embryos being discarded for mild and benign conditions and that selection based on disease reinforces existing discrimination against the disabled by expressing the view that a person living with a disability has a life not worth living. As with sex selection, the decision to offer PGD for medical selection, either as a threshold matter or mediated across the genetic disease pool, is largely a matter of physician choice. Unlike regimes in other countries that specifically control access to PGD according to codified standards, US ART providers are free (or burdened) to make these decisions as a matter of professional conscience.[82]

Individuals or couples seeking PGD often seek screening out of a desire to detect (and typically discard) embryos containing an anomaly that has plagued their family line for one or more generations. Case 5 introduces us to a single woman who is colorblind. Her particular type of vision deficiency is blue-yellow colorblindness, an autosomal dominant genetic trait. She intends to conceive using donor sperm and IVF, even though her primary care physician has advised that she is a good candidate for home insemination. Her goal is to test for and eliminate any embryos with colorblindness, explaining that she has suffered tremendously from this condition during her life. When pressed, she clarifies that her suffering arises mostly in having a limited wardrobe and being teased in grammar school. While no law currently prevents a physician from detecting and discarding embryos that are destined to yield colorblind offspring, is such conduct advisable? Should the provider's assessment that being colorblind is a benign condition posing no health risk to a child trump the patient's desire to shield her future family from the perceived difficulties she experiences in her life as a result of the condition?

In all likelihood, the patient in Case 5 would be able to obtain this desired treatment within the US system, perhaps by a provider who recognizes the woman has the legal right to learn the vision status of her child through prenatal testing and elect to abort an affected fetus. A benefits/burdens analysis could steer a provider in the treatment direction as a way of preferring embryo discard over fetal demise. If abortion providers do not (and cannot in most states) query patients about their reasons for seeking treatment, it is understandable that ART providers might take a similar "don't ask, don't tell" position. On the other hand, providing IVF to an otherwise fertile patient in which a likely outcome is the creation and subsequent destruction of embryos that are widely regarded as healthy seems somehow wrong and to be avoided. Again, thoughtful and written policies can help providers think through these scenarios, while giving notice to prospective patients about each practice's clinical and ethical limits.

Selection of the Number of Embryos for Transfer

A third dilemma providers face once a patient undergoes IVF and embryos await transfer is disagreement over the number of embryos to transfer into the uterus. This dilemma arises primarily in a financial context, owing to the high cost and low insurance reimbursement rate surrounding fertility care. Since the average cost for a single round of IVF hovers around $12,000 and an estimated 85% of ART care is paid out of pocket by patients, many who undergo this high-price procedure can afford only a single cycle.[83] Anecdotal evidence abounds that patients often request their physician to exceed recommended practice standards for embryo transfer in order to increase the odds that a pregnancy will result.[84] Importantly, transferring more embryos than are recommended for a patient's age and diagnosis may increase the chances of pregnancy, but it likewise swells the likelihood that a multiple birth will result. Birth of multiples, particularly triplets or higher, poses significant risk to the woman and her babies compared to a singleton birth.

One suspects that this bedside tug-of-war is extremely difficult for both the physician and the patient. Physicians want their patients to "succeed," which to the provider means the birth of a healthy single infant. Patients, however, may describe success as the birth of *any* baby, whether multiples and even whether or not completely healthy. Physicians are guided by industry-recommended guidelines for embryo transfer as well as tort-based standards of care.[85] Patients are often guided by years of infertility and limited economic, emotional, and psychological resources to withstand a failed IVF cycle. If a physician cedes to a patient's plea to transfer excess embryos, is she showing compassion, recklessness, or something in between? If a physician steadfastly adheres to recommended guidelines, is he showing wisdom or disregard for the patient's well-being? If a patient demands and receives excess embryos, can she hold the physician legally accountable for failing to meet the standard of care in reproductive medical practice? Even if the patient does not pursue a claim for a high-order multiple birth, can the state's licensing authority investigate and charge the provider with regulatory violations?[86] In reality, the threat of legal liability, whether from private or public enforcers, plays a significant role in the lives of physicians, and ART providers are no less anxious to avoid legal entanglement than any other medical professional. The hard truth is that in the practice of ART, physician risk-aversion can sometimes translate into offspring deprivation for some patients. ART providers hold the power to control whether and which child will be born, a power that comes with great responsibility.

CONCLUSION

Doctors who specialize in reproductive medicine experience a range of practice-related emotions, from the joy of helping an infertile person welcome a healthy child into the world to the agony of seeing that same child die or suffer as the result of parental maltreatment.[87] The natural inclination to embrace the "good" reproductive outcomes and avert the "bad" ones means that physician discretion inevitably plays a role in whether and how ART is dispensed at the bedside. Infertility, whether medically or socially based, leaves prospective patients vulnerable to this exercise of physician autonomy, with structural prohibitions against unlawful conduct often proving porous and ineffectual. This chapter outlines the key time frames in which provider and patient interests have the potential to clash, offering legal and ethical analysis of how these clashes might be resolved. Recognizing that both those who provide treatment and those who need treatment can have legitimate concerns and suspicions about the others' motivation and goals is essential to building greater trust into the doctor–patient relationship. With so much at stake, improving communication, transparency, and accessibility in reproductive medicine are worthy goals as we brace for the unthinkable discoveries that lie ahead.

Notes

1. In this chapter, ART refers to the various medical techniques used to achieve pregnancy by means other than sexual intercourse, most commonly in vitro fertilization (IVF) and artificial insemination by donor (AID). For a report on international efforts to tally the number of children born worldwide using IVF, see Suzanne Elvidge, "Five Million Births From IVF: Study Published," *BioNews*, October 21, 2013, http://www.bionews.org.uk/page_ 354987.asp. (accessed October 15, 2014).
2. See, for example, Chiara Sbaregli et al., "Infertility and Psychiatric Morbidity," *Fertility & Sterility* 90 (2008): 2107 (noting higher levels of anxiety, depressed moods, and eating disorders among infertile v. fertile subjects); also see "Trying IVF Again?" at http://www. sharedjourney.com/trying-ivf-again.html (describing men who experience the IVF process as humiliating) (accessed October 15, 2014).
3. See Centers for Disease Control, 2012, *Assisted Reproductive Technology Fertility Clinic Success Rates Report* 23 (August 2014) (reporting that approximately 88% of all ART cycles initiated in 2012 did not involve donor eggs), http://www.cdc.gov/art/ART2012/PDF/ ART_2012_Clinic_Report-Full.pdf (accessed October 15, 2014).
4. See Bryan Murray, "Informed Consent: What Must a Physician Disclose to a Patient?" *Virtual Mentor* 14 (2012): 563, http://virtualmentor.ama-assn.org/2012/07/pdf/hlaw1-1207. pdf (accessed October 16, 2014).
5. Valerie Blake, *When Is a Patient-Physician Relationship Established? Virtual Mentor* 14 (2012): 403 (citations omitted), http://virtualmentor.ama-assn.org/2012/05/pdf/hlaw1- 1205.pdf (accessed October 16, 2014).
6. For a description of the anonymous sperm donation process, visit the California Cryobank website at http://www.cryobank.com/ (accessed October 16, 2014).
7. See Rajasingam S. Jeyendran (ed.), *Sperm Collection and Processing Methods* (2003).
8. See, for example, *Baskette v. Atlanta Center for Reproductive Medicine*, 648 S.E.2d 100 (Ct. App. Ga. 2007) (characterizing claim of mishandling stored sperm as medical malpractice but dismissing under the statute of limitations).
9. See, for example, *Shin v. Kong*, 80 Cal. App. 4th 498 (2000) (physician who inseminated married woman with his own sperm rather than husband's owed no duty of care to husband because the men were not in a doctor–patient relationship).

10. See, for example, *Tarasoff v. Regents of the University of California*, 17 Cal. 3d 425, 551 P.2d 334 (Cal. 1976) (psychiatrist had duty to warn readily identifiable victim murdered by patient); *Safer v. Estate of Pack*, 291 NJ Super 619, 677 A.2d 1188 (NJ App 1996) (physician had duty to warn patient's daughter of genetic transmissibility of patient's disease); but see *Byrd v. WCW*, 868 SW2d 767 (Tex. 1994) (physician no owed no duty to child patient's father whom he wrongly accused of sexual abuse).

11. Barry R. Furrow et al., *Health Law*, 529 (5th ed. 2004).

12. *Skinner v. Oklahoma*, 316 U.S. 535, 541 (1942) (striking down a state law mandating sexual sterilization of repeat felons).

13. For a discussion of federal and state civil rights laws that apply to ART treatment refusals, see Judith Daar, "Accessing Reproductive Technologies: Invisible Barriers, Indelible Harms," *Berkeley Journal of Gender, Law, & Justice* 23 (2008): 18.

14. A companion value to this concern is the provider's certainty that the child is better off by never being born, rather than suffering whatever ill health befalls the born child. For a thorough analysis of legal regimes grounded on these and other child welfare rationales, see I. Glenn Cohen, "Beyond Best Interests," *Minnesota Law Review* 96 (2012): 1187 (arguing child-protective justifications for regulating reproduction are "vacuous and pernicious").

15. See Huntington Disease Society of America, http://www.hdsa.org/ (accessed October 16, 2014).

16. See Mark Sauer et al., "Providing Fertility Care to Men Seropositive for Human Immunodeficiency Virus: Reviewing 10 Years of Experience and 420 Consecutive Cycles of In Vitro Fertilization and Intracytoplasmic Sperm Injection," *Fertility & Sterility* 91 (2009): 2455.

17. Americans With Disabilities Act of 1990, 42 U.S.C. §12101 et seq.

18. *Bragdon v. Abbott*, 524 U.S. 624 (1998).

19. See, for example, Kimberly Mutcherson, "Disabling Dreams of Parenthood: The Fertility Industry, Anti-Discrimination, and Parents With Disabilities," *Law & Inequality* 27 (2009): 311; John Y. Phelps, "Restricting Access to Human Immunodeficiency Virus (HIV)-Seropositive Patients to Infertility Services: A Legal of the Rights of Reproductive Endocrinologists and of HIV-Seropositive Patients," *Fertility & Sterility* 88 (2008): 1483; Carl H. Coleman, "HIV, ARTs, and the ADA," *American Journal of Bioethics* 3 (2003): 43.

20. In a more thorough, elegant, and detailed analysis of HIV and ART, Professor Kimberly Mutcherson reaches essentially the same conclusion, but provides a useful step-by-step approach to how a court would likely resolve a plaintiff's claim. See Mutcherson, supra note 19.

21. See Mark Sauer, "American Physicians Remain Slow to Embrace the Reproductive Needs of Human Immunodeficiency Virus–Infected Patients," *Fertility & Sterility* 85 (2006): 295.

22. Centers for Disease Control and Prevention, "HIV-1 Infection and Artificial Insemination with Processed Semen," *Morbidity Mortality Weekly Report* 39 (1990): 249, 255–256.

23. See D. Cohan et al., "CDC Should Reverse Its Recommendation Against Sperm Washing-Intrauterine Insemination for HIV Serodifferent Couples," *American Journal of Obstetrics and Gynecology* 209 (2013): 284.

24. Practice Committee of American Society for Reproductive Medicine, "Recommendations for Reducing the Risk of Viral Transmission During Fertility Treatment with the Use of Autologous Gametes: A Committee Opinion," *Fertility & Sterility* 99 (2013): 340, 341.

25. Ethics Committee of the American Society for Reproductive Medicine, "Human Immunodeficiency Virus and Infertility Treatment," *Fertility & Sterility* 94 (2010): 11.
26. Centers for Disease Control and Prevention, "Achievements in Public Health. Reduction of Perinatal Transmission of HIV Infection: United States 1985–2005," *Morbidity Mortality Weekly Report* 55 (2006): 592.
27. Americans With Disabilities Act, Title III Regulations, Sec. 36-104.
28. See, for example, Brian R. Gin, "Genetic Discrimination: Huntington's Disease and the Americans With Disabilities Act," *Columbia Law Review* 97 (1997): 1406. Counterarguments to the position that asymptomatic HIV and presymptomatic Huntington's should be regarded identically under the ADA focus on the clinical aspects of both syndromes. While HIV immediately and persistently impairs the immune system, Huntington's impact on the body occurs concurrently with the appearance of symptoms.
29. 28 C.F.R. §36.208 (2004).
30. Mutcherson, supra note 19, at 347–348 (citations omitted).
31. Ibid. at 353. See also F. Shenfield et al., "Taskforce 8: Ethics of Medically Assisted Fertility Treatment for HIV Positive Men and Women," *Human Reproduction* 19 (2004): 2454, 2456 (when potential fertility patient living with HIV possesses "lifestyle risks . . . which may compromise parental competence and/or jeopardize the welfare of the child, such as non-compliance to HIV treatment," physicians may ethically refuse to work with the patient).
32. Andrea D. Gurmankin, Arthur L. Caplan, & Andrea M. Braverman, "Screening Practices and Beliefs of Assisted Reproductive Technology Programs," *Fertility & Sterility* 83 (2005): 61 (reporting 81% of survey respondents unlikely to treat man who was physically abusive to existing child).
33. Ethics Committee of the American Society for Reproductive Medicine, "Child-Rearing Ability and the Provision of Fertility Services: A Committee Opinion," *Fertility & Sterility* 100 (2013): 50.
34. Ibid. at 52.
35. See *Skinner v. Oklahoma*, supra note 12 (declaring the right to reproduce "fundamental," which later case law subjected to infringement of strict scrutiny requiring the government to show a compelling state interest).
36. Ethics Committee *Child-Rearing*, supra note 33, at 53.
37. See, for example, Cal. Civil Code §51 et seq. (the Unruh Civil Rights Act prohibiting discrimination in public accommodations on the basis of disability).
38. See Mutcherson, supra note 19.
39. Alicia Ouellette, "Selection Against Disability: Abortion, ART, and Access," *Journal of Law, Medicine, & Ethics* 43 (forthcoming 2015) (manuscript on file with author).
40. Portions of this section are based on the forthcoming book, Judith Daar, *The New Eugenics: Selective Breeding in an Era of Reproductive Technologies* (Yale University Press, manuscript on file with author).
41. Institute of Medicine of the National Academies, *Unequal Treatment: Confronting Racial and Ethnic Disparities in Health Care* (2002): 80–214.
42. Dayna Bowen Matthew, "A New Strategy to Combat Racial Inequality in American Health Care Delivery," *DePaul Journal of Health Care Law* 9 (2006): 793, 794.
43. See, for example, Anjani Chandra et al., National Health Statistics Reports, *Infertility and Impaired Fecundity in the United States, 1982–2010: Data from the National Survey of Family Growth*, No. 67 (August 14, 2013), at 18 (reporting racial disparities in incidence of infertility); Arthur L. Greil, Julia McQuillan, and Karina M. Shreffler, "Race-Ethnicity

and Medical Services for Infertility: Stratified Reproduction in a Population-Based Sample of U.S. Women" *Journal of Health & Social Behavior* 52 (2011): 1 (documenting disparities in treatment seeking); K. S. Richter et al., "Racial/Ethnic Disparities in Assisted Reproductive Technology (ART) Outcomes: An Analysis of 10,413 Patients From a Single Fertility Practice," *Fertility & Sterility* 96 (2011): S64.

44. See generally, Judith Daar, "Accessing Reproductive Technologies: Invisible Barriers, Indelible Harms," *Berkeley Journal of Gender, Law, & Justice* 23 (2008): 18.

45. Marcia C. Inhorn and Michael Hassan Fakid, "Arab Americans, African Americans, and Infertility: Barriers to Reproduction and Medical Care," *Fertility & Sterility* 85 (2006): 844, 845–846.

46. Dorothy E. Roberts, "Race and the New Reproduction," *Hastings Law Journal* 47 (1996): 935.

47. Ibid. at 940 (reporting in one study 20% of Black patients diagnosed with PID actually suffered from endometriosis).

48. See Vega, the brokenbrownegg website, at http://thebrokenbrownegg.org/about/mrs-tiye/ (reporting one Black woman's frustration over unsuccessful attempts to get a referral to an infertility specialist) (accessed October 2, 2014).

49. http://thebrokenbrownegg.org/about/mrs-tiye/ (accessed October 2, 2014).

50. http://www.ihr.com/infertility/provider/ivf-fertility-clinics-california-los-angeles.html (accessed October 8, 2014).

51. Mapping L.A. Neighborhoods, *Los Angeles Times*, available at http://maps.latimes.com/ neighborhoods/ (accessed October 8, 2014).

52. Ariel Weissman et al., "Use of the Internet by Infertile Couples" *Fertility & Sterility* 73 (2000): 1179.

53. Jim Hawkins, "Selling ART: An Empirical Assessment of Advertising on Fertility Clinics' Websites," *Indiana Law Journal* 88 (2013): 1147.

54. Ibid. at 1170.

55. Ibid., citing Leslie Bender, "Genes, Parents, and Assisted Reproductive Technologies: ARTs, Mistakes, Sex, Race & Law," *Columbia Journal of Gender & Law* 12 (2003): 1.

56. Marcia C. Inhorn, Rosario Ceballo, and Robert Nachtigall, "Marginalized, Invisible, and Unwanted: American Minority Struggles with Infertility and Assisted Conception," in Lorraine Culley, Nicky Hudson, and Floor van Rooij (eds.), *Marginalized Reproduction* (2009), 185.

57. See Tarun Jain & Mark D. Hornstein, "Disparities in Access to Infertility Services in a State with Mandated Coverage," *Fertility & Sterility* 84 (2005): 221.

58. Gurmankin, supra note 32, at 65 (47% saying they were "not at all or slightly likely to turn away" a couple on welfare, who wants to pay for ART with Social Security checks).

59. See, for example, US Department of Health & Human Services, "Characteristics and Financial Circumstances of TANF Recipients, Fiscal Year 2010" (setting out the recipient demographics of temporary assistance for needy families, with Whites, Blacks, and Latinos each sharing about one third of all aid), available at http://www.acf.hhs.gov/programs/ofa/resource/character/fy2010/fy2010-chap10-ys-final (accessed October 8, 2014).

60. See Centers for Disease Control & Prevention, US Department of Health and Human Services, Unmarried Childbearing (2012), available at http://www.cdc.gov/nchs/fastats/ unmarried-childbearing.htm (accessed August 26, 2014) (reporting 40.7% of US births in 2012 to unmarried women).

61. Gurmankin, supra note 32, at 65.

62. See. for example, *North Coast Women's Care Medical Group, Inc. v. San Diego Superior Court*, 44 Cal. 4th 1145, 189 P.3d 959 (2008) (upholding state law prohibiting discrimination on the basis of sexual orientation as applied to ART physician who refused service to lesbian as an expression of religious belief).

63. See, for example,American Psychological Association, Sexual Orientation, Parents & Children (2004) (finding no scientific evidence that parenting effectiveness is related to parental sexual orientation); F. Maccallum and S. Golombok, "Children Raised in Fatherless Families from Infancy: A Follow-Up of Children of Lesbian and Single Heterosexual Mothers at Early Adolescence," *Journal of Child Psychology Psychiatry* 45 (2004): 1407 (being raised in a fatherless home does not have negative consequences for children).

64. Civil Rights Act of 1964, 42 U.S.C. §2000d et seq. (2014).

65. See, for example, the federal Fair Housing Act of 1968, 42 U.S.C. §3600 et seq. (2014) (prohibits discrimination in the sale, rental, and financing of housing based on race, color, national origin, religion, sex, familial status, and disability).

66. See Daar, supra note 13, at p, 65, fn 175 (listing states that protect against marital status and sexual orientation discrimination).

67. Ethics Committee of the American Society for Reproductive Medicine, "Access to Fertility Treatment by Gays, Lesbians and Unmarried Persons: A Committee Opinion," *Fertility & Sterility* 100 (2013): 1524.

68. See Va. House Bill 187 (2006) (prohibiting physicians from performing any reproduction-assisting technique on an unmarried woman); Mary Beth Schneider, "Assisted Reproduction Bill Dropped," *Indiana Star*, October 6, 2005, at 2B (describing Indiana bill that would have required all ART-seeking patients to be married to each other).

69. Human Fertilisation and Embryology Act of 1990, Sec. 13(5).

70. Human Fertilisation and Embryology Act of 1990 (as amended in 2008), Sec. 13(5).

71. HFEA Code of Practice (8th ed.), Sec. 8.11 (2009).

72. See Jessie R. Cardinale, "The Injustice of Infertility Insurance Coverage: An Examination of Marital Status Restrictions Under State Law," *Albany Law Review* 75 (2011-12): 2133 (listing Arkansas, Hawaii, Maryland, Rhode Island, and Texas as limiting insurance coverage for infertility treatment to married patients; discussing states that require a medical indication for coverage).

73. A. H. Handyside et al., "Biopsy of Human Preimplantation Embryos and Sexing by DNA Amplification," *Lancet* 347 (1989): 49.

74. PGD can be performed either on Day 3 in which one of the embryo's 4–8 cells, called blastomeres, can be removed, or on Day 5 in which around 10–20 cells are removed from the trophectoderm or outer layer of the developing embryos, called a blastocyst. See Ruthi B. Lathi et al., *Outcomes of Trophectoderm Biopsies on Cryopreserved Blastocysts: A Case Series, Reproductive Biomedicine Online* 25 (2012): 504, http://www.rbmojournal.com/article/S1472-6483(12)00414-2/abstract.

75. The United States is one of a few countries that permit sex selection for nonmedical reasons using PGD. According to the Center for Genetics and Society, at least 36 countries ban the practice, including 25 European nations and 8 countries in Asia. The long list of countries with bans includes Australia, New Zealand, Germany, India, Israel, Spain, Turkey, and the United Kingdom. See Center for Genetics and Society, *Countries with Laws or Policies on Sex Selection* (2009), available at http://geneticsandsociety.org/downloads/200904_sex_selection_memo.pdf (accessed November 26, 2014).

76. In contrast, laws in at least eight states prohibit women from procuring an abortion for reasons related to the sex of the fetus. See International Human Rights Clinic, University of Chicago Law School, *Replacing Myths with Facts: Sex-Selective Abortion Laws in the United States* (2014).

77. Susannah Baruch, David Kaufman, and Kathy L. Hudson, "Genetic Testing of Embryos: Practices and Perspectives of US In Vitro Fertilization Clinics," *Fertility & Sterility* 89 (2008): 1053.

78. Ibid. at 1056. A 2011 study found that 17% of all PGD cycles over a two-year period were for elective sex selection. Elizabeth S. Ginsburg, et al., "Use of Preimplantation Genetic Diagnosis and Preimplantation Genetic Screening in the United States: A Society for Assisted Reproductive Techology Writing Group Paper," *Fertility & Sterility* 96 (2011): 865.

79. Sunita Pari and Robert Nachtigall, "The Ethics of Sex Selection: A Comparison of the Attitudes and Experiences of Primary Care Physicians and Physician Providers of Clinical Sex Selection Services," *Fertility & Sterility* 93 (2010): 2107.

80. Ibid. at 2112–2113.

81. See, for example, S. Puri, et al., " 'There Is Such a Thing as Too Many Daughters, but Not Too Many Sons.' A Qualitative Study of Son Preference and Fetal Sex Selection Among Indian Immigrants in the United States," *Social Science & Medicine* 72 (2011): 1169.

82. For example, in the United Kingdom access to PGD is controlled by the Human Fertilisation & Embryology Authority that limits its use to serious genetic conditions. See http://www.hfea.gov.uk/preimplantation-genetic-diagnosis.html (accessed October 31, 2014).

83. See Rosalind Berkowitz King & Joan Davis, "Introduction: Health Disparities in Infertility," *Fertility & Sterility* 85 (2006): 842.

84. See Deborah L. Forman, "When 'Bad' Mothers Make Worse Law: A Critique of Legislative Limits on Embryo Transfer," *University of Pennsylvania Journal of Law & Social Change* 14 (2011): 273, 297–298. See also Tara Siegel Bernard, "Insurance Coverage for Fertility Treatments Varies Widely," *The New York Times*, July 25, 2014 (reporting patient desires to exceed recommended embryo transfer guidelines to save money on later cycles).

85. See The Practice Committee of the Society for Assisted Reproductive Technology and the Practice Committee of the American Society for Assisted Reproductive Medicine, "Guidelines on the Number of Embryos Transferred," *Fertility & Sterility* 86 (2006): S51.

86. Such was the case of the infamous Octomom physician who transferred 12 embryos at the alleged behest of his patient, Nadya Suleman, who gave birth to octuplets. While Suleman did not sue her physician, the California licensing authority suspended the doctor's medical license.

87. See, for example, *Huddleston v. Infertility Center of America*, 700 A.2d 453 (Superior Ct. Pa. 1997) (traditional surrogate sued the agency that matched her with the genetic/intended father after he murdered the one-month-old boy).

CHAPTER 11

···

ETHICAL ISSUES IN
NEWBORN SCREENING

···

JEFFREY R. BOTKIN

MANY new parents have little awareness of the battery of screening tests that are routinely conducted on newborns in the United States and the developed world. A band-aid on the infant's heel is the most tangible sign to parents that newborn screening was done. Often referred to, inaccurately, as the "PKU test" by parents and providers alike, newborn screening actually targets a whole host of conditions through complex public health programs that represent the single largest application of genetic testing in modern medicine. Newborn screening is one of the most significant achievements in public health over the past 50 years (CDC 2011). Despite this success, the programs invite ongoing debate over a number of ethical and legal issues that have been part of the newborn screening landscape since the inception of the programs in the 1960s. This chapter will review the history of newborn screening, outline some of the key ethical and legal issues raised by these programs, and offer a prediction about how new technology may change these systems over the next few decades.

The purpose of newborn screening is to identify infants affected with a range of genetic, endocrine, and infectious diseases before the conditions cause irreversible morbidity or mortality for the child. Ideally, early detection allows preventive or therapeutic interventions before the child becomes sick. The first condition amenable to newborn screening was phenylketonuria (PKU), a condition that remains the paradigm condition for this approach to preventive health care. PKU is a genetic condition that is caused by a decrease in the function of a key enzyme in the body that metabolizes the amino acid phenylalanine to tyrosine. In the absence of the enzyme, phenylalanine accumulates in the body to high levels, causing progressive brain damage. Prior to birth, the mother's body metabolizes phenylalanine for her fetus, but following birth, the infant's body must handle this task. Infants with PKU appear entirely healthy at birth, but become progressively and irreversibly delayed within several months. However, if a diet low in phenylalanine is introduced when the infant is a few weeks of age, and continued through a lifetime, the adverse effects of the disease can be almost entirely prevented.

Screening followed by dietary treatment for PKU can have an almost miraculous effect on the health of the child and the welfare of the family.

PKU was first identified by a physician, Asbørn Folling, in 1934 after a mother of two developmentally delayed children noticed a strong smell to their urine. PKU was subsequently identified as one of the most common causes of developmental delay at the time. The capability for screening for PKU was developed in the early 1960s by Robert Guthrie (Lewis 2014). Key to population screening was the ability to detect high levels of phenylalanine in dried bloodspots on filter paper cards. This enabled drops of blood to be obtained from a heelstick of the newborn, dried on filter paper, and sent through the mail in regular batches to a central laboratory. Although the test technology has evolved considerably since the early 1960s, heelsticks and bloodspots on filter paper cards remain basic elements of the programs throughout the world. The filter paper cards are called "Guthrie Cards" in honor of the inventor of this screening capability. (Currently, newborn screening programs also include hearing screening and screening for cyanotic congenital heart disease—approaches that do not involve blood tests. The focus of this discussion will be bloodspot screening.)

Once the ability to conduct screening and treat affected infants was developed, advocacy groups for individuals with developmental delay pushed for population screening. Advocates had a receptive ear in the Kennedy administration at the federal level (Brosco 2011). However, the medical profession, and the American Academy of Pediatrics specifically, were not supportive initially of population screening (Paul and Brosco 2013). The concern was that scientists and clinicians did not know enough about PKU and the about potential benefits and risks of screening. In response to the reluctance of pediatricians and hospitals to support PKU screening, advocates successfully convinced state health departments to adopt newborn screening as a public health measure. Massachusetts was the first state to adopt PKU screening in 1963, and other states came onboard with screening within the following decade.

The conduct of newborn screening as state-based public health programs has had a number of important ramifications. This is an unusual approach to medical testing or screening, tests that are usually conducted by clinicians using hospital or commercial laboratories and with the charges for testing being covered by the patient or a third party payer. The ramifications of the state-based approach are severalfold:

- Screening is provided for all newborns regardless of the family's ability to pay.
- Until the last decade, the state-based approach permitted substantial variation from state to state on what conditions were targeted.
- Newborn screening is "mandatory" in most states, meaning that parental permission is not required for screening.
- The mandatory approach to screening, and other factors, has led to poor family and professional education about newborn screening.
- The state-based, public health approach to screening has not fostered the development of a national infrastructure for research on screening for these rare conditions.

The following sections will address each of these features in turn.

Provision of Services Regardless of the Ability to Pay

A great strength of the newborn screening system is that the screening services are provided for every infant in the United States regardless of the parent's ability to pay. This was an important element of the programs since their inception and has remained a key feature ever since. States vary in how newborn screening is funded (American Academy of Pediatrics 2000). The majority of states charge the birthing facilities for the newborn screening "kits" that provide the Guthrie cards and cover the laboratory testing and short-term follow-up for infants who test positive. Currently, the state charges birthing facilities about $100 for the kit. Birthing facilities typically then charge new parents (or their third-party payers) for the kit and for obtaining and managing the bloodspot sample. These facilities typically charge parents more than $100, although these charges are bundled in the overall delivery charges. If the parents are not insured, the cost of newborn screening will be covered by the hospital and the state. The net result of this system is that parents are not aware that they are being billed for this service and every newborn is provided service without attention to cost issues.

Most states will cover services for infants who screen positive until a definitive diagnosis is made and the child is entered into a professional relationship with a generalist or specialist who will provide long-term services. Long-term services are not provided through the system, meaning that parents and affected children are subject to the potential gaps and inequities of the US health system. Clearly the efficacy of the newborn screening system itself will only be as good as the services provided for affected children. For many conditions like PKU, the primary intervention is dietary and special foods are poorly covered by many health insurance providers. Inadequate coverage of special foods for children affected with rare metabolic conditions remains a major challenge for these families (Camp, Lloyd-Puryear, and Huntington 2012).

Variation from State to State

Within a few years, states began to add additional tests to the newborn screening panel, including congenital hypothyroidism, galactosemia, and hemoglobinopathies, including sickle cell disease. States made these determinations largely independently with the well-known Wilson and Jungner criteria for population screening as the guiding standard for most states. (See Figure 11.1) These criteria were articulated in 1968 to address population screening in general, but the concepts were relevant to newborn screening (Wilson and Jungner 1968).

However, the criteria are subjective enough that, over time, state screening programs diverged in the nature and number of tests conducted. What does it mean to say, for example, that a condition is an "important health problem"? Many conditions for which

1. The condition sought should be an important health problem
2. There should be an accepted treatment for patients with recognized disease
3. Facilities for diagnosis and treatment should be available
4. There should be a recognizable latent or early symptomatic stage
5. There should be a suitable test or examination
6. The test should be acceptable to the population
7. The natural history of the condition, including the development from latent to declared disease, should be adequately understood
8. There should be an agreed policy on whom to treat as patients
9. The cost of case finding (including diagnosis and treatment of patients diagnosed) should be economically balanced in relation to possible expenditure on medical care as a whole
10. Case-finding should be a continuing process and not a "once and for all" project

FIGURE 11.1 Wilson and Jungner Classic Screening Criteria

screening is conducted are relatively rare, with a population prevalence in the range of 1 in 10,000 to 1 in 100,000 infants. Obviously these diseases represent important health problems to the families affected. Furthermore, state populations vary in racial makeup, and some heritable conditions have substantially different frequencies in different racial groups. If a state has a small proportion of, say, African Americans in the population, would it be appropriate to conclude that sickle cell disease is not "an important health problem" in the state? Due to considerations of justice, states have implemented screening for rare conditions and conditions for which only a small subpopulation in the state is at increased risk.

By 2000, the variation between states in newborn screening programs had become substantial and lay and professional advocates successfully pushed for a uniform screening panel (American Academy of Pediatrics 2000). In 2004, the American College of Medical Genetics (ACMG) published a recommended list for a uniform panel (ACMG 2006) and, at about that same time, the Secretary of HHS, pursuant to federal legislation, established an advisory panel to make recommendations for the addition of new conditions to state panels. Subsequently, the Secretary's Advisory Committee on Heritable Diseases in Newborns and Children has conducted evidence reviews and made recommendations for states (Secretary's Advisory Committee 2015). Although the Secretary of HHS must approve the recommendations of the Advisory Committee, states remain free to add new conditions as they think appropriate. This system has resulted in substantially more uniformity between states in how newborn screening is conducted.

Mandatory Screening

In all areas of the United States but the State of Wyoming and the District of Columbia, newborn screening is considered "mandatory." That is, screening can be conducted without the explicit consent of the parents. Most states permit parents to opt out of screening for religious or philosophical reasons, although there are no major religious traditions that have doctrines that preclude newborn screening. Approximately eight states do not permit parents to opt out under state law, but, in practice, parents are almost never forced to accept screening over their objections. The single exception was a recent case in Nebraska in which state officials brought charges of child neglect against a family who refused newborn screening based on their idiosyncratic religious beliefs (Harrell 2009). The state took physical custody of the child for several days in order to conduct screening (with normal results). Subsequently, the Nebraska Supreme Court determined that a failure to permit newborn screening was not, in and of itself, sufficient to uphold a determination of child neglect. The actual number of parents who object to newborn screening is extremely low, both because a large majority of parents support newborn screening and because parents are not effectively informed of their ability to opt out in many states.

Mandatory screening has been a feature of newborn screening programs since their inception in the 1960s and has been controversial since that time. The justification has been that screening for conditions like PKU provides such substantial benefit to affected children that our traditional respect for parental authority over health care decisions for their children need not be honored in this context. However, in 1994, the Institute of Medicine recommended a consent model for newborn screening (Andrews et al. 1994) and in 2013, the American Academy of Pediatrics along with the American College of Medical Genetics recommended that parents provide permission for newborn screening, although they did not necessarily advocate for use of a signed consent form (American Academy of Pediatrics 2013). The primary arguments in favor of parental permission include a respect for parental authority, the role of informed consent in enhancing parental knowledge about newborn screening, and low probability that any particular newborn, absent a family history, will be affected by a targeted condition. There is also the clear expectation that the large majority of parents will provide permission for screening, meaning that mandates are not necessary.

Arguments in support of the current "opt-out" approach were presented by the American Society of Human Genetics in a 2015 statement on ethical and legal issues in genetic testing in children (Botkin et al. 2015). A key point is that newborn screening is rather complex in some respects and that fostering a truly informed decision in the context of the hectic environment of postpartum care is not feasible. The suggestion is that neither the staff nor new parents are likely to attend to informed decision making when many other issues about the care of a new baby and postdelivery mothers have higher priority. The consent process and signature on a form are likely to become perfunctory, undermining the primary value in the informed consent process. Surveys that have asked members of the lay public about this issue have found that respondents are largely split over whether an opt-in or opt-out approach is most appropriate (Botkin et al. 2012).

An emerging element in the debate over parental permission is the perception that some conditions being added to the state newborn screening panels do not clearly fit the original criteria promoted for mandatory, state-based screening. The benefits from screening for PKU are substantial and the risks are minimal, arguably justifying a mandatory state policy. But the benefits associated with screening for some conditions being considered for newborn screening are much less dramatic. Fragile X disease is a good example (Bailey et al. 2008). Fragile X is a genetic condition that is manifest primarily in boys as developmental delay. However, there are some implications for girls who may have some developmental delay and who may have health problems like ovarian dysfunction decades later. There is no definitive treatment for Fragile X, although early intervention may help families address social and behavioral challenges at a younger age for the child, potentially enhancing their efficacy. Furthermore, parents, if informed of an affected newborn, will be forewarned of their risk of bearing an affected child with future pregnancies. Third, parents may benefit from eliminating the so-called "diagnostic odyssey," the difficult path many parents follow from provider to provider in their attempt to find a diagnosis for their child's rare and unfamiliar condition. So there are benefits to screening newborns and to their parents even in the absence of a definitive treatment, but these benefits are much less compelling than those for PKU, congenital hypothyroidism, or sickle cell disease. Furthermore, Fragile X is a complex condition, and screening can yield information that is hard to interpret. Should conditions like Fragile X be on newborn screening panels and, if so, should the state mandate such testing along with all the other conditions on the newborn screening panels?

One consideration is to create a "second tier" of conditions amenable to newborn screening but not mandated by the state. These conditions would be offered to parents but not mandated by the state. This approach was endorsed by the President's Council on Bioethics in its 2008 statement on newborn screening (President's Council on Bioethics 2008; Fleischman, Lin & Howse 2009). Other scholars are pursing this concept (Bailey and Gehtland 2015). Whether these second-tier tests would be administered through state programs or be purchased separately on the commercial market is an open question. Clearly this approach raises some justice issues because if these tests are not covered under the state program, access for families with limited means would be reduced. This lack of access may not be of critical concern if screening for these conditions is not associated with clear and substantial benefits, however.

PARENT AND PROFESSIONAL EDUCATION ABOUT NEWBORN SCREENING

The education of both clinicians and parents is seen as an important component of newborn screening systems that may enhance the efficacy of programs and reduce adverse impacts. Yet it has been broadly recognized that current approaches to parental education are largely ineffective (Arnold, Davis, and Ohene-Frempong et al. 2006). The lack of effective education for parents is an important problem in the United States for several reasons. Of primary significance is the parents' role as key participants in state newborn screening programs. Prompt collaboration between professionals and parents is critical to providing initial screening, confirmatory testing and evaluation, and follow-up services for affected children. In addition, the literature clearly documents that some parents and families are harmed through an inadequate understanding of false-positive test results (Waisbren 2003). Second, as recognized by the American Academy of Pediatrics, parents have a right to basic information about medical interventions conducted on their children, regardless of the mandatory nature of newborn screening in almost all states (American Academy of Pediatrics 2000). Third, surveys and focus groups document that, when made better aware of newborn screening programs, parents indicate a strong preference for better education about newborn screening and for this information to be provided prenatally (Davis et al. 2006; Botkin et al. 2014). Fourth, 21 states require parental education through their newborn screening legislation, and all states prepare educational materials for parents. Fifth, the research use of residual specimens cannot be justified under state mandates for clinical screening, so there is a new expectation, established by federal law, that parents be offered information and choice about this practice at least for research funded by the federal government (Lewis 2015).

All newborn screening programs offer information to parents, primarily through printed material provided in the newborn nursery. However, as noted, most states do not have an informed permission requirement for newborn screening services, meaning that informational requirements for screening can be met through passive mechanisms such as brochures. That is, there is no requirement that parents understand the nature of newborn screening services or approve the testing of their child. The literature clearly documents the limited efficacy of this traditional approach (Arnold et al. 2006). Recognizing this problem, the American Academy of Pediatrics Task Force on Newborn Screening outlined a national agenda for strengthening state newborn screening systems and specifically called for the development and assessment of new educational tools for parents and professionals (American Academy of Pediatrics 2000). Subsequent research has shown that parents do not need or expect a detailed explanation of the conditions targeted or the complexities of the screening program. A set of simple facts about the program and what to expect regarding results is sufficient (Davis, Humiston, and Arnold et al. 2006).

Given the problems in effectively engaging parents in the immediate postpartum time period, there is a growing consensus that education of parents regarding newborn screening and residual specimens should occur as a part of prenatal care, rather than in the postpartum period alone (Farrell and Mischler 1992; Campbell and Ross 2004; Botkin 2005). The prenatal period is a potentially more effective time for education due to a longer timeframe and the parents' eagerness to learn about anything related to the health of their future child (Diem 2004; Rothwell et al. 2013).

Our own research group conducted a randomized, controlled trial of two computer tablet–based educational videos for pregnant women at about 36 weeks gestation. Women were recruited in three US cities and included a diverse set of participants with respect to income, education, and racial/ethnic heritage. Whereas the educational interventions improved knowledge of newborn screening when measured post delivery of the infant, the more remarkable finding was that the educational interventions enhanced the support of parents for newborn screening programs. Our findings were similar with respect to mothers' knowledge and support for research uses of residual dried bloodspots, a practice that has been controversial in several states in recent years (Botkin et al. 2016). Whereas educational interventions appear to be effective in such controlled circumstances, there are substantial challenges to implementing effective education about a complex topic on a population-wide basis. However, the almost universal use of tools like smartphones, tablets, and computers offers the possibility of innovative approaches to education that are not dependent on the time and expertise of clinicians in busy office or hospital settings.

Research Relevant
to Newborn Screening

As noted earlier, the original introduction of the PKU screening program was controversial and was not supported by many professionals because many felt that the condition was not adequately understood. Most of the conditions targeted by newborn screening are quite rare, posing serious challenges to gaining an adequate understanding of the condition and its treatment. Even clinicians at referral centers are likely to see only a limited number of affected children during the course of a career, and these patients will be spaced over time. This means it is virtually impossible to undertake a controlled clinical trial of a treatment intervention at only one or a few centers. This results in substantial variation between centers in treatment strategies and, often, assessments of efficacy by comparison to historical controls (Botkin 2005).

This same set of challenges pertains to research on screening programs to determine whether early detection and intervention improve the outcomes for affected children. Carefully designed trials of screening are particularly important due to the way in which population screening changes the known clinical spectrum of the conditions targeted. Most medical conditions have a wide range of severity. When conditions are first identified and characterized by clinicians, they describe individuals who tend to be more severely affected. This is simply because mild cases tend to go unnoticed or not recognized as distinctly different from other conditions. However, when population screening is conducted, affected individuals across the range of severity are found because they are identified through a biochemical abnormality and not by clinical symptoms. Therefore, screening programs identify many more "affected" individuals that are detected from clinical symptoms alone. This creates an "ascertainment bias" when comparing outcomes of individuals identified through screening to those identified by clinical presentation. If we compare the outcomes of these two groups (screening identification vs. clinical identification), the outcomes of the screened group will appear better simply because the screened group is enriched with less severe cases. A result may be that professionals and public policy experts will falsely conclude that screening improves outcomes.

Ascertainment bias creates serious challenges in conducting research on newborn screening. From a scientific perspective, it would be ideal to randomize newborns to screening versus clinical identification when there is equipoise about the efficacy of screening, and then to compare the outcomes of these two groups. Yet if there is reasonable confidence that early detection and intervention will improve the lives of affected children and their families, it becomes an ethical challenge to randomize children to a clinical detection group. Lay advocacy groups that are organized around certain conditions are often convinced of the value of population screening before the professional community, raising a political challenge to conducting a randomized trial, in addition to the barriers of cost and complexity.

To date, the only newborn screening research project that randomized population screening was the cystic fibrosis trial in Wisconsin started in the 1980s (Farrell and Mischler 1992). In this project, all newborns were screened for cystic fibrosis at birth, but investigators only looked at a random half of the results. Infants with cystic fibrosis in the group with early results were identified early and treatment begun. The other half of infants had their results read at 4 years of age. Children with a positive cystic fibrosis result were tracked down, families were informed of the result (if the children had not been clinically diagnosed already), and treatment was initiated. By comparing the early detection group with the later detection group, critical data were obtained on the efficacy and impact of newborn screening for cystic fibrosis. However, the ethics of this trial were much debated, and one set of parents entered a lawsuit against the state because they had a second child born with cystic fibrosis before the trial read the results of their first affected child. This suit was unsuccessful because of the extensive review and approval of the trial design. Nevertheless, due to these types of ethical concerns, randomized controlled trials of screening will be difficult to perform. As screening capabilities evolve and become more powerful and accurate, public health programs may be stuck with making critical decisions regarding population screening using comparisons of outcomes from screened infants with historical controls—a poor evidence base for programs that impact 4 million children per year.

THE FUTURE

Virtually all of the tests used for bloodspot screening at the present time target metabolic products that are variously found at increased or decreased concentration in affected infants. Given the fact that most conditions detected through newborn screening are genetic, theoretically, newborn screening could transition to DNA-based tests. However, the genetics of such conditions are often complex with gene dysfunction arising from numerous different variants in different individuals. The CF gene, for example, has thousands of mutations that cause the disease, some of which are common but many of which have been found in only one or a few individuals. So while DNA-based analysis for the common CF mutations is used in newborn screening programs, the definitive test remains the sweat test. For these reasons, at the present time, tests for metabolic abnormalities remain the test of choice for these rare conditions because testing for these end products reflects a final common pathway for hundreds of different mutations and interactions between multiple genes. It is certainly possible that, with time and research, we will know enough about the underlying genetics of these conditions to target DNA variants directly. If so, it is possible that the rapid, automated analysis of DNA will move the analysis from public health laboratories to hospital-based or even bedside testing.

Consider the scene in the 1997 movie *GATTACA* when, from a drop of blood, the technician reads out predictions for the future health of the baby when he is only minutes old. This scenario is appearing to be less a science fiction story and more a realistic possibility if we choose to pursue this course. Such a change in technology could have profound impacts on various aspects of the programs, including the central role of public health programs and the features that flow from that foundation, including universal access as well as mandatory implementation.

The rapid expansion of newborn screening has occurred because new tests can be efficiently added to the existing program infrastructure. Yet as the number of tests expands, the original justifications for the program infrastructure weaken. That is, when the benefits to the child become less compelling, the justification for the mandatory, public health approach to screening becomes more difficult to maintain (Gross et al. 2006). At the same time, a stronger justification for individual parental choice about screening is challenged by the enormous difficulty of adequately educating each and every new parent about these complex choices. Making public policy in the context of such value trade-offs requires much more transparency and public engagement than has been a feature of newborn screening programs traditionally.

BIBLIOGRAPHY

American Academy of Pediatrics, Committee on Bioethics, Committee on Genetics, and the American College of Medical Genetics and Genomics, Social, Ethical and Legal Issues Committee. 2013. *Pediatrics* 131: 620.

American Academy of Pediatrics, Newborn Screening Task Force. 2000. Serving the family from birth to the medical home: Newborn screening: A blueprint for the future: a call for a national agenda on state newborn screening programs. *Pediatrics* 106: 389–422.

American College of Medical Genetics. 2006. Newborn screening: Toward a uniform screening panel and system. *Genetic Medicine* 8 (Suppl.): 1S–252S.

Andrews, Lori B., Jane E. Fullarton, Neil A. Holtzman, and Arno G. Motulsky, eds. 1994. *Assessing Genetic Risks: Implications for Health and Social Policy.* Washington, DC: National Academy Press.

Arnold, Connie L., Terry C. Davis, Janet Ohene Frempong, Sharon G. Humiston, Anna Bocchini, Estela M. Kennen, and Michele Lloyd-Puryear. 2006. Assessment of newborn screening parent education materials. *Pediatrics* 117, no. 3: s320–s325.

Bailey, Donald B., Jr., and Lisa Gehtland. 2015. "Newborn Screening: Evolving Challenges in an Era of Rapid Discovery." *Journal of the American Medical Association* 313: 1511–1512.

Bailey, Donald B., Jr., Debra Skinner, Arlene M. Davis, Ian Whitmarsh, and Cynthia Powell. 2008. Ethical, legal, and social concerns about expanded newborn screening: Fragile X Syndrome as a prototype for emerging issues. *Pediatrics* 121: e693–e704.

Botkin, Jeffrey R. 2005. Research for newborn screening: developing a national framework. *Pediatrics* 116: 862–871.

Botkin, Jeffrey R., John W. Belmont, Jonathan S. Berg, Benjamin E. Berkman, Yvonne Bombard, Ingrid A. Holm, Howard P. Levy, Kelly E. Ormond, Howard M. Saal, Nancy B. Spinner, Benjamin S. Wilfond, and Joseph D. McInerney. 2015. ASHG position statement: Points to consider: Ethical, legal, and psychosocial implications of genetic testing in children and adolescents. *American Journal of Human Genetics* 97: 6–21.

Botkin, Jeffrey R, Erin Rothwell, Rebecca A. Anderson, Nancy C. Rose, Siobhan M. Dolan, Miriam Kuppermann, Louisa A. Stark, Aaron Goldenberg, and Bob Wong B. 2016. Prenatal education of parents about newborn screening and residual dried bloodspots. *JAMA Pediatrics* 170, no. 6: 543–549.

Botkin, Jeffrey R., Erin Rothwell, Rebecca A. Anderson, Aaron Goldenberg, Miriam Kupperman, Siobhan M. Dolan, Nancy C. Rose, and Louisa Stark. 2014. What parents want to know about the storage and use of residual newborn bloodspots. *American Journal of Medical Genetics Part A*. 164: 2739–2744.

Botkin, Jeffrey R., Erin Rothwell, Rebecca Anderson, Louisa Stark, Aaron Goldenberg, Michelle Lewis, Matthew Burbank, and Bob Wong. 2012. Public attitudes regarding the use of residual newborn screening specimens for research. *Pediatrics* 129: 231–238.

Brosco, Jeffrey P. 2011. Hidden in the sixties: Newborn screening programs and state authority. *Archives of Pediatric and Adolescent Medicine* 165: 589–591.

Camp, Kathryn M., Michele A. Lloyd-Puryear, and Kathleen L. Huntington. 2012. Nutritional treatment for inborn errors of metabolism: indications, regulations, and availability of medical food and dietary supplements using phenylketonuria as an example. *Molecular Genetics and Metabolism* 107: 3–9.

Campbell, Elizabeth D., and Lainie Friedman Ross. 2004. Incorporating newborn screening into prenatal care. *American Journal Obstetrics and Gynecology* 190: 876–877.

Centers for Disease Control and Prevention (CDC). 2011. Ten great public health achievements—United States, 2001–2010. *Morbidity and Mortality Weekly Report* 60, no. 19: 619–623.

Committee on Assessing Genetic Risks, Institute of Medicine. 1994. *Assessing genetic risks: Implications for health and social policy*, Lori B. Andrews, Jane E. Fullerton, Neil A. Holtzman, and Arno G. Motulsky, eds. Washington, D.C.: National Academies Press.

Davis, Terry C., Sharon G. Humiston, Connie L. Arnold, Joseph A. Bocchini, Jr., Pat F. Bass III, Estela M. Kennen, Anna Bocchini, Donna Williams, Penny Kyler, and Michele Lloyd-Puryear. 2006. Recommendations for effective newborn screening communication: Results of focus groups with parents, providers, and experts. *Pediatrics* 117: S326–S340.

Diem, Klaus. 2004. Newborn screening—should it be part of prenatal care? *American Journal of Obstetrics and Gynecology* 190, no. 4: 874.

Farrell, Philip M., and Elaine H. Mischler. 1992. Newborn screening for cystic fibrosis. The Cystic Fibrosis Neonatal Screening Study Group. *Advances in Pediatrics* 39: 35–70.

Fleischman, Alan R., Lin, Bruce K., and Jennifer L. Howse. 2009. A commentary on the President's Council on Bioethics Report: The changing moral focus of newborn screening. *Genetics in Medicine* 11: 507–509.

Gross, Scott D., Coleen A. Boyle, Aileen Kenneson, Muin J. Khoury, and Ben S. Wilfond. 2006. Public health emergency to public health service: The implications of evolving criteria for newborn screening panels. *Pediatrics* 117, no. 3: 923–929.

Harrell, Heather. 2009. The role of parents in expanded newborn screening. *Journal of Law, Medicine & Ethics* 37: 846–851.

Lewis, Michelle H. 2014. Newborn screening controversy: Past, present, and future. *Journal of the American Medical Association Pediatrics* 168, no. 3: 199–200.

Lewis, Michelle H. 2015. Lessons from the residual newborn screening dried bloodspot litigation. *Journal of Law, Medicine & Ethics* 43 (Suppl. 1): 32–35.

Paul, Diane B., and Jeffrey P. Brosco. 2013. *The PKU paradox: A short history of a genetic disease.* Baltimore, MD: Johns Hopkins University Press.

President's Council on Bioethics. 2008. *The changing moral focus of newborn screening.* Washington DC: Author. Available at https://bioethicsarchive.georgetown.edu/pcbe/reports/newborn_screening/.

Rothwell, Erin, Lauren Clark, Rebecca Anderson, and Jeffrey R. Botkin. 2013. Residual newborn screening samples for research: Parental information decision needs. *Journal of Specialists in Pediatric Nursing* 18, no. 2: 115–122.

US Department of Health and Human Services, Advisory Committee on Heritable Disorders in Newborns and Children. 2015. Available at http://www.hrsa.gov/advisorycommittees/mchbadvisory/heritabledisorders/.

Waisbren, Susan E., Simone Albers, Steve Amato, Mary Ampola, Thomas G. Brewster, Laurie Demmer, Roger B. Eaton, Robert Greenstein, Mark Korson, Cecilia Larson, Deborah Marsden, Michael Msall, Edwin W. Naylor, Siegfried Pueschel, Margretta Seashore, Vivian E. Shih, and Harvey L. Levy. 2003. Effect of expanded newborn screening for biochemical disorders on child outcomes and parental stress. *Journal of the American Medical Association* 290: 2564–2572.

Wilson, James Maxwell Glover, and Gunnar Jungner. 1968. *Principles and practice of screening for disease.* Geneva: World Health Organization. Available at http://apps.who.int/iris/handle/10665/37650.

PART III

PARENTS

CHAPTER 12

HOW WE ACQUIRE PARENTAL RIGHTS

NORVIN RICHARDS

THOSE who serve as parents to a child have a special set of moral rights and responsibilities where that child is concerned. What those rights and responsibilities are varies somewhat with the culture, but they always identify an important way in which this child is *your* child rather than someone else's, or a child who (in this sense) has no parents. Of course, there is more to being a parent than just rights and responsibilities. There are also opportunities, again varying with the culture but often including the chance to have an intimate relationship of a unique kind. The relationship can be imbued with love that is at least as deep as romantic love, and often much more durable. Moreover, parenthood can be richly illuminating and formative, not only for the child but also for the parent. Clearly, it can be one of the great goods in a person's life.[1]

What would entitle someone to have this potential good? More specifically, what would entitle a person to be a parent to a particular child *right from the start*, as it were? This would be as opposed to adopting the child, or joining what had been a single-parent family as a welcome second parent. What puts the first people who are entitled to be parents to a particular child in that position?

One answer is that *creating* the child is what does the trick. That requires us to work out who it is that creates a child, however, especially when the technology of assisted reproduction is employed, but also when it is not. In cases of both kinds, a number of people play causal roles without which the child would not exist. Does that make all of them creators of the child who therefore have parental rights, as Avery Kolers and Tim Bayne believe it might?[2] If not, what distinguishes the ones who have acquired parental rights from the ones who have not?

A second question is, why would it be *parental* rights that were acquired by creating the child? Those are not rights of ownership, since our children are not our property. So, even if building something out of material that belongs to us does make what we have built our property, it needn't also be true that building a child out of our bodies gives us *parental* rights to that child. It still has to be explained how this works, if that is to be the account we should accept.

Perhaps the key is that the child will carry your genetic code. Perhaps that is what identifies you as one of his creators, and also what entitles you to be a parent to him in the years to come. Once again, however, it would be necessary to explain why this should be true. According to Joseph Millum, "it is hard to see what justificatory connection there might be between stretches of DNA and moral standing."[3] Moreover, here are Kolers and Bayne again: "The extent to which the genetic parents' gametes compose even a newborn infant is already miniscule. The genetic material is a negligible part of the *material* constitution of the child or even the foetus . . . the newborn's body is almost wholly composed of material that was previously part of the gestational mother."[4] They conclude that "the defender of genetic constitution owes us reasons for thinking that genetic constitution is somehow more important or deeper than material constitution."[5] They think those reasons can't be provided, and thus that to say a child belongs to whoever *made* that child leaves it unclear whether this means she belongs to her genetic parents or to her gestational mother, who might be a third person. If a third party were the gestational mother, Kolers and Bayne would say that the child would belong to all three people, and to anyone else who played a causal role of the right sort in creating her—but they haven't settled upon what the right sort of causal role is. They agree that "being causally implicated in the creation of a child is the key basis for being its parent,"[6] and they favor a "pluralistic" view, according to which a great many parties "should be regarded as having *prima facie* responsibilities and rights as parents."[7]

I will argue for a narrower view than theirs. I begin, however, by arguing against a new and highly interesting approach that has been offered by Joseph Millum. His idea is that the way a child's first parents acquire their parental rights is by *earning* those rights, through behavior that is an investment in the child. He calls this an instance of "the investment principle," and he remarks that "The investment principle is a straightforward way to understand the principle of justice that says that reward should be proportional to work."[8] In the first section, I offer arguments against this way of understanding the matter. In the second and third sections, I develop a different way of doing so. In the fourth section, I explain how the theory I have offered applies to cases in which a child has been created with the help of assisted reproductive technology.

MILLUM'S INVESTMENT PRINCIPLE

Here is the heart of Joseph Millum's view:

> *The investment principle: Ceteris paribus*, the extent of an agent's stake in an object is proportional to the amount of appropriate work he or she has put into that object.
>
> *Object* is a placeholder for anything over which people can acquire rights. A person's *stake* is some set of rights over the object. The nature of these rights will be determined by the nature of the object. The *appropriate work* for producing any object of type O is (morally permissible) work that leads to a good O. This work may vary across

environments and there may be more than one way to produce a good O. Finally, all of this applies *ceteris paribus*, since there could be other moral principles whose rulings conflict with those of the investment principle and may outweigh them.[9]

Suppose we agree that appropriate work always earns the worker a stake in the object that the work helps produce, at least if the worker has not freely agreed to work for compensation instead. Here the object is supposed to be a child, and the stake earned by the appropriate work is supposed to be "rights over" that child.

A first point is that there is no reason why the rights a worker earned would have to be *parental* ones, all of which have to do with playing a certain central role in the child's life. For example, suppose a child is conceived through in vitro fertilization, and that the technicians involved go well beyond their contractual obligations to help ensure that everything goes well. If that extra work earns them a stake either in the conceptus or the child, it's not at all clear that this must take the form of parental standing. Perhaps what they have earned is the right to be kept informed about the child in the years to come, the right to have him sometimes available to them for noninvasive studies, or some other form of special access to him. Those would be rights they had earned by the work they did, but not ways in which they had become what Millum calls "moral parents" to the child, with parental rights and responsibilities. We need a way to distinguish work that earns parental rights from work that earns rights of a different kind.[10]

In addition, since it is *work* that matters, according to Millum, it is important what he means by the term. In a footnote, he says, "I am ignoring here a separate issue, which is how to distinguish work from nonwork. My inclination is to include all activity as potential work, and assign it a nonzero value when it is expected to produce something of value."[11] Things get clearer in the body of the text: "We have established that effort directed at expected value is work."[12]

If there is effort, it's not obvious when this *wouldn't* be directed at expected value. If I am making an effort, isn't this because I think it is worth doing so? The contrasting term seems to be "aimless activity." That is a minor complaint, however; here is a more serious one. For Millum, "effort directed at expected value is work," presumably regardless of what value it is that the worker expects to produce. That means having sex would count as work, regardless of what those who were having sex expected to get out of it. The sex wouldn't ordinarily be *much* work, in terms of the effort required, but it would be work. Here is Millum, again: "the act of coitus leading to conception normally involves very little work . . . "[13]

Now, if coitus leading to conception is even *very little* work, and what earns a person rights over something is putting work into it, do we earn rights over the child if our coitus results in one being conceived? I think Millum means for this to be true only if we had the sex with the intention of conceiving a child, or at least in the hope of doing so. It is hard to be sure because he does not say what it is to put one's work *into* a particular object. However, it is plausible to think that putting one's work into something is a matter of working with the intention of producing it or helping produce it, or at least in the hope that one's work will do so.

Suppose, for example, that you and I are digging a well. As we dig, we take care to avoid large rocks. We strike one anyway. Surely neither of us has put any work into finding rocks or into finding this rock in particular. We were putting our work into digging a well. On Millum's principle, then, we have acquired no rights to the large rock that was only the by-product of our labors, even if it turns out to be something of great value, because it is not an object into which we were putting our work.

That seems wrong, assuming no one else had the mineral rights to the land where we were digging the well, or a prior claim to anything unearthed on this particular dig. Otherwise, it seems as if digging up the rock *would* give us a claim to keep it. Finding the rock was just lucky, rather than a return on work invested in finding such things, but so what? We are still the ones who found it, when it was out there for the finding. That seems enough to entitle us to keep it, contrary to Millum's principle that we acquire rights to something only by investing our work into producing it.

Suppose next that two people who are having sex do not even hope that they will conceive a child. Of course, if they do conceive they won't have *found* the child, unlike the people who were digging a well and found a rock. They will have created the conceptus, but they will have done so despite not having put their work into that but into whatever other "expected value" they hoped the sex would bring. On Millum's principle, it follows that they would not have acquired any rights to the conceptus, when they conceived. It would only be a by-product of their labors, like the rock that you and I found when we were digging a well.

The intuition to the contrary is that they would have acquired rights to this by-product of their sexual activity, if certain further conditions are met. For example, suppose they had longed for a pregnancy but had given up hope. They thought the male's sperm count was too low, or that the woman's fallopian tubes or eggs were too damaged, or that they were both too old to conceive. They continue to have sex for other reasons. To their astonishment and delight, the woman does become pregnant. Millum's principle denies that this gives them a right to go on to be parents to the child, since they were not putting their "work" into conceiving one. The contrary intuition is that it does.

Note too that most pregnancies are unplanned. This means that most of the time, the conceptus is only a by-product of the work the couple did, not something they put their work into producing. So, for Millum, most of the time when someone becomes pregnant there is a period during which those who conceived the child have no right to be parents to him or her. No one does, since no one has put work into producing a child, and (on his view) it is by putting work into something that rights over it are earned.

That might be unsettling only to a philosopher. It doesn't mean that a couple who conceive a child without meaning to do so can *never* acquire rights to that child. They can do so at a later stage. Millum thinks women do this by investing the work of gestation and childbirth (presumably with the aim of producing a child, since only then will it be work they have put into that object).

> Gestational accounts of parenthood claim that moral parenthood, and therefore parental rights, arises in the first instance through gestation. The investment theory supports this claim. Indeed, one of the more plausible justifications for gestationalism is that women perform considerable labor during pregnancy.[14]

When Millum says that parental rights arise "in the first instance through gestation," he appears to contradict his earlier line of argument. After all, (a) people can have coitus in order to have a child, (b) their coitus is at least a *very little* work that they have put into that object, and (c) putting work into an object is supposed to earn the worker rights to that object. It ought to follow that parental rights arise "in the first instance" when people have coitus, if they meant to conceive and did so, rather than always arising "in the first instance through gestation."

Much deeper concerns emerge when Millum explains how he thinks rights would be acquired at the stage of gestation.

> A key question for assessing the size of a contributor's stake is how to measure the amount of morally deserving work (henceforth just 'work'). Two main factors appear relevant: the effort expended and the value created.[15]
>
> Around the time of conception, a number of individuals may have a stake in the fetus, especially in cases of assisted reproduction. However, over the course of pregnancy and childbirth, the work of the gestational mother will substantially outweigh this other work. Thus, at birth, the gestational mother will generally have a massive majority stake in the child. Amongst other things, this implies that she has the power to decide which other people will invest parental work, and therefore who else will become a moral parent.[16]

Notice that these points are not restricted to cases in which the gestational mother hadn't intended to become pregnant: Clearly, pregnancy would have been her intention "in cases of assisted reproduction." Rather, on this view women *always* acquire their parental rights after they have become pregnant, by doing the hard and valuable work of completing the pregnancy. What about men? In particular, what about the biological father of the child?

> If other people, such as the child's biological father, are not substantially involved during a woman's pregnancy, then their parental rights can be acquired only by sharing caregiving after birth. However, fathers (and others) need not be so excluded. Through their relationship with the mother during pregnancy, they may be able to provide support that constitutes a parental contribution. Further, the gestational mother may have given her partner reason to think that he or she would get to be a parent, and this may give the partner a legitimate claim to be allowed to parent.[17]

Those are very different paths to parental rights than the gestational mother's own. The last of the paths open to others, that of being given reason to believe one will get to be a parent to the child, isn't even a way in which one would earn the rights by putting in work. The other two paths do involve putting in work—being supportive during pregnancy, and sharing caregiving after birth. However, that work would certainly be far less taxing than the work the gestational mother does in carrying the child to term and giving birth. It would also be vastly inferior in "value created," the other main variable Millum sees as determining the amount of work a person put in.[18] (Surely properly looking after yourself during pregnancy and then giving birth contributes more substantially to the birth of a healthy child than being supportive during pregnancy.) In sum, these other ways of acquiring parental rights would make one only a minor claimant, compared to the gestational mother, if parental rights were determined by the work one had put in relative to the work someone else did. No wonder Millum thinks gestational mothers ordinarily have "a massive majority stake in the child" once that child is born.

Notice next that gestational mothers do not have this advantage because the minor claimants simply chose not to do work that would have been on a par with hers. They couldn't have done work of that order, given certain facts of biology. Too bad for them, if they would like to have just as strong a claim to be a parent to the child as the gestational mother does. After all, parental rights are to be determined according to "the principle of justice that says that reward should be proportional to work,"[19] and their work just doesn't measure up.

That seems deeply unfair, in a way Millum contemplates on a much smaller scale.

> . . . if two tailors both have a choice between machine-sewing and hand-sewing and one chooses the former, she may deserve a greater reward for her greater productivity; however, if one cannot afford a machine, but must sew by hand, it would be unfair if he is penalized . . . only if I am responsible for the difference in expected value does this affect what I deserve, that is, the amount of work I do . . . I suggest therefore that work is best assessed as the amount of appropriately directed effort, where appropriateness is defined as the ratio of the effectiveness of the means taken to the most effective means the agent could have taken.[20]

According to this paragraph, what matters is how close each of you came to working as effectively as you could. If so, and if everyone has an equal opportunity to work as effectively as he or she can, then everyone has an equal opportunity to earn equal standing regarding the child.

That might ease the concern that on Millum's account the way in which we acquire parental rights is deeply unfair to those who cannot perform gestation and give birth. However, it does so by undercutting his assertion that gestational mothers more or less automatically deserve far greater rewards in parental rights than anyone else.[21] There is also a deeper problem: Everyone *doesn't* have an equal opportunity to acquire parental rights, on Millum's account. This is because rights of that kind are acquired only after the woman knows she is pregnant, and she has the authority to decide who acquires them. Let me explain.

The gestational mother acquires her own parental rights by putting in the work of pregnancy and childbirth. The first of the ways in which others can acquire them is by having her give them "reason to think [they] would get to be a parent" after the child was born. Millum says only that the gestational mother *may* have given her partner this encouragement; evidently, it is up to her whether she does so. That means it is up to her whether someone earns parental rights in this first way.

The second way others can acquire parental rights is by giving the pregnant woman "support [during pregnancy] that constitutes a parental contribution." But surely it would be up to her whose support she accepted. Certainly the biological father is not entitled to insist that she accept his, on the ground that this will be his child biologically, since "the investment theory gives no weight to genetic relationships per se."[22]

The third way for others to acquire parental rights is by sharing caregiving after birth. By then, of course, the gestational mother would have acquired her own parental rights. Those would surely include a right to decide whether someone else joined her in caregiving. The exception would be for someone who already had parental rights of his or her own, and was therefore entitled to do this. But, as noted, no one can be in that position unless the gestational mother permits it, either by accepting this person's support during pregnancy or by giving "reason to think he or she would get to be a parent" after the child was born. So this third route to parental rights is also hers to give or to withhold. We are back to biology determining that one worker is far better off where parental rights are concerned than another. If it is unacceptable for differences beyond the parties' control to determine their rewards, as Millum holds in connection with the two tailors who cannot work equally effectively, then his own theory of how they are acquired is also unacceptable.

Finally, it is striking that Millum appears always to think of the parties who produce a child as investing their work separately, with their individual stake determined by how large an investment they made compared to that which others made, and with those who make a massive later investment entitled to throw the lesser workers off the job. If we must think of what is done as investments people make, surely there are times when we should think of them as making a *joint* investment. When there is a joint investment, it needn't be true that one of the investors gains an upper hand (a "massive majority stake") upon playing his part or her part, even when that part is a larger contribution. Instead, each might retain an equal right to the returns from their joint investment: in this case, an equal right to be a parent to the child. That picture seems truer to the facts, when the couple has agreed explicitly to try to have a child together. When else it might apply is the interesting question, which Millum does not address.

The key, I suggest, is not how the work that one person has put into having a child compares with the work that someone else has put into this. The key instead is what these people were *doing*, at that time. That includes whether what they were doing was making a joint effort to create a child, but it also includes much more than that. The next two sections will develop this line of thought.

RIGHTS WHEN A CHILD IS CONCEIVED INTENTIONALLY

The idea central to Millum's account is that we sometimes act in ways that deserve a reward. A more basic idea is that we are at liberty to act in those ways, as well as others. Indeed, we are at liberty to do anything we choose, as long as it is not morally wrong.

This means in part that we are free to begin any innocent action we like. It also means we are entitled to continue any morally innocent action we have underway, as long as it continues to be morally innocent, just because it is what we are doing. It needn't also be deserving of reward. We are entitled to continue it just because we were free to start it, and we did, and continuing wouldn't be morally wrong.

Without this entitlement to continue what we begin, our liberty to act as we choose would amount to very little. It wouldn't quite be true that others would always be free to make us stop whatever we began. They would only be free to *begin* to stop us, not to continue until they had succeeded. They would have to hope they could stop us in one fell swoop, and we too might be inclined to limit our public actions to what could be completed very quickly. This has comic possibilities, but no appeal whatever as an account of moral life. Better to take our liberty to do as we choose to include an entitlement to continue any morally innocent action we have begun and are not wrong to continue, just because we have it underway.

One standard way to identify what a person has underway is in terms of the intentions with which she is acting. As an illustration, recall the couple who had decided together that they would have a baby, to whom they would be parents in the years to come. Suppose that each of them reached this conclusion of his or her own free will, and that there was nothing else that made it morally wrong for them to embark upon such a project. In short, they were at liberty to begin it. Suppose they began it by having sex with the intention of creating a child to whom they would later be parents, and that they succeeded in conceiving one. That would entitle them to continue with their project, as long as it is not morally wrong for them to do so: in her case, to be the gestational mother of the child; in his, to be "supportive" during the pregnancy.

This is true regardless of whether children are created at the moment of conception, or only later in the process. The reason is that continuing what we have begun includes both completing our first step in it and taking the next one. On either view about conception, then, when the couple we are imagining have sex that results in conception, this entitles them to continue their project of creating a child whose parents they will be in the years to come. Part of being parents to the child is having parental rights regarding her. So, for them to be entitled to continue this project is for them to be entitled to those rights. There is no difference between being entitled to moral rights and having those rights. So this is a couple who have acquired parental rights, by having sex that resulted in conception. Joseph Millum would sharply disagree.

Here is one last point of comparison. Millum does not think that conceiving a child could ever be enough to provide one a fully robust claim to parental rights, akin to that acquired by gestation, with any later "nurturing" being something one had acquired the right to do. I think that is exactly what happens when two people intentionally conceive a child of their own free will, as the first step in a morally innocent joint project of having "a child of their own." They are the easy case, however. As we know, many pregnancies are unintended by either party. Neither party would have acquired parental rights in the way described. The next section will describe other ways in which parental rights can be acquired when a pregnancy is unintended.

Unintentional Pregnancies
and Legitimate Expectations

Suppose a woman finds herself pregnant, though she had not intended to be. Since it is she who is pregnant, whatever happens next in this matter must be something she does with her body (for example, manage the pregnancy so as to deliver a healthy child), something she allows her body to do without her direction (allow the pregnancy to continue or to end in miscarriage), or something that she does or allows to have done to her body (have an abortion.) That fact gives her a prima facie right to decide what it is to be. Of course, she can't choose something that would be morally wrong to do. However, it would almost never be wrong to choose to go ahead with the pregnancy and be a parent to the child in the years to come. So, that is almost always something a pregnant woman is entitled to do. She needn't also have intended to be pregnant. Rather, she is entitled to be a parent to the child she has conceived just by virtue of being pregnant with that child. What brought her these parental rights would be the actions that resulted in her being pregnant.

Of course, the story can't be the same for the man who was involved in the unintended pregnancy. The key where he is concerned is that in addition to having certain intentions when we do something with another person, we also act in the context of our previous actions with that person. That can be the basis for legitimate expectations about what the other person will do if certain unintended consequences occur.

For example, suppose A promises B that if things don't go as planned, A will pick up the pieces in a certain way. This entitles B to have A do exactly that if the time comes, assuming the promise was freely made and clearly not in jest. It needn't also be true that A had actually intended things to go in this way. Ordinarily, he won't have intended that they should, but will have meant only to cover a contingency he hoped would not arise. When it does arise, his promise of what he would do if it did entitles B to have him act as he said he would.

In the case of an unintended pregnancy, this is going to mean that the woman would be entitled to have the man be a father to the child whom neither of them meant to conceive, if he promised that he would do this if she ever did conceive. Suppose next that it had been she who had promised him this. As noted, being pregnant gives her considerable authority over what happens next. It is a domain over which she can make some promises in advance. Those include promising that the man with whom she is having sex could be a father to the child if they were to conceive one. Having made that promise, she wouldn't then be perfectly free to choose not to inform him that she was pregnant, to choose a different partner for the next stage, or to choose to go it alone. Instead, he would be entitled to be a father to the child, and to the parental rights that entailed, and she would need a justification for such actions. This wouldn't be because the two of them had intended to conceive a child to whom they would be parents. It would be because this is what she had promised would happen if she became pregnant on some occasion when they had not intended her to, and that is a promise she has the authority to make.

No doubt it is far more common for there to have been no promises. Sometimes, what there will have been instead includes delighted conversations of a future in which the couple are parents to their children. If that is how things have gone, for the woman to make a solemn promise that the man would be the father to the child if they conceived one would be jarring, and the same would be true of his asking for such a promise. Both actions are out of keeping with the kind of relationship they have. Unless there has been something substantially to the contrary, the conversations they have had about their future as parents to their children license expectations to be a parent to a child if one were to be conceived. The conversations do this no less effectively than a promise. This is partly because the expectation is one the other party has nourished, in various ways, rather than one a person has formed and harbored on his or her own.

Exactly what expectation has been licensed by their conversations is a matter of how it was reasonable for them to understand what they were saying to each other. Sometimes, the reasonable understanding would have been that it didn't matter when the child was conceived, that whenever that happened, if it did, it would begin the new stage of their lives together. Other times, the reasonable understanding would have been a different one. For example, suppose the two are high school sweethearts or college sophomores. They don't intend to conceive when they have sex, but they do talk happily about a future in which they have children. Ordinarily, this won't be the only kind of conversation they have about the future, and each will also have given other indications of his or her plans for the life that lies ahead. Those might make it obvious that she plans to be a physician, and that he plans to be an attorney. These careers wouldn't rule out their having a baby right away and being a mother to the child or a father to the child, but it would be surprising for that to be part of what either of them had in mind when they talked about having children together. Instead, the reasonable belief for them is that the children they are picturing won't come into the picture until considerably later. If so, what each of them has entitled the other to expect is that that they would have children together some day, years ahead. The question is whether that would also make it reasonable to believe they would be parents together at this earlier one, if she became pregnant.

It's easy to imagine versions of the story in which it does not. Ordinarily, giving birth to a child and being a parent to that child when you are this young either derails any plan to be a physician or an attorney, or makes that plan much harder to carry out. So, it isn't reasonable to believe you are committing yourself to early parenthood, when you commit yourself to having children together some day, unless it is also reasonable to believe that having children together has primacy over those goals, in your personal scheme of things. It could be reasonable to believe that about you, but not solely because you had clearly indicated that you wanted to have children together some time years ahead, as well as indicating that you had those other plans for your future.

If that is all there is to go on, it is reasonable to expect that the present pregnancy will be important to both of you, since you want to have children together some day. That entitles each of you to be treated as if it were important to you. The young man is entitled to be told of the accidental pregnancy. However, what they've said to each other doesn't entitle either of them to be a parent to a child who would be born now, this early in their lives, because (in this context) what they've said to each other about it doesn't make it reasonable to expect that this is how things would go if she became pregnant now. I think the young woman would do the boy a prima facie wrong if she quietly had an abortion on her own, but only because he would be entitled to know they had conceived, not because he would be entitled to be a father to that child.

There could also be a different version of their case, in which the reasonable expectation was the opposite one: that if their current sexual activity resulted in pregnancy, the male would be a father to the child and the female a mother. For example, it might be that in their culture, that's just what a person does if somebody gets pregnant. If someone were to give a career higher priority, jaws would drop all over town. If so, that is the reasonable expectation in the absence of any conversations to the contrary. In addition, the broader conversations a particular couple have had about their future lives could make it reasonable to think that having children together matters more to them than anything else. Then a young woman who terminated the pregnancy on her own would do the biological father a prima facie wrong, by acting contrary to an expectation she had nourished that he would be a father to any child they conceived even right away.

In each variation, expectations are licensed by the reasonable understanding of conversations the couple has had. It would be a prima facie wrong to disappoint such an expectation, once the woman had indeed become pregnant. There needn't also have been an intention to conceive. Rather, each party acquires parental rights when they conceive without intending to do so, when that is what they are entitled to expect. As noted, there are also other reasons why the woman acquires parental rights. The point of interest is that the man acquires them as well, if they have a history together of the kind I described.

Imagine next a couple who have a continuing sexual life, but have never discussed what they would do if she became pregnant, let alone pictured this as a time when they would share familial bliss. There might be nothing else in their history that would entitle either of them to any expectations about what would happen. However, the story can also be a different one. For example, suppose that they had been through thick and thin together in a variety of ways, supporting each other in times of need and sharing in each other's good fortune. That would encourage each of them to believe the same would be true if a child should be conceived. The belief might be false. Having a child together is something new, of its own kind. However, it could be more reasonable than the belief that they would go their separate ways, or that she would keep the matter to herself and have an abortion. It would also be a belief that neither of them had discouraged the other from having, despite understanding that a day might very well come when it would either have to be honored or disappointed. I think that can be enough to give the woman in the story a prima facie claim to expect the man to be a father to the child, if she finds that she is pregnant. By the same token, it can also give him a prima facie claim to be offered this opportunity. If so, parental rights would be his for the taking because the couple freely chose to have sex that resulted in pregnancy, and they did so in the context of the blended and supportive kind of life they were having together.

Finally, there are the many unplanned pregnancies that lack any of these back-grounds. In them, neither party has made a credible promise about what will happen if the woman becomes pregnant. Moreover, the couple have no history together at all, or none that supports beliefs about who would be a parent to a child if one were conceived. All that happens is that this time when they have sex it results in a pregnancy that nei-ther of them intended.

I argued earlier that the pregnant woman would almost always be entitled to go on to be a parent to the child, and thus to have parental rights. To reiterate, this is because whatever happens next in this matter must be something she does with her body, some-thing she allows her body to do without her direction, or something that is done to her. That entitles her to decide what it is to be, and becoming a parent to the child is one of the options she would almost always be free to choose. So, becoming pregnant in this casual way entitles her to choose to have parental rights.

Once again, that wouldn't be true of the man in this story, on the view I have offered. Since he isn't pregnant, he doesn't have her kind of claim to the choice. Nor was the man we are imagining entitled to expect he would get to be a father to the child if they were to conceive one. He hasn't been promised this, there have been no background discussions that meant an explicit promise was not needed, and they have had no history together that makes it a reasonable belief that she has encouraged him to have. On the view I am offering, there is no other reason to see him as having acquired parental rights when they had sex. He has simply chosen to act in a way that brings him none.

It is important that it does not follow he has also acquired no responsibilities of any kind. This is because his actions helped cause the pregnancy, and he is responsible for the consequences of his actions. He and his sexual partner played an equal causal role in bringing that one about, and they played this role simultaneously. They each ran the same risk that she would become pregnant, and they each did so of their own free will. That gives each of them the same causal responsibility for the pregnancy. The intriguing question is what this responsibility requires them to do.[23]

One mistaken answer is that it requires very little of the man, and a great deal of the woman. The reasoning would be that all they did when they acted *together* was to get her pregnant, so the only costs they should split equally are the costs of any tests that are needed to confirm that she is. On this view what the woman does *about* being pregnant is a new course of action that *she* carries out, rather than something the two of them did together back when they had sex, or are doing together now. So if, for example, she chooses to complete the pregnancy and give birth, he doesn't owe half the costs of that. It is something she brought about later when she chose to do it, so the costs fall entirely to her.

This reasoning is fundamentally mistaken. What the woman does about being preg-nant is not independent of what the couple did together when they had sex. Granted, what they did together does not force her to deal with the pregnancy in the way she does. She has other options. However, because what they did together got her pregnant, it does force her to choose among those options. In the cultures with which I'll begin, these fall into two broad categories: complete the pregnancy, or bring it to an end. The fact that she must choose between these is something for which the man and the woman are equally responsible.

Each of the options has its costs. So, to do what forces her to choose between them (by having sex that results in her becoming pregnant) is to force her to do something that will have the costs of one option, or something that will have the costs of the other. To say the man and the woman are equally responsible for this disjunction of costs means that they are equally responsible for the costs that are required by the disjunct it was reasonable to expect that she would choose.

Suppose she chooses the disjunct in which she completes the pregnancy, carrying the child to term and giving birth. If that is the option the man should have expected she would choose, he is equally responsible for its costs, but here is a complication. What those costs actually are depends on the way in which she carries it out. For example, suppose she could hire the obstetrician-to-the-stars to attend to her, and give birth in the luxurious hospital that this obstetrician uses, or she could hire someone who is perfectly competent but also undistinguished, and give birth in the city hospital. Obviously, the first way of completing the pregnancy is much more expensive. What does it mean, then, to say that since the man should have expected she would complete the pregnancy, he is equally responsible for "the costs" of doing so?

Ordinarily, it means he is equally responsible for the lower set of costs. The reason is that those are the costs that must be paid in order to complete the pregnancy. The higher costs exceed that and are the costs not of completing the pregnancy but of doing so in a special way. What the man and the woman did together when they had sex forces her to choose between completing the pregnancy and bringing it to an end, but it does not also force her to choose between the luxury pregnancy and the ordinary one. What forces her to choose between those is her own choice to complete the pregnancy. That means the man is not equally responsible for her having to choose between the two ways of completing the pregnancy, and *that* means he is not equally responsible for the costs of the luxury pregnancy if she chooses to go that route.

Here is an exception. Suppose the reasonable belief for him to have had when they had sex was that if this woman were to become pregnant, she would not only compete the pregnancy but would use Dr. A rather than the much cheaper but perfectly competent Dr. B. (Perhaps she has used Dr. A for past pregnancies and often says this is the doctor any woman should use.) In that case, part of the risk the man who has sex with her is accepting is that she will become pregnant *and use Dr. A.* Since he should have known that, the costs he should share equally with her if she does become pregnant are the costs of using Dr. A, not the lower costs only of completing the pregnancy in a perfectly competent way.

It might be asked why she is the one who gets to choose what to do about the pregnancy that resulted from their causal sex, instead of this being a decision that she and the man must make together. The reason, once again, is that she is the one who is pregnant. That means the decision that must be made is a choice about what she is to do with her body, or to her body. That is hers to decide. The man has no similar claim to decide it on the ground that he had as much to do with the need to decide it as she did.

Suppose next that after the child is born, the woman wants also to keep him for her own, rather than allowing him to be adopted. In the cultures with which I've begun, those are not options between which she is forced to choose because the sex she had with the man got her pregnant. Rather, she is forced to choose between them because she chose to complete the pregnancy rather than to end it. The man with whom she conceived the child bears no responsibility for what she chose in that regard. It wasn't a choice they made together, and (assuming a social setting in which this is true) completing the pregnancy was not something she had to do because of what they did do together. So he bears no responsibility for the costs of going on to raise the child to whom she gives birth, or for any costs of putting that child up for adoption. His only responsibility is for half the costs that must be paid if she is to successfully complete the pregnancy and give birth (or half the costs of the more costly Dr. A, if that should have been his expectation).

There are cultures in which an unmarried woman who has become pregnant is much less free to do as she chooses than I've described. In some of them, she would have no choice but to end the pregnancy, and if she were to complete it she would have no choice but to part ways with the child and allow others to raise him. That is, if she acted differently she would be so vilified and her outcast life so miserable that it is unreasonable to expect her not to take a course that saves her from this. Here is a variation.

In this culture, women who give their children to others to raise are so vilified that a woman's only reasonable choice is to keep any child to whom she gives birth. Then to be pregnant is not to face a choice between ending the pregnancy and completing it, but a choice between ending the pregnancy and completing it *and keeping the child*. Those are the genuine alternatives, and the choice she has to make is between them. Suppose she chooses to complete the pregnancy, thereby choosing also to keep the child. In this setting, that means her sexual partner is equally responsible for the costs of raising the child, since he is equally responsible for her having to make this choice and thereby equally responsible for the costs of whichever alternative she chooses. My earlier argument applies only to cultures in which the woman's genuine alternatives include completing the pregnancy and then either keeping the child or giving the child up.

A different concern is that I have also written as if the only costs of an unintended pregnancy were financial and were limited to the costs of obstetric care. Clearly there can be great emotional costs as well. Suppose it were terribly distressing for a woman to find that she was pregnant after casual sex. Her sexual partner is equally responsible for that distress. Similarly, some of the cultures I've been imagining will impose harsh costs on the woman who becomes pregnant under the circumstances imagined, but not on the man. It isn't possible for him to shoulder half the cultural costs imposed upon her. The way to hold him equally responsible for the emotional and cultural costs of their having conceived a child is to say he should pay half of any financial costs *those* impose. This is unsatisfying, but I think it is the best we can do.

Earlier, I also argued that the man we are imagining would not be entitled to be a father to the child in the years to come. This is because of the circumstances under which the two of them had the sex that resulted in pregnancy. They had it with no assurances on either side. Neither of them had made any promises, or nurtured any expectations, or left in place a reasonable belief that he would be a father to the child if one were conceived. If he had had those assurances from her, he would be entitled to parental rights, and also responsible for half the costs of being a parent to the child. If she had had those assurances from him, she would be entitled to have him be a father to the child, or, if he was unwilling to do so, to pay half the costs of the pregnancy and childbirth and half the costs of being a parent to the child.

That concerns people who conceive a child when they have sex. It is now possible to conceive one without anyone having sex, of course, through the use of assisted reproductive technology. The closing section will apply the approach I have offered to that way of acquiring parental rights.

INTENTIONS AND ASSISTED REPRODUCTIVE TECHNOLOGY

The Center for Disease Control defines assisted reproductive technology as "all fertility treatments in which both eggs and sperm are handled. In general, they involve surgically removing eggs from a woman's ovaries, combining them with sperm in a laboratory, and returning them to the woman's body or donating them to another woman."[24] The version of interest is the one in which the fertilized egg is placed in the body of a different woman than the one from whom they were taken. That will mean there are two women who might seem to have parental rights, rather than only one: the woman who contributed the genes, and the woman who carried out the gestation.

It is also possible to have two women contribute the genes. The first step would be to remove the nucleus of a woman's egg but not the mitochondria, replacing the nucleus with genetic material from the egg of a different woman. Since the mitochondria have DNA of their own, any child produced using this egg would have two genetic mothers, rather than only one. Finally, the sperm used could be that of a man who was the partner of one of the women involved in the process, or it could be that of a different man.

In all of these variations, who is entitled to be a parent to the child? Since the point of the process is to create a child, the analogue is not that of an unintended pregnancy but an intended one. According to my earlier reasoning, when people have sex with the intention of creating a child to whom they will be parents in the years to come, this entitles them to continue their project and thus to have the rights that are part of parenthood. The only restriction is that their project must be morally innocent; it cannot begin with a rape, for example, or by tampering with the birth control so as to trick the other party.[25] The same is true in this context. As long as their project is morally innocent, when people employ reproductive technology with the intention of creating a child they will serve as parents, this entitles them to continue their project and have those parental rights.

To get further, it must first be settled whose project it is, when the technology is employed. This is not the same as asking whose idea it is to use the technology. That person might have nothing further to do with the project, having only suggested it to those who then carried it out. Since she wouldn't have the project underway, she couldn't have a right to continue it and thereby acquire parental rights.

A different answer takes the project to be that of whoever engages in it with the intention of creating a child to whom he or she will be a parent. This has the advantage of excluding the person who only made the suggestion, but it does not capture what is central to a project being *your* project. The person whose project it is would be the one who is in charge: the one who has the authority to alter the project once it is underway or to bring it to an early end. He or she differs in that way from those who are only contributing to the project, regardless of what form their contribution takes. Of course, a project can be the project of more than one person. That happens when they share the authority I have described.

The intentions that can bring parental rights are those of the person whose project it is. That is, if she employs the technology in order to create a child to whom she will be a parent, doing so entitles her to continue that project, as long as her project is morally innocent. None of those who are only contributing to her project are similarly entitled to continue it in a way that will lead to *their* being parents to the child, because it isn't their project that has begun. It's hers, not because she intended it to work out in a certain way but because she is in charge of it, and it is morally innocent. This makes it hers to continue in her way, not theirs to continue in their way.

But what if they had joined her project with the secret intention of ending up as parents to the child, or they had initially meant only to contribute but had changed their minds along the way and now intended it to end with them as the parents? Those would not be ways in which it had become their project, since their intentions wouldn't make them the one who were in charge of what was being done. So, the project would remain one that they were not entitled to continue in the way they wished.

Of course, they would be people who had a different project underway, when they played their part in this one. It too would be a project in which they intended to end up as parents to the child. Why wouldn't they be just as entitled to continue theirs? The reason is that their projects are not morally innocent, and it is only morally innocent projects that we are entitled to continue just by virtue of having them underway. The people we are now imagining began their projects by joining another person's project under false pretenses or are now seeking to subvert the project of someone who is entitled to continue. Since those things are wrong to do, they bring no entitlement to continue what one has underway. In short, the only person or persons who would be entitled to go on to be a parent to a child created by means of assisted reproductive technology would be the person or persons whose project it was to use the technology for that purpose.[26]

Who that would be admits of a great many possibilities, though some are more likely than others. Often, it is the project of a heterosexual couple who employ someone else to contribute the sperm or the egg, or to serve as the gestational mother. It can also be the project of a same-sex couple in any of those same ways. It could also be the project of a single person or that of a group of people with the intention that all of them would be parents to the child they created. Finally, although those whose project it is ordinarily play one of the biological parts in it, that is not logically necessary. Instead, the entire biological cast could be in the employ of the person or persons whose project it was.

As noted, it is only morally innocent projects that we are entitled to continue just by virtue of having them underway. It is easy to imagine versions that would not meet this condition, in which some of the parties were forced to contribute rather than doing so of their own free will. There has been a great deal of careful argument about whether it is always wrong to employ a surrogate as a gestational mother.[27] If it is, this can't bring parental rights to those who employ one in order to become parents to a child. Perhaps some would say the same of a project whose director plays no biological part himself or herself, having hired others to donate the sperm and the egg and carry out the gestation. If so, that can't be a way to acquire parental rights. I think it can be, and that this depends in particular on why it is being done. However, issues of that kind are rightly resolved; on the view I have offered, there is nothing that restricts initial parental rights to whomever contributes the sperm that provides half of the child's genes and whomever contributes the egg that delivers half of them, or to whomever carries out the gestation and gives birth. In and of themselves, none of those entitle a person to be a parent to the child, and none are needed in order to have that entitlement.

Instead, I have argued, men and women acquire initial parental rights in the following ways. Assuming what they do is morally innocent:

1. Women acquire parental rights by becoming pregnant, regardless of whether that was their intention.
2. Men acquire parental rights when they and their partners intentionally conceive a child of their own free will, as the first step in a morally innocent joint project of having "a child of their own." This is true regardless of whether the child is conceived through coitus or through assisted reproductive technology.
3. Men also acquire parental rights when a pregnancy was unintended, but only if there was a previous promise that if a child were to be conceived then they would be a father to that child, their sexual partner nourished reasonable expectations to that effect, or their history with that person made this a reasonable belief that she did not discourage.

When that context is absent, having sex in which a child is conceived does not entitle a man to continue as a father to that child, but it does obligate him to bear half of certain costs.

ACKNOWLEDGMENTS

I am grateful to Robert Young for his extensive help with this paper, and to Leslie Francis for several very insightful suggestions.

Notes

1. For an excellent discussion of the value of parenthood, see Christine Overall, *Why Have Children?* (Cambridge, MA: The MIT Press, 2013).
2. Avery Kolers and Tim Bayne, "'Are You My Mommy?' On the Genetic Basis of Parenthood," *Journal of Applied Philosophy*, 18, no. 3 (2001): 273–285; Tim Bayne and Avery Kolers, "Toward a Pluralist Account of Parenthood," *Bioethics* 17, no. 3 (2003): 221–241.
3. Joseph Millum, "How Do We Acquire Parental Rights?" *Social Theory and Practice*, 36, no. 1 (January 2010): 112–132, at 127.
4. Kolers and Bayne, "'Are You My Mommy?' On the Genetic Basis of Parenthood," *Journal of Applied Philosophy*, 18, no. 3 (2001), 276.
5. Kolers and Bayne (2001), 277.
6. Bayne and Kolers, "Toward a Pluralist Account of Parenthood," *Bioethics* 17, no. 3 (2003), 241.
7. Bayne and Kolers (2003), 240.
8. Millum, 114.
9. Millum, 114, his italics.
10. This is not the point Millum acknowledges when he says that "Exactly what divides parental work and nonparental work will be contentious" (Millum, 120). According to him, "parental work will be whatever work is appropriate to assisting the child's development at its particular life-stage," and what he acknowledges would be contentious is whether a bit of work is indeed "appropriate to assisting the child's development at its particular life-stage." What I think must be shown is that there is no further distinction within the category of work that does so, between work that earns a distinctively *parental* stake and work that earns a stake of a different kind.
11. Millum, 116, fn 6.
12. Millum, 116.
13. Millum, 117.
14. Millum, 128.
15. Millum, 116.
16. Millum, 123.
17. Millum, 123–124.
18. "A key question for assessing the size of a contributor's stake is how to measure the amount of morally deserving work (henceforth just 'work.') Two main factors appear relevant: the effort expended and the value created" (Millum, 116).
19. Millum, 114.
20. Millum, 117.
21. Millum wouldn't avoid this conclusion on the ground that the results of the "natural lottery" cannot be unjust: "I am ruling out certain forms of luck (e.g. resultant and constitutive luck) as relevant to desert . . . " (Millum 116, fn 7). It would be constitutive luck that enables women to be gestational mothers and not men, so this isn't supposed to lie at the heart of differences between the parental rights a gestational mother deserves and the ones deserved by the biological father of the child.
22. Millum, 125.
23. There is also a further question, which I thank Leslie Francis for raising. Suppose that although both of the couple are acting freely, one of them is acting on false assumptions.

For example, the man might mistakenly think that the woman is "on the pill," and thus that the risk of pregnancy is very low. It is not that she has deceived him about this; he is just wrong about it. When they have sex, both of them run the same risk that it will result in pregnancy, but she runs that risk knowingly and he runs it in ignorance. Do they bear the same responsibility for the outcome if she does become pregnant?

I think that depends on whether his mistake was reckless. I would say we have the same responsibility for what we do recklessly as we have for what we do knowingly, less responsibility for errors that were not reckless but that we should have known better than to make, and still less responsibility for errors for which we are blameless but which have important costs to others.

24. CDC Assisted Reproductive Technology, http://www.cdc/gov/art/, accessed December 2, 2013. The contrast is to "procedures in which only sperm are handled (i.e., intrauterine— or artificial—insemination) or procedures in which a woman takes medication only to stimulate egg production without the intention of having eggs retrieved."

25. There are harder questions concerning when a project is morally innocent that I cannot pursue here. One would be whether it is morally innocent to employ a surrogate who is in difficult economic circumstances due to social injustice. The answer determines whether that is a way of acquiring parental rights, on the view I am offering.

26. This escapes the criticisms raised against the simpler view that "a child's first parents are just those persons who first intended to raise the child" (Melinda A. Roberts, "Good Intentions and a Great Divide: Having Babies by Intending Them," *Law and Philosophy* 12 [1993]: 287–317, at 288.) That is her characterization of the view defended by John Hill in "What Does It Mean To Be a 'Parent'?: The Claims of Biology as the Basis for Parental Rights," *NYU Law Review* 66 (May 1991). For her trenchant criticisms of that view, see her pages 288–298. For further criticisms of the Intentionalist view, see Bayne and Kolers, "Toward a Pluralist Account of Parenthood," *Bioethics* 17, no. 3 (2003): 236–238.

27. See, for example, Elizabeth S. Anderson, "Is Women's Labor a Commodity?" *Philosophy and Public Affairs* 71 (1990); Diana Tietjens Meyers, *Kindred Matters: Rethinking the Philosophy of the Family*, ed. Diana Tietjens Meyers, Kenneth Kipnis, and Cornelius F. Murphy, Jr. (Ithaca, NY: Cornell University Press, 1993); Norvin Richards, *The Ethics of Parenthood* (Oxford: Oxford University Press, 2010).

BIBLIOGRAPHY

Austin, Michael. 2004. The Failure of Biological Accounts of Parenthood. *The Journal of Value Inquiry* 38: 499–510.

Bayne, Tim and Avery Kolers. 2003. Toward a Pluralist Account of Parenthood, *Bioethics* 17, no. 3: 221–241.

Feldman, S. 1992. Multiple Biological Mothers: The Case for Gestation, *Journal of Social Philosophy* 23: 98–104.

Gheaus, Anca. 2012. The Right to Parent One's Biological Baby, *Journal of Political Philosophy* 20, no. 4: 432–455.

Hall, Barbara. 1999. The Origin of Parental Rights, *Public Affairs Quarterly* 13: 73–82.

Kolers, Avery, and Tim Bayne. 2001. 'Are You My Mommy?' On the Genetic Basis of Parenthood, *Journal of Applied Philosophy* 18, no. 3: 273–285.

Millum, Joseph. (January 2010). How Do We Acquire Parental Rights? *Social Theory and Practice* 36, no. 1: 112–132.

Millum, Joseph, and Elizabeth Brake. 2013. Parenthood and Procreation, in *The Stanford Encyclopedia of Philosophy*. http://plato.stanford.edu/entries/parenthood.

Roberts, Melinda A. 1993. Good Intentions and a Great Divide: Having Babies by Intending Them, *Law and Philosophy* 12: 287–317.

CHAPTER 13

MOTHERS AND OTHERS

Relational Autonomy in Parenting

SARA GOERING

BECOMING a mother was, for me, a transformative experience.[1] Overnight I became a person intimately connected to an expected but in most ways completely unknown human being who was tiny, fragile, and completely dependent. She needed to be fed, cleaned, and soothed, and our doctors told us we needed to monitor her to make sure her physiological systems were all functioning appropriately. Things I imagined would happen for her as a matter of natural course—basics like breastfeeding and sleeping—took practice and required great patience. Walking out of the hospital felt like entering a whole new world, suffused with responsibility and thick with love. Her goods and my goods were intricately bound together, not simply as a physical matter (now that we were physically separable), but socially, emotionally, perhaps even cognitively. I was utterly preoccupied. I wanted her to be healthy and happy, and my happiness now felt almost entirely dependent on hers. As we walked to the car, I was immediately aware of the daunting challenge ahead of me. It would require far more than just wrangling her into a car seat and getting her home safely; I was her *mother*, and I was going to need to figure some things out—she was depending on me.[2]

Of course, that's a bit of hyperbole. She also depended on her father, our family and friends, her health care providers, and an institutional system that allowed me to have a little time off from work to give my wholehearted attention to her. I didn't do my mothering alone, couldn't imagine having done it alone, but I nonetheless felt immense awe at this new role I had taken on.

In this chapter, I want to explore some of the ways in which motherhood, or perhaps more precisely, mothering,[3] affects autonomy. In particular, I will argue that the attention to mothering can (1) make us more aware of the relational nature of our selves, (2) give us insight into how a relational view of the self need not *trap* us in existing relations that constitute us, and (3) help us reimagine social structures around childrearing that influence what relationships are possible, and thus how mothering is performed; doing so should help to enhance the autonomy of mothers.[4]

These relational features of the self are common to us all—even nonmothers—but we too commonly overlook them, given a particularly American but more broadly Western emphasis on individualism and individual autonomy. Mothering, because it inevitably involves the social and emotional entanglement that results from hands-on caring, highlights the ways in which humans self-define through our relationships.[5] Using the concept that feminist theorists have understood as *relational autonomy*, I show how mothering reveals the relational aspects of our autonomy and our selves *over time* and through changes. Additionally, I consider how recognizing and responding to that relationality more fully may productively alter the sometimes overwhelming situation of contemporary motherhood.

A wide variety of feminist scholars have already helpfully analyzed the practice of motherhood as well as its injustices (for instance, Noddings 1984; Ruddick 1989; Held 1993; Willett 1995; Lindemann-Nelson 1997; DiQuinzio 1999; Kittay 1999; Meyers 2001; Mullin 2005; Lintott 2010; Lewiecki-Wilson and Cellio 2011). My aim here is to contribute to and extend this literature by showing how the relationality that defines us need not constrain us. One of the worries about relational theories of the self is that on such views, we are literally stuck in our relations; if they not only causally influence but also help to constitute us,[6] then to what extent can we ever escape them, or reinvent ourselves? Motherhood shows us not only how relationally intertwined we are but also how we can separate ourselves and redefine new constitutive relations.

SETTING THE STAGE

In the United States and much of contemporary Western culture, our mainstream conception of motherhood sets a very high standard. Mothers are the presumptive primary caretakers of children, but not only that. They are also widely expected to be "self-sacrificial, unconditionally loving, and totally identified with their children—the prototype of a gladly nonautonomous being" (Meyers 2004, 257). In her book *Perfect Madness: Motherhood in an Age of Anxiety*, Judith Warner (2005, 3) describes contemporary American motherhood as involving a "caught-by-the-throat feeling ... of *always* doing something wrong" given the oppressive culture of motherhood that urges mothers, whether working or not, to do all in their power to make their children "winners" and to feel guilty when they do not. From the earliest stages of pregnancy we are warned, for instance, to consider before taking a bite of cake: "Is this the best bite I can give my baby? If it will benefit your baby, chew away. If it'll only benefit your sweet tooth or appease your appetite, put your fork down" (from *What to Expect When You're Expecting*, quoted in Kukla 2008, 81). The pressure continues through choices about sleeping arrangements, pacifier use, providing enrichment opportunities versus overscheduling, and so on. Throughout, mothers are directly (and often solely) attributed responsibility for the well-being of their children. Feminist theorists have identified this as the troubling "ideology of motherhood" and rightly criticized it from many angles (e.g., Mullin 2005; Lewiecki-Wilson and Cellio 2011). As Mullin notes, "In broad strokes, according to the ideology of motherhood, with the exception of the necessary provision of material resources, mothers are thought to be necessary and sufficient for the happiness of their young children, and young children are thought to be necessary and sufficient for the happiness of their mothers" (Mullin 2005, 121). The ideology is damaging not simply because it individualizes responsibility, sets an unattainable standard, and treats women from different classes and ethnicities unfairly (see, e.g., Collins 1994; Romero 1997; Nedelsky 1999; Tronto 2002; Roberts 2005) but also because it is difficult to resist even for many staunch feminists. It infects our thinking even as we try to resist it. It's impossible to achieve, but it has us in its grips.

I want to avoid contributing to this unfortunate ideology by romanticizing the connection between mothers and their children.[7] But I also do not want to downplay the depth of connection and joy that can be experienced through the mother–child bond.[8] In fact, I think attention to the kinds of bonds and relationships that typically form between mothers and their children, and the effects those bonds have on the mother's autonomy, will be productive for thinking about what it means to be relationally autonomous, how we can maintain autonomy even as our relationships grow and change, and how we might reimagine the social structures and policies that encourage certain kinds of caring relationships around childrearing.

THE TRANSFORMATIVE EFFECTS OF BECOMING A MOTHER

Becoming a parent (by giving birth, adopting, or marrying into a family with children) is typically a transformative experience that can radically alter one's conception of oneself, and likewise, one's autonomy. In becoming parents, we do not merely gain loved ones; we expand our selves. This may be because of our tightly intertwined goods and the shared sense of vulnerability: "having a child is 'to decide forever to have your heart go walking around outside your body'" (Elizabeth Stone, quoted in LaChance Adams 2014, 57). Or perhaps it is simply because our notions of ourselves metaphorically open up, to get "big . . . and deep and wide . . . when I stretched out my arms all my children could get in between. I was *that* wide" (Weir 2008, 16, quoting Toni Morrison's character Sethe, in *Beloved*).[9]

In becoming mothers, the significance of our relationality becomes more apparent, even impossible to ignore. Choosing what to want and do is no longer a matter of simply assessing our individual internal preferences but also of consulting the needs and desires of those who are fully dependent on us, needs and desires that are intertwined with our own, sometimes almost indistinguishably so. Eva Kittay describes the paradigmatic caregiver as having a "transparent" self—a self that sees through its own needs to focus on the needs of its charge (Kittay 1999, 51).[10] But the physical and emotional labor of caregiving, and the bond developed from that closeness and investment of the self, often alters the aims and desires of the caregiver. She doesn't so much fade to transparency; rather, herself is expanded to include the child. Even though we can identify ourselves as individual entities, distinct spatially from our children, our identities become connected in ways that make us become more fully a plural subject, a "we" that matters together. Becoming a parent adds constraints on autonomy for sure, but it also expands and enables more complex exercises of autonomy and offers a vivid illustration of how socially entwined we all are.

Becoming a mother is what L. A. Paul (2014) calls a "life-changing experience. . . . Your preferences change. The way you live your life will change. What and who you care about will change" (81). The typical attachments you form to your child[11] alter the very way you are in the world, indeed alter *who* you are. You *become* a mother. And in that becoming, what it means for you to act autonomously changes. As an example, consider what Jennifer Nedelsky says about her life with a new son: "At least in the early years, I was able to attend deeply to his needs by following my own heartfelt desires. My wants were not, of course, identical to his, but they were intertwined. My need to be with him was related to his need for me. But I did not experience myself as giving up my needs for his, but as following a thread of passionate desire in my relationship to him" (1999, 310). She says caring for her son this fully did not feel like selflessness—or sacrifice—but more like absorption, a relationship unlike most others, because she had no issues with what she would be "getting back."

This kind of transformation, from "I" to "we," obviously extends to other circumstances. We develop deep bonds to partners and spouses, and start speaking in terms of what "we" need, what career and life paths would be good for "us" in addition to how "we" plan to spend the holidays. When we speak of this plural subject (Gilbert 2000) and the collective activities it undertakes, we typically do not presume that one party in the "we" is controlled by the other (as in heteronomy) or simply that both parties are (perhaps coincidentally) making the same choices autonomously. Rather, we understand them to be intentionally choosing together on the basis of shared interests, aims, or values. Members of the "we" are not entirely self-ruling, nor are they ruled by others. They occupy, instead, a middle space, deciding together for the sake of the unit. They may each have a good of their own, but there is also a good for the couple and when they act as a "we," they aim for that shared good.

In the case of mothering, the other party in the "we"—the infant or child—is much more fully dependent on the mother and clearly contributes less (at least in the early years) to the choices about what "we" will do. But the child's desires and needs are nonetheless at the heart of the "we": "we need to get home in time for a nap" or "we need to stop for a snack" or even "we need to let mommy rest now so we'll survive the birthday party later." The interests of the two overlap and combine. When a mother makes decisions, she makes them as the part of the "we" that can most successfully identify and articulate needs for the larger entity. Of course, sometimes mothers come up short in assessing these interests. Mothering teaches and requires patience and flexibility. We may think that getting to the birthday party is in "our" interest, but the child may insist that studying the ants on the sidewalk is vastly more important, or that finding the favored red shoes is a requirement for getting out the door at all. The best laid plans— ones *we* seem to have agreed to in advance—often go up in flames when the appointed hour arrives. In managing the expanded self, mothers have to negotiate competing demands and interests in the service of achieving what is good for the "we" that includes child and mother.

In the earliest stages of life, infants spend much of their time being held, fed, admired and soothed. They are intimately connected with those who mother them. When breastfed, they are quite literally attached to the mother, still sharing her nutrition, her warmth, and her stresses. They are carried everywhere, lovingly adored, and gently socialized. Some psychological theories suggest that infants do not fully consider them- selves separate from their mothers until roughly age 15 months. The two, while sepa- rable, have significant overlap in identity. But all is not necessarily rosy and peaceful, of course. Babies also cry. They are needy. They demand attention. Mothers needn't delight in every moment or feel fully connected to each expression of an infant's desire. What mother has not wanted to scream "Go to sleep!" to the infant who deceptively appears to be soundly asleep but cries as soon as the mother stands up or so much as removes her hand from his body? But the connection—wanting what is best for the baby, taking it as one's own end, and sometimes actually seeming to feel what the baby feels—is evidence of our participation in a greater "we" that broadly has its own good.

As children grow and develop, they typically develop skills in articulating their own interests, and they explore their differences from their mothers.[12] They become more adamant about what they want, more willing to contradict the wisdom of the elder in the shared "we." Of course, they sometimes still check in for security: "Mom, do I even like asparagus?" is asked because the mother is the repository for memories of likes and dislikes that are not etched forever in memory after just one try. Children begin to acknowledge not only the existence of a time before their birth (a truly perplexing rev- elation for many young children) but also the reality that their mother may have some interests fully separable from their own ("Why did you go on that work trip without me?" or "Why don't you want to play Go Fish again?"). Eventually—at least for most children—they may not even want their mother around regularly. They learn to separate their identities to some extent, to intertwine their identities with others around them (friends, teachers, grandparents, etc.), and so to diminish the mother's role. The moth- er's journey, then, moves from being almost fully aligned with her offspring to ultimately letting them go—not to be cast away entirely, but rather to be released into their own networks of relationships. LaChance Adams sums it up well: "From the time one begins to care for a child, whether through pregnancy or adoption, he is taking steps away. Even as the mother longs for independence, her child is already leaving. The 'secret code of the mother's mourning' is that the relationship with her child, even when it is expected as an invasion, is already an uneasy letting go" (2014, 55–56).

So how do we theorize this intimate relationship, one that begins with a transforma- tion of the mother's self into an expanded "we," which then grows in complexity and richness, and (with luck) eventually ends with a diminishment of relatedness, as chosen others move in to replace the centrality of the given mother?[13] Understanding that process is, I think, key for understanding how any of us can be relationally autonomous—even relationally constituted—without being *trapped* in our existing networks of relationships.[14]

RELATIONAL IDENTITIES: BEING DEFINED BY RELATIONSHIPS WITHOUT BEING CONFINED BY RELATIONSHIPS

What is it to be relationally autonomous? At the very least, it means recognizing that all of us are dependent and fully reliant on caregivers to help us get to the point where we can be autonomous. As Annette Baier notes, we are all "second persons" who only achieve personhood through being in relation to others who help to create and define us (Baier 1985). Yet the relationality is not only a precondition of achieving autonomy but also a simultaneous influence on autonomy. That is, our relationships—both personal and more broadly social—contribute directly to who we are, and as a consequence, to our capacity to exercise autonomy; "agents' identities are formed within the context of social relationships, and shaped by a complex intersection of social determinants, such as race, class, gender and ethnicity" (Mackenzie and Stoljar 2000, 4). Although most theories of autonomy include conditions of voluntariness and prohibit undue influence on choice, and highlight the importance of internal integration of desires, relational autonomy theorists highlight the ways in which our autonomous choices arise in the context of social structures and norms (Mackenzie and Stoljar 2000) and from active engagement with our closest loved ones. We don't want them to be controlling, but we typically think their input is *part of* rather than *in opposition to* our capacity to make autonomous choices. In making a difficult choice about my future, for instance, I don't simply want to get away from everyone and introspect about what will be best for me; I want to hear from my closest family and friends how they interpret my options and have conversations that explore how my different options fit with their understandings of me. I am not completely bound by their views, of course, but their views inform my own self-understanding; they allow me to try out my views on who I am and want to be, and how to get there, with my Aristotelian "other selves." (Nelsen notes that "Paradoxical though it may seem, individual autonomy may be enhanced when individuals inquire with others" [2010, 347]).

I am, in other words, defined not simply by my own story about who I am but also by the stories told by others about who I am. Who I really am—now, given that my identity is likely to be dynamic—may be something like an equilibrium between the story I tell about myself and the stories told by others about me (Schechtman 2009; Baylis 2013; Lindemann 2014). Our relationality is deep and constitutive, in other words, and it is part of how we come to know ourselves in a way that allows us to be autonomous. "It is only in and through our relationships and interactions with others that we acquire suf-ficient self-understanding to work out which of our desires should constitute reasons for us, which commitments are most important, which emotional responses we should attend to, how to reconcile inner conflicts arising from the obligations of different social roles, and so on" (Mackenzie 2008, 527). To be autonomous, we must know our own minds, and as the relational autonomy theorists have shown, to do that, we rely in part on others. The Socratic recommendation to "know thyself"—reinterpreted and handed down through the ages—requires, for most of us,[15] the help of friends.

Knowing that we are dependent in this way on the recognition and responsiveness of others makes us vulnerable to them. Others may fully deny me the identity that I want to claim—that is, I might have what Lindemann calls an "impossible identity" (2014, 140–143) such as being a transgender person in certain communities where there is a refusal to recognize the validity of such an experience. But even in less tragic circumstances, my friends and family may have difficulty recognizing an aspect of me that I try to express or want to develop. Perhaps I want to get uptake for my efforts at making myself more even-tempered, but my family refuses to let go of their conception of me as the hot-headed youth I once was. I may in fact be acting in a way that supports my own self-conception, but it will be difficult for me to solidify my new identity if no one around me recognizes it. As Lindemann argues, we are dependent on others to help hold us in our identities, but we are also dependent on them to let go of certain aspects of our identities that we have repudiated (Lindemann 2014).

So one of the worries of acknowledging relational selves and noting their importance for developing and exercising our autonomy (through helping us with autonomy com-petency skills such as self-understanding or self-definition; Meyers 2000), is accounting for our ability to autonomously reshape or change our identities—and thus our relation-ships. If my close others help to define me, are in fact part of me (as my relation of being mother to a child is an integral part of who I am), then how do I avoid being trapped by the web of relations that is me? The idea of a web of relations holding me in my identity might sound comforting, but only if the relations are good. Otherwise, the stickiness of the web (remember, those others actually partially constitute me) could overwhelm my autonomy. What if my relations are stifling, overbearing, or demeaning?

Lindemann argues that we have moral duties to let go of others' repudiated identities, to be responsive to individuals' self-definitions when possible, recognizing some reality constraints (2014, 135–136). But not everyone will uphold such duties. Let's say that my mothering—developed in the context of the ideology of motherhood—has led me to be the one who always sacrifices, who is last to the table, who takes the smaller or less attractive portion each time.[16] I might have willingly taken on this role at first, but now find myself stuck as the family's sacrificial caregiver. My children and partner expect it of me, and the culture around me supports this kind of sacrifice on the part of mothers. But maybe I'm feeling frustrated and annoyed. I don't really want to continue in this role, but I also feel guilty when I don't do it. In this case, the context of my self-understanding, combined with the oppressive norms governing my role as a mother, make me "feel crazy" (Benson 2000) for not wanting what I think I'm supposed to want, for seeming to undermine my very relational identity. And in this case, if I turn to the others who are purportedly there to help me in *being* autonomous, they are likely to reflect back to me the vision of who I have been (caregiving mother) and what the culture holds I am supposed to be (happily sacrificing mother). It appears to be a relational trap.

But consider again the typical relationship between mother and child, which starts with extensively overlapping interests and engagement, and slowly, over time, and as the child gets to know others, transitions into a different kind of relation. The child's relational web expands to include the grandparents, the day care providers, the neighbors, friends, and so on. The child's interactions with these intimate others offers the opportunity for self-examination and self-expansion for the child; she becomes not just daughter, but granddaughter, student, friend. And as her identity stretches to include these new relations, the connection to the mother can become less significant, less indispensable. My point is not to say that it must, that the role of mothers *inevitably* diminishes with time; rather, I only want to point out that the distribution of support across multiple others decreases the reliance on any one connection. A child who is widely cherished and cared for can have a strong bond with her mother, but she also has the opportunity to try on different possibilities for herself, to have others help her create and reflect back different aspects of her identity.

TRANSFORMING THE STRUCTURES
AND EXPECTATIONS AROUND MOTHERHOOD

If a child's typical course leads to a self expanded through relationships to nonparental others, and this expansion serves to distribute the opportunities and responsibilities for holding her in her identity (indeed, for helping to define her identity), then we can also apply this idea back to the mother herself. Mothers who are beleaguered by their responsibilities—who struggle to be "good enough" mothers, much less achieve motherhood ideals—may feel trapped in their roles, bound by their family status. Their capacity to be autonomous may be constrained. Wanting to be a good mother—in a context in which doing so is a fairly unachievable ideal; "one of the darkest, deepest shames so many of us mothers feel nowadays is our fear that we are Bad Mothers, that we are failing our children and falling short of our own ideals" (Waldman 2009, 3)—but feeling unable to do so may shatter women's sense of self-worth, an important part of autonomy competency (Mackenzie 2000). To be clear, this feeling of failure can coexist with the feeling of joy from having the expanded self of motherhood. In the context of the rigid ideology of motherhood, the joy of the bond is simultaneously cast with a weight of responsibility, and a fear of not living up to social (and our own) expectations.

Changing those expectations likely will not be feasible simply through attention to our internal psychology. Ayelet Waldman's book *Bad Mother* is a humorous call for mothers to be realistic about our obligations, to claim, in a way, our failures to meet the unreasonable standard, and so to start to break down that standard. But the problem is not simply in the heads of women. It's out there in the structures and practice norms of the world. A system that distributes caregiving duties, that gives mothers the opportunity to build relations outside the family, ones that can reflect different aspects of their interests and commitments, could enable mothers to keep or make the same kind of expansion moves that their children usually make as a matter of course. That is, in a differently structured system (with more effective family leave policies and more available day care), mothers too might more easily hold on to their premotherhood identity relations or build new relations that expand their self-conceptions and allow them opportunities to develop new communities of support. Too often, at least for many mothers (both those who work outside the home and those who do not), the motherhood relation almost entirely takes over the woman's identity. "One sometimes forgets that one is actually a person other than [the child's] mother" (quoted in LaChance 2014, 50).

Many women do describe motherhood as a time of transformation that involves loss as well as expansion. Consider how Naomi Wolf describes the loss of her former self after motherhood: "An 'I' would go forward, swept irrevocably on by the tide of the natural order.... And the 'I' would reconfigure eventually around [the baby's] need, and take joy in it, and spin a new identity. But it would never again be the 'I' it had been before" (Wolf 2001, 106). In critiquing this expectation of self-sacrifice, LaChance Adams worries that for many mothers, being "self-sacrificing" means not only that they put their children's needs ahead of their own, but also that they have sacrificed the self they once were, because the current mothering self "has been transformed in ways in which self and other are integrated" (McMahon quoted in LaChance 2014, 53).

But integrating the self and other (i.e., the child) need not mean fully *sacrificing* the former self. Transformative changes by their nature involve significant change; our former selves will be altered in important respects. Our time is limited, and we can only maintain so many close relationships and parts of our identities, given the required commitments of attention, energy, and time. But adding new relationships—even transformative ones like mother–child relations—need not eliminate key aspects of the former self, even as they transform it. That this turns out to be true so often may be more a sign of our existing expectations, practices, and norms of motherhood rather than a requirement of caring for an infant or young child.

So what would increase a mother's autonomy, relationally conceived? In our current system of practice, parenting is typically done in relative isolation—often away from extended family, and without good child care options or supports (Boyd 2010, 141). But if we encouraged and supported a more communal approach to childrearing—spreading the responsibility for the child's care as well as the emotional and social connections that make up the child's identity—we could ensure that mothering is more fully "distributed" (to use Kittay's phrase, 1999).

This idea aligns with practices described by hooks and Hill Collins as common in African American communities (hooks 1984; Collins 1994). "Other-mothers" and "fictive kin" make caring for children and working outside the home part of the routine for many mothers who need to work outside the home to make ends meet but who cannot afford or find high-quality day care. These others take pressure off the birth mother or primary rearing mother, and also offer the child important additional adult relationships of care. Although the other-mothers are often found through close networks of family and friends, they needn't be private but could also be made available through publicly funded day care centers and preschools. Nesting our children in a wider set of loving relationships provides support for both child and mother.

Some might worry that this model of more distributed caregiving and relationality will undermine the child's stability or make her uncertain which adults she can expect to care for her. But having a wide variety of caring adults does not confuse children; it protects them. The ideology of motherhood makes us feel guilty when we drop our children off for day care (at least at the beginning), and we fear our children may lose track of who their mother is, given all the caregivers. But they do not. They learn to love their teachers and classmates, sometimes even begging to stay longer when we arrive for pickup. And when they have problems, we have a community of people who care and know our child well. Distributing some of the mothering labor allows a wider variety of maternal thinkers to share their insights and help to address problems when they arise. As Mullin (2005) and Kittay (1999) both point out, this may be necessary for children with significant impairments, but it also offers significant advantages in respect to caregiving for any child.

Mothers who feel guilty about sending our children off to day care may have internalized commonly held assumptions about private mothering. That is, we may wrongly "assume that there is only one person who is the real mother, such that if we accept that stepmothers and fathers and adoptive parents can be the real maternal thinkers, we seem to have denied the role of mothers and maternal thinkers to birthgivers. . . . If we disabuse ourselves of the notion that one and only one person must be recognized as a child's mother, then we can recognize that there are no legitimate reasons to argue that only biological mothers can be maternal thinkers" (Mullin 2005, 127). Her point is not simply about family created in nontraditional ways but also about caregiving support systems built outside the private family home.

None of this is to claim that individual mothers should be made to feel guilty about doing most of the caregiving labor themselves if they so prefer. Rather, my emphasis is on providing real options for mothers, ensuring that their relational networks of support are robust enough to protect and support not just their children but also their own identities. Rather than only meeting this constraint with the provision of day care, we can also help to ensure it by changing laws and/or public attitudes about children in public. Having the ability to breastfeed children in public, ensuring there are safe public parks to allow children to play and parents to meet, and generally providing a welcoming attitude to children on public transportation and in public buildings will allow mothers to avoid being cut off from potential relationships of support. Too often we do our mothering relatively alone. Nedelsky notes the difficulty of mothering in isolation and laments the ways in which we have even privatized the way we address problems in childrearing; mothers she knows go to psychotherapy to talk about their problems rather than talking with friends or other mothers and offering reciprocal listening and shared strategies (Nedelsky 1999, 327).

Critics might worry that sharing mothering labor will obscure important differences between the parents—who are understood to be ultimately responsible for the child's welfare—and the growing cadre of other caregivers, perhaps in a way that ultimately undermines the mother's autonomy. What if my child starts behaving somewhat strangely at day care (e.g., biting or having meltdowns), and the day care providers disagree with me about the likely causes and significance of the new behavior? Who gets to diagnose the problem and determine the best course of action? Although I suspect many people want to say, in unqualified terms, that it should be the mother (or parents more generally), I think the situation is actually more complicated. Some of the child's experience will be unknown to the parents, given the time spent apart, and the perspectives of the child care workers are important components of understanding the child and her best interests. In the best scenario, the adult parties will negotiate a plan together, pooling their knowledge and using their shared care for the child as motivation. Legally, the mother may remove the child from that day care arrangement, of course, but doing so should involve attention to impact of the loss of those caring relationships on the child, and it would inevitably also involve recognition of the impact on the mother herself.

In considering how child care might be structured more effectively and fairly, Mullin describes a model of "coordinated care" shared by several caregivers. "The mothers and the paid providers work together, learn from one another, and see themselves as socializing children as well as seeing to their emotional and physical safety" (Mullin, 2005, 148). This model addresses the best interests of children and women—whether as mothers or paid caregivers—but does so in the context of understanding that parents are likely to expect a much longer term relationship with their child than can be expected from other child care providers. This model is not, it should be noted, particularly different from the relationship between teacher and student. Students come to expect different teachers each year in school, but that does not interfere with their ability to bond with, learn from, and discover parts of themselves through interacting with each teacher.

This picture may sound excessively rosy. What about cases where relationships are not worth maintaining? Boyd (2010) discusses constraints on mother's autonomy in the context of legal decisions that encourage co-parenting and involvement of both parents (even where the father—e.g., a sperm donor—may not have intended to be involved, or where the one of the parents creates difficulties for the mother and child but difficulties short of legal definitions of harm). As Boyd notes, there's an irony that the shared parenting emphasis that may be intended to free mothers in more typical co-parenting situations may constrain mothers who either prefer to raise children on their own or who need to be able to move, with a child, in order to maintain employment. "A mother-caregiver is, then, responsible for both childcare and ensuring the involvement of the father. In a supportive, non-conflicted relationship between adults who prioritise the interests of the child, this model can work well for women and even give them more flexibility to pursue their interests outside parenting. In other less supportive circumstances, the joint decision-making limits a mother's potential to make decisions she may deem to be in her child's or her own best interests. . . . Mothers who raise what may be legitimate concerns about the safety of contact arrangements can be vilified as 'no contact' mothers. In some cases, they lose their custody as a result" (Boyd 2010, 144).

If such mothers try to move in order to be nearer to extended family and caregiving supports (or for better jobs, or to be with new partners), they are often not legally permitted to do so, in order to preserve access to the child's father; this may be true even if the father is not providing much or any material support for the child. Here is a case where the relational web of the child seems to trap the mother in a situation that is not particularly good for her, or perhaps even good for the child. We need a way to allow women to distance themselves from problematic relationships (Ball 2005, 95; Boyd 2010) and encourage them as well as judges to question their own views about what is in the child's bests interests (e.g., to resist the ideologies of motherhood and the gendered norms of caregiving).

What might that look like? If being autonomous starts with being in a relational network, and being responsive to others, women—given social norms and practices that gender caregiving—are likely to do more of the labor of holding others in their identities. So women may feel more pressed to give up their career aspirations, their new partnerships, and so on in the name of securing the well-being of their child (which in the court's estimation may require regular access to even a relatively uninvolved or merely biological father). Boyd's recommendation is to encourage both women and judges to "focus on the nature and quality of the relationships surrounding a mother's parenting. . . . Parenting a child might ideally involve multiple adults and/or greater societal involvement in care for children, so that the onerous responsibilities do not fall on one individual (usually a woman), thereby unduly limiting her autonomy" (2010, 150). The child's best interests, in other words, might be filled by a wider array of adult others, rather than only the biologically related ones. This is not to dismiss the claims of fathers who are involved with the child but do not any longer share an intimate relationship with the child's mother. Their relationships matter, and they form part of the child's identity. But the decision to maintain, disconnect, or at least stretch the distance in the relationship should perhaps be based more on a history of care and quality interaction with the child than on mere relatedness.

Conclusion

Feminists and others have made great progress in theorizing relational autonomy, and showing how personal relationships and social norms and oppressions both create and constrain our ability to make choices that reflect our dear selves. Reflecting on the experience of mothering shows us how these relational selves are developed, but also how they change over time, and how we might think about the difficult but all-too-human task of trying to maintain good relationships while exiting difficult ones. Lindemann's call to attend more carefully to the moral realm of personal identities—of our obligations to hold others in their identities, as well as knowing when to let them go—has a particular salience in the realm of mothering, and it can show us possibilities for holding mothers in identities they can gladly endorse, even as we learn how to let go of our growing children.

Notes

1. Others also use this phrasing. See L. A. Paul's (2014) *Transformative Experience*, a book that develops a thesis started in her wonderful essay "What you can't expect when you're expecting" about the ways ourselves and preferences change in unexpected ways through transformative experience. See also Lindemann, this volume, ch. 23.
2. I believe this kind of experience is shared whether one gives birth or receives a young child via adoption. The enormity of the challenge facing new parents is the same, despite differences in how one becomes a parent.
3. As Sara Ruddick (1989) points out in *Maternal Thinking*, the act of mothering—involving "maternal thinking"—can be done by a wide variety of actors, including men, hired nannies, and others not traditionally thought of as fulfilling the role of mother. Mothering involves the everyday practices of caring for children, including physical, emotional, and social labor, and it typically leads to a bond that extends beyond any contract for care. See also Kittay (1999), *Love's Labor*, for discussions of distributed mothering.
4. As an aside, having this piece in a volume on reproductive ethics is fitting, even though it does not deal with the topics most paradigmatically grouped under that heading. As Kukla (2008) argues, "Consider how the phrase *reproductive ethics* has come to refer almost exclusively to ethical analyses of discrete choices faced during pregnancy or even earlier. Key topics in reproductive ethics include abortion, pre-implantation genetic diagnosis, and fertility medicine. This ought to strike us as strange. Reproduction is the process of creating new people and building families and communities. . . . This is a process that extends across the life span" (69). My own previous work on "postnatal reproductive autonomy" also aims to help fill this gap (Goering 2009).
5. Hilde Lindemann's wonderful book *Holding and Letting Go* (2014) offers a valuable discussion of the social practices of personhood and personal identity in arenas not focused solely on motherhood. I draw from her book in making my argument in respect to motherhood. See also Lindemann's work on damaging master narratives of pregnancy in this volume (chapter 23).
6. See the discussion of this distinction in the introduction to Mackenzie and Stoljar (eds.) (2000) *Relational Autonomy*.
7. This worry is explored extensively in Sarah LaChance Adam's book that explores the ambivalence mothers sometimes feel toward their children, and the reality that some mothers harm their children: *Mad Mothers, Bad Mothers, and the Ethics of Ambivalence* (2014). She quotes Jane Lazarre (from *The Mother Knot*): "The only thing which seems to me to be eternal and natural in motherhood is ambivalence and its manifestation in the ever ongoing cycles of separation and unification with our children" (p. xxii, quote on p. 29 in LaChance).
8. Nedelsky (1999, 311–312) expresses "anger and resentment" about what she took to be "the collective betrayal by my feminist sisters" who had written primarily about the oppressive obligations of motherhood, rather than any of its joys and pleasures.

9. Weir notes that "This understanding of freedom goes *beyond situating freedom in the context of relationships* (the project of most theorists of relational autonomy) to argue that *freedom is precisely the capacity to be in relationships that one desires: to love whom and what you choose to love.*"

10. To be clear, Kittay recognizes that such a transparent self is unachievable, but sees it as the "benchmark for the self-conception of the dependency worker, qua dependency worker ... It is a regulatory ideal ... It is an altruistic ideal. But while altruism is often seen as morally supererogatory, this ideal is *required* of the labor I have called dependency work" (1999, 52).

11. I say typical, though I recognize that others may disagree. LaChance Adams (2014) suggests that most women are more ambivalent about motherhood.

12. I think it is important to note that this seems to happen even for children who, in other respects, are not developing typically. See Kittay, 1999, also 2011.

13. The intimacy is often the easy part, relative to letting go. As poet Rainer Maria Rilke notes, "We need, in love, to practice only this; letting each other go. For holding comes easily; we do not need to learn it" (quoted in Lindemann 2014, 160).

14. See Barclay (2000) for an argument that the socially constituted self or strongly socially determined self cannot be autonomous.

15. I want to recognize that there may be hermits or antisocial people who choose not to be around others. My aim is not to suggest that they cannot be autonomous or have self-understanding, but rather to point to the ways that most of us achieve self-understanding.

16. I think here of Kittay's remark about her own mother: "My mother has been serving us dinner. My father and I are nearly finished eating. She alone remains unfed. A sigh announces the completion of her task and a well-deserved respite. She sits down to eat. With a shrug and a smile, and with a touch of ironic humor, she says, 'After all, *I'm* also a mother's child'" (Kittay 1999, 23).

Bibliography

Baier, A. 1985. Cartesian persons. In *Postures of the mind: Essays on mind and morals*, 74–92. Minneapolis: University of Minnesota Press.

Ball, C. 2005. This is not your father's autonomy: Lesbian and gay rights from a feminist and relational perspective. *Harvard Journal of Law and Gender* 28: 345–379.

Barclay, L. 2000. Autonomy and the social self. In *Relational autonomy*, ed. Catriona Mackenzie and Natalie Stoljar, 52–71. New York: Oxford University Press.

Baylis, F. 2013. "I am who I am": On the perceived threat to personal identity from deep brain stimulation. *Neuroethics* 6, no. 3: 513–526.

Benson, P. 2000. Feeling crazy: Self-worth and the social character of responsibility In *Relational Autonomy*, ed. Catriona Mackenzie and Natalie Stoljar, 72–93. New York: Oxford University Press.

Boyd, S. 2010. Autonomy for mothers? Relational theory and parenting apart. *Feminist Legal Studies* 18: 137–158.

Collins, P. H. 1994. Shifting the center: Race, class and feminist theorizing about motherhood. In *Representations of motherhood*, ed. Donna Bassin, Margaret Honey, and Meryle Mahrer Kaplan, 56–74. New Haven, CT: Yale University Press.

DiQuinzio, P. 1999. *The impossibility of motherhood: Feminism, individualism and the problem of mothering*. New York: Routledge.

Friedman, M. 2000. Autonomy, social disruption and women. In *Relational autonomy*, eds. Catriona Mackenzie and Natalie Stoljar, 35–51. New York: Oxford University Press.

Gilbert, M. 2000. *Sociality and responsibility: New essays in plural subject theory*. Lanham, MD: Rowman & Littlefield.

Goering, S. 2009. Postnatal reproductive autonomy: Promoting relational autonomy and self-trust in new parents. *Bioethics* 23, no. 1: 9–19.

Held, V. 1993. *Feminist morality*. Chicago: Chicago University Press.

hooks, b. 1984 *Feminist theory from margin to center*. Boston: Beacon Press.

Kittay, E. 1999. *Love's labor: Essays on women, equality and democracy*. New York: Routledge.

Kittay, E. 2011. Forever small: The strange case of Ashley X. *Hypatia* 26, no. 3: 610–631.

Kukla, R. 2008. Measuring mothering. *International Journal of Feminist Approaches to Bioethics* 1, no, 1: 67–90.

LaChance Adams, S. 2014. *Mad mothers, bad mothers and what a "good" mother would do: The ethics of ambivalence*. New York: Columbia University Press.

Lewiecki-Wilson, C., and J. Cellio, eds. 2011. *Disability and mothering: Liminal spaces of embodied knowledge*. Syracuse, NY: Syracuse University Press.

Lindemann, H. 2014. *Holding and letting go: The social practice of personal identities*. New York: Oxford University Press.

Lindemann-Nelson, H, ed. 1997. *Feminism and families*. New York: Routledge.

Lintott, S, ed. 2010. *Motherhood: The birth of wisdom*. Malden, MA: Blackwell.

Mackenzie, C. 2008. Relational autonomy, normative authority, and perfectionism. *Journal of Social Philosophy* 39, no. 4: 512–533.

Mackenzie, C. 2000. Imagining oneself otherwise. In *Relational Autonomy*, ed. Catriona Mackenzie and Natalie Stoljar, 124–150. New York: Oxford University Press.

Mackenzie, C., and N. Stoljar, eds. 2000. *Relational autonomy: Feminist perspectives on autonomy, agency and the social self*. New York: Oxford University Press.

McMahon, M. 1995. *Engendering motherhood: Identity and self-transformation in women's lives*. New York: Guilford.

Meyers, D. 2000. Intersectional identity and the authentic self: Opposites attract! In *Relational autonomy*, ed. Catriona Mackenzie and Natalie Stoljar, 151–180. New York: Oxford University Press.

Meyers, D. 2001. The rush to motherhood: Pronatalist discourse and women's autonomy. *Signs* 26, no. 3: 735–773.

Meyers, D. 2004. Gendered work and individual autonomy. In *Being yourself: Essays on identity, action and social life*, ed. D. Meyers, 257–273. Lanham, MD: Rowman & Littlefield.

Mullin, A. 2005. *Reconceiving pregnancy and childcare: Ethics, experience and reproductive labor*. New York: Cambridge University Press.

Mullin, A. 2007. Children, autonomy and care. *Journal of Social Philosophy* 38, no. 4: 536–553.

Nedelsky, J. 1999. Dilemmas of passion, privilege and isolation: Reflections on mothering in a white, middle class nuclear family. In *Mother troubles: Rethinking contemporary maternal dilemmas*, ed. J. Hanigsberg and S. Ruddick, 304–334. Boston: Beacon Press.

Nelsen, P. 2010. Oppression, autonomy and the impossibility of the inner citadel. *Studies in Philosophy and Education* 29: 333–349.

Noddings, N. 1984. *Caring: A feminine approach to ethics and moral education*. Berkeley: University of California Press.

Paul, L. A. 2014. *Transformative experience*. New York: Oxford University Press.

Paul, L. A. 2015. What you can't expect when you're expecting. *Res Philosophica* 92, no, 2: 1–23.

Roberts, D. 2005. Feminism, race and adoption policy. In *Adoption matters: Philosophical and feminist essays*, ed. Sally Haslanger and Charlotte Witt, 234–246. Ithaca, NY: Cornell University Press.

Romero, M. 1997. Who takes care of the maid's children? Exploring the costs of domestic service. In *Feminism and families*, ed. Hilde Lindemann Nelson, 151–169. New York: Routledge.

Ruddick, S. 1989. *Maternal thinking*. Boston: Beacon Press.

Schechtman, M. 2009. Getting our stories straight: Self-narratives and personal identity. In *Personal identity and fractured selves*, ed. Debra Mathews, Hilary Bok, and Peter Rabins, 65–92. Baltimore, MD: Johns Hopkins University Press.

Tronto, J. 2002. The "nanny" question in feminism. *Hypatia* 17, no. 7: 34–51.

Waldman, A. 2009. *Bad mother*. New York: Anchor Books/Random House.

Warner, J. 2005. *Perfect madness: Motherhood in the age of anxiety*. New York: Riverhead Books.

Weir, A. 2008. Home and identity: In memory of Iris Marion Young. *Hypatia* 23, no. 3: 4–21.

Willett, C. 1995. *Maternal ethics and other slave moralities*. New York: Routledge.

Wolf, N. 2001. *Misconceptions: Truth, lies, and the unexpected journey to motherhood*. New York: Doubleday.

CHAPTER 14

....

PROCREATORS' DUTIES

Sexual Asymmetries

....

DON HUBIN

PARENTS typically have many moral responsibilities to, and with regard to, their children. At least some of these—and, in particular, a duty to support and nurture—stem from the causal role parents usually play in the creation of the new life. To examine this parental obligation and to explore the sexual asymmetries involved, we will engage a series of fanciful cases[1] that separates this responsibility from others typically associated with parenthood.[2] But first, it is worth making explicit several points that are pertinent, even if prosaic.

RESPONSIBILITY FOR DEPENDENT LIFE

....

Humans begin life in a fragile and dependent state. This is universally, even if not necessarily, true. The period of dependency for humans is the longest of any animal and it has increased with the increasing complexity of human social life. Even normal, healthy adults are dependent on one another, of course, but typically this dependency takes the form of *inter*dependency. Infants and toddlers are dependent for their day-to-day existence on assistance from older humans. As children age, they typically become less dependent on others for such assistance, but it is not until near adulthood that most humans would manage to fare reasonably well for themselves functioning as interdependent equals among other humans.

Were it otherwise—were humans to spring into existence fully developed and educated in the ways of the world—the obligations we incur by creating them would be quite different. This is not to say that we would have no moral obligations arising from our creation of such fully developed humans. If we created such people in a situation in which they would suffer, we would owe them, at a minimum, what assistance we could to alleviate that suffering, and this obligation would spring from our being causally and morally responsible for their existence.[3]

Our obligations with respect to the humans we actually create are far more extensive than this. Those who voluntarily engage in actions they know, or should know, will result in the creation of a dependent human being have, I shall argue, a special obligation to provide for that human being. This obligation includes a requirement to take reasonable steps to ensure the nurturance, protection, education, and development of the dependent human being.

Before trying to state the moral principle in play here, let's illustrate this obligation with a fanciful case. Imagine a scientist, Jok Odudu—named after the African creator and rain god who presides over childbirth—has set for himself the task of making a human baby "from scratch." I mean by this that he plans to sequence the genetic material from molecules that are clearly nonliving. He will create an entire artificially produced conceptus from inanimate materials and then incubate this organism in an artificial womb. Suppose that all goes well and the result of this process is a healthy living child, indistinguishable from any other child except by its history.

Jok is not the child's genetic father. Let us suppose that there is no causal connection between the genetic make-up of Jok and that of the child and, furthermore, that there is no greater genetic similarity between these two than there is between any two arbitrary unrelated humans. Jok, we will suppose, is driven only by the desire to *create* human life artificially. When he creates the life, he has no desire to function as a social parent and, consequently, does not. Finally, he never develops feelings of affection toward the child once the child exists, nor does the child develop such feelings for him.

Whatever else is missing from the bundle of elements that constitute the typical parent–child relationship,[4] there is one respect in which Jok is like a typical parent. He is causally and morally responsible for acts that he knows could lead to, and in fact do lead to, the creation of a new human life.

In the case as described, Jok not only voluntarily undertook an action he was aware might result in the creation of a new human life; he did this with the specific intention of creating a new life. It is, of course, not always true of typical parents that their procreative actions were undertaken with the intent of creating a life. Frequently, as is evidenced by the existence of a market for contraceptives, they intended that the act *not* create a new life. In these cases, a parent's responsibility for the new human life does not result from the same sort of intentional creation of dependent life that Jok undertakes. But the parent normally has responsibility, nonetheless—typically both causal and moral responsibility.

We can modify the story of Jok to capture this point of analogy. Imagine that Jok has no desire to create a baby. What he enjoys doing is producing an artificial conceptus. But let us imagine that Jok lives in a world where the gestation of humans is not a delicate matter. In his world, fertilized human ova will develop normally in a wide variety of environments in much the way that many common bacteria colonies can in ours. A human conceptus, casually tossed on the laboratory counter, will frequently develop into a healthy infant so long as no one interferes. Jok knows all of this—or at least he *should* know all of this given the evidence available to him.

Because he does not want to produce a human infant, he may take some precautions to avoid this outcome. Perhaps he tries to ensure that the conceptus is disposed of in a way that prevents its development. However, Jok also knows that his procedures for preventing development are fallible—sometimes a conceptus he creates will develop notwithstanding his efforts to prevent this. Despite these risks, he intentionally engages in an action that he knows (or should know) could result in the creation of a new human life. We are imagining that he does this without coercive influences or other factors that would interfere with our attributing moral responsibility to him for the outcome of his action.

Now, with respect to causal and moral responsibility, Jok might be thought to be a better analog of those parents, considered as a couple, who engage in intercourse without the intention of creating a new human life—indeed, with the intention of avoiding this outcome.

The developing humans in Jok's lab, if any, are in all other respects completely ordinary. They have the customary physical and emotional needs. For normal physical development, they need food, air, heat, and protection from disease and other harmful environmental factors. For normal psychological development, they need affection, appropriate interaction with adults and other children, appropriate stimuli, and more. If these needs are not met, these infants will suffer physically, psychologically, or in both ways.

Should such suffering occur, the infants (or, later, children) would be innocent of any wrongdoing that merited or caused the suffering. The suffering would not be the result of the voluntary actions of any agent other than Jok. Jok has voluntarily engaged in an action that he knows, or should know, could make it the case that some innocent individual will suffer unless someone provides for that individual. And, in fact, the action has had that consequence. In the absence of any special arrangements or justified social conventions that impose this obligation on others, it seems plausible to hold that Jok has a special obligation, based on his causal role in the creation of the new life, to provide for that new life.

These considerations lead rather clearly to an attractive principle that I shall call "the Responsibility for Dependent Life Principle"—the RDLP, for short. Before attempting to state the principle, several important caveats must be made. Though I will speak of "dependent life" generally, I mean to refer only to dependent *sentient* life. Ultimately, we will focus on forms of life that have the moral status typically thought appropriate to normal humans. I do not believe that anything of moral significance turns directly on the biological classification of the organism in question. Nevertheless, since our ultimate concern is the moral responsibility human parents have for their children, we are not concerned here with dependent life forms that have a significantly different moral status than that of humans.[5]

A second set of caveats concerns the moral-theoretic status of principles like the RDLP. It is, perhaps obviously, not to be understood as a fundamental moral principle.

I intend it as a derivative moral principle that, I hope, will be plausible to people who have markedly different opinions on foundational moral questions. Furthermore, in part *because* it is not intended as a fundamental moral truth, it is best understood as a prima facie moral principle.

The term "prima facie" has caused more than a little confusion in moral and legal philosophy.[6] When applied to an obligation, it has been used in two quite distinct senses. The first is the evidential/epistemic sense. In this sense, to say that there is a prima facie obligation to perform an action is to say only that, in the absence of further considerations, there is a reason to believe that an actual obligation exists. These further considerations can either *undermine* or *override* the prima facie obligation. They undermine it if they entail that there is, in the particular case, no actual obligation at all. These further considerations override the prima facie obligation if they entail that, despite the moral factors on which the prima facie obligation is premised, weightier moral considerations determine that one's all-things-considered obligation is to act contrary to the prima facie obligation. In the second sense, all prima facie obligations are actual obligations, though they may be overridden by other considerations and, hence, exist but not determine the overall obligation in a particular case. They will show their existence, nonetheless, by their "moral residue."[7] For clarity, I use "pro tanto moral obligation" to pick out this second sense of "prima facie obligation" and refer to the corresponding moral principles as "pro tanto moral principles."[8]

In calling the RDLP a "prima facie" moral principle, I do not mean to imply that it always applies and generates a moral reason. I do not claim that it is a pro tanto moral principle; it is a prima facie principle only in the first of the two senses described earlier. Countervailing moral considerations may either *override* it or *undermine* its application. And undermining considerations need not be of the form of countervailing moral obligations or, indeed, any countervailing moral considerations at all.

With those cautionary comments in place, then, here the plausible principle I propose:

> *Responsibility for Dependent Life Principle (RDLP):* If an agent voluntarily engages in actions that the agent knows (or should know) might produce a morally significant dependent life without wrongdoing of others that the agent can't reasonably be expected to anticipate and, in fact, these actions *do* produce such a dependent life without wrongful actions of others, then, in the absence of special arrangements or justified social conventions that impose this duty on others, the agent has a special duty to promote the well-being of that dependent life and, a fortiori, to prevent its suffering.

Because I rely on this principle, it would clearly be desirable to demonstrate its truth. My desire to do this is, however, tempered by an appreciation of the difficulty of producing such a proof. In lieu of a demonstration, I hope to offer considerations that render the principle plausible and to respond to objections to the principle. My goal here is to offer a prima facie case for the truth of a principle that generates duties only prima facie. This is a rather modest ambition, but one that is still worth achieving, as will be evident upon exploring some of its implications.

The RDLP does not, itself, specify the strength of the duty to provide for the well-being of the dependent life; it does not indicate what level of sacrifice is required on the part of the creator of the dependent life. One could hold that those who create dependent life (of the right sort) owe that life everything within their power to give. In William Rose's screenplay of *Guess Who's Coming to Dinner*,[9] one central character, John Prentice (played by Sidney Poitier in the film), responds to his father's suggestion that he owes it to his parents not to marry a Caucasian woman because of the sacrifices his father and mother made in raising him. In particular, his father alludes to the miles he had carried a mailbag so that his son could become a doctor. John Prentice tells his father: "If you carried that bag a *million* miles—you did what you were *supposed* to do! Because you brought me into this world and from that day, you owed me everything you could ever *do* for me."[10]

Alternatively, one could hold that the special obligations of the creator of dependent life are weak and easily overridden by other moral considerations—or even, depending on one's moral views about such things, by considerations of personal convenience. I shall be assuming that the prima facie duty to provide for the well-being of the dependent life, given the sort of life we are discussing, is not trivial. When the duty actually arises, it plays a strong role in determining one's "all-things-considered" obligation. However, I will not attempt to be more precise than this.

The RDLP assigns responsibility for dependent life to an agent only when the potential procreative consequences arise in the absence of wrongdoing by others that the agent can't reasonably be expected to anticipate. This limits its applicability, perhaps excessively. But some limitation along these lines is clearly necessary. As Judith Thomson points out, a woman's innocent walk outside might be a necessary casual contributor to her being raped and impregnated. To avoid responsibility for a dependent life, it is not true that a woman must "never leav[e] home without a (reliable!) army."[11]

Though the RDLP is modest in its ambitions and initially plausible to many, it is not uncontroversial. It grounds a special moral obligation concerning the well-being of another individual on an agent's voluntarily playing a causal role in that individual's creation and holds that this obligation can arise: (a) in the absence of any social conventions; and (b) without the agent voluntarily accepting the obligation. We will look at some of the objections that have been raised to these two aspects of the RLDP.

The RDLP asserts what some would consider a *natural* duty to support children. While it recognizes and allows for the operation of "justified social conventions" that can impose the primary duty for rearing children on others, the RDLP asserts that, in the absence of such conventions, procreators acting under the specified conditions have a special duty—and one not grounded on social conventions—to provide for and raise their children.

Joseph Millum denies the existence of special, *natural* responsibilities to support and rear children. On Millum's view, parental responsibilities are to be explained *entirely* on a "*conventional-acts* account, according to which parental duties are taken on by individuals through acts whose meaning is determined by social convention."[12] This implies that parental responsibilities "can be acquired only because of social conventions regarding their acquisition."[13]

In telling the story of Jok Odudu, we made no reference to any social conventions. Indeed, the story is consistent with Jok being the lone inhabitant of an otherwise deserted island. Nevertheless, we are led to the plausible—almost inescapable, I think— conclusion that Jok has a duty to provide for and support the products of his procreative activity. Millum is aware of the potential threat posed by the implications of his theory in cases where there is no social convention concerning parenting responsibility. His response is that, were a community to lack such conventions, the responsibility for providing for the well-being of children "falls on the community as a whole, just as it does for the well-being of other dependent persons with morally important needs."[14] And, presumably, if Jok is on that desert island beloved of philosophers, he constitutes a community of one (plus however many infants he produces).[15] This would allow Millum to conclude that Jok does, indeed, have special duties to provide for and support the infants he creates, but ground this duty on proximity and capacity or shared community instead of on Jok's procreative activities.

Millum's denial that procreators have a *special* and *natural* duty to provide for the well-being of the morally significant beings they produce has, though, unattractive implications. Imagine that Jok works remotely to create his conceptuses on a distant well-populated island using a three-dimensional biological printer he previously installed there. After being gestated in artificial wombs, the products of his experiments are left in baskets outside the gates of his remote facility. The residents of this island have, no doubt, a responsibility to provide for the well-being of the dependent products of Jok's activities. They are, after all, in a position to alleviate the suffering of innocent, morally significant beings. But Jok has the primary responsibility for providing for their needs. He acts wrongly by failing to provide for them precisely because he is the cause of their existence in a dependent state and there is no morally justified social convention assigning this responsibility to others. Millum's purely conventional account of parental duties—and, in particular, his denial of a natural duty based on procreative activities— cannot account for this duty.

Millum is correct to recognize that social conventions have a very important role to play in understanding responsibilities for rearing children.[16] There are societies where these responsibilities fall, by social convention, primarily to both parents' extended families, to the extended family of the mother, or to the society as a whole. The RDLP acknowledges this phenomenon and allows that, when these arrangements are morally justified, they can diminish or eliminate the specific, day-to-day moral responsibilities of procreators. But Millum is wrong to think that procreators have no *special natural* duty to provide for their offspring under appropriate conditions. Natural duties of procreators play an important part in the explanation of parental responsibilities. They manifest this role most clearly, perhaps, when there are no social conventions concerning responsibility for dependent life. Plausibly, though, they do not absent themselves from the stage even where such social conventions involve a complete reassignment of day-to-day parental responsibilities to someone other than the procreators.[17]

The RDLP requires a voluntary act on the part of an agent to incur the special obliga-tions concerning the well-being of the created individual. It does not, though, make the existence of the obligations dependent on voluntary acceptance of them. This sort of causal account of the special duties of procreators is notoriously denied by Judith Jarvis Thomson in what is without doubt the best-known philosophical article on abortion, "A Defense of Abortion."[18] A detailed critique of Thomson's somewhat enigmatic, and often misunderstood, argument and its progeny is beyond the present project.[19] However, a few remarks about this issue are in order.

Thomson argues that even granting, *arguendo*, that the fetus has a right to life and that the right to life is weightier than the right to control one's body, abortion is a permissible act. In her view, this is because of the content (or, as some say, the "shape" or "scope") of the right to life. The famous "unconscious violinist" case shows this. Thomson asks us to imagine that you are kidnapped and wake up in a hospital to find your body function-ing as a life-support system for an unconscious violinist, who must remain hooked up to your body for the next 9 months in order to survive. The unconscious violinist has a right to life, like any other person. We can grant, furthermore, that the right to life is morally weightier than the right to control one's body. (At least, the infringement on your right to control your body that is threatened here is a less serious infringement than an infringement on a person's right to life.) Still, Thomson argues, the violinist does not have a right to use your body and you act permissibly if you unhook yourself from the violinist, with the anticipated result that he dies.

The RDLP provides a basis for what has come to be called "the responsibility objec-tion" to Thomson's defense of abortion. There is a rich and often intricate literature defending and criticizing different versions of this objection.[20] The core idea, though, is an obvious one and one that Thomson, herself, recognized: There is a rather obvi-ous difference between Thomson's unconscious violinist case and the case of abortion of pregnancies not resulting from rape. In the latter, but not the former, the woman is at least partly responsible for the fetus's dependence on her body. Thomson and her later champions have offered ingenious examples designed to show that voluntarily engaging in an action that predictably causes someone to be in need of assistance from you does not, in itself, generate an obligation to provide that assistance.

The case of Jok Odudu, though, shows that it can do so, even when the act that causes the need of assistance is the very act that causes the existence of the needy individual. The intuition is straightforward and compelling. Jok's voluntary action—an action that he knew could result in the production of a dependent life (of the relevant significant sort) and in fact did so—brought about a situation in which, unless he provides care for that dependent being, either that being will suffer or others will have to bear unchosen costs to prevent that suffering. It is pro tanto wrong to bring about unnecessary suffer-ing in the world or to impose unchosen costs on others to avoid that suffering. In the absence of morally justified practices that assign to others the responsibility to provide for the dependent being, it is pro tanto wrong to fail to provide care for a dependent being that has been brought into existence by your voluntary actions when the possibil-ity of procreation was reasonably foreseeable.

COMPLICATIONS: SEX AND GESTATION

What we have tried to illustrate with the story of Jok is how causal and moral responsibility for an innocent dependent life can create moral obligations to provide the necessary care for that life. While the story selectively presents some causal features that are common elements of parenthood, crucial disanalogies remain. The most obvious disanalogy stems from this mundane observation: Humans reproduce sexually and doing so normally involves two people—typically, though as we are painfully aware, not always—two agents who are capable of free and responsible choice. As we shall see, this is one factor that complicates the assignment of moral responsibility for supporting and nurturing dependent life.

Where a new life results from sexual activities of adults under conditions of moral responsibility, the individual moral responsibility for the creation of a new dependent life is not nearly as clear as it is in the story of Jok. The parties may have different intentions in engaging in sex, different desires concerning reproduction, and different moral commitments concerning the termination of a pregnancy resulting from the sexual activity. The shared causal responsibility in the context of these differences may result in judgments of differing moral responsibility for the creation of a dependent life and, as a result, differing moral duties to support and provide for the product of procreation.

The possibility of terminating the pregnancy raises additional complications—ones we have ignored in the preceding stories about Jok. The nature of these complications is determined, to a very large degree, by the nature and moral status of the fetus and the moral permissibility of abortion. If, as some believe, the human fetus is a person with a right to life from the moment of conception, then the further moral complications added by the possibility of abortion are not obvious. The moment conception takes place, the conceptus is a person with a right to life, and it is completely dependent on others to sustain its life. In cases where sexual intercourse was voluntary on the part of both parties, it seems initially plausible to hold that each parent has a moral responsibility to provide for what we could, on this assumption, correctly call an "unborn child."[21] However, if the conceptus is not a person with a right to life from the point of conception, then the act of intercourse does not represent the last opportunity for (relevant) action before the creation of the dependent being with the requisite moral standing. As we shall see, this can complicate the matter of the moral responsibility of the two parents.[22]

Sex

It does not take competent adults to make a baby. It is so easy that even a child can do it, unfortunately.[23] When a child becomes a parent at a very early age, we have doubts about whether the child meets the general requirements for moral responsibility. If the child does not, then regardless of the child's causal role in the pregnancy, we should not hold him or her morally responsible for the dependent life that results.[24]

Even when the parents are adults, they might not be morally competent or, more frequently, they might not be willing participants in the act that created the dependent life. Adults with serious mental impairments might lack the capacities necessary for moral responsibility. Furthermore, in cases of rape, one of the parties is not a willing party to the sex act. When the rape takes the form of brute force, as opposed to a threat of force, or when it takes place while the victim is unconscious, the victim is not even a causal agent in the act and clearly has no special moral responsibility for any dependent human being created by such an act—at least none based on the RDLP.[25] When the rape involves a coercive threat of force, the victim may be a causal agent but, because of this threat, not be morally responsible for the actions involved in the rape or for the consequences of the rape, including (if it *is* a consequence of the rape) a new dependent human life.

A variety of factors, including various incapacities (either general or specific, temporary or permanent) or coercion, can diminish responsibility for the production of dependent life—in the limiting case, undermine any claim of responsibility at all. Nevertheless, in the typical case in which an innocent dependent human life results from sexual intercourse, both parties meet the minimal general conditions for moral responsibility and both are voluntarily and intentionally engaging in behavior that they know, or should know, can result in the creation of an innocent dependent human life. That is why we concluded before that, *considered as a couple*, they are relevantly similar to Jok and, so, have a special duty under the RDLP to support and provide for any child that results from their actions.

The existence of multiple agents complicates issues of moral responsibility for the consequences of actions. In the case of human pregnancies created in the stereotypical way, through the consensual actions of normal adults, we confront cases where each agent is necessary for the consequence to occur. Initially, it is plausible to think that in these cases, at least when the choice of each agent to have sexual relations is adequately informed and voluntary, responsibility for the pregnancy is shared equally by the two agents.[26]

Where both parties are sufficiently knowledgeable about the potential consequences of sexual intercourse, including the likelihood of these consequences, and both are acting in a fully voluntary way, the complications introduced solely by the existence of two co-creators of the dependent life do not generate any great difficulties. We can illustrate the situation with a slight modification of the story of Jok.

Imagine that Jok works with Ala, who draws her name from the Igbo myth of the highest goddess, the Earth Mother. In fact, Ala works together with Jok in his lab on the activities that create the artificially produced conceptus; neither could do this alone. We shall assume and both know that, given the sort of work they are doing in the lab, a conceptus could be produced and that the environment might be "friendly enough" for this conceptus to develop into a dependent life of a morally significant sort. Assuming that both Jok and Ala meet the conditions for moral responsibility, the RDLP assigns them each a special obligation to promote the well-being of that dependent life once that dependent life is of the proper sort.

This seems like a reasonable outcome even where their intentions and desires differ. To illustrate: let us change our previous assumption concerning Jok's desire to produce a child. Suppose that Ala does not intend or desire to produce a child, but Jok does. Despite the divergent intentions and desires, absent the special arrangements alluded to in the RDLP, Ala has a special obligation to provide for any children resulting from their joint activities.

There are many problems with the assignment of individual responsibility for participation in joint ventures. And these problems certainly arise with respect to typical human reproduction. Furthermore, matters become significantly more complex, as we shall see, with the introduction of the other complicating factor we will discuss.

Gestation

Human development, both pre- and postnatal, is a gradual process and there is great controversy over the question of when, during a normal human organism's development, it becomes the sort of being whose interests are properly protected by the RDLP. Some believe that the fetus is a morally significant entity—indeed, a person with right to life—right from the point of conception.[27]

We will not attempt to settle here the question of when, in the process of development, the life of a human organism takes on the special moral status that most of us believe normal adult humans have. But that thorny question is intimately intertwined with the issues we face of responsibility for dependent life and, in particular, *paternal* responsibility for dependent life. Here is why.

If the conceptus is not the sort of life that is covered by the RDLP, then those who create a conceptus do not, in virtue of that act and the principle, have a special obligation to promote the well-being of the conceptus. In many cases, if they take no actions to end the pregnancy, the fetus will develop and be born.[28] If it develops into a normal infant and child, at some point it will have a moral status that results in its having interests that are protected by the RDLP. However, some people hold that terminating a pregnancy, at least in the early stages, is morally permissible under most conditions—even for purposes of the mere convenience of the parents. If that is true, then, one way of avoiding the special obligations arising from the RDLP is to abort the pregnancy. And this option, in conjunction with obvious sexual asymmetries, alters the situation in important ways.

Let us suppose that the developing fetus is not the sort of life that is protected by the RDLP at early stages of the pregnancy but is by the latest stages of pregnancy.[29] Furthermore, let's suppose that the killing of the fetus prior to this time is not a significant moral wrong.[30] Now, a man and a woman who bear responsibility for the creation of a fetus will not have the duties imposed by the RDLP if the fetus is aborted prior to its achieving the moral status required by that principle. There may be other moral considerations that bear on their actions of conceiving, and then aborting, the fetus, but the parents cannot run afoul of the RDLP when they abort early enough.

So, the assumption that the fetus does not have the requisite moral status to be covered by the RDLP at the point of conception bears importantly on the issues that concern us here. If the assumption is correct, abortion could allow a *couple* to permissibly avoid the duties imposed by the RDLP after conceiving a fetus. It is a trickier matter, though, to determine how this assumption bears on the *individual* responsibility of the two co-creators of the fetus.

Nature might have been kinder to modern humans—at least allowing us to avoid some thorny moral problems—if the continued development of the fetus to the point where it was covered by the RDLP required positive, conscious actions from *both* genetic parents. But nature has its own purposes and those do not always make the world an easier place for us. In fact, nature does not require any special positive actions of *either* genetic parent to bring a significant proportion of pregnancies to term. However, a pregnancy coming to term does require the *absence* of certain actions. In particular, a relevant requirement is that no form of artificial abortion be performed. Because nature has determined that the fetus will develop in only one parent's body, there is a significant asymmetry between the two genetic parents. Furthermore, nature has determined that if the fetus develops, it will always be in the female's body. And because the asymmetry is related to sex, it can function as a basis for asymmetries in gender roles.[31] It is a further matter, though, to determine the implications of these sexual asymmetries on the rights and obligations of the two parents.[32]

Let us return to Jok and Ala to get some distance from, and hence perspective on, the issue. If we try to modify our fanciful case to make it more similar in the relevant respects to the way in which humans typically reproduce, we will have to make a number of amendments. As suggested earlier, the activity that produces the dependent human life must take place in Jok's lab.[33] In addition, what develops immediately from their collaborative work is an organism that is not protected by the RDLP but, absent any interference, has a significant probability of developing into an organism that is. Finally, we must assume that Jok has a morally and legally permissible way to prevent the organism from developing into a being that is protected by the RDLP. There are, of course, many ways to fill in the gaps in this scenario. Some of these are clearly morally relevant in ways that lead us to different answers about the individual responsibility of Jok and Ala. What we are setting in place now, though, is just the skeletal elements of the story. How we flesh out this skeleton will be crucial. As Judith Thomson says concerning abortion, "there are cases and cases, and the details make a difference."[34]

There are some ways of fleshing out our story of Jok and Ala that lead to relatively uncontroversial moral conclusions. Suppose, for example, that Jok and Ala have discussed the possibility that one of the products of their experiment will begin to develop as a normal human fetus does. Jok has expressed his unwillingness to terminate the developing organism. Ala has agreed to share in providing for the future needs of any such dependent being, should it develop and their plan for sharing these responsibilities is adequate for the needs of the protected life. In this case, Jok and Ala have made an agreement about what will be done if the products of their experiments begin to develop into dependent beings. Assuming both are competent, adequately informed, and not operating under any sort of coercion, they are each morally responsible to share in providing for the dependent life (if one develops) in accordance with their plan. Antecedent agreement makes for an easy case—at least when it is not followed by reversals in the parties' commitments.

Would that the real world were so morally simple! In modern, Western industrialized nations, people frequently engage in potentially procreative acts with little communication of their intentions, desires, or moral and religious principles. The two parties may have very different understandings of the significance of the sex act, the nature of the relationship, and what each will do if a pregnancy results. Sometimes misunderstandings between the parties are innocent—or at least innocent of active deception or reliance on a known misunderstanding of the other person. But this is not always so. People sometimes mislead their sexual partners about their level of commitment, their intentions and desires with respect to the other person and with respect to a possible pregnancy or child. This deception can be verbal, involving overt lies or misleading statements, or nonverbal—a touch or a glance at an appropriate time can convey information, sometimes misleading information, about one's intentions, desires, and beliefs. Problems are caused not only by deception, verbal or not, but by one party's reliance on misconceptions about the other's intentions, desires, and moral commitments.

The problem is not always a failure to communicate. People are often unclear about their own values, expectations, and beliefs in these areas. They do not know what they expect from the other person or what they, themselves, intend to do in response to the various possible outcomes of their sexual activity. Indeed, they often do not *have* any settled values, expectations, and beliefs about important matters that may arise from their sexual activity.

Assigning responsibility for dependent life under "real-world" conditions—even when both parties were voluntary participants in activities that they knew, or should have known, could result in a pregnancy—is a more difficult task than we have so far modeled. Under what conditions, if any, is the responsibility of one party significantly diminished or removed completely? When one party to the sexual act has intentionally deceived the other party about the possibility of a pregnancy—leading them to engage in an action they would not otherwise perform—what effect, if any, does this have on the responsibility of the deceived party for a resulting dependent life? If one party has been reckless with respect to providing relevant information to the other, is the responsibility of the other party diminished?

Caveat Copulator?

These are difficult questions—so difficult that it is tempting to look for a way around them. Perhaps, one might argue for a sexual-activity version of the caveat emptor principle: *caveat copulator*. Such a principle would say that, if you voluntarily engage in sexual relations with another person, you are responsible for any dependent life that results ... period—a moral strict-liability-with-respect-to-the-consequences-of-sexual-activity approach. But, other than providing a simple answer to difficult questions, there is little to be said in favor of this approach and much to be said against it.

In the first place, it is not consonant with our moral evaluation of other sorts of actions. We do not generally hold people morally responsible for the consequences of actions they performed as a result of wrongful deception, at least when their reliance on the misrepresentations was reasonable. Imagine that I gave a person what appeared to be, and what I describe to her as, a starter pistol—apparently loaded with blanks and having a plugged barrel—and this happens in a context where she has no reason to suspect deception. If, when she fires it to start a race, a real bullet discharges from the gun and kills an innocent bystander, we do not hold her responsible for the death. In this context, she acted reasonably in firing the gun on the assumption that it was firing blanks. What could it be about sexual intercourse that would justify moral evaluation so different from other activities?[35]

Surely, were Jok or Ala to intentionally mislead the other about the possibility of a dependent life being created by their activities in a context where it is reasonable for the other to rely on these misrepresentations, it would diminish or vitiate the responsibility of the deceived party for any resulting dependent life. Suppose that Jok lies to Ala, insisting that his lab cannot support the development of a conceptus they will jointly create, possibly even providing her with evidence for this. Suppose the history of the relationship between Jok and Ala make it reasonable for Ala to believe, based on Jok's statements, that there is virtually no chance of a conceptus developing to the point where it is morally significant. It seems, at least initially then, that it is reasonable for Ala to rely on this in making her decision about whether to engage in the activity with Jok. If a conceptus were to develop, Jok, and not Ala, bears primary moral responsibility for the support of the resultant dependent life. Because of the seriousness of procreation, failure to disclose information you believe to be relevant to a potential partner's decision about whether to engage in activities that are normally potentially procreative is wrong. It is even more clearly a serious moral wrong to engage in an intentional, positive act of deception about such matters.[36] The clearly wrongful actions of Jok make us more willing to assign to him full responsibility for the dependent lives resulting from his joint activity with Ala.

This conclusion is not inescapable. We could hold that the activities of Jok and Ala are "inherently dangerous" and that the decision to engage in them exposes one to moral responsibility for the consequences of those activities despite the presence of factors that normally mitigate responsibility. Some might think that this is an appropriate stance to take with respect to sexual behavior. This is the driving thought behind the caveat copulator approach.

We do not, though, accept a caveat copulator approach with respect to all the possible consequences of sexual activities. Consider, first, the legal issue. In some jurisdictions, HIV-positive individuals are guilty of criminal acts if they have unprotected sexual intercourse with another person without disclosing their HIV status.[37] Even when criminal sanctions are not available, failure to disclose one's HIV status could be the basis of civil liability were the other participant to contract HIV as a result of the sexual activity. Surely sexual intercourse is "inherently dangerous" with respect to the possibility of contracting sexually transmitted diseases. Nevertheless, the law does not take a caveat copulator stance with respect to these risks.

The moral case is clearer. Certainly people can, and do, act irresponsibly with respect to the possible contraction of sexually transmitted diseases. But we do not hold people morally responsible for contracting a disease as a result of reasonable reliance on the representation of others that the activity in question does not risk transmitting a disease.

Secondly, the caveat copulator approach encourages irresponsible and immoral behavior. This is, perhaps, ironic. It is likely that the caveat copulator approach toward the unintended consequences of sexual activities was attractive to previous generations precisely because it was thought to discourage what was considered to be irresponsible and immoral behavior: engaging in nonmarital sexual relations. Whatever effect strict liability for the consequences of sexual activities might have had on suppressing such activities in the past, there is little reason to think that it is having such effects now. More to the point, though, many now do not believe that nonmarital sexual relations are, in themselves, irresponsible and immoral.

The caveat copulator approach encourages the behavior of wrongfully misleading one's sexual partners about important aspects of one's desires, intentions, and values and, thus, about the likelihood of various possible consequences of the sexual activity.[38] The effects of such deception for one's sexual partners may be extremely serious. So, an individual who does not seek to become a parent may engage in sexual intercourse with an individual only as a result of the other person representing that she or he is positively infertile.[39] This representation may be made knowing that it is false and with the specific intention of securing compliance with a sex act that would be otherwise unattainable, something that is clearly pro tanto morally wrong.[40]

Finally, the caveat copulator approach with respect to sex acts encounters difficulty defining "sex act" in a manner that makes the principle plausible. For there are sex acts and there are sex acts, and it matters how we formulate the caveat copulator principle. Sex acts that one of the participants could not reasonably foresee would lead to the creation of a new life may yet be essential causal factors in this outcome. The case of Emile Frisard is instructive.[41] Late in 1983, Frisard was frequently at the East Jefferson General Hospital to help take care of his parents who were patients there. A nursing aide at the hospital, Debra Rojas, became "abnormally friendly" (as one witness described it) with the family, visiting Frisard's parents' room frequently "to the point of being bothersome" (as another testified). Frisard was with his parents practically every night and Rojas often visited when he was there. According to Frisard's unchallenged testimony, on one of these visits Rojas offered to perform oral sex on Frisard provided he used a condom. He agreed and, after he left, Rojas apparently inseminated herself with the sperm in the condom. Frisard denied that he ever had vaginal intercourse with Rojas, and he apparently had no indication that Rojas would use his sperm in this way. A witness testified that she saw Rojas in a storeroom using a medical device to insert something in her vagina. Frisard engaged in a sex act with Debra Rojas under the very reasonable presumption that pregnancy could not result from that action. But Rojas did become pregnant, and DNA testing proved that it was Frisard's genetic child. Frisard's sex act with Rojas was a causal contributor to the pregnancy.

A true caveat copulator approach with respect to sex acts that causally contribute to the creation of dependent life, if applied to sex acts in general, would declare Frisard's reasonable belief that he was not engaging in a potentially procreative act as irrelevant to Frisard's responsibilities. But this is ludicrous.[42] There is nothing about the fact that it was specifically a *sex act* that led to Rojas's ability to use his sperm to impregnate herself that justifies taking a strict liability approach to Frisard's actions. The purloined sperm could as easily have been taken from a semen specimen that Frisard had left for analysis, even if it was extracted surgically. Why should those who engage in sex acts have a special responsibility to beware of what might be done with their sperm? One might speculate that there is a puritanical "pay to piper" attitude at work on some people's intuitions in cases like Frisard's. But surely any reasonable principle would base a duty to support dependent life on the reasonably expected likelihood that the act could produce such a life, not on whether the act involved sexual pleasure or was anticipated by the participants to do so.

We could, of course, restrict a caveat copulator principle to acts of genital intercourse. It's difficult to see, though, why the *type* of sexual activity is relevant except to the degree that it affects the agents' reasonable expectations of a resultant pregnancy. Caveat principles are focused on an agent's responsibilities for inherently risky conduct; they should be pegged to the level of risk. If a man has had a vasectomy and been tested multiple times with a sperm count of zero, genital intercourse may have no greater procreative probability than Frisard faced. If a woman *reasonably* relies on a man's representation that he is such a man, why should greater caution be required for vaginal sex than other forms of sexual contact?

Our current concern is not with misappropriated sperm but with sexual intercourse that is induced on a representation that it cannot be procreative. There are, though, important points of analogy. In both instances, one party induces another to engage in a sex act that the second party has every reason to believe cannot lead to a pregnancy. While it is true that the "turkey baster" cases require a further act on the part of the deceiver, after sexual intercourse, it is hard to see how this makes a relevant difference to the moral responsibility of the deceived party.[43]

Attempting to avoid the problem of determining when and how much a person's responsibility for dependent life is diminished or vitiated when the person has been the victim of fraud or deception about the possibility of pregnancy by adopting a moral *caveat copulator* approach is unacceptable. People do have a diminished responsibility when they are reasonably led, by the wrongful actions of others, to misunderstand the likely consequences of their actions. This is not to deny that each partner has a responsibility to control his or her own fertility. Doing so is prudent, in any event. However, blaming one party for not doing so in the presence of a credible but fraudulent representation by the other that such control is unnecessary is an instance of blaming the victim.

It does not follow from what has been said that any person deceived into engaging in sexual activity by fraudulent representations that the sex cannot result in pregnancy has no responsibility for a resultant child. It is one thing to rely on the assurances of a long-time, intimate partner about his or her fertility; quite another to rely on such assurances from a near stranger. In the latter case, the deceived party certainly has a legitimate grievance against the deceiver. And the deceiver is not exonerated. Casual relationships are not a license to deceive. But it is not an instance of "blaming the victim" to expect all individuals to take reasonable precautions to avoid something as serious as unintended procreation and to hold them responsible for the consequences of not taking such precautions.

What has been said earlier is frustratingly unsatisfactory with respect to the vast majority of cases where responsibility for dependent life is problematic. In most cases, there is not active, or even passive, deception about such factors as one's fertility, contingency plans in case a pregnancy does ensue, and so forth. These are vexed issues and they require detailed, context-dependent analysis. My primary point here is that such analysis is needed; the thorny issues cannot be dodged by an appeal to a simple caveat copulator approach.

SEXUAL ASYMMETRIES

The discussion of the previous section did not explore the sexual asymmetries of human reproduction mentioned earlier. Either party can be a victim of deception with regard to the fertility of their partner and, so, with regard to the procreative potential of the activities. The rejection of a caveat copulator approach does, however, support the RDLP's restriction to cases that do not involve, in the indicated manner, the wrongful conduct of others. And this element of the RDLP has moral implications grounded in these sexual asymmetries.

Because pregnancy takes place in the woman's body and, we are assuming *arguendo*, that abortion is morally permissible, the responsibility for dependent life assigned by the RDLP can exhibit sexual asymmetries. I assume that the pregnant woman has the sole moral authority to terminate or continue a pregnancy. The question of whether the RDLP assigns asymmetric responsibility for the dependent life created by voluntary sexual activities depends on whether the woman's failure to get an abortion could count as wrongful conduct that the man cannot reasonably be expected to anticipate.

Let us, one last time, try to attain the distance for real-life cases afforded by our fanciful example of Jok and Ala. Imagine now that our two scientists have had detailed discussions about the potential of their activities to produce a developing fetus, the interests of which, if no action is taken, will be protected by the RDLP. They take actions to prevent their conceptuses from beginning to develop, but Jok assures Ala that, if one does begin to develop, he will destroy it before it becomes morally significant. Ala makes it clear that Jok's commitment is a necessary condition for her participation with Jok in their joint activities. Furthermore, just to get an extremely clear case, let us suppose that Jok is making a *lying* promise. Finally, imagine that terminating the developing fetus would not be physically or psychologically harmful to Jok, nor contrary to his moral or religious commitments.

If, in such a scenario, Jok declines to terminate a developing fetus, I think Jok acts wrongly and, indeed, wrongs Ala. If it was reasonable for Ala to believe Jok's promises, then I believe, Jok has responsibility for the resulting dependent life, but Ala does not—at least in the case where Jok can fulfill the obligations.[44]

The case described is extreme. I do not claim that wrongful failure to terminate a pregnancy arises only in such an extreme case, but I do not attempt here to determine the conditions under which failure to abort is wrong. There are many complexities. My point here is merely that there are such cases and they affect the division of moral responsibility for dependent life of the two procreators.[45] When a woman acts wrongly in choosing not to terminate a pregnancy, this can affect the responsibility of the father for the child resulting from their procreative activities. While they are similarly situated with respect to the sexual activity that began the pregnancy, the parity is broken in morally relevant ways by the sexual asymmetries of human reproduction.

Conclusion

Contra what defenders of a purely voluntaristic theory of procreators' duties assert, the procreative act itself, under specified conditions, can create special moral duties to provide for dependent life even in the absence of any act of voluntary acceptance of such duties. The conditions on the existence of this causally based duty of procreators, in the presence of the biological asymmetries of human reproduction, can under certain conditions give rise to asymmetric moral responsibilities for the dependent life created. This does not entail the so-called choice for men position—that a man does not have a responsibility to support a child if he declines to do so at some point early in the pregnancy.[46] But it does suggest that a man's special obligation to support a child that he fathers can, again under certain conditions, fail to arise simply from his voluntary engaging in potentially procreative activities.

Notes

1. Opinions differ on the philosophical value of fanciful speculations. While there is reason to be cautious of the verdicts of our moral "intuitions" when presented with strange scenarios, there is great value, I believe, in employing radical thought experiments. Henry David Thoreau says:

   When you are starting away, leaving your more familiar fields, for a little adventure like a walk, you look at every object with a traveler's, or at least with historical, eyes; you pause on the first bridge, where an ordinary walk hardly commences, and begin to observe and moralize like a traveler. It is worth the while to see your native village thus sometimes, as if you were a traveler passing through it, commenting on your neighbors as strangers. (*The Journal of Henry David Thoreau*, Vol. II. Boston: Houghton Mifflin and Company, 1906, 452).

   Similarly, it is worth the while to see our conceptual village with a traveler's eyes. Fanciful thought experiments help us to do that.

2. With a focus on paternity, I separate some of the rights and obligations of parenthood and the empirical elements of stereotypical parenthood in "Daddy Dilemmas: Untangling the Puzzles of Paternity," *The Cornell Journal of Law and Public Policy*, 13 (2003), and "Fatherhood," *International Encyclopedia of Ethics* (Hoboken, NJ: Wiley-Blackwell, 2013).

3. I set aside here a host of fascinating questions concerning the moral evaluation of the act of creating life of a morally significant sort. Our concern here is with the obligations owed as a result of a procreative act.

4. Stereotypical parents have not only causal responsibility for the children they produce but, as well, are genetically related and have psychological bonds with their children. For further discussion of the various elements of stereotypical paternity, in particular, see Donald Hubin, "Daddy Dilemmas: Untangling the Puzzles of Paternity" (*op. cit.*) and "Fatherhood" (*op. cit.*).

5. Complications arise from the fact that not all offspring of humans have the moral status of normal humans. In the United States every year, about 1,000 anencephalic babies are born. (But for prenatal testing and availability of abortion, the number would be far higher.) These babies lack a cerebellum and a cerebrum; they will never achieve the capacities that are essential for the moral status of normal humans. The parents of these infants may well have special duties based on their responsibility for dependent life that results from their procreative action, but the actions required by such duties will be significantly different from those required by parents of more normal infants. For simplicity, I ignore these complications in the text.

6. See M. B. E. Smith's "Is There a Prima Facie Obligation to Obey the Law?" for helpful discussion of the two distinct senses in which "prima facie" has been used in philosophical discourse.

7. See Judith Thomson's discussion of moral residues in *The Realm of Rights* (Cambridge, MA: Harvard University Press, 1992): 84ff.

8. See Andrew Reisner, "Prima Facie and Pro Tanto Oughts," in *International Encyclopedia of Ethics*, edited by Hugh LaFollette (Hoboken, NJ: Wiley-Blackwell, 2013).

9. William Rose, *Guess Who's Coming to Dinner*, Film. Directed by Stanley Kramer. Columbia Pictures, 1967.

10. Ibid., p. 98 (emphasis in original). The character holds not only that parental duties are enormously demanding, but also that there are no corresponding filial duties. Just prior to the passage quoted in the text, the character says, "I owe you *nothing!*" Perhaps both Prentice's denial of a filial duty and what many will see as his exaggeration of the parental duty should be considered rhetorical excess in defense of the plausible claim that a child does not owe his or her parents what Prentice's father was asking of him.

11. Judith Thomson, "A Defense of Abortion," *Philosophy and Public Affairs* 1(1971): 59.

12. Joseph Millum, "How Do We Acquire Parental Responsibilities?" *Social Theory and Practice* 34, no. 1 (2008): 71.

13. Ibid., p. 79

14. Ibid., p. 83.

15. It is not clear whether Millum grounds the nonconventional duty to provide for children on co-membership in a community, in a sociologically significant sense of that term, or on the mere fact that an individual is in a position to render support. Presumably, there is a duty to provide for the well-being of dependent persons even if they are not members of our community (in any sociologically significant sense of "community"). But some believe that there is a more stringent duty to provide for members of our community.

16. Appeal to the cultural variability of childrearing obligations is also raised by Elizabeth Brake as a serious problem for causal theories of parental obligations ("Willing Parents: A Voluntarist Account of Parental Role Obligation," in *Procreation and Parenthood: The Ethics of Bearing and Rearing Children*, ed. David Archard and David Benatar (Oxford: Oxford University Press, 2011), 151–177). Brake allows that there could be procreative costs that are the responsibility of the causal parents to bear but denies that these constitute parental duties, which she takes to be much more demanding. Parental duties, Brake believes, arise in virtue of an individual voluntarily taking them on. Brake's criticism of causal theories of parental duties is challenged by Lindsey Porter ("Why and How to Prefer a Causal Account of Parenthood," *Journal of Social Philosophy* 45 (2014): 182–202). See also, Bernard Puskar, "Breaking the Bond: Abortion and the Grounds of Parental Obligation," *Social Theory and Practice* 37, no. 2 (2011): 311–332, and "The Costs of Procreation," *Journal of Social Philosophy* 42, no. 1 (2011): 65–71.

17. Lindsey Porter (*op. cit.*) argues that procreator's obligations, what she calls "maker's obligations" include a pro tanto obligation to take on parental responsibilities. Elsewhere, Porter argues that procreators have a lifelong obligation to the children they create even when they have given them up for adoption ("Adoption Is Not Abortion-Lite," *Journal of Applied Philosophy* 29 (2012): 63–78).

18. See Judith Thomson, "A Defense of Abortion," *op. cit.* Thomson's argument is cast in terms of the right of a fetus to sustenance from the mother but, given plausible assumptions about the relationship between rights and obligations—assumptions Thomson would likely accept—her view entails a rejection of the RDLP. I do not believe Thomson's challenge is successful but cannot take up this challenge here.

19. I discuss Thomson's argument and the challenge it presents to the RDLP in depth in *Parsing Paternity* (manuscript).

20. For a relatively early statement of the objection, see Michael Tooley's *Abortion and Infanticide* (Oxford: Clarendon Press, 1983), 45. For critiques of the objection, see Harry S. Silverstein's "On a Woman's 'Responsibility' for the Fetus," *Social Theory and Practice* 13, no. 1 (1987) and David Boonin-Vail's "A Defense of 'A Defense of Abortion': On the Responsibility Objection to Thomson's Argument," *Ethics* 107, no. 2 (1997): 286–313). Defenses of versions of the objection can be found in Richard Langer's "Silverstein and the 'Responsibility Objection'," *Social Theory and Practice* 19, no. 3 (1993): 345–358 and Gerald Lang's "Nudging the Responsibility Objection," *Journal of Applied Philosophy* 25, no. 1 (2008): 56–71.

21. Though this is initially plausible and, in many cases, correct, we will examine later further conditions that must hold for it to be true.

22. This is potentially misleading. The complications we will examine are, in fact, present even if the fetus is assumed to be a person with a right to life and covered by the RDLP from the point of conception. Because of the ever-present lag between sexual intercourse and conception, there is always the possibility of preventing the pregnancy by actions taken after sexual intercourse and prior to conception. In principle, this possibility is sufficient to create the complications we will examine in connection with the possibility of terminating a pregnancy.

23. Though the pregnancy rate of US teenagers (ages 15–19 years) has been dropping steadily since the early 1990s, the National Center for Health Statistics estimates that in 2012, 305,388 babies were born to females in this age group. (See "Teen Pregnancy in the United States," available at http://www.cdc.gov/teenpregnancy/aboutteenpreg.htm#TeenPregnancyUS, accessed September 16, 2014.)

24. The rather obvious, and in most cases uncontroversial, moral observation that a young child often does not meet the general requirements for moral responsibility, if correct, indicts our current legal practices. Surprisingly, when minor males become fathers as the result of an act of statutory rape by an adult female, courts have consistently enforced child support obligations against these boys and such decisions have been upheld by state appellate courts and even state supreme courts. For a discussion of this, see my "Daddy Dilemmas: Untangling the Puzzles of Paternity," *The Cornell Journal of Law and Public Policy* 13 (2003): 51.

25. Here, too, court decisions sometimes astonish. Courts have found that a paternal responsibility to support exists even when the pregnancy results from rape by incapacitation of the biological father. I discuss a case of this sort in "Daddy Dilemmas" (*op. cit.*): 54–55.

26. This is probably best understood on the analogy to "joint and several" liability in the law. Each party has an equal responsibility, but if one party fails in this responsibility, the entire responsibility can fall to the other party.

27. Most of us, including many who claim to believe this, do not accept the moral consequences of such a view. For example, few believe that the *same* efforts are morally required to save the life of an aborted fetus as that of a child, and there is no call among those who are "pro-life" to expend the billions of dollars necessary to lessen the natural abortion rate, often estimated at between one-half and two-thirds of all pregnancies. If one really believes that the fetus has the same moral status as a normal adult human (or a normal human child), then our failure to address the high natural abortion rate should be viewed as a very serious indictment of our health system. Furthermore, though it is not logically related to the moral issue, few people have the very same emotional reaction to the loss of early-stage fetal life that they do to the loss of a child's life. To the couple, the loss of a fetus can be devastating, to be sure. However, we do not typically have funerals for fetuses that naturally abort within a couple of weeks of conception; we do not name the fetuses, engage in religious rites with respect to them, and so forth.

28. It is estimated, though, that the majority of pregnancies are terminated by spontaneous (natural) abortions. Given that pregnancy is defined in terms of the implantation of the embryo in the woman's body, the rate of spontaneous termination of developing conceptuses is even higher.

29. We shall assume here that the developing human organism is covered by the RDLP at birth, at least when the infant is normal (and, of course, if that is true, then also in many cases of abnormal fetuses). This is not uncontroversial. For example, the view defended by Mary Ann Warren, "Status of Abortion" (*The Monist* 57 (1973): 43–61), Michael Tooley,

Abortion and Infanticide (Oxford: Clarendon Press, 1983), and others about the basis of membership in the moral community or of a right to life might lead one to deny this. I do not mean to dismiss this position or these authors' arguments for it. For ease of exposition, I ignore the complications raised by this viewpoint.

30. For all we have said, the time at which the developing human is "covered by" the RDLP need not coincide with the time at which the killing of the fetus becomes seriously morally wrong. For simplicity, though, we shall assume here that they coincide.

31. It is interesting to speculate on how social relations and moral views of intelligent beings, otherwise like us, would be altered if these natural facts were different. This is largely the province of science fiction writers and some bold evolutionary biologists. For example, Ursula Le Guin explores the social implications of hermaphroditic reproduction in *The Left Hand of Darkness* (New York: ACE Books, 1976) and E. O. Wilson illustrates in a fanciful way some of the biological foundations of our moral views and our emotional reactions in *Consilience: The Unity of Knowledge* (New York: Vintage, 1998), 148.

32. In 1981, the US Supreme Court upheld a California statutory rape law that was not neutral with respect to the sex of the victim partly on the grounds that "young men and young women are not similarly situated with respect to the problems and the risks of sexual intercourse. Only women may become pregnant, and they suffer disproportionately the profound physical, emotional, and psychological consequences of sexual activity" (*Michael M. v. Superior Court of Sonoma County*, 450 U.S. (1981), 464).

33. Constructing the case in a way that reverses the roles of the two parties in the development of the fetus provides an additional dimension to the "distance" we achieve by employment of our thought experiment. The moral analysis is, presumably, neutral with respect to the sex of the participants.

34. Judith Thomson, "A Defense of Abortion," *op. cit.*, p. 58.

35. Courts have used a variety of mechanisms to deny relief to those involved in sexual relations with each other for breach of promise, fraud, and intentional infliction of emotional distress connected with the sexual activity. The right to privacy and the unseemliness of litigation of private matters, among other things, have been cited as grounds holding participants in sexual actions responsible for the consequences of those actions despite factors that typically diminish or exclude legal responsibility. Jill Evans explores the problems with many of these arguments in "In Search of Paternal Equity: A Father's Right to Pursue a Claim of Misrepresentation of Fertility," *Loyola University Chicago Law Journal* 36 (2005): 1045–1109. The assignment of legal responsibility where there is no moral responsibility is always morally problematic but sometimes justified nonetheless. Our concern here, though, is with the *moral* evaluation of the responsibility of the parties.

36. Tom Dougherty ("Sex, Lies, and Consent" *Ethics* 123, no. 4 (2013): 717–744) argues that consent to sexual relations requires knowledge of any facts that would be "deal breakers"— facts which, if known, would lead the person not to have sex. All sex with a person who is ignorant of any "deal breaker" is nonconsensual sex. As a result, deception about deal-breaking fact counts as deceiving someone into having sex. On Dougherty's view, lying or intentionally misleading a sexual partner about your fertility, for example, or even withholding information about it, if that information would affect his or her decision to have sex, would count as "deceiving someone into sex" and be a serious moral wrong.

37. For example, the Michigan Criminal Code (MCLS § 333.5210) states that: "[a] person who knows that he or she has or has been diagnosed as having acquired immunodeficiency syndrome or acquired immunodeficiency syndrome related complex, or who knows that

he or she is HIV infected, and who engages in sexual penetration with another person without having first informed the other person that he or she has acquired immunodeficiency syndrome or acquired immunodeficiency syndrome related complex or is HIV infected, is guilty of a felony." In December, 1998, the Canadian Supreme Court ruled that Henry Courrier was guilty of criminal assault for engaging in unprotected sexual penetration without first informing his partners that he was HIV-positive (R. v. Courrier. 1998. S.C.J. No. 64. SCC). The Court held that Courrier's partners' "consent" was obtained through fraud as a result of his failure to disclose his HIV status.

38. To say that the caveat copulator approach *encourages* irresponsible and immoral behavior might appear to be an exaggeration; at most, one might allege, it *fails* to discourage such behavior. However, taken in the context of other obligations and expectations, the failure to discourage behavior may result in actual encouragement of the behavior. If rewards, or what some individuals may see as rewards, are conferred on some basis other than the irresponsible behavior but *despite* its presence and the basis for the reward would not exist but for the irresponsible behavior, the overall effect of ignoring the irresponsible behavior in determining an agent's responsibilities is positive encouragement of the bad behavior.

39. This was the situation alleged in the case of *Wallis v. Smith*, 22 P. 3d 682, 683 (NM: Ct. App. 2001). Peter Wallis maintained that he and Kellie Smith had a serious discussion of possible reproductive consequences of engaging in sexual intercourse, during which he declared his desire not to become a father at that time. He alleges that he agreed to have sex with Smith only on the condition that she was using birth control pills; that Smith represented that she was, indeed, using birth control pills; and that, after their sexual relationship began, Smith stopped using birth control without telling Wallis. Smith subsequently became pregnant.

40. Courts sometimes say, when dismissing "wrongful birth" cases, that children are never a wrong or a harm. But this is false. Though children, when desired, are a source of great joy, even if it is invariably conjoined with frustration and aggravation, this does not show that unchosen parenthood is not at least sometimes a harm. Both Andrew Kopelman ("Forced Labor: A Thirteenth Amendment Defense of Abortion," *Northwestern University Law Review* 84 (1990): 480–535) and Margaret Little ("Abortion, Intimacy, and the Duty to Gestate," *Ethical Theory and Moral Practice* 2 (1999): 295–312) make this point very convincingly about pregnancy itself.

41. Similar issues are raised by the *Phillips v. Irons*, 354 Ill. App. 3d 1164 (Ill. App. Ct. 1st Dist., 2005), discussed in my paper, "Human Reproductive Interests: Puzzles at the Periphery of the Property Paradigm," *Social Philosophy & Policy* 29 (2012): 117–119.

42. Ludicrous, but not inconsistent with legal practice in the United States. Based on DNA testing, the court determined that Frisard was the father and ordered him to pay child support retroactively, resulting in an immediate arrearage of almost $18,000. This decision was upheld on appeal, though the trial court's specific determination of the amount of child support was remanded for further consideration on grounds unrelated to the unusual genesis of the pregnancy.

43. It is clear how this difference can affect the moral evaluation of the deceiving party. In cases of purloined sperm used for the purposes of impregnation, the creation of the dependent being is the intended outcome of the course of conduct. In cases of deception about birth control, this is not always the case. Though the deceiver is behaving irresponsibly, the mens rea of the potentially harmful conduct could be negligence or recklessness, not intentional wrongdoing.

44. I set aside here the question of whether Ala has responsibility to support the dependent life in the case where Jok is incapable of doing so.

45. See Ezio Di Nucci ("Fathers and Abortion," *Journal of Medicine and Philosophy* 39 (2014): 444–458) for an argument that a woman's failure to abort a pregnancy can wrong a man apart from the pecuniary responsibilities of child support.

46. For defenses of this position, see Steven Hales, "Abortion and Fathers' Rights," in *Reproduction, Technology, and Rights: Biomedical Ethics Reviews*, edited by James M. Humber (Clifton, NJ: Humana Press, 1996): 5–26; Steven Hales, "More on Fathers' Rights," in *Reproduction, Technology, and Rights: Biomedical Ethics Reviews*, edited by James M. Humber (Clifton, NJ: Humana Press, 1996): 43–49; and Elizabeth Brake, "Fatherhood and Child Support: Do Men Have a Right to Choose?" *Journal of Applied Philosophy* 22 (2005): 55–73.

BIBLIOGRAPHY

Boonin-Vail, David. "A Defense of 'A Defense of Abortion': On the Responsibility Objection." *Ethics* 107, no. 2 (1977): 286–313.

Brake, Elizabeth. "Fatherhood and Child Support: Do Men Have a Right to Choose?" *Journal of Applied Philosophy* 22 (2005): 55–73.

Brake, Elizabeth. "Willing Parents: A Voluntarist Account of Parental Role Obligation." In *Procreation and Parenthood: The Ethics of Bearing and Rearing Children*, edited by David Archard and David Benatar, 151–177. Oxford: Oxford University Press, 2011.

Di Nucci, Ezio, "Fathers and Abortion," *Journal of Medicine and Philosophy* 39 (2014): 444–458.

Hales, Steven D. "Abortion and Fathers' Rights." In *Reproduction, Technology, and Rights: Biomedical Ethics Reviews*, edited by James M. Humber, 5–26. Clifton, NJ: Humana Press, 1996.

Hales, Steven D. "More on Fathers' Rights." In *Reproduction, Technology, and Rights: Biomedical Ethics Reviews*, edited by James M. Humber, 43–49. Clifton, NJ: Humana Press, 1996.

Hubin, Donald. "Fatherhood." In *International Encyclopedia of Ethics*, edited by Hugh LaFollette. Hoboken, NJ: Wiley-Blackwell, 2013.

Hubin, Donald. "Reproductive Interests: Puzzles at the Periphery of the Property Paradigm." *Social Philosophy and Policy* 29 (2012): 106–125.

Hubin, Donald. "Daddy Dilemmas: Untangling the Puzzles of Paternity." *The Cornell Journal of Law and Public Policy* 13 (2003): 29–80.

Humber, James M 1996. "Maternity, Paternity, and Equality." In *Reproduction, Technology, and Rights: Biomedical Ethics Reviews*, edited by James M. Humber, 27–41. Clifton, NJ: Humana Press, 1996.

Kopelman, Andrew. "Forced Labor: A Thirteenth Amendment Defense of Abortion." *Northwestern University Law Review* 84 (1990): 480–535.

Lang, Gerald. "Nudging the Responsibility Objection." *Journal of Applied Philosophy* 25, no. 1 (2008): 56–71.

Little, Margaret. "Abortion, Intimacy, and the Duty to Gestate." *Ethical Theory and Moral Practice* 2 (1999): 295–312.

Porter, Lindsey. "Why and How to Prefer a Causal Account of Parenthood." *Journal of Social Philosophy* 45 (2014): 182–202.

Puskar, Bernard. "Breaking the Bond: Abortion and the Grounds of Parental Obligation." *Social Theory and Practice* 37, no. 2 (2011): 311–332.

Puskar, Bernard. "The Costs of Procreation." *Journal of Social Philosophy* 42, no. 1 (2011): 61–75.

Reisner, Andrew. "Prima Facie and Pro Tanto Oughts." *International Encyclopedia of Ethics*, edited by Hugh LaFollette. Hoboken, NJ: Wiley-Blackwell, 2013.

Schrage, Laurie. "Is Forced Fatherhood Fair?" *New York Times*, accessed September 5, 2014. http://opinionator.blogs.nytimes.com/2013/06/12/is-forced-fatherhood-fair/.

Silverstein, Harry S. "On a Woman's 'Responsibility' for the Fetus." *Social Theory and Practice* 13, no. 1 (1987): 103–119.

Smith, M.B.E. "Is There a Prima Facie Obligation to Obey the Law?" *The Yale Law Journal* 82, no. 5 (1973): 950–976.

Thomson, Judith. "A Defense of Abortion." *Philosophy and Public Affairs* 1 (1971): 47–66.

Thomson, Judith. *The Realm of Rights*. Cambridge, MA: Harvard University Press, 1992.

Tooley, Michael. *Abortion and Infanticide*. Oxford: Clarendon Press, 1983.

Warren, Mary Ann. "On the Moral and Legal Status of Abortion." *The Monist* 57 (1973): 43–61.

....

CHAPTER 15

REPRODUCTIVE CONTROL FOR MEN

For *Men?*

....

MARGARET P. BATTIN

LET us suppose that modern male contraception becomes available sometime in the near future and is as good as the best of the modern female contraceptives already available now. What difference would it make? What issues of rights, obligations, gender roles and equity, and much more would arise?

MODERN CONTRACEPTION, FEMALE AND MALE

....

If we take a look at the current array of contraceptive methods available in the contemporary world, we see dramatic female–male inequality. Females can choose from a vast array of different methods: pills, patches, rings, gels, foams, diaphragms, cervical caps, female condoms, injectables, subdermal implants, intrauterine devices (IUDs), and various forms of sterilization, including tubal ligation, tubal blockage, and, if all else fails, after-the-fact methods like the morning-after pill. Sexually active males with a female partner, in contrast, have just three methods of fertility control: the condom; withdrawal or other forms of interrupted contact or noncontact, including scheduled abstinence; and sterilization, usually by means of vasectomy.

That's it, guys.

Furthermore, females have a vast range of effectiveness in the modalities from which they can choose. Of these various modalities, the gels, foams, sponges, female condoms, the diaphragm, the cap, and similar modalities that need to be applied at or near the time of intercourse—what we can call "time-of-need" methods—all have fairly high failure rates in ordinary usage. In contrast, the "hybrid" methods—the pill, the patch, the 3-month injectable, modern modalities that have sustained biochemical activity but require repeated dosing—have moderate failure rates but require attention and scheduled redosing. And in even greater contrast, the "automatics," called LARC, for long-acting reversible contraception—the subdermal implant and the IUD—require no attention once in place and are effective for 3 to 12 years, depending on the specific type, yet are immediately reversible. The LARC contraceptives, unlike the time-of-need ones, have very low failure rates. These LARC contraceptives are, as David Grimes says, "forgettable."[1]

To be sure, some religious groups, notably the Catholic Church, prohibit all "artificial" contraception for both males and females, including barrier methods, modern contraception, and sterilization, but they do permit natural family planning. The various forms of natural family planning, as modern forms of "rhythm method" or scheduled abstinence are called, rely on slightly different methods of calculating the window in a woman's menstrual cycle when conception can occur. Natural family planning can work well for mutually committed couples, but it is unreliable in other situations.

Permanent sterilization is available to both men and women, but it is not a method of choice for anyone young or middle-aged who may want to begin or continue childbearing. Reversal of vasectomy is sometimes possible but is never guaranteed, and in any case it requires complex, expensive microsurgery. Freezing of sperm before vasectomy or using in vitro fertilization after female tubal ligation is sometimes also advanced as a form of contraception—sterilize now, but use fertility technologies later to decide in favor of procreation—but of course itself introduces risks of expense and failure. It is the reversible contraceptives that are of particular interest here, those that prevent pregnancy now but still keep open the possibility of future reproduction.

There is research in the pipeline on long-acting, highly effective reversible male contraception, much like what women already have—but it is not here yet. In other words, men who may wish to have children at a later date have virtually nothing they can rely on for secure, "forgettable," failure-proof fertility control.

Reproductive Inequality

Let's get more serious: There is a real problem with reproductive control here.

Perhaps the most striking feature of this contraceptive picture, both in the United States and around the world, is the pronounced inequality between women and men in protecting themselves against a pregnancy they do not want to occur. Of course, both women and men can maintain (near) perfect contraceptive security by abstaining from sexual intercourse in the first place or by having themselves permanently sterilized. Both women and men can be made to risk contributing to conception by being forced, manipulated, or seduced into intercourse when that is not their choice. Once sex is actually taking place, it is women who in general retain by far the greater control over the reproductive outcome of the act of sex, at least where contraceptive use is a possibility at all. At the root of this male–female inequality, I believe, is the assumption that contraception is primarily a "women's issue," and that it is sufficient if women take care of this matter. Particularly in the developed world, the notion that birth control is the responsibility primarily of women has gathered increasing strength from the mid-1960s on, with the development of effective methods of female contraception like the Pill.[2] Of course, withdrawal, a method quintessentially under male control, has still remained a primary method of fertility regulation in much of the world, especially eastern Europe during the Soviet period, and the condom is also a widely used male contraceptive method, though, like withdrawal and sterilization, its acceptability varies widely among different cultures. Men may perceive themselves to have substantial, even equal say with women in matters of sexual and contraceptive decision making.[3] Yet, especially in the developed world, as far more effective female contraceptive methods have become available and the social roles of women have begun to change from childbearing alone to work-oriented roles, cultural conceptions have evolved away from those considering pregnancy initiation or avoidance a matter of male privilege, a male or joint matter rather than primarily a female one. This view is reinforced by the claim, argued by many and especially by feminists, that reproductive control appropriately goes to women, since it is within the bodies of women that reproduction takes place. After all, this view holds, the consequences of pregnancy are far greater for women than for men. Feminists and others have celebrated women's new capacity for reproductive control, even if it is not always reliably exercised; it is regarded as one of the technological triumphs of the twentieth century.

SEX AND RESPONSIBILITY—
OR WHO IS TO BLAME?

In popular opinion and political disputes over social issues, considerable emphasis is often placed on "responsibility" in sex—or, more precisely, on responsibility for sex's reproductive outcomes. People who engage in sex are expected to be "responsible" for contributing to pregnancy and to assume responsibility for any children their activities may bring into the world. Along with these expectations also comes a good deal of blame for outcomes perceived as the product of irresponsible behavior.

This popular talk of responsibility and its failures can be divided into two loose camps—what might be called "male-blaming" and "female-blaming" accounts. In male-blaming accounts, attention is typically directed at the sexual behavior of the male, who is seen as seeking copulation opportunities whenever possible. The assumption behind such views is that males are biologically driven to impregnate females wherever possible; they are ready to procreate without regard for the interests or concerns of either the woman or any future children. Because, on the male-blaming view, males do not succeed in overcoming these precivilized biological strategies, they are to be blamed for their lack of reproductive responsibility. On this view, it is only within marriage, an institutional structure of civilization, where the male acquires a long-term interest in the welfare of his wife and is in a position to provide a home for any future children, that this natural irresponsibility can be suitably contained, or so it is said. As the psychologist and feminist Martha Burk writes, "The problem of unwanted pregnancy is largely one of uncontrolled sperm."[4] Yet what is now called "irresponsible" male behavior has often been excused in the past: the old-fashioned, amiably tolerant view was that young, bachelor men were understandably likely to "sow wild oats."

But there is popular female-blaming responsibility talk, too. Here the charge is that males are victimized by females' reproductive irresponsibility, some of which is inadvertent but much of which is deliberate. Males are vulnerable to seduction by predatory females, on this view; they are victimized by women who lie about their intentions or ambitions in a relationship.[5] Males are particularly subject to reproductive trickery by women who claim to be using contraceptives but in fact are not. This trickery, so the female-blaming charge goes, takes several forms: the female on the prowl who views a particular man as a "good catch," and, taking advantage of his biological readiness to engage in sexual intercourse when a willing female presents herself, entraps him into marriage by letting herself become pregnant. She may not even want the relationship, just the child, or just the child and the child support. A variant of the entrapment strategy is the maneuver, said to be especially common among teenagers, of the girl who lets herself get pregnant in order to keep a threatened relationship from breaking apart; or of the married woman who tries to obligate the husband to remain at home, if he shows signs of restlessness, by having another child. These stereotyped, conflicting views are at the heart of contemporary social debate over reproductive responsibility in all its many forms, including responsibility for avoiding a pregnancy, for decisions about whether to continue a pregnancy, and for the child's welfare after birth. They are at the heart of the popular rhetoric of blame. But their significance can be seen more clearly if we look at the actual circumstances of male and female reproductive control: here, as we will see, because women have vastly greater opportunities for contraceptive control than do men (even if not all women take advantage of these opportunities), views about responsibility take on new weight, though in different ways, in both the male-blaming and female-blaming views.[6] She can avoid pregnancy if she wants; she can let a pregnancy happen if she wants, and in either case can do so without the consent of the male. This disparity may be reduced, or on the other hand may paradoxically be exacerbated, as new forms of male contraception appear on the market and he gains greater reproductive control himself. Of course, to say that women currently have greater opportunities than men for reproductive control is not to say that they have greater interpersonal control or greater power within a relationship, nor that they have greater control within a larger social structure. Nevertheless, *reproductive* control—our focus here—is crucial in determining the consequences of sex.

REPRODUCTIVE CONTROL,
MALE AND FEMALE

Male reproductive control? Are you kidding? How?

Reproductive control can be achieved by either the male or the female in one of several ways: by abstinence from sexual intercourse altogether, by permanent sterilization, by cooperation in scheduled abstinence and timing strategies such as *coitus interruptus* and the various forms of rhythm method, or by use of what are referred to as "modern" or sometimes "artificial" contraceptives. But these different modalities distribute reproductive control quite unequally.

Male Control: Abstinence

Abstinence is effective in reproductive control for either male or female if neither party is forced, manipulated, or seduced into sexual activity by the other, and if both parties adhere to their commitments toward abstinence. These circumstances, of course, cannot be entirely guaranteed. The *intention* to remain abstinent, no matter how firm, cannot guarantee absolute reproductive control, whether in the face of rape or unwilling seduction, or just because one changes one's mind.[7] Reliance on abstinence as a method of reproductive control is usually held to give greater power to men since, it is assumed, men rape women more frequently than women rape or forcibly seduce men, and men are therefore more frequently able to assert their will over the female's resistance. Rape is, of course, not the only kind of force men can exert over women, though it is the most conspicuous; what is true here of rape—that an armed or physically stronger male can, in general, exert his will over an unarmed or physically weaker female—may be reversed in some cases, but whether for men or for women is in an enormous variety of ways also true of psychological and physical power struggles within a relationship. Abstinence may be sincerely intended, but it doesn't always work.

Male Control: Partial Abstinence

When we notice, however, that certain other contraceptive strategies also depend on partial abstinence, it becomes evident that there may be more at issue here. Both *coitus interruptus* and rhythm or natural family planning methods rely on scheduled abstinence: They permit intercourse but depend on abstinence from that component of it which can lead to conception, whether ejaculation only or any intercourse during the female's fertile period. Other forms of sexual contact are sometimes used as alternative means of sexual gratification: oral sex, anal sex, and mutual masturbation; whether these make restraint from full intercourse more or less difficult is open to question. In any case, partial abstinence methods have poor efficacy rates: The US failure rate for withdrawal is 22% in ordinary practice.[8] (In some countries where withdrawal is widely used as the primary means of fertility control, as in many of the post-Soviet countries, abortion has been routinely used as a backup.) The overall failure rate for periodic abstinence involving fertility-awareness based methods, including the standard days method, the 2-day method, the cervical mucus method, body-temperature method, symptothermal method, and lactational method, is about 24% in the first year of use.[9] It is not entirely clear what accounts for couples' contraceptive failures with these partial-abstinence methods.[10] In any case, whether men or women do or do not retain equal degrees of control in attempting to remain abstinent or use timing methods involving periodic abstinence is a highly politicized issue, tied to the issue of whether male- or female-blaming explanations of reproductive irresponsibility are invoked.

Male Control: The Condom

The condom is the male's only currently available form of nonpermanent contraception—his closest approach to a "modern contraceptive technology." The modern condom is certainly an improvement over the linen sheaths associated with the eighteenth-century adventurer and womanizer Casanova, and over many sorts of historically earlier versions; it has been continuously improved in modern times. The modern condom has unparalleled importance in preventing sexually transmitted disease; while vaccines are available for some sexually transmitted diseases (STDs), such as human papillomavirus (HPV), the condom remains the most effective method of preventing the transmission of chlamydia, syphilis, gonorrhea, HIV, and other diseases. It has no adverse physical effects. However, as a method of contraception, the condom, with its much higher failure rates—18% in the first year of typical use (as distinct from 2% in the lab) and vastly less convenience (application required with each act of intercourse)—remains a distant second to the much more effective hybrid and LARC technologies. Yet the condom still remains the male's only choice of a reversible contraceptive technology.

Male Control: Vasectomy

To be sure, permanent sterilization is an option; some 13% of married men in the United States have had vasectomies.[11] However, it is not a reliably reversible option for men who might want children in the future. Yet it is the only (nearly) foolproof method of fertility control for males—there are very infrequent failures, less than 1%, usually in the period right after surgery—but it comes at a cost that is unacceptable to many men, the cost of being unable to change one's mind about reproduction at a later date.

There's not much out there for you, guys. Is that fair? Just think about all the good stuff women have got.

MALE AND FEMALE METHOD DIFFERENCES

There are four particularly substantial differences between the contraceptive methods open to a woman and those open to her male partner. The female, as we have seen, has at her disposal a very wide array of contraceptive choices: in addition to acquiescence in *coitus interruptus* and cooperation in the management of rhythm schedules or natural family planning, as well as permanent sterilization, she also has the entire array of contraceptives catalogued earlier: foams, gels, films, the diaphragm, the female condom, the sponge, the ring, the cap, the patch, the shot, the pill, the implant, and the IUD—a whole smorgasbord of "time-of-need," "hybrid," and "automatic" types. They involve different rates of efficacy, different costs, different side effects and risks, different challenges in access, and are variously appropriate or contraindicated in some situations. But almost all of the female methods provide advantages in ordinary conditions of use that make them better than any method of nonpermanent contraception available to men. In virtually every case, the advantage goes to the woman.

Indetectability

Although the application of some forms of female contraception can be fairly readily observed or detected, such as the diaphragm and various spermicides, these procedures can be more or less discreetly performed. Some forms of female contraception are invisible and impalpable; for example, oral contraceptives cannot be detected except by watching a user swallow them or finding them hidden in a drawer somewhere. The IUD can only be inadvertently detected during intercourse by penile contact with or digital inspection of its tail or string. The subdermal implant, the smaller-than-a-matchstick single-rod Nexplanon, is inconspicuous to the touch. And injectables like Depo-Provera cannot be detected at all. They are private. In contrast, except for surgical sterilization, there is little possibility of privacy in current methods of nonpermanent contraception for men. The only reliably nonpermanent male methods of reproductive control—withdrawal, periodic abstinence, and the condom—are entirely evident at the time of sexual intercourse, far more so than *any* female method except rhythm-dictated abstinence and the female condom. Women have privacy that men do not, though in this respect, it is easier for women to cheat.

Unobtrusiveness in Sex

Closely related to indetectability, female forms of contraception all interfere with the sexual act less than the male's only available reversible technology, the condom, except, of course, for the female condom. Although some female contraceptives interfere with the spontaneity of the sexual act, as spermicides and the diaphragm may do, many hybrids and all long-acting female contraceptives—the Pill, the depot injection, the IUD (except perhaps for the string), and the subdermal implant—are not obtrusive at all in the sexual act. Although the presence or absence of contraceptive protection may have psychological consequences for the sexual act, these technologies have no physical effect on the sexual act and for that reason may be more likely to be used.[12] The obtrusiveness of the male condom, in contrast, is one reason it is not always reliably used: It can interfere with spontaneity and pleasure, and many men say they do not like it.

Effectiveness

Hybrid and LARC female contraceptive methods are far more effective than the nonpermanent male methods.[13] As we have seen, withdrawal and traditional rhythm-method forms of periodic abstinence have failure rates as high as 22% and 24%, respectively; the male condom has a failure rate in typical first-year usage of 18%, much of which is due to inconsistent and or incorrect usage.[14] Some female methods also have high failure rates: The diaphragm has a failure rate in first-year use of 12%,[15] and the original Reality female condom, a whopping 21%. But the female's most effective reversible methods—the IUD and the subdermal implant—have failure rates that are very much lower, between 0.8% and .05%.[16] A couple relying on the male condom alone, without spermicides and with typical (rather than laboratory-perfect) use, with its failure rate of 18% during the first year, is about 360 times as likely to sustain a pregnancy as the same couple using the subdermal implant, with its failure rate of between 0.8% and .05%.

Furthermore, these rates are failure rates *per year*. The condom's 18% failure rate per year taken over 60 or 70 years of a man's sexual life would mean many failures during the course of that lifetime, though the declining fecundity and occurrence of menopause in an older man's partner and his own decreasing frequency of sexual activity may make the likelihood of conception smaller in later years.

After-the-Fact Control

Further reinforcing this inequality in reproductive control, males have no analog of emergency contraception, "morning-after" pills, ullipristal, or mifepristone, or other drugs or procedures that prevent fertilization, prevent implantation, or interrupt the continuance of pregnancy—beyond the crude and violent attempt some men occasionally make to destroy a fetus by beating a pregnant woman in the abdomen. With emergency contraception or abortifacient drugs, the woman can change her mind after intercourse, or after conception, or after implantation and pregnancy is underway; but this last-ditch option in reproductive control is not available to the male. Thus, men have not only less current control, but no acceptable retroactive control as well. Of course, he can respond: He can support her in getting an abortion, pay for the abortion, protest it, implore her or try to force her to have an abortion, but he does not really have control. He can always leave the scene, or beat her up, or even kill her, but with more aggressive paternity laws at least in some countries[17] and the new possibility of genetic identification, he cannot really escape.

Aren't hers better than yours? She has control before and after, but you don't have either one. Tough luck, guys

Little wonder if some males resent the position this imbalance places them in. Males, at least in the popular "male-blaming" view, are perceived as "irresponsible," especially if unmarried and, furthermore, of minority status; but the technology available to them unavoidably places them in a position quite disadvantageous vis-à-vis that of women. Even the man who tries to be responsible in using the condom may still end up being resented if a failure occurs. The female-blaming view coincides with explanations of how women can be capable of maneuvering men into reproductive situations they do not want: Because many female methods of contraception can be undetectable and the male is forced to take claims about them on faith, women are thus capable of deceit in a way that the male is not—not because he is more virtuous, but because his contraceptive behavior is more obvious. Except for the male who might falsely claim to have had a vasectomy, or promises to withdraw, or in some anecdotal reports, takes off the condom during sex, males cannot dissemble about whether they are or are not practicing reversible birth control. Of course, males can lie about other things in a sexual encounter— "it'll be alright," "I love you," and "I'll take care of you" are classic examples. Indeed, in one study of college students in Southern California, as many as 47% of males (and 42% of females) said they would lie in order to have sex.[18] But this is not possible for the male concerning contraception: Once intercourse is underway, he usually cannot hide his use or nonuse of reversible contraception from his sexual partner.

MALE LEGAL AND POLICY INEQUALITY

The resentment this inequality can generate among males may be especially strong, and indeed well justified, in the context of political calls for greater "responsibility" on their part and legal enforcement of such views. The demand seems to be that unmarried males ought to refrain from sexual activity altogether or at least be prepared to assume financial liability for any children they produce if they engage in sex; but there seems to be no accompanying demand for equalizing males' and females' reproductive control. Indeed, except for the couple that uses no contraception at all, there is no way, given currently available contraceptive technologies, that the male and the female can secure equal control, yet they are assigned equal responsibility for supporting the child. Indeed, although couples' access to contraception has been incrementally protected since the 1965 privacy case *Griswold v. Connecticut*,[19] it was not until 1997 that Title X began to fund male family planning services and research.[20] Family planning clinics now typically provide male contraceptive information, both about their partner's methods and about options open to them,[21] yet while this information may provide men with knowledge about how to make more effective use of the modalities they have available—the condom, vasectomy, natural family planning, or withdrawal—it does not provide them with better methods. Women now have the lion's share of contraceptive control, at least if they have access to reliable, long-acting methods; but men as well as women get the blame. Of course, that the modalities available to the female are both more effective and more private than those available to the male does not excuse him from using what modalities are available to him, but it is clear that blame is not always fully appropriate.

After all, US law has insisted that the male is financially responsible for the reproductive outcomes of his sexual activity even if he attempts to practice birth control or believes he cannot be contributing to conception. Although the father's child support obligations have often been only erratically enforced (and often could not be, prior to the possibility of establishing paternity by means of genetic identification), nevertheless in a number of cases men have been held liable for child support and other costs even though, at the time of sexual intercourse, they used contraception that proved ineffective or were lied to by their partners about their contraceptive use.[22] In the 1981 New York case *Pamela P. v. Frank S.*,[23] the lower court found in the father's favor and excused him from child support payments, but the Court of Appeals reversed this decision 2 years later: yes, he would have to pay. In the 1984 Michigan case *Faske v. Bonanno*, the court ruled that fraud and misrepresentation were not defenses that the father could use.[24] In another Michigan case in 1990, *Beard v. Skipper*, misrepresentation about contraception was held not to be a mitigating factor in determining the father's child support payments.[25] In Arkansas, the 1993 case *Erwin L.D. v. Myla Jean L.* held that the mother's agreement to not pursue paternity charges to get financial support was not a defense for the father, and that "birth control fraud" is also not a defense; the father was required to pay child support.[26]

To be sure, many of these cases happened 20 or more years ago; it is not clear why there are apparently no more recent reported decisions. Problematic cases do still occur: Recently a 24-year-old man was informed by the state of Arizona that he was being held responsible for support for his daughter, now aged 6 years, from the time of her birth to adulthood. He was 14 years old at the time he had a brief affair with a woman then 20 years old; they had broken up not long afterward, and he knew nothing of the pregnancy or existence of the child. Nor, in the view of the state, did it make any difference that this could have been prosecuted as a case of statutory rape, because he was under the age of 15 years at the time of conception; as the biological father, he was still responsible for support of the child unless the woman seeking child support had been convicted of sexual assault.[27] Some legal scholars, for example Myrisha Lewis,[28] object to the position men are placed in, but in the United States at present it remains the law. Men are also held responsible for child support in cases where the woman decides to have the child despite the man not wanting to, and there is no contraceptive fraud involved. The overall message of these decisions is clear: Once conception through sexual intercourse has occurred, the father has no further reproductive control.

Bad news indeed. If you get someone pregnant, guys, you may always have to pay, no matter what you actually intended.

CONTRACEPTIVE TECHNOLOGIES UNDER DEVELOPMENT FOR MEN

But wait a minute, guys. Maybe there's something good on the way. Imagine: real male fertility control, maybe even as good as yours, ladies.

Modern contraceptives are not yet available for men. But some fairly promising male technologies are under development, both in the United States and especially India and China, and some are already in premarket testing phases. Some of these involve male time-of-need and hybrid contraceptives, but, if the research goes well, several may be true LARC "automatics": They will be long-acting, user-independent, coitus-independent, noninterfering with sexual activity, and immediately reversible; that is, they will have the same essential characteristics that the true "automatic" technologies for women already have.

Current technologies under development for males[29] fall into approximately five major groups: those that involve blockage or occlusion of the vas deferens, the tubule through which sperm move from the testes to ejaculation; hormonal methods, including those that interrupt signaling that controls spermatogenesis; nonhormonal "male pills," of which there are a number of possibilities; those that involve testicular toxicants, including heat, killing or damaging sperm as they are produced; and those that employ vaccine strategies. With new research, there may well be others. None is fully successful yet, and none is on the market yet; but research in male contraception is now beginning to attract real interest.

One ubiquitous explanation of why research in male contraception has not been pursued as vigorously as research in female contraception holds that it is far harder to stop male sperm production, which may reach as high as 100–150 million or more a day, than to stop the production or implantation of a single egg per month, occasionally two. Yet spermatogenesis is an extremely complex physiological process, involving a 74-day period for the development of fully mature sperm. This provides numerous opportunities for interference in male reproductive capacity: intervention in the formation, maturation, storage, transport, motility, and other functioning of sperm. However, none of these are easy to achieve without disrupting other characteristics of male sexual identity.

The list that follows includes a selection of some of the male contraceptive technologies that are currently in development or are anticipated for development in the near future. Not all of them will prove safe or efficacious; not all of them will make it to market; and not all of them will win users' favor once they are openly available. Dozens of others have been pursued through various stages of research but failed or were abandoned. Yet this partial list of male methods under development[30] does serve to show something of the active research now going on, methods some of which can reasonably aim for the same characteristics already available in some LARC female contraceptives: contraceptives that are highly effective, long-acting, user-independent, noninterfering in the sexual act, and immediately reversible. These represent, one might say, our initial attempts to achieve for men what is already possible for women, to "reverse the default" so that siring a pregnancy is not the possible outcome of sexual intercourse unless something is done to prevent it, either by oneself or one's female partner.

Vas-Occlusive Methods

RISUG (reversible inhibition of sperm under guidance), formerly called SMA and, in a related version, known as Vasalgel, is a polymer, powdered stryrene maleic anhydride, combined with dimethyl sulfoxide (DMSO). The resulting gel is injected percutaneously or by the no-scalpel method into the vas deferens, where it forms a coating around the inside of this tubule. RISUG partially blocks the vas and lowers the pH of the environment just enough to kill sperm that do pass through; it is effective almost immediately. To reverse the contraceptive effect, it can be flushed out by an injection of a solution of sodium bicarbonate or by using noninvasive methods involving massage, vibration, and low electrical current. RISUG has been tested for over 25 years in rats and monkeys and has been in advanced human trials in India; it was said to show excellent effectiveness, with no evidence of toxicity or teratogenicity. Some human volunteers received injections 10 or 15 years ago, though research standards have been challenged. Vasalgel, the variant being developed by the Parsemus Foundation, has now been approved for human trials in the United States, to begin late in 2016. However, reversibility had not been successfully shown in animal trials in the United States and a recent study with a single baboon failed, but initial studies with rabbits have been promising. The Male Contraception Initiative predicts that if all goes well, Vasalgel could be available as early as 2018.[31]

Hormonal Methods

1. Testosterone injections. Male hormonal contraceptives involve the administration of some form of testosterone. Because this alone will not completely suppress sperm production in a minority of men, testosterone is therefore combined with progestins for greater efficacy.[32] Under development since the 1980s, testosterone enanthate injections have undergone trials in nine countries. High contraceptive efficacy is achieved even without complete azoospermia. The weekly testosterone enanthate injections were considered a proof of concept, and more recent research has focused on longer lasting injections given monthly or every 6 weeks. China completed a Phase III clinical trial[33] of testosterone undecanoate injections, which were effective and well tolerated. There appear, however, to be differences in

efficacy in different populations: East Asian men respond better than Caucasian men, for reasons not yet well understood.[34] Multiple other formulations[35] of injections have been tested in more than a dozen countries; so far none of these formulations has gone beyond Phase II clinical trials. However, although the progestins can be taken orally, testosterone cannot because it clears the body too quickly to be administered as a once-a-day pill.

2. Implant system. The male implant system is possible with either crystalline testosterone pellets (tested in Australia) or a synthetic androgen known as MENT. One type of implant being tested has two components: one implant, containing an analog of gonadotropin hormone–releasing hormone (GnRH), suppresses spermatogenesis; the other supplies a synthetic androgen, MENT, as a replacement for testosterone to ensure normal libido and sexual behavior.[36]

3. Other hormonal modalities. Researchers are also investigating other ways of delivering a male hormonal contraceptive, including a two-gel once-daily regimen applied to the skin, patches, and pills. At the moment, there is no orally available form of testosterone that would make a hormonal "male pill" product commercially feasible.[37]

Nonhormonal "Male Pills"

1. Drugs that interfere with sperm maturation. A number of drugs in early clinical trials or in proof-of-concept stages offer male contraception by changing the way sperm mature in the testes. These drugs interfere with the creation of fully functional sperm, resulting in sperm that cannot swim or fuse with an egg.

   In 2016, a research team at the University of Minnesota announced that progress in developing a basic compound for a male Pill, a molecule that is more selective and potent, involving a different scaffold, than previous attempts. It works by undermining sperm development through the target of a receptor called retinoic acid receptor alpha, one of three receptors that affect sperm development. However, contraceptive strategies that work by affecting sperm development involve a substantial delay before they are effective—that's because normal sperm development takes 90 days—and also substantial delay in return to fertility. The aim was also to develop a water-soluble form that could be taken orally rather than requiring injection. This new compound is, however, not yet ready for testing in animals.[38] In a related approach, the research team was able to get fertility to return after a month, and the rodent offspring that resulted were healthy.

2. Drugs that interfere with ejaculation. These would take effect within several hours of ingestion and wear off within 24 hours. Dubbed the "clean sheets pill," it blocks the longitudinal muscles of the vas deferens from contracting so that sperm are not pushed forward, resulting in no ejaculate, although the circular muscles remain active and the male experience is identical to orgasm. As one volunteer put it, "all of the twitch but none of the spurt."[39]

Testicular Toxicant Methods, Including Heat

Drawing on the long-known fact that sperm production declines if the testes are too warm, even as warm as ordinary body temperature, heat-based methods recently or currently under exploration include scrotal immersion in hot water, artificial cryptorchidism (difficult), underwear that holds the testes snug against the body (ineffective) or tucked in the inguinal canal (effective), and ultrasound. These methods are intended to reduce sperm counts below fertility levels for up to several months. Work pioneered by Dr. Marthe Vogeli, a Swiss physician who practiced in India from 1930 to 1950, found that a 116°F testes-only water bath for 45 minutes a day for 3 weeks every 6 months will yield reliable contraception.[40] Soaking in hot tubs, of course, can jeopardize male fertility, but it is by no means a reliable form of contraception.

Male Contraceptive Vaccines

Immunization by injection against some aspect of the male reproductive system is also on the drawing boards. One vaccine inoculates against gonadotropin-releasing hormone (GnRH) that stimulates sperm production. Another that has been successfully tested in primates inoculates against Eppin, a molecule in semen that is required for sperm motility. The ideal immunocontraceptive would provide continuous yet reversible contraception for up to 1 year.[41]

None of these male methods are proven to work yet, and you cannot buy them yet. A principal exception is RISUG, being developed by the Parsemus Foundation under the name Vasalgel, which in studies in India really works as a contraceptive, but reversibility in men has not yet been proven.

Furthermore, the safety and side-effect profiles of these various methods under exploration are not yet well understood. Some may turn out to pose risks to the general health, reproductive health, or psychological health of men who use them. To be sure, FDA clearance would require that these risks be minimized, but an issue open to discussion is whether these risks would have to be as low, or lower, than the early versions of modern contraception for women—the original (high-dose) Pill, for instance. It liberated many many women from unwanted pregnancy, but it posed a substantial cost in risk of stroke for some.

Almost none of these new male methods, even if they did work, would be true "forgettables," that is, forms of long-acting, highly effective, reversible contraception. RISUG/Vasalgel would indeed be a "forgettable" and is perhaps closest to market, but reversibility has not been established, as recent failures in baboons have shown. Just the same, these new methods offer men the eventual prospect of reliable reproductive control in a way never possible before: This will be a big, big gain for men. But at the same time these new male contraceptives may pose new issues of reproductive control—a source of perennial tension between women and men—unless, I shall argue, we see them in the right way.

Reasons for Male Concern

But, guys, does any of this stuff about long-acting male contraception make you uneasy?

We might expect, for a start, at least three major sources of resistance to modern male contraception.

Safety and Efficacy Concerns

Concerns about safety and efficacy will be paramount, at least initially. None of the male technologies under development has yet been proven fully safe, either safe with respect to the overall health of the man or safe with respect to his fertility. Of course, there have always been concerns about the safety and efficacy of women's methods; they too may have side effects, may affect fertility, may delay return to fertility, and may not be perfectly effective. Despite these "risk–benefit" issues, the majority of women still contracept, and the question here is whether male methods need to meet or exceed the safety and efficacy levels of female methods.

Concerns about efficacy in male contraception affect even the most promising current candidate, RISUG, and indeed all of the male methods under development. One challenge is that the FDA has no standards regarding what it would consider sufficiently efficacious for a male contraceptive designed to suppress spermatogenesis. An effort to develop such standards with an eye toward eventual adoption by regulatory agencies determined that 100% suppression of spermatogenesis is not necessary for contraceptive efficacy, and estimated that reducing sperm to 1 million or fewer per milliliter of ejaculate would provide >99% effective contraception,[42] but complete azoospermia cannot be promised.

These concerns are perfectly appropriate at the moment. Indeed, it will be some time, even many years, before we can have adequate safety data, whether over 10,000–20,000 cycles as the FDA requests for female contraception, or over two or more generations as some voices of caution will insist. But we can imagine that technologies will be developed that are known to be safe and highly effective.

How men's responsibilities with respect to the reproductive outcomes of sex might differ if the new male contraceptives were, for example, safe but with poor efficacy profiles—that is, with high failure rates—or, conversely, were highly effective but not very safe, are questions that are likely to arise as these contraceptives actually come onto the market. Questions will also arise concerning male and female obligations to control fertility if the new male contraceptives are much less effective than female ones, or much less safe, or, perhaps, the other way around, both more effective and safer. These issues may resemble current ones in female reproductive control: Does a woman have a moral obligation to her partner, assuming he does not wish to have a child, to use the most effective and safest contraceptive means available?—that would be the LARC methods—or is she entitled to choose from among the smorgasbord currently available to her, including methods of lower efficacy and/or safety, like, say, the Pill or even the female condom, even though by doing so she would put her male partner at risk for rearing obligations or financial support for a child he does not want? These questions are not much discussed with reference to female contraception; it is hard to predict how vigorously they might be pursued with reference to modern male contraception.

Interfering with Sexual Drive

A substantial source of resistance for males would no doubt be the fear that any such long-acting contraceptive device would interfere with male sexual drive or the capacity for sexual performance. Certainly some of the technologies explored in the past have produced this side effect. This is an issue with which women have already been concerned for a long time, though maintenance of libido and sexual arousability is sometimes assumed to be not quite as important to female identity as it is to that of the male.[43]

But the surprising news is that at least some of the male technologies may work the other way around. Early reports on testosterone injections and the "male pill" then under development in England suggested that libido and potency may be enhanced, not diminished, by some of these contraceptive modalities. One of the first men to test the male pill (actually a series of testosterone injections) in Britain—this was in 1994-34-year-old Pete Lethaby, was reported in the popular press as saying that "It increased my sex drive, put more hair on my chest and built up the muscles on my upper body."[44] Kevin McQuaide, a 38-year-old subject in the same study, said that the minor side effects of acne on his back and weight gain did not bother him; if anything, he said, he feels more virile on the drug. "My voice is deeper, I need to shave more often and it has increased my sex drive."[45] Of course, such effects would occur only with hormonal methods; but the general point is that such technologies must not seriously interfere with male drive or performance.

But suppose it were the reverse? This has been the case for many of the female methods as they were developed—especially for some, like the Pill, in that their original dose sizes interfered somewhat with female libido and had other undesirable side effects, but were welcome anyway for the huge gain in reproductive control they provided.

Interfering with the Capacity to Impregnate

Seemingly closely related and equally entrenched is resistance to any technology that would interfere with the capacity to fertilize or impregnate. This is a much more subtle issue, having to do not with male sexual performance but with what is seen as male sexual *achievement*: impregnation of the female.

The two notions of male sexual performance and male sexual achievement are ubiquitously conflated in much of our thinking and indeed subconscious awareness, as they are in that of many cultures around the world. For example, in English, both "virility" and "potency" are often used in ordinary language to refer both to the capacity to ejaculate and to the capacity to fertilize; we do not distinguish clearly between them. Although there is fairly widespread male acceptance of some forms of fertilization limitation, these may also at the same time be more fully accepted when they are not perceived to interfere with the underlying male *capacity* to fertilize. Males do use condoms; these do limit fertility. But they do so only by withholding the semen, which itself remains "potent" or fertile, and the user retains immediate control over his fertility by being able to remove the device at any time. Likewise, withdrawal and scheduled-abstinence methods do not render the male infertile; they simply prevent contact between his still-fertile semen and the female. In contrast, some of the long-term methods under development would limit fertility in ways that cannot be observed or immediately overridden by the user, and hence would be, one might suspect, more likely the focus of male unease and suspicion. The man who wears a condom is still capable of impregnating a female, if he takes the thing off; the man who takes the pill is not.

To be sure, resistance to limitations of the capacity to fertilize has been widely explored in connection with vasectomy. But vasectomy is most frequently used by older men who have already had children—that is, who have already proved their capacity to fertilize. Contraceptives that limit the capacity for fertility might be viewed as much more problematic by younger men, even though the very point of a contraceptive is to limit fertility.

Reasons for Male Enthusiasm

As entrenched as some forms of resistance to the possibility of male contraception can be expected to be, several other considerations might seem to offer support. Could modern male contraception eventually be accepted, enthusiastically—perhaps even demanded—by men for themselves?

Sharing the Responsibility for Contraception with One's Partner

Some men in today's world, even where access to modern contraceptive technologies is good, report a sense of guilt or futility because they are unable to share the burden of contraception with their partners. They observe their wives or girlfriends taking the pill, inserting a diaphragm, using an IUD, and recognize that it is the woman in the relationship who does all the contraceptive work and sustains whatever nuisance and side effects there may be. Sharing the contraceptive burden is a primary consideration for many men who now have vasectomies. Some men say, for instance, that if long-term contraceptives were available to them, they would be eager to trade off with their partners, so that she used some form of contraceptive for, say, a couple of years, and then he took his turn.

Enhancing Sexual Freedom

Some men (as well as some women) may welcome long-term contraception because it gives them greater liberty in a variety of sexual situations, including nonmarital and extramarital ones. In the United States, the average age at first intercourse is 17 years; the age at first marriage is now 27 years for females and 29 years for males. As the interval between first sex and first marriage has lengthened—in 1960, the age at first marriage was 20 years for females and 22 years for males—the average period of nonmarital or premarital sexual activity has increased to a decade or more.

Obviating Political and Legal Controls

That males—especially young, unmarried males—might welcome the availability of effective, long-term contraception points to what the alternatives might be in a political climate determined to control what it regards as inappropriate reproduction. This is an issue of gaining personal control oneself, before political and policy-driven legal controls might intervene.

SHIFTING CONTRACEPTIVE RESPONSIBILITY FROM FEMALE TO MALE?

But to shift contraceptive responsibility from the female to the male would not solve the reproductive control problems at issue here; it would merely shift part of the problem while creating new difficulties. Because women would lose a substantial measure of reproductive control if males rather than females became responsible for contraception, but, as gestators as well as primary caregivers, women would still bear the principal biological burdens of unwanted pregnancy, this shift would by no means create a more just arrangement.

After all, there is no reason to suppose that men could be trusted more in contraceptive activity than women can. As Charlotte Owen of the Family Planning Association told *Esquire* magazine, "We support the development of a male contraceptive, but we have reservations about making it available to younger men. A lot of girls wouldn't trust a new boyfriend who said he was taking it."[46] And as one reporter warned, "There will, of course, be the danger of condom-shy men resorting to: 'It's OK, I'm on the pill.' "[47]

DOUBLE COVERAGE: GENDER-EQUAL CONTRACEPTIVE CONTROL

But a shift of contraceptive responsibility from women to men is not the only alternative. Suppose, instead, a conjecture that reflects, I think, the right way to see the new modern male contraceptives. Suppose such contraceptive methods, especially the long-term, high-efficacy types like implants and reversible vaccines, the LARC methods, were to become available to men but remain in use by women as well. Then *both* parties would have them, so that "double coverage" would be possible. Of course, in the real world, effective, long-term male contraception will no doubt become available and be accepted gradually, in different contexts, different cultures, in line with the cultural patterns and preferences of or pressures on different users, and double coverage may take hold as a social norm in some groups before others, thus raising additional issues of contraceptive inequality.

Nevertheless, in order to see what is really at stake in the underlying ethical issues in male contraception, we can explore a generalized conjecture, universalizing LARC to both women in general and men in general. This is the thought experiment I call *M's Conjecture*, about reversing the default in human reproduction, *what if everybody routinely used automatic, LARC contraception, except when they wanted to have a child?* I have been exploring this conjecture with respect to women in the various contexts of global population growth and decline, teen pregnancy, pregnancy after rape and mass rape, pregnancy in maternal chronic illness and environmental exposure, and abortion.[48] Although the universality of use imagined is indeed a thought experiment, the technologies that would make this possible for women are not science fiction—they are available *now*. But now we can expand this conjecture to include men, not just that versions of LARC contraception had become available to men, but that use of them had become accepted, normal, routine: *what if everybody used automatic contraception* would really mean *everybody*, not only women but also men? What if men had equally effective contraceptive modalities available to them as women do, and actually, routinely, as a matter of course, used them?

M's Conjecture

What if *everybody*, women and men, routinely used one form or another of long-acting reversible LARC contraception all the time, so that all sexual intercourse involved "double coverage," except where both partners wished to have a child?

This thought experiment exposes one of a number of fundamental, mistaken assumptions we characteristically make in thinking about contraception.[49] We might call this a "no overkill" or "unnecessary duplication of effort" assumption—the central, problematic assumption that "one's enough," that contraception need only be pursued by either the male or the female. This mistaken assumption is, of course, factually inadequate—after all, in the United States today, about 50% of unplanned pregnancies occur in women who are using some form of contraception. But this mistaken assumption, that for both male and female to use contraception would be redundant, superfluous, a kind of excess incurring additional risks and side effects, but biologically unnecessary to avoid pregnancy is also unethical, in that it will be seriously destructive to reproductive rights if it survives into an era of modern male contraception.

Indeed, the "one's enough" assumption is a flat, stupid, shortsighted mistake, already a central culprit in issues about reproductive control. This assumption is harmless in some situations, as perhaps in long-term monogamous couples who agree about their reproductive choices; but, I want to show, this assumption is genuinely damaging and ethically unsupportable as a general position. It is the assumption we *must* correct before modern male contraception comes online.

Some erosion of the "one's enough" unnecessary-duplication-of-effort assumption has been taking place since the beginning of the AIDS epidemic in the early 1980s. Some couples already in effect have double coverage, or what is called "dual use" in the medical literature, where the male uses a condom for sexually transmitted disease prevention and the female uses a spermicide, diaphragm, oral contraceptive, implant, IUD, or other modality for contraception—about 8% of all couples in the United States, and about 20% of those involving young (15–24 year olds) and never-married women.[50] But the conjecture we are exploring here involves something still more thorough: What if both parties were routinely using long-acting, reversible, automatic LARC methods for contraceptive purposes? What if this were seen as normal, routine, something both parties just automatically do? In addition, depending on the degree of monogamy or other features of their relationship, they might also use a condom, vaccine, multipurpose prevention technology, or other modality for the prevention of disease transmission. Whereas disease control is an important consideration in nonmonogamous sexual relationships between parties with prior sexual experience, *M's Conjecture* is concerned with *reproductive* outcome, and it is *reproductive* control that "double coverage" with highly effective, long-acting reversible contraception grants.

As I have said, it is a virtually unchallenged assumption of modern contraception usage that "one's enough"—if either the female or the male does it, that is sufficient.[51] There are various reasons, of course, why the "one's enough" assumption seems plausible. After all, double coverage would mean duplication of expense, duplication of effort in the mechanics of procurement, application, and storage of whatever contraceptive methods the couple employs, and duplication of exposure to any risks or side effects the various modalities might impose. But to assume that "one's enough" is to fail to notice that there are important benefits to be had in this seeming duplication of effort, benefits that cannot be achieved with single coverage alone. These benefits are particularly evident in the matter of reproductive control. These are great enough, I think, to claim that support for single coverage, although harmless in its practical consequences in some situations, is destructive of a gender-balanced conception of reproductive rights as a general position and, thus, I think we should recognize, ethically unsupportable. Our real support should be for double coverage all the time, a full reversal of the default in human reproduction and a position that requires positive choice by each of the prospective parents, followed by discontinuation of their contraceptive modality by each of them, for conception to occur.

Now imagine—to continue the conjecture being explored here—what would it be like if there were universal double coverage: that is, if *both* females and males *routinely* used automatic LARC contraception? The conjecture assumes, not unrealistically, that such methods for males can be sufficiently developed and tested so that they can be known to be safe, effective, free from substantial side effects, rapidly reversible, and that furthermore they will be inexpensive, easy to emplace, and will not interfere with sexual performance or satisfaction. This is still science fiction at the moment, but I think not for long, and it could eventually be that some of the male methods will be cheaper, easier to emplace, of higher efficacy, and safer than even the best female methods now available.

So imagine *M's Conjecture* in actual practice: *Everybody* uses automatic, background contraception—*all* fertile females and *all* fertile males, *all* the time, except when they want to have a child. This would produce a full, complete reversal of the default mechanism: Conception would require a positive choice on the part of both the male and the female, plus a positive act on the part of each to self-remove his or her respective device or have them removed or neutralized to make conception possible. It would take two to tango, so to speak. Except in those cases in which one party had been coerced, either by the partner or by some third party, into removing or having his or her contraceptive device removed, there would be no nonvoluntary contribution to conception either on the part of men or on the part of women, and virtually every child born would be the product of a deliberate choice on the part of both its parents.

The contemporary world is one of toughness about responsibility in sexual matters and for the consequences of sex, in which both male-blaming and female-blaming political agendas are openly pursued. To sort out whether male-blaming or female-blaming views are the more justified, and whether public policies should be based more heavily on one than the other, would, of course, embroil us in endless political dispute. But in the conjectural world explored here, there would be no need to disentangle these issues or to try to answer the old questions about whether men or women actually have the greater degree of reproductive control. Except for preventing coercion, there would be no need to determine whether women are more likely to be victimized by men— especially (as the male-blaming view would have it) those dangerous unmarried males always ready to impregnate without regard to the consequences for the woman or for any future offspring; or whether (as the female-blaming view would hold) men are more likely to be victimized by scheming women bent on entrapping any man who seems to be a good catch. This age-old debate—familiar stock in literature, poetry, and drama, and indeed much of popular culture (not to mention the law)—would become almost entirely irrelevant, because with genuine double coverage each individual now would have the capacity to make *independent* choices concerning control over his or her own contribution to conception. This is the fullest expression of reproductive rights. Paternity issues, buttressed by the sort of genetic identification already routinely performed in these cases, would virtually disappear: The birth of a child would not merely permit identification of the father (whether or not the father was the official partner of the mother) but would entail that he had knowingly and willingly contributed to its conception. In a world in which *everybody* did it—in which the default outcome in human reproduction were fully reversed and each individual would need to make a positive choice in order to contribute to conception—there would be no need to indulge in globalizing, stereotyping, and unproductive generalizations about whether men or women are less to be trusted; in this double-coverage future world, no one would be put in the position of *having* to trust someone else in so basic a matter as deciding whether to have a child.

There are some obvious practical advantages to double coverage. With universal automatic contraception for males as well as females, whether or not genetic identification is involved, the seemingly intractable problem of abortion, we may speculate, could be reduced. This could be expected to occur in two ways. First, their number would be reduced: About half of all pregnancies in the Unites States are unintended,[52] and of these unintended pregnancies, nearly half are terminated in abortion. Some 48% of all unintended pregnancies in the United States are the result of contraceptive failure, virtually all of it associated with user-controlled time-of-need or hybrid methods,[53] and 51% of abortions are performed in women who had been using contraception—most commonly condoms (27%) or a hormonal method (17%)—in the month they became pregnant.[54] Clearly, at least half of the abortions that now take place would not occur. But the decline would presumably be even greater: In *M's Conjecture*, there would be no cases in which a woman was not using contraception but nevertheless did not want a child; thus many of the most problematic situations in the reproductive landscape would not occur, whether or not they might have resulted in abortion.

Furthermore, with double coverage for both partners with modern, automatic LARC contraception or the more reliable forms of hybrid contraception with very low failure rates, the likelihood of contraceptive failure for that couple is the product of the failure rates of those two different forms of contraception, and hence much lower. (Here too, like safety officers, we value redundancy.) If both male and female were to use hybrid contraception with a 1% failure rate, for example, their joint failure rate would be .01%, 100 times lower. If both the male and female used technologies that had failure rates equivalent to that of Nexplanon, 0.05% per year, the failure rate would be 0.0025% or 25 per million couples per year. There are now about 70,000 abortions annually associated with contraceptive failure[55]; this would reduce that rate to close to zero.

Second, double coverage might reduce principled resistance to abortifacient or potentially abortifacient automatic female methods—the IUD, and others that may theoretically prevent implantation of a fertilized egg.[56] Because with double coverage that includes a highly effective male method, no or virtually no sperm can get through to fertilize the egg in the first place, the fact that the female methods might have been abortifacient becomes irrelevant, except for the very few failures of the male's technology—failures that would need to coincide with failures of the female's highly effective technology as well, thus making the likelihood of conception occurring very small.

But this is not yet to address the central issue: What about reproductive control in general, and the gender inequalities that current methods of fertility management have seemed to produce so far? That's what *M's Conjecture* allows us to explore.

WOULD DOUBLE COVERAGE REALLY EQUALIZE MALE AND FEMALE REPRODUCTIVE CONTROL?

Changing the default mechanism by means of universal automatic reversible contraceptive use, however, has another distinctive consequence for reproductive control, both female and male. When each individual, male and female, is protected from involuntary or semivoluntary contribution to conception by needing to make a positive decision to do so, it also becomes the case that any individual wishing to conceive or father a conception must have a willing partner. This is a new situation, and it may challenge deep-seated current assumptions.

After all, it has always been possible for both sexes to reproduce without a willing partner. For women, this can involve sustaining pregnancy by means of deceit, seduction, or perhaps forced intercourse, or even attending enough wild parties or raves. For men, it can involve a range of possibilities from sowing wild oats to rape. For some men and women without partners, for whatever social reasons, the possibilities of force and deceit have meant that hope of childsiring or childbearing has never been completely closed off.

To be sure, institutions have developed to supply such desires in less aggressive ways. For instance, some sperm banks are willing to inseminate single or lesbian women without male partners[57]; some surrogate mothers have accepted contracts from single or gay men. No doubt such institutions would survive. So would a variety of far less formal arrangements: men who donate sperm to single or lesbian women; women who volunteer as surrogates for male friends. However, the traditionally tolerated institution of sowing wild oats would be closed off to men; men could no longer expect to sire children in a more or less random, unplanned, one-night-stand sort of way, without making a positive choice to do so, and the image of the wild man—the wild sexual man (or more accurately, the wild reproductive man)—would become extinct. In this new world, complete reproductive autonomy means complete autonomy to refrain from having children one does not elect, but where a willing partner is lacking it cannot guarantee complete autonomy to choose to have a child by oneself. Reproductive control, for both females and males, is limited in this important sense.

REPRODUCTIVE CONTROL AND EQUALITY

Thus, although at first sight double coverage seemed to work to equalize reproductive control, and thus produce a shift in the appropriate assignment of responsibility to both females and males in equal ways, the issue may not be so clear. After all, it could be argued that even a seemingly egalitarian arrangement such as this, in which men and women would have equal control over their own reproductive choices, would only exacerbate longstanding inequities in social situations in which, as is true of many real-world situations in a wide variety of cultures, men and women are quite unequal in power.[58] In most social situations, men have greater privilege and greater power than women; men have power over the women with whom they are involved in reproductive relationships; and men in these relationships can physically harm women, can financially limit women, can physically or socially isolate women from the larger world, and so on. Nevertheless, this argument continues, there is one sphere in which women can exercise greater power: the domestic and especially reproductive sphere. In traditional relationships, this is often the woman's only sphere of influence, and hence it can be argued that it is appropriate that she exercise greater power here. This is a traditional view, in that it assumes that the woman's sphere of influence is domestic and that her identity centers around childbearing; but it is also a feminist view in that it assumes that a woman's preferences really matter. Traditional or not, this picture of a restricted sphere describes the circumstances of a great many women, both in contemporary America and in the rest of the world. What must not be taken away from a woman whose world is like this, this argument holds, is her greater degree of control in the matter of whether the couple shall have children.

Consider the following example[59]:

> A couple, both teachers and both 34 years old, are considering whether to have children; they do not have any so far. She, both because of her basic values and because she hears her biological clock already ticking, wants children. He does not. Indeed, he does not know whether he will ever want to have children; but he is quite sure he does not want them now. They care for each other; they have a happy life together; but they do not agree about children.

With double coverage, assuming both he and she use automatic contraception and neither persuades the other to change his or her mind about the issue at hand, this couple will not have children: His refusal trumps her desire. Double coverage is a mutual-veto arrangement. But it could be argued that because of the centrality of childbearing to the identity of women, much more so than to men, this apparent equality is not really *equality* at all: He is able to perpetrate much greater harm to her by refusing to have children than she could to him by having children he did not want. This is true, it could be maintained, even though, in this example, they are the same age, have similar jobs, and in other ways are able to exercise nearly equal autonomy in their dealings with the world.

But children are not just another consumer item in the world; they are something different, and of particularly central importance to the woman.

Of course, one might argue that it is not in the interests of the child to be born into a relationship in which the father—or for that matter either member of the couple—did not want a child. It is certainly true that the consequences can be bad for the child who is born unwanted and remains unwanted; but it can also be the case that although the father or the mother did not want the child prior to conception, as the gestation period progresses and the child is finally born, it comes to be wanted and loved. Though this is by no means always the case, unwanted children may well become wanted ones.

Now consider a couple whose circumstances are far less privileged. This couple is poor, there is a greater age difference between them, and the woman has little education and work experience. She cherishes deeply traditional values. She is far more dependent on her husband, much more within his control. She wants children badly—that is the one sphere within which she could fully bloom—but he does not want them at all. In this situation of far less equal background power, should his wishes still trump hers? Of course, he can already control her reproductive options by using a condom, avoiding sex, or getting a vasectomy without her knowledge or consent; but the ways she may currently have of maneuvering him into siring a child he does not want would be more firmly closed off to her if he were using automatic contraception. But now, in this more difficult case, her options for changing this circumstance are still more limited: Although there are plenty of men out there presumably ready to sow their seed, her options for extricating herself from the current relationship—she has no power, no independence, no money, no resources for surviving in the world—are far more limited, and she cannot realistically hope to have a child fathered by somebody else. What might have given this deeply traditional woman's life real meaning, of the only sort that is available to her, is closed off.

One ready reply to these concerns is that people who disagree so profoundly and inflexibly about whether to have children should not get married in the first place. If such basic disagreement erupts after they are already married, they should divorce and find more compatible partners who share their respective views about childbearing—after all, it will be an easy divorce, uncomplicated by children. Of course, in some cultures and religious communities this is not a realistic option. Even where divorce is a possibility, there will be variants of these cases in which the couple already have children, but she wants more and he does not; these are less compelling morally, however, in that the woman in these cases already has the children that are, on this view, the central source of her identity.

There are other objections to this argument. For example, since it appears to hold that the husband ought to accede to his wife's wishes for a child because that is a central source of identity for her, it bears an uncanny resemblance to arguments of just a century or two earlier: then, it was held to be the wife's duty to provide the husband with the children he wished and that reflected his own position and prestige, the source of his identity, regardless of her preferences in the matter. (This, of course, is still the view in much of the world.) But these rejoinders do not defeat the argument; they only reinforce the importance, for future discussion, of exploring the consequences of using double-coverage, mutual-veto LARC contraception, and of being clear about whether apparent equality in reproductive control is really the case.

There will also be questions concerning male and female obligations to control fertility, as we said earlier, if the new male contraceptives are much less effective than female ones, or much less safe, or, perhaps, the other way around, both more effective and safer. As we said, there will also be issues analogous to current ones in female reproductive control: Does a woman have a moral obligation to use the most effective and safest contraceptive means available, or is she entitled to choose from among the smorgasbord currently available to her, even though by choosing methods of lower efficacy she would put her male partner at risk for rearing obligations or financial support for a child he did not want? Would the question be the same for men? But *M's Conjecture*, as we said, will in effect provide an answer to these questions: In this universal LARC thought experiment, both male and female are using methods of highest efficacy, and thus neither partner puts the other at risk of having a child he or she did not want.

However, there might be one other consequence of the universal LARC use by both men and women, so that the default would be fully reversed and that it would take two independent decisions to remove the device so that conception could occur. It would, as we said earlier, take two to tango. But in a conjectural world like this, where everybody routinely used automatic contraception as a matter of course, it would come as no surprise to anyone that both parties hold a reproductive veto. Thus, exploration of whether they wanted to have children, or would instead exercise their veto, would presumably play a major role in courtship and premarital discussion, even in arranged marriages, same-sex marriages, and various unconventional arrangements. Indeed, this might be a healthy contribution to the quality of marital and other sexual relationships, to have these things understood in advance rather than have them fought out—with all the various weapons of dissembling and trickery—after the relationship has already begun.

Alternatively, one can imagine societies in which marriage really only begins with the initiation of pregnancy or the birth of a child—the living proof that a couple has made a joint, child-affirming choice—as, for instance, among the Amazonian Shuar or, to some extent, in traditional and contemporary Sweden. I see no reason to doubt that a change in the default mechanism so that contribution to conception requires a positive choice, and furthermore a change for both men and women, would bring about profound changes in the nature of intimate relationships, but I see many reasons to think these changes would be constructive ones. Most important, it seems to me, is to recognize that these gains in each person's right not to have children he or she does not want outweigh what might seem to be one person's "right" to have children with a partner who does not willingly do so.

Of course, we may assume, there will be exceptional cases, ones where partners are not or cannot be on the same page about whether to have children. The very existence of universal LARC, used by both men and women, would, however, tend to encourage sexually entwined couples to be on the same page in the first place, because both of them would know what the stakes are right from the start.

"Trust me, I'm taking the pill," isn't a good excuse from either side; this is about *each* sexual partner assuming responsibility for reproductive outcome, each exercising reproductive control. There may be arguments, disagreements, extended negotiations, but neither party can at least in principle force the other to capitulate. Yet, more happily, love can play a big role here, too, where both parties are sensitive to what the other wants as well as their own desires, and—as is already the case for many many couples—it can make beautiful music when they agree in jointly electing to have a child.

What the Future Holds

This chapter may have seemed like a science-fiction intrusion in an otherwise real-life book, but the development of modern male contraception is not very far-fetched science fiction, something maybe just a decade or so—perhaps less—away. Indeed, some research groups suggest that RISUG/Vasalgel and perhaps a male pill may be available within just a few years—that is, if research proceeds at an adequate rate; and some technologies are already in human trials.

In general, the pharmaceutical companies make the same error as we all have: Failing to see that double coverage offers not just greater contraceptive security, but far greater personal security in a climate insisting on reproductive responsibility. Double coverage enhances reproductive rights in a way that single coverage, in which one party must either rely on or assume control over the contraceptive efforts of the other, cannot.

A recent World Health Organization study found that 41%–75% of males worldwide would welcome nonsurgical male contraceptives that could be used apart from intercourse[60]; that is, contraceptives much more like those women already have. Yet this perception still only envisions male contraception as an alternative, not as an overlapping addition. If the failure to see that double coverage is not redundant but offers a number of crucial benefits ends up discouraging basic and commercial research in male automatic contraceptives, as it seems to have been doing, this unwarranted assumption may be a particularly important one to isolate and challenge.

That should be easy. After all, its most concrete commercial application is that "double coverage" would mean "double markets." In any case, it is clear that double-coverage use of "automatic," "forgettable" LARC reversible contraception would have a major effect in solving many large-scale, global problems that are the consequences of sex, in a way that is, most important, fundamentally consistent with respect for basic reproductive rights for *both* women and men.

Acknowledgments

Thanks to Kirsten M. Thompson, Bixby Center for Global Reproductive Issues, UCSF; Elaine Lissner, director, Male Contraception Information Project (MCIP); Mel Leverich; Steve Capone; Blake Vernon; David Turok, MD, and Kirtly Parker Jones, MD, of the Family Planning Research Group at the University of Utah Department of Obstetrics and Gynecology; Lisa Kearn; and Anikka Hoidal Knight.

Notes

1. David A. Grimes. "Forgettable Contraception." *Contraception* 80, no. 6 (2009): 497–499.
2. Julie Lynn Fennell, "Men Bring Condoms, Women Take Pills. Men's and Women's Roles in Contraceptive Decision Making." *Gender & Society* 25, no. 4 (2011): 496–521.
3. William R. Grady, Koray Tanfer, John O. G. Billy, and Jennifer Lincoln-Hanson. "Men's Perceptions of Their Roles and Responsibilities Regarding Sex, Contraception and Childrearing." *Family Planning Perspectives* 28, no. 5: 221–226.
4. Martha Burk, "The Sperm Stops Here," *MS* Nov.–Dec. (1997), p. 18.
5. See Donald Hubin, "Procreator's Duties," Chapter 14 of this volume, for consideration of some of these hypotheticals in a series of thought experiments. Hubin also considers whether male/female differences in reproductive control underwrite arguments for differences in resulting responsibilities.
6. For an illustrative example of the tension between male-blaming and female-blaming accounts in the context of contraception, see, for example, the comments to an interview of Elaine Lissner in "Priceonomics on the Economics of Male Birth Control," Oct. 19, 2015, http://priceonomics.com/the-economics-of-male-birth-control/.
7. For a meta-analysis of data about abstinence-only education among young people, see John S. Santelli, Mary A. Ott, Maureen Lyon, Jennifer Rogers, Daniel Summers, and Rebecca Schleifer, "Abstinence and Abstinence-Only Education: A Review of U.S. Policies and Programs." *Journal of Adolescent Health* 38 (2006): 72–81.
8. Our information about withdrawal is minimal because many physicians in the United States refuse to consider it a true method of contraception, and there is no funding for research about it. Use of withdrawal is quite prevalent; it is hidden because most tabulations of contraceptive prevalence take the most effective method used per woman and drop all other methods. See Rachel K. Jones, Julie Fennell, Jenny A. Higgins, and Kelly Blanchard. "Better Than Nothing of Savvy Risk-Reduction Practice? The Importance of Withdrawal." *Contraception* 79 (2009): 407–410.
9. James Trussell, "Contraceptive Efficacy," in Robert A. Hatcher et al., eds. *Contraceptive Technology*, 19th revised edition. New York: Irvington Publishers, 2007, table 27-1, p. 759; James Trussell, "Contraceptive Failure in the United States." *Contraception* 83, no. 5 (2011): 397–404.
10. Our information about withdrawal is minimal because many physicians in the United States refuse to consider it a true method of contraception, and there is no funding for research about it. Use of withdrawal is quite prevalent; it is hidden because most tabulations of contraceptive prevalence take the most effective method used per woman and drop all other methods. See Rachel K. Jones, Julie Fennell, Jenny A. Higgins, and Kelly Blanchard. "Better Than Nothing of Savvy Risk-Reduction Practice? The Importance of Withdrawal." *Contraception* 79 (2009): 407–410.
11. Vasectomy prevalence numbers from the 2006–2008 cycle of the National Survey of Family Growth, NSFG: 10% of US couples practicing contraception do so by means of vasectomy; 6% of US couples in which the woman is aged 15–44 years; 13% of sexually active women report *ever* having a partner with a vasectomy; 13% of married men have had a vasectomy. W. D. Mosher and J. Jones. "Use of Contraception in the United States: 1982–2008." *Vital Health Statistics* 23 (2010): 1–44.
12. J. A. Higgins and Y. Wang. "The Role of Young Adults' Pleasure Attitudes in Shaping Condom Use." *American Journal of Public Health* 105, no. 7 (2015): 1329–1332.

13. Information provided for public use on effectiveness of various types of contraception is available in many places, including, for instance, the Centers for Disease Control at http://www.cdc.gov/nchs/nsfg.htm and the Bedsider Birth Control Support Network, at https://bedsider.org, which also offers information by telephone at (888) 321–0383.

14. The condom's failure rate in laboratory situations is comparatively low, 2%; in ordinary bedroom usage, it is 18% during the first year of use. However, a 2% failure rate does not mean that 2 out of every 100 condoms used will lead to unintended pregnancy; the rate is based on computations using couples, rather than condoms, as the measured denominator. A 2% failure rate means that of 100 couples who use condoms perfectly for 1 year, two couples will experience an accidental pregnancy. Robert A. Hatcher, *Contraceptive Technology*, 20th ed., p. 154.

15. There is little reliable research on the effectiveness of the diaphragm without spermicides, mostly because the studies have been statistically underpowered to calculate 12-month failure rates. Lynley A. Cook, Kavita Nanda, David A. Grimes, and Laureen M. Lopez. "Diaphragm Versus Diaphragm With Spermicides for Contraception." *The Cochrane Library* (2003, updated 2011), http://onlinelibrary.wiley.com/doi/10.1002/14651858. CD002031/abstract;jsessionid=3C4145811951D848C6E5A3BC5BFC65AE.f04t02.

16. See O. Graesslin and T. Korver. "The Contraceptive Efficacy of Implanon: A Review of Clinical Trials and Marketing Experience." *European Journal of Contraception and Reproductive Health Care* 13, Suppl. 1 (2008): 4–12. The first-year failure rate is sometimes stated as 0.2%, but this figure is inflated by the inclusion of pregnancies that had been initiated but were not detected before implantation.

17. See, for example, US Department of State. "Notice of Declaration of Foreign Countries as Reciprocating Countries for the Enforcement of Family Support (Maintenance) Obligations." *Federal Register* 79, no. 161 (August 20, 2014): 49368–49369; European Parliament, Directorate-General for Internal Policies. Child maintenance systems in EU member states from a gender perspective. http://www.europarl.europa.eu/RegData/etudes/note/join/2014/474407/IPOL-FEMM_NT(2014)474407_EN.pdf.

18. Robert A. Hatcher, *Contraceptive Technology*, 20th ed., p. 10, citing Susan D. Cochran and Vickie M. Mays, "Sex, Lies, and HIV." *New England Journal of Medicine* 322, no. 11 (1990): 774–775.

19. *Griswold v. Connecticut*, 381 U.S. 479 (1965).

20. US Department of Health and Human Services, Office of Population Affairs. "Male Family Planning Services." http://www.hhs.gov/opa/title-x-family-planning/initiatives-and-resources/male-services/.

21. See Margaret M. Schulte and Freya L. Sonenstein, "Men at Family Planning Clinics: The New Patients?," *Family Planning Perspectives* 27 (1995): 212–216, 225.

22. For the imposition of child support obligations on men who had been assured by the woman that pregnancy could not result from their act of intercourse, see *Hughes v. Hutt*, 500 Pa. 209, 455 A.2d 623 (1982); *Stephen K. v. Roni L.*, 105 Cal. App. 3d 604, 164 Cal. Rptr. 618 (1980). These cases are cited by John A. Robertson in his classic work *Children of Choice: Freedom and the New Reproductive Technologies*. Princeton, NJ: Princeton University Press, 1994, p. 239, fn. 29.

23. *Pamela P. v. Frank S.*, 110 Misc. 2d 978, 443 N.Y.S.2d 343 (Fam. Ct. 1981) *modified sub nom. L. Pamela P. v. Frank S.*, 88 A.D.2d 865, 451 N.Y.S.2d 766 (1982) *aff'd*, 59 N.Y.2d 1, 449 N.E.2d 713 (1983). New Hampshire and Minnesota courts have also made similar rulings: *Welzenbach v. Powers*, 660 A.2d 1133 (N.H. 1995) (finding that public policy

bars misrepresentation about contraception as a cause of action); *Murphy v. Myers*, 560 N.W.2d 752 (Minn. Ct. App. 1997) (finding fraud and misrepresentation cannot be affirmative defenses in paternity actions). See also *Wallis v. Smith*, 22 P.3d 682, 683 (N.M. Ct. App. 2001) (finding that an unwed father could not assert actions for fraud, breach of contract, and tort actions to recoup child support paid to the child's mother).

24. *Faske v. Bonanno*, 137 Mich. App. 202, 357 N.W.2d 860 (1984).

25. *Beard v. Skipper*, 182 Mich. App. 352, 451 N.W.2d 614 (1990).

26. *Erwin L.D. v. Myla Jean L.*, 41 Ark. App. 16, 847 S.W.2d 45 (1993).

27. Alia Beard Rau, "Statutory Rape Victim Forced to Pay Child Support." *USA Today* (Sept. 3, 2014), http://www.usatoday.com/story/news/nation/2014/09/02/statutory-rape-victim-child-support/14953965/.

28. Myrisha S. Lewis, "Making Sex the Same: Ending the Unfair Treatment of Males in Family Law." *Wisconsin Journal of Law, Gender & Society* 27 (2012): 257–280.

29. Nancy J. Alexander and Norman B. Hecht, "Male Contraception: Future Possibilities," Office of Technology Transfer, National Institutes of Health, Bethesda, MD; Elaine Lissner, "Frontiers in Nonhormonal Male Contraceptive Research," Male Contraception Information Project, Santa Cruz, California; Eunice Kennedy Shriver National Institute of Child Health and Human Development, "New Research on Male Contraceptive Methods," http://m.nichd.nih.gov/news/spotlights/Pages/062314-male-contraception.aspx; David E. Cummings and William J. Bremner, "Prospects for New Hormonal Male Contraceptives," *Endocrinology Metabolism Clinics of North America* 23, no. 4 (1994): 893–922.

30. For a more comprehensive account, see Paul Kogan and Moshe Wald, "Male Contraception." *Urologic Clinics of North America* 41, no. 1 (2014): 145–161.

31. "RISUG," http://malecontraceptives.org/methods/risug.php. "Vasagel," http://www.parsemusfoundation.org/projects/vasalgel/.

32. John K. Amory, "Progress and Prospects in Male Hormonal Contraception," *Current Opinion in Endocrinology Diabetes Obesity* 15, no. 3 (2008): 255–260.

33. Y, Gu et al. "Multicenter Contraceptive Efficacy Trial of Injectable Testosterone Undecanoate in Chinese Men." *Journal of Clinical Endocrinology & Metabolism* 94, no. 6 (2009): 1910–1915.

34. Paul Kogan and Moshe Wald, "Male Contraception." *Urologic Clinics of North America* 41, no. 1 (2014): 145–161.

35. See the bar charts and studies cited here: "Experimental MCH Formulations," http://male-contraceptives.org/methods/hormonal_form.php.

36. Under development by the Population Council, New York, "Product Licensing," http://www.popcouncil.org/about/product-licensing.

37. Bill Bremner and John Amory's study was a proof of concept. The testosterone required taking a pill three times a day, and even then the pharmacodynamics were not tolerable for the volunteers. John Amory has since tested nano-milled testosterone and has decided that is not a viable contraceptive product either. Kirsten Thompson, personal communication.

38. Male Contraceptive Initiative, Two Updates In Male Contraception, Aaron Hamlin, March 31, 2016 https://www.malecontraceptive.org/two-updates-male-contraception/.

39. Parsemus Foundation, "Contraception With Protection From HIV," https://www.parsemusfoundation.org/projects/clean-sheets-pill/; Male Contraception Initiative, "Clean Sheets Pill," http://www.malecontraceptive.org/#!clean-sheets-pill/c1u8o.

40. Elaine Lissner in Priceonomics on The Economics of Male Birth Control, Oct. 19, 2015, http://priceonomics.com/the-economics-of-male-birth-control/.

41. Under development by the Population Council, New York, http://www.popcouncil.org/about/product-licensing.

42. The effort was spearheaded by Eberhard Nieschlag, who attended the Seattle FOCI meeting. Kirsten Thompson, personal communication, October/November 2011.

43. Some female technologies do have some impact on these matters, for instance, as oral contraceptives are found to slightly decrease the frequency with which women initiate sexual activity though they continue to have orgasm with the same frequency and report the same amount of sexual pleasure. (This finding has seemed of little significance in the medical literature because it is the male who initiates sexual activity in the vast majority of cases.)

44. Denna Allen, "It Pepped Up My Sex Drive, Gave Me a Hairy Chest and Turned Me Into a Hunk, But Would You Trust a Man to Take the Pill?; Masculine Side-Effects of Taking the Male Contraceptive Pill," *Daily Mirror*, August 23, 1994, p. 7. Of course, most steroids do this; they also increase the risk of heart disease and the possibility of testicular atrophy.

45. Elizabeth Sweetenham, "Male Pill Made Me More Virile," *Daily Mail*, April 26, 1994, p. 37.

46. David Thomas, "Health: United Y-Front for the Pill," *The Daily Telegraph*, August 23, 1994, p. 12.

47. Denna Allen, "It Pepped Up My Sex Drive, Gave Me a Hairy Chest and Turned Me Into a Hunk, But Would You Trust a Man to Take the Pill?; Masculine Side-Effects of Taking the Male Contraceptive Pill," *Daily Mirror*, August 23, 1994, p. 7.

48. See my book in progress: Margaret P. Battin, *Sex & Consequences: "Automatic" Contraception and the Reproductive Problems of the Globe.*

49. A number of other unwarranted assumptions in our thinking about contraception are developed in my book in progress, *Sex & Consequences: "Automatic" Contraception and the Reproductive Problems of the Globe.*

50. In a 1991 study, the male used a condom while the female used a concomitant method of birth control for 54% of women using foam, 52% of women using the sponge, 42% of women using the diaphragm, and 21% of women using oral contraceptives. Robert A. Hatcher, *Contraceptive Technology*, 20th ed., p. 155. The Ortho Study was of 7,805 women aged 15–50 years.

51. Klaas Heinemann, Farid Saad, Martin Wiesemes, Steven White, and Lothar Heinemann, "Attitudes Toward Male Fertility Control: Results of a Multinational Survey on Four Continents," *Human Reproduction* 20, no. 2 (2005): 543–548. Table III in this article shows percentages regarding who decides on birth control and attitudes toward a new male fertility control disaggregated by country.

52. Information provided for public use on pregnancy rates is available from the Centers for Disease Control, covering unintended pregnancy rates from 1982 to 2010. William D. Mosher, Jo Jones, and Joyce C. Abma, "Intended and Unintended Births in the United States: 1982–2010," *National Health Statistics Reports* 55 (2012), http://www.cdc.gov/nchs/data/nhsr/nhsr055.pdf.

53. All data on failure rates in this paragraph are from Trussell 2011, op. cit.

54. Guttmacher Institute, "Induced Abortion in the United States," (2014), http://www.guttmacher.org/pubs/fb_induced_abortion.html#7a.

55. Based on the Guttmacher Institute's estimated 1,313,000 abortions in the United States in 2000, with 53.7% of women obtaining abortions reporting the use of any contraceptive method.

56. In medical terminology, pregnancy first begins with implantation; hence, methods like the IUD that can prevent implantation are not abortifacient. However, some popular and religious usage considers pregnancy to begin with conception.

57. For example, Pacific Reproductive Services, https://www.pacrepro.com; and the Chicago Women's Health Center, http://www.chicagowomenshealthcenter.org/services-page/alternative-insemination.
58. I owe this point to Leslie Francis.
59. I owe this example to the late David Green, MD.
60. Elaine Lissner in "Priceonomics on the Economics of Male Birth Control," Oct. 19, 2015, http://priceonomics.com/the-economics-of-male-birth-control/.

CHAPTER 16

....

SOCIETAL DISREGARD FOR THE NEEDS OF THE INFERTILE

....

DAVID ORENTLICHER

It is often thought that public policies favor families and foster childbearing. And in many ways, that is the case. The federal and state governments give tax deductions to households with dependent children; health insurance policies cover the costs of pre-natal care, labor, and delivery; and states invest more money in K–12 education than in any other program. Parents often encourage their adult children to procreate, pregnancies are celebrated with baby showers, and births are marked with baptisms and other religious rites.

But there is another side to the family-oriented ethic in the United States. When it comes to the desire of infertile persons to have children, health care funding policy, legal rules, and popular sentiments often are not very sympathetic. Infertile couples typically must rely on their own resources to procreate, without reimbursement by their health care insurance; the law may erect barriers to assisted reproductive services; and infertile couples may not find much concern for their plight from friends or even some family members.

In this chapter, I will illustrate the indifference of society to the needs of the infertile through the examples of in vitro fertilization (IVF), surrogate motherhood, and uterus transplantation.

INFERTILITY

....

Infertility is defined as occurring when a couple engages in unprotected intercourse for 1 year without being able to conceive a child, and it is estimated to affect 15%–20% of couples in the United States.[1] Although it often is thought that environmental factors or high-risk behaviors have increased the likelihood of infertility, that does not seem to be the case. Rather, there is greater awareness of the condition and therefore a greater likelihood that couples will seek treatment for their inability to reproduce and be diagnosed as infertile.[2] In addition, a person's chances of creating a pregnancy decline after age 25. Men and women at age 25 have twice the likelihood of conceiving a child in a particular month as men and women at age 35.[3] Thus, as many couples have postponed efforts to have children until their 30s or 40s, their likelihood of becoming pregnant has become less than if they tried to have children in their 20s.[4]

Infertility can result from a number of different abnormalities in the male or female reproductive system. For example, because of sexually transmitted disease, chemotherapy, mumps during adolescence, testicular injury, or other reasons, a man may produce low levels of sperm or the sperm may be dysfunctional. Women may have trouble ovulating, or their fallopian tubes may be scarred from infection and not allow passage of eggs from the ovaries to the uterus. Female infertility also may result from a ruptured appendix, abdominal or pelvic surgery, or endometriosis (uterine cells growing outside the uterus). In many cases, the cause of infertility is unknown.[5]

In Vitro Fertilization

A number of treatments are available for infertility. For example, if a woman does not have viable eggs, she can obtain eggs from a donor (really a seller). For women whose fertility is blocked by fallopian tube dysfunction, IVF is often successful. With IVF, doctors retrieve eggs from a woman after hormonal stimulation of the ovaries, fertilize the eggs with sperm in a petri dish, and transfer some of the embryos to the woman's uterus. The remaining embryos are frozen for future use.[6] Male infertility can be overcome much more easily today than in past decades. While sperm donation is still an important option, the development of intracytoplasmic sperm injection (ICSI) has made sperm donation less necessary. With ICSI, the doctor injects a single sperm into each of the women's eggs that have been retrieved as part of IVF, and men who produce even very low levels of functioning sperm can procreate with their partners.[7]

But treatment can be very expensive. Consider the financial realities facing an infertile couple in the United States that wants to have a baby through IVF. For just one cycle of IVF, the couple will have to pay $15,000–$25,000.[8] If the couple lived in France, Israel, Sweden, or a number of other countries, their health insurance would cover the costs of the procedure.[9] But in the United States, health insurance plans typically do not pay for the costs of IVF.[10] According to a 2013 survey of employers by the consulting firm Mercer, only 27% of large employers (those with 500 or more employees) provide coverage for IVF.[11] Moreover, even when coverage is provided, it often has strict coverage caps. The policy might reimburse costs only up to a maximum amount, or it might cover only a limited number of IVF cycles.[12] Coverage for employers with fewer than 500 employees is even more spartan. Health insurance plans might cover some infertility services, such as evaluation by a specialist, but the policies usually exclude coverage for IVF or other assisted reproductive technologies that can treat the infertility.[13]

My own health care coverage through Indiana University is typical. I have an Anthem preferred provider plan with a high deductible and health savings account, and the coverage is generally quite good (free preventive care; the same coverage for mental health problems and substance abuse as for heart disease, cancer, or other illnesses; and a $2,500 cap on out-of-pocket expenses for in-network services[14]). However, the plan does not cover IVF or other therapies for infertility, nor does it cover diagnostic testing or prescription drugs for infertility.[15] Another Indiana University preferred provider plan with a $500 deductible and a $2,400 annual cap on out-of-pocket expenses has the same coverage exclusions for infertility treatment.[16]

Interestingly, coverage for abortion has been much more common than coverage for infertility treatments. In a survey of private health insurance plans in Washington State, researchers estimated the percentage of enrollees aged 15–44 years who were covered for various reproductive services. They projected that only 2% of enrollees were covered for infertility services while 47% of female enrollees were covered for elective abortion.[17] Moreover, none of the plans that covered infertility services included coverage of IVF or other assisted reproductive technologies. Coverage for reversible contraception exceeds coverage for abortion. Even before the Affordable Care Act imposed a contraceptive insurance mandate, a high percentage of health insurers provided coverage. A national study in 2002 found that 89% of plans included reimbursement for contraception.[18]

It also is useful to compare coverage of infertility treatments with coverage for other medical needs. Some scholars question whether it makes sense to view IVF and other methods of assisted reproduction as medical treatments since they bypass rather than correct the causes of infertility.[19] IVF may help an infertile couple have a child, but it does not address the reasons for the infertility. According to this argument, insurance coverage should be available for treatments like antibiotics that eliminate the underlying problem but not for treatments that leave the underlying cause alone.

But as other scholars have observed, many medical treatments restore lost function without correcting the underlying problem, as when insulin is prescribed for diabetes.[20] Moreover, it turns out that coverage for infertility pales even when compared with coverage for medical equipment or devices that compensate for a disability such as paraplegia or amputation without correcting the underlying cause of the disability. My insurance plan is typical. Although it provides no coverage for IVF or other infertility treatments, it covers 80% of the costs of medical equipment and devices, once the deductible is satisfied. After a person's out-of-pocket spending for all medical treatment reaches $2,500 for the year, the plan picks up 100% of the costs of medical equipment and devices.[21]

Advocates for infertility treatment coverage have had some success in getting legislation passed to support their cause.[22] Thirteen states mandate insurance coverage for infertility treatments,[23] and two states require that coverage be offered.[24]

However, even when legislation exists, it may not provide much help. California, Louisiana, and New York expressly exclude IVF from the mandate to cover or to offer coverage,[25] and Hawaii's mandate provides a "one-time-only benefit" for married couples using their own sperm and eggs and only if their infertility is associated with endometriosis, exposure in utero to DES, blockage or surgical removal of one or both fallopian tubes, or abnormal male factors contributing to infertility.[26] Moreover, the Employee Retirement Income Security Act of 1974 (ERISA) overrides the infertility coverage mandates as part of its general preemption of state insurance mandates when an employer self-insures for employee health care insurance,[27] and the Affordable Care Act does not include infertility treatments in its package of essential benefits that health insurers must provide.

The limited success with efforts to pass legislative mandates for infertility coverage contrasts with efforts to require coverage when people want to evade parenting. More than half of the states require private insurers to cover contraceptive services, and the Affordable Care Act now requires most insurers to cover contraceptive services with no sharing of costs by the user of the services.[28]

Can one defend the absence of coverage for IVF or other treatments by pointing to costs and benefits? Some critics have cited high costs and poor results of IVF. While it is true that an average IVF cycle costs between $15,000 and 25,000, that many couples will need multiple cycles of IVF before they give birth to a child, and that many other couples will never reproduce with IVF, the success rates have risen considerably, and the costs are actually quite manageable.

Although IVF resulted in live births at a low rate in the past,[29] its effectiveness is much improved. According to data from 2011, a live birth resulted from 29% of IVF cycles using fresh embryos, with women under 35 giving birth about 46% of the time.[30]

Data from Massachusetts indicate that IVF coverage is an affordable component of health care insurance policies. In 1987, Massachusetts enacted a mandate for coverage of infertility services, including IVF, and researchers examined the impact on insurance premiums from the mandate. The researchers found that premiums increased by about four-tenths of a percent to cover infertility services.[31]

Experience in other countries also illustrates the affordability of coverage for IVF. France provides full coverage for IVF,[32] and Israel also has shown that IVF can be covered with a much smaller budget for health care. In Israel, the national health service covers IVF (and other assisted reproductive services) for all women up to age 45 until a woman has had two children with her current partner. Moreover, the two-children limit is not strictly applied in practice, and women can still receive substantial funding for treatment to have more than two children.[33]

More important, if the absence of coverage for IVF were simply a matter of costs, then one would expect that insurers would cover the costs of artificial insemination, which are quite low. But while it is covered more often than IVF, it still is not typically covered either.

Upon close examination, then, the claims that infertility treatments cost too much money do not seem persuasive. However, the existence of such claims is consistent with a societal indifference to the problem of infertility. If the public does not view childlessness as a significant loss, then it will not support even modest expenditures to foster procreation among the infertile. Indeed, this is the whole point of a cost argument. The cost argument against IVF coverage essentially boils down to the sentiment that helping people have children has little value. As a result, infertile persons are unable to secure support when it comes to having a key health care need met.

Funding for IVF may be unavailable, but couples are not prohibited from using their own dollars for the treatment. With surrogacy and uterus transplants, however, there has been considerable opposition to the practices entirely.

Surrogate Motherhood

When Mary Beth Whitehead decided to maintain her maternal relationship after agreeing to serve as a surrogate mother for Elizabeth and William Stern, the ensuing litigation resulted in a landmark decision by the New Jersey Supreme Court[34] and much commentary about the propriety of surrogate motherhood.

Surrogacy of any kind can be controversial, but it is especially so when the surrogate mother not only carries the pregnancy to term but also is the genetic mother ("traditional surrogacy"). In such cases, the surrogate is impregnated with the father's sperm—or that of a sperm donor—and the resulting embryo is a combination of the sperm and the surrogate's egg. To many observers, traditional surrogacy seems like baby selling.[35]

As a result, legal limitations on traditional surrogacy are common. In a number of states, paid traditional surrogacy is prohibited, sometimes with penalties for participation.[36] In other states, traditional surrogacy contracts are not prohibited, but they also are not enforceable. If the surrogate wants to claim her parental status, she may do so.[37]

In contrast, a number of states permit and enforce contracts for "gestational surrogacy," in which the surrogate carries the pregnancy but does not have a genetic relationship with the child.[38] In gestational surrogacy, an embryo is created via IVF with an egg from the intended mother or an egg donor rather than from the surrogate. Still, even though gestational surrogacy is permitted in many states, it is prohibited in other states.[39]

To be sure, the use of surrogate motherhood raises more complicated questions than does the use of IVF or other assisted reproduction services. When a couple has a child through IVF after supplying the sperm and eggs and having the pregnancy carried by the female partner, no one else can claim parental status. In surrogacy, on the other hand, more than one woman has served a maternal role, and competing parental claims can emerge. In Mary Beth Whitehead's case, for example, she was the genetic mother and the gestational mother of the child, and many observers believed she should be able to assert her parental status even though she had agreed to relinquish her parental rights in favor of Elizabeth Stern, the intended mother. Hence, opposition to surrogacy reflects in large part concerns about the interests of the surrogate.

Nevertheless, there also is good reason to believe that opposition to surrogacy also reflects a discounting of the interests of the infertile couple that has retained the surrogate. For example, philosophy professor Elizabeth Anderson has criticized surrogacy[40]—and argued that it should be prohibited when performed for pay[41]—on the ground that commercial surrogacy degrades and exploits the surrogate.[42] Anderson's objections to surrogacy are important and provide good reasons to question a role for commercial surrogacy. Yet in an article that runs more than 20 pages, Anderson devotes roughly a paragraph to the concerns of the infertile couples that would like to retain a surrogate. She observes that "the option of adoption is still available" and that opportunities for adoption should be increased for couples who might be disqualified because of age or other standard adoption eligibility rules.[43] Anderson also suggests that racist and eugenic motivations may drive the interest in surrogacy—surrogacy allows couples to have healthy, White infants when "there is no shortage of children of other races" or of "older and handicapped children who desperately need to be adopted."[44]

But as philosophy professor Heidi Malm has observed, we do not expect fertile couples to forgo biological parenting in favor of adoption.[45] We also do not suggest that the desire of fertile couples to have genetically related children reflects racist or eugenic motivations.

Law professor Margaret Radin writes less critically of the interest in surrogacy among infertile couples, coming to a rejection of paid surrogacy more tentatively. But she is rather dismissive of the interest among infertile couples and potential surrogates in the practice of surrogacy. Radin observes that "some surrogates *believe* their actions to be altruistic" and that "people *seem to believe* that they need genetic offspring in order to fulfill themselves."[46]

While it is admirable when people are willing to adopt children who currently lack a family, there are very good reasons why people desire biologically related offspring. To some extent, the desire for a genetic connection reflects an interest in preserving one's family line, to extend the legacy of one's parents and other ancestors. There are more practical considerations as well. Adopted children may suffer from significant developmental problems that would not be detected before the adoption. In addition, people care very much whom they include in their families, whether through marriage or other relationships, and that is no less true for parenting relationships.[47] Spouses may want to have children only with their chosen partners and without involving other people in the parenting process. Adoption entails parenting with two other people, typically strangers, and that greatly interferes with the ability of individuals to shape their most intimate relationships between their partners and themselves. Suggesting that infertile couples can simply adopt gives inadequate consideration to their interests in a biological relationship with their children.

The debates over surrogacy illustrate in another way the sense that the infertile couple's interests are given insufficient consideration. Opposition to surrogacy in large part reflects the view that the surrogate's interests in maintaining her relationship with the child outweigh the couple's interests in assuming full parenthood.[48] Yet much of the concern about the surrogate's interests is not substantiated by the empirical evidence.

To be sure, the data are not definitive. More research needs to be done. But the data to data are consistently reassuring. While an occasional surrogate, such as Mary Beth

Whitehead, is psychologically devastated at the prospect of relinquishing her parent–child relationship, almost all surrogates are comfortable with their roles. In one study of 34 surrogates, all of them were happy about their decision to serve as a surrogate, and none had any doubts about the decision to hand over the child to the couple or difficulties with the handover.[49] Over the next year, a few experienced difficulties with their surrogate role, but at the end of the year, only two had some difficulties, and those were minor in nature (i.e., "the surrogate mother described having been or being upset but believed that the feelings were short term").[50] The typical surrogate is motivated in large part by the desire to help the infertile couple have a child,[51] and she generally maintains a psychological distance from her fetus and does not form close bonds with it.[52] Thus, it is the unusual surrogacy arrangement that leads to litigation. According to one commonly cited estimate, less than one-tenth of 1% of surrogacy cases lead to court battles.[53]

Critics of surrogacy also have worried that infertile couples will exploit the economic insecurity of poor women, who will be induced to serve as surrogates because of their financial desperation.[54] But as other observers have pointed out, infertile couples would likely not want to share parenting with impoverished women,[55] and empirical studies find that while surrogates are not wealthy, they come from stable, working-class homes that earn modest incomes.[56] The data do not indicate that surrogates are pressured into their roles because of financial difficulties.[57]

In short, characterizations of surrogacy often misjudge the balance between the competing interests, giving too little weight to the couple's interests and therefore making it too easy for those interests to be trumped by the surrogate's interests.

For many infertile couples, there is no alternative to involving other women in their efforts to procreate. Surrogacy will continue to play an important role in procreation even if only in some states and even if primarily in the form of gestational surrogacy.[58]

For some infertile couples, however, recent developments in organ transplantation may overcome the obstacles facing women who are infertile because they do not have sufficient uterine function to carry a pregnancy. Uterus transplants may save these women the need to resort to gestational surrogacy. But there is opposition to the possibility.

Uterus Transplants

The procedure of uterus transplantation is still in its infancy. Only a handful of uterus transplants have been reported worldwide, including nine in Sweden, one in Turkey, and one in Saudi Arabia,[59] and the first birth did not occur until October 2014,[60] but advances in technique and assurances about safety may make the transplants available more widely. Some women are born without a functioning uterus; others have hysterectomies for cancer, postpartum hemorrhage, or other reasons. Many of these women want to become mothers and carry their own pregnancies.

However, the prospect of uterus transplantation has elicited sharp criticism. According to philosophy professor Rebecca Kukla, the surgery is not, "in any traditional sense, therapeutic."[61] But surgeons routinely transplant hearts, lungs, livers, and kidneys. If a woman can receive a new kidney, why not a new uterus? Ethicists have raised a number of objections. On close examination, none seems persuasive.

Some scholars have distinguished life-extending organs from life-enhancing body parts such as faces and hands. As long as transplant recipients have their new organs, they must take drugs to prevent their immune systems from rejecting the transplanted organs. The risks can be substantial. For example, the immunosuppressive drugs put people at an increased risk of cancer. While it often makes sense to assume serious health risks for the possibility of a longer life, does it make sense to assume the risks of organ transplantation to realize improvements in the *quality* of life?[62]

We always should worry about risks from novel treatments, but the risks seem quite tolerable for uterus transplantation. Over time, scientific advances have reduced the side effects from immunosuppression. The risks are not as serious as they used to be. In addition, a transplanted uterus can be removed after childbirth, avoiding the need for long-term immunosuppression that exists with other kinds of transplants. Finally, we generally allow patients to weigh the benefits and risks of medical treatment for themselves. Absent a disproportionate balance between risks and benefits, it is not appropriate for society to usurp health care decision making from patients. Hence, face and hand transplants are becoming more common, even though they do not prolong life.[63]

Critics of uterus transplants also worry about the health risks to others. Perhaps women can weigh for themselves whether the benefits of uterus transplantation outweigh the risks. But they are not the only people whose health might be jeopardized. If a woman is taking immunosuppressive drugs during her pregnancy, there may be serious risks to the child-to-be.[64]

Although no woman has yet given birth after a uterus transplant, we still have some important evidence regarding the risks to fetuses from immunosuppressive drugs. Recipients of kidneys, livers, and other organs take the same immunosuppressive drugs as would recipients of a uterus transplant, and more than 15,000 children have been born to transplant recipients since the 1950s.

Though not definitive, the data are generally reassuring. While children exposed to immunosuppressive drugs during pregnancy are more likely to have a premature birth and low birth weight, they do not appear to be at elevated risk of physical malformations or other serious side effects.[65] Moreover, it is generally difficult to argue that people should not reproduce because of the health risks to their offspring. Procreation is a right of fundamental importance and should be recognized for all persons, even if they may pass a serious disease to their children. Thus, for example, it is acceptable for women to reproduce when they are infected with HIV or carry the gene for a severe inherited disorder.

Of course, steps often can be taken to minimize the risk that an infectious or genetic disease will be transmitted from women to child, but risks often remain, and the right to reproduce is preserved nevertheless.

Still, there may be an important difference between women with uterus transplants and women with an infectious or genetic disease. These other women often cannot have genetically related children without exposing their children to their health risks. The woman wanting a uterus transplant can have genetically related children by creating embryos with her partner through IVF and then arranging with another woman to serve as a gestational surrogate for the pregnancy. Thus, the women can have genetic ties to their children and also protect them from exposure to immunosuppressive drugs. As Kukla has observed, "tons of people have perfectly normal lives without gestating a biological child."[66]

While many women may be perfectly happy parenting children without going through pregnancy, that should not lead us to dismiss the interests of those women who very much want to become mothers after pregnancy. Indeed, there are serious disadvantages if a woman lacking a functioning uterus tries to have children without a transplant.

Adoption allows for parenting, but as discussed earlier, it comes without a biological connection between mother and child. In addition, adopted children may suffer from undetected health problems.

Gestational surrogacy can ensure a genetic relationship with children, but it has serious drawbacks, too. As discussed, in some states, it is prohibited by law. In addition, the genetic mother loses the ability to develop gestational ties with her child. As illustrated by the disputes over parental rights between surrogates and intended mothers,[67] gestational ties play a significant role in forming motherhood. Some gestational surrogates come to view themselves as the child's mother, just as a woman who delivers a child with a donated egg comes to see herself as the child's mother. Genetic and gestational ties both can be important in the development of the mother–child relationship. Hence, for many women, becoming a parent without carrying the fetus during pregnancy will leave a significant void.

To be sure, the uterus transplant recipient will not experience pregnancy in the same way as other women. Pelvic nerve connections cannot be restored during uterus transplantation, so the recipient will have different sensations.[68] But women generally vary in the way they experience pregnancy, and many aspects of pregnancy do not depend on the pelvic nerves.[69]

Gestational surrogacy—and indeed all alternatives to uterus transplants—require the intended mother to share her parenthood with another woman, who typically will be a stranger to the intended mother's family. As discussed earlier, people have strong interests in having children only with their chosen partners and without involving other women in the parenting process.

If the arguments against uterus transplants seem weak, we should consider whether other factors are at work. What else might explain the objections to uterus transplants? To some extent, the opposition may reflect the usual tendency for new forms of assisted reproduction to provoke concern. People worried much more about artificial insemination and IVF when they were first introduced than they do today.[70] But there probably is another important factor at work. As indicated in the cases of IVF and surrogacy, society appears to discount the interests of infertile couples in having children. I explore this phenomenon in greater depth in the next section.

SOCIETY AND THE INTERESTS
OF THE INFERTILE

Public policy in the United States gives insufficient attention to the interests of infertile persons because infertility does not seem to be viewed as a serious enough problem. Rather than viewing infertility as a significant disability and infertile persons as deserving assistance in their efforts to procreate, many Americans dismiss the idea that infertility is disabling.

To be sure, as discussed later, the law will protect infertile people from some forms of discrimination. For example, if an employer refused to hire an infertile person, the Americans With Disabilities Act (ADA) would make the employer's refusal unlawful. But that is not the kind of discrimination that infertile persons face.[71] Rather, they face barriers to receiving medical treatment that will overcome their infertility, barriers that people with other medical problems do not face. And these barriers reflect a common view that being infertile is not really disabling.

There is much evidence for the view that people do not see infertility as really disabling in the way emphysema, heart disease, paraplegia, or blindness is seen as disabling, that fertile persons frequently dismiss the idea that infertility is a significant problem. Before discussing the evidence, I will explain why infertility is a disability.

Infertility Is a Disability

"Disability" refers to the existence of substantial limitations on a person's "major life activities."[72] Major life activities include functions like seeing, hearing, walking, speaking, learning, and working.[73] Commonly, disability is caused by an impairment, which is defined as a "physical or mental anomaly."[74] If a person has the impairment of paralyzed legs, then the person is disabled with respect to the major life activity of walking. A person with the impairment of advanced emphysema may be disabled with respect to the major life activities of walking or working.

Infertile persons generally meet the definition of a disability because they have an impairment of their reproductive tracts that substantially limits the major life activity of procreation. Having children is an interest of fundamental importance to many people; for many people, it is the most important endeavor they undertake in their lives. Indeed, it would be odd to identify working at a job as a major life activity but not similarly recognize bearing and raising children as a major life activity. Because of the central role that reproduction plays in the lives of so many individuals, the Supreme Court has held both that procreation is a constitutionally protected right[75] and that reproduction is a major life activity.[76]

To be sure, some would argue that infertility is an inevitable result of aging and therefore represents a natural state, not a disabling condition. But many infertile persons are of normal childbearing age and have lost their reproductive capacity through illness or injury. Moreover, many well-recognized disabilities, including osteoporosis, are a common result of aging.[77] If we are willing to provide hip replacements for seniors with reduced bone density to overcome their disabilities, we also should be willing to provide treatments to people with infertility to overcome that disability.[78]

Infertility has psychological, as well as physical, implications—the emotional impact of infertility can be substantial, particularly for women. For people who want to reproduce, but cannot, the loss can be devastating.[79] In one study, nearly half of the women in an infertility treatment program reported that their infertility was the most upsetting experience of their lives.[80] In another study, participants were asked to rate their most stressful experiences, and infertility rated as high as the death of a spouse or child.[81] And when infertility is a consequence of cancer or its treatment, some cancer survivors describe the loss of fertility as causing as much emotional pain as the cancer itself.[82] As one woman who had been diagnosed with Hodgkin's lymphoma said, "When I was first diagnosed with cancer, my friends couldn't believe how well I took the news. But the one fear that continued to haunt me was the thought that I might become infertile."[83]

Infertility Is not Seen as Disabling

Despite the disabling nature of infertility, it often is not seen as disabling. Studies of infertile couples by academic scholars are illustrative. For example, in her research on infertility, Elizabeth Britt found that "the infertile often feel as if the seriousness of their condition is trivialized." Disclosure of infertility might elicit "jokes about the couple not knowing how to have sex or about the fun the couple must be having trying to conceive a child." Other people "might suggest that infertility is a blessing in disguise" or that it is not as bad as other medical conditions since reproduction "supposedly is so optional." Or they might say something like "Oh well, so what, so you don't have to have a baby, so what, just adopt."[84]

Margarete Sandelowski found that infertility "is too often dismissed as an unfortunate physical impairment, but one perfectly compatible with good health and life." An infertile woman might be reminded that there are far worse problems, and be told by relatives that "'At least you've got a nice husband and a nice house and plenty of food. . . . At least you don't have cancer.'"[85] Couples in her study of infertility "complained that infertility was not viewed as a 'serious disease' worthy of the resources people afflicted with other diseases can get."[86]

Similarly, Arthur Greil found from his interviews with infertile couples that they criticized fertile people for "treating the plight of the infertile as if trivial and inconsequential."[87] The infertile also were troubled that fertile individuals "acted as if . . . infertility were a small and relatively easy problem to solve."[88] As one woman reported, her friends might say, "'Why don't you go on a cruise?' Or 'Why don't you just relax? And then you'll get pregnant.'"[89] According to Greil, infertile couples do not feel like they are viewed as inferior because of their infertility. Rather, the discrimination they feel arises out of a "failure of others to acknowledge the seriousness of infertility."[90] In one typical remark, an infertile person observed, "I think [fertile people] discriminate by making light of the problem."[91]

Discussion of IVF by legal and other scholars also indicates that infertility may not be seen as a real disability. In the constitutional context, law professors Carl Coleman and Radhika Rao have considered whether a ban on access to IVF or other infertility treatments would violate an infertile couple's constitutional right to procreate. Both of them quickly dismiss the interests of infertile couples in constitutional protection and conclude that restrictions on access to infertility treatments would be constitutionally valid.[92] In his analysis, Coleman observes that the Constitution cannot protect every interest that people assert as deeply important to them and gives the smoking of marijuana as an example of an asserted interest that should not be given constitutional protection.[93] The idea that the desire to have children and the desire to smoke marijuana are comparable is troubling.

Or consider an argument against IVF that biology professor Ruth Hubbard articulated in the early days of assisted reproduction. In response to the view that women have a right to bear children, Hubbard wrote that it "had never occurred to [her] that every woman has a right to bear a baby any more than that every woman has a 'right' to a 34 inch bustline or a 24 inch waist."[94] Hubbard went on to acknowledge that many women genuinely suffer from their inability to have children but that the answer is not to provide IVF, which she viewed "to be a path to disaster," but to engage in "strong, deep, feminist, consciousness raising."[95] Anthropology professor Eric Hirsch reported a similar perspective from a British woman who participated in his discussions of assisted reproduction. As Hirsch described it, the woman worried that "children just become the next thing in the long list of material possessions one is supposed to have." Or as the woman put it, "it's like you get a car, a dishwasher and then a dog and then you think what next."[96] The view that infertile couples are selfish and materialistic is a common one.[97]

Some scholars are even harsher in their critiques of women who pursue assisted reproductive technologies. A number of feminist writers have rejected the possibility that an infertile woman's desire to reproduce reflects a genuine expression of autonomy and instead attributed the desire to "nothing more than the result of the patriarchal mandate that she reproduce."[98] Not only do these scholars deny the authenticity of the infertile woman's desire to procreate, they also portray her efforts to reproduce as harmful to other, poorer women—when the privileged woman undertakes expensive assisted reproduction treatments, she depletes resources that could be used to meet basic health care needs of underprivileged women.[99] Moreover, it is argued, infertile women are racist, eugenic, and selfish when they exhibit a preference for a White, biologically related infant over an orphaned, older, minority child—even though fertile couples exhibit the same preferences.[100]

In the tax context, legal academics have debated the question whether expenses for fertility treatments are deductible as medical expenses. In her analysis of the issue, Katherine Pratt described an exchange among tax specialists on a law professors' listserv. One leading expert argued against the deductibility of fertility treatment costs on the ground that reproductive dysfunction does "not involve the sort of catastrophic losses that justify a medical expense deduction."[101] But the costs of prescription drugs for diabetes and high blood pressure are deductible, even though there is no catastrophic loss involved. Another leading expert rejected the deductibility of fertility treatment costs on the ground that the treatments do not constitute health care. Rather, in his view, reproduction is an optional activity, a lifestyle choice.[102]

In short, public attitudes toward infertile couples and views of academic writers indicate that infertility often is not seen as a disabling condition in the United States.

Infertility May Even Be Seen as Enabling

Moreover, in the view of many people, the infertile person is better off than the fertile person. Having children, it is said, places one at a disadvantage when it comes to opportunities for a fulfilling life, whether in the professional world or with one's partner. In Elaine Tyler May's study of childless persons in the United States, she recounts a number of representative comments. According to one voluntarily childless woman, she and her husband chose not to have children because "we like the freedom." And she prefers to call herself "child-free" rather than "childless" because child-free suggests the absence of something undesirable.[103] Another woman said that she and her husband did not care to have children interfere in their relationship. A man reported that he "simply did not want the troubles and commitment associated with raising children."[104] While some voluntarily childless couples explain their decision in terms of a desire to devote more time to careers or civic endeavors, it is far more common for the voluntarily childless to talk about their preference for a private life without children over a private life with children. A private life without children allows them more time with their partner for love, intimacy, and enjoyable pursuits.[105]

In a British study, common reasons given by persons who were certain that they did not want children include the increased and permanent responsibility that parenthood entails, the sacrifice of spontaneity and freedom that goes along with the increased responsibility, and the greater opportunities for self-fulfillment without children.[106] Representative comments from that study include a man citing the advantages of a freer schedule and the time that he could spend enjoying his wife's company. A woman spoke of the independence she enjoyed and the freedom from the constraints of parenthood.[107]

There are many social practices that reflect a less than enthusiastic view of children in society. Consider this excerpt from *Sex and Destiny:*

> At the heart of our insistence upon the child's parasitic role in the family lurks the conviction that children must be banished from adult society. . . . The heinousness of taking an infant or a toddler to an adult social gathering is practically unimaginable. . . . Restaurants, cinemas, offices, supermarkets, even Harrods auction rooms, are all no places for children. In England, restaurants mentioned in *The Good Food Guide* boldly advise parents to "leave under-fourteens and dogs at home."[108]

Scholars who write on reproductive issues reflect the increasingly prevalent sense that a life without children may be preferable to a life with children. Consider, for example, the vision of parenting of law professor Jed Rubenfeld in his discussion of why the right to privacy should invalidate laws that prohibit abortion:

> For a period of months and quite possibly years, . . . motherhood shapes women's occupations and preoccupations in the minutest detail; it creates a perceived identity for women and confines them to it; and it gathers up a multiplicity of approaches to the problem of being a woman and reduces them all to the single norm of motherhood.[109]

Rubenfeld also worries that becoming a mother directs women into "singular, normalized" lives that are "rigidly directed."[110]

But parents commonly believe their lives have been greatly enriched by their children and that parenting expands their options in life. As one friend and single mother said to me, "My child gives me a purpose in life, something that is lacking in the lives of my single friends who don't have children." Oddly, Rubenfeld considers it a greater constitutional concern if the state were to ban abortion than if the state were to prohibit parents from having more than two children.[111]

Janice Raymond warns of the dangers of technological advances that allow infertile women to have children. Raymond writes, "[n]ew reproductive arrangements are presented as a woman's private choice. But they are publicly sanctioned violence against women."[112] Raymond also says this about IVF: "Represented as expanding women's choices, IVF technology, for example, actually narrows the life choices of women who consume the technology."[113]

The point is not that Rubenfeld and Raymond raise insignificant issues. Rather, the concern is that they worry more about the consequences of encouraging parenting than the consequences of discouraging parenting. For Rubenfeld, it is worse to deny the option of abortion than to deny the option of procreation. Raymond sees more danger to women in giving them the opportunity to procreate when infertile than in withholding new reproductive options.

All of this is not to suggest that infertility is never felt or seen by others as disabling. Indeed, studies have found that infertile persons often experience a sense of stigma from their infertility.[114] This is particularly the case for persons from cultural backgrounds that highly value procreation. And there are articles and books in both popular and academic publications that praise assisted reproduction for infertile persons.[115] Nevertheless, childlessness does not provoke the levels of social disadvantage that it once did or that other disabilities currently do.

And public attitudes have changed most for people of higher education and greater wealth,[116] arguably people with more influence in shaping public policy. Indeed, past changes in attitude about family and procreation have been driven by a small part of the population. In the nineteenth century, the newly developing urban middle class led the way in the decline of fertility rates.[117]

If infertility has become a condition that is viewed by many as not disabling, and even enabling, we might expect those sentiments to be reflected in legal doctrine. That is the case. Although some law recognizes the disabling nature of infertility, infertile persons generally do not enjoy much protection under the law. For the most part, public policy does not reflect the view that infertility is a meaningful disability.

INFERTILITY AND THE FAILURE
OF ANTIDISCRIMINATION LAW

The Law's Recognition of Infertility as a Disability

The U.S. Supreme Court recognized in the case of *Bragdon v. Abbott* that the inability to reproduce can count as a disability and therefore trigger the protections of the Americans With Disabilities Act of 1990 (ADA).[118] However, the extent of protection is quite limited. Indeed, in *Bragdon*, Sidney Abbott invoked the ADA because of discrimination that resulted from her HIV infection rather than from her compromised ability to reproduce.[119]

Under *Bragdon*, the ADA appears to protect infertile persons from denials of health care under the ADA. If a doctor refused to dialyze or operate on a patient because of the patient's infertility, the patient could seek redress under the ADA.

But the main discrimination that infertile persons face in the health care system does not involve denials of treatment for kidney disease, heart disease, or cancer. Rather, as discussed earlier, the infertile generally cannot obtain coverage for the costs of medical treatments that allow them to overcome their infertility and reproduce—unlike persons with other disabling conditions like heart disease, arthritis, emphysema, or paraplegia who enjoy recourse to health care insurance when they need medical services. For the most part, infertile persons are uninsured for the costs of having children. And, as the next section indicates, the ADA offers no help in remedying this differential treatment by health care insurers.[120]

The Law's Insufficient Protection for the Infertile

Even though *Bragdon* held that infertility is a disability under the ADA, judges have concluded that insurers do not violate the ADA when they fail to cover the costs of treatments for infertility. According to the courts, there is no discrimination on the basis of disability since coverage is denied for all persons, not just for persons who are disabled.[121]

Saks v. Franklin Covey[122] is illustrative. In that case, Rochelle Saks received health insurance benefits through her employer, the Franklin Covey Co. Because of infertility,

Ms. Saks underwent numerous tests and tried various drugs and procedures to become pregnant, including intrauterine insemination (IUI) and IVF. When Franklin Covey refused to cover the costs of her infertility care, Ms. Saks sued under the ADA to recover those costs,[123] and the district court found no ADA violation. The court observed that the insurance plan treated all employees the same. Franklin Covey did not provide less fertility-related benefits to infertile workers than it did to fertile workers. The court then cited decisions by federal courts of appeals, according to which "insurance distinctions that apply equally to all insured employees do not discriminate on the basis of disability."[124]

Although the *Saks* court gave the impression that its hands were tied and that it could not find discrimination under the ADA, the law was uncertain enough that the court could have found discrimination on the basis of disability. The precedents cited by the court involved cases in which insurance plans provided higher coverage for some disabilities than for other disabilities. But the Supreme Court had earlier drawn a distinction under disability law between providing no coverage and a meaningful level of coverage. In *Alexander v. Choate*, the Court upheld Tennessee's cap on hospital coverage of 14 days per year, even though it disfavored persons with disabilities, on the ground that the disabled still had meaningful access to hospital coverage.[125] The *Saks* court could have distinguished the differential treatment of fertile and infertile persons in its case from the differential treatment in other cases on the ground that persons claiming discrimination in the other cases still had meaningful access to coverage from their employers, while infertile persons employed at Franklin Covey had no access to treatment for their infertility.[126]

To be sure, even if the *Saks* court had concluded that Franklin Covey discriminated against infertile persons, it had other bases for rejecting Ms. Saks' claims. The ADA includes two exemptions from its provisions for insurers. First, the ADA does not limit the ability of an employer to establish and administer its own health care plan that is exempt from state regulation under the Employee Retirement Income Security Act of 1974 (ERISA).[127] Since Franklin Covey ran a self-insured health care plan, it was exempt from state regulation under ERISA; and since the company operated a bona fide plan, it also was not subject to the dictates of the ADA.[128]

In addition, even if Franklin Covey had not self-insured its employees, its health insurance plan would have enjoyed an exemption from the ADA. The act allows health insurers to employ their usual practices of classifying risks, as long as the practices are actuarially sound.[129] The ADA withdraws the protection of the insurance provisions when they are used as a subterfuge to escape the requirements of the Act, but Franklin Covey's exclusion of coverage for IUI and IVF preceded the enactment of the ADA.[130]

But whether the infertile lack protection from discrimination because of the way courts interpret the ADA or because of the way Congress wrote the ADA, the law does not ensure that the infertile are given adequate access to treatments for their infertility. Antidiscrimination law falls short when it comes to the needs of the infertile.

Some scholars have suggested that it may be appropriate for courts to deny claims of discrimination by infertile persons, that the infertile should not have recourse to the courts to protect themselves from discrimination in access to medical care for their infertility. In this view, it is not a problem that the law fails to help the infertile. Rather, principles of judicial review explain why antidiscrimination law should be reserved for other persons, those who belong to a stigmatized class.

The judicial review argument draws on the work of John Hart Ely and his important theory of judicial authority.[131] In this view, our governmental system relies primarily on the political process to resolve disputes and allocate benefits and burdens, with majority preferences being decisive. If courts were to intervene, judges would be substituting their own preferences for those of the majority, and that normally would entail an improper exercise of judicial power. But sometimes, the political process operates in an unfair manner. In particular, when the interests of a stigmatized minority are at stake, the majority is likely to disfavor the minority out of prejudice or other illegitimate motives and fail to give due recognition to the minority's interests. In such circumstances, courts should intervene. Judges ought to thwart the majority on behalf of a minority when the political process does not treat the minority fairly. On the other hand, when the political process gives a particular group a fair chance to advocate for its interests, then the group is not entitled to a judicial rescue simply because it lost in the political process.

Under this view of the role of courts, write Carl Coleman and Radhika Rao, the infertile do not quality for judicial protection. The infertile enjoy sufficient influence in the political process. People using fertility treatments are disproportionately White and wealthy, and they are able to mobilize the support of other influential interest groups, such as the medical community and the pharmaceutical industry to avoid unfair treatment by legislatures.[132]

While initially appealing, the judicial review argument ultimately fails. As Rao recognizes, infertility crosses racial and economic lines.[133] In fact, Blacks and other minorities are more likely than Whites, and the poor are more likely than the wealthy, to be infertile.[134] Moreover, while Coleman and Rao observe that the users of infertility treatments are overwhelmingly White and wealthy, that simply reflects the fact that discrimination against the infertile has its biggest impact on minority and poor persons who often cannot afford the high costs of fertility treatments. As a number of scholars have argued, this disparate impact may be intentional—the denial of insurance coverage for infertility treatments may reflect a social sentiment against reproduction by Blacks, the poor, and other disfavored minorities. In other words, eugenic motivations likely play an important role in shaping public policy on treatment for infertility, as they have historically.[135] Reproductive policies in the United States have long favored procreation by Whites and wealthier persons and disfavored procreation by minorities and poor individuals.[136] When health care insurance does not cover infertility treatments and couples (or individuals) must pay out-of-pocket for the treatments, then the significant costs of those treatments mean that the treatments tend to be reserved for wealthier, White couples who can fund their treatments out of personal resources.[137]

Costs are not the only factor in explaining higher use of infertility treatments by Whites. Minorities often feel more stigmatized by their infertility and may be less willing to identify themselves as infertile and seek treatment for it, minorities are more likely to distrust the health care system because of past racist experiences, and White physicians may be less likely to recommend assisted reproductive technologies for infertile Black patients.[138] Nevertheless, the financial barriers are important and a useful strategy for limiting access to care.

Most fundamentally, the judicial review argument is not persuasive because it does not account for discrimination on the basis of societal indifference. When the majority does not view a group's interests as important, the group will not fare well in the political process.

The Deficiencies of Antidiscrimination Theory

It is not surprising that antidiscrimination law would fall short when it comes to infertility. Antidiscrimination law rests heavily on an "anticaste" principle that does not take into account the kind of discrimination faced by the infertile.

The anticaste principle reflects the view that a key justification for antidiscrimination law lies in the desire to maintain a truly egalitarian society, one that is free of classes of persons who are relegated to a second-class level of citizenship. The principle animates leading Supreme Court decisions regarding discrimination, dating as far back as the Court's first case interpreting the Fourteenth Amendment's application to claims of discrimination on the basis of race. In *Strauder v. West Virginia*, the Court considered a challenge to a state law disqualifying Blacks from eligibility to serve on juries.[139] A unanimous Court struck down the disqualification, writing that the Fourteenth Amendment provides protection to Blacks "from legal discriminations, implying inferiority in civil society" and those "discriminations which are steps towards reducing [Blacks] to the condition of a subject race."[140]

More recent Court decisions regarding discrimination on the basis of race, gender, or sexual orientation have reinforced the law's anticaste principle. In *Brown v. Board of Education*, the Court found "separate but equal" public school education unconstitutional because it "generates a feeling of inferiority as to [children's] status in the community that may affect their hearts and minds in a way unlikely ever to be undone."[141] Similarly, in *Frontiero v. Richardson*, the Court worried about "statutory distinctions ... [that] often have the effect of invidiously relegating the entire class of females to inferior legal status."[142] And in *U.S. v. Windsor*, the Court struck down the federal Defense of Marriage Act because it imposed "a disadvantage, a separate status, and so a stigma upon all" who were validly married under state law and gave them "second-class marriages."[143]

Just as the anticaste principle explains antidiscrimination law in the context of race, gender, or sexual orientation, so does it explain legal protection from discrimination on the basis of disability. Indeed, the legislative history of the ADA emphasizes the need to overcome the second-class status that persons with disabilities endure. According to the Congress that adopted the ADA, for example, "studies have documented that people with disabilities, as a group, occupy an inferior status in our society."[144] Congress also found that persons with disabilities have been "relegated to a position of political powerlessness in our society."[145]

The anticaste principle reaches many forms of societal bias, but it does not reach the bias that results from societal indifference. Infertile persons do not suffer from a second-class citizenship in the way that Blacks, women, and other disfavored groups once did. Hence, the infertile have not been successful when invoking antidiscrimination law to ensure adequate access to treatments for their infertility.

Does Indifference to Infertility Reflect Invidious Bias?

Although indifference to the problem of infertility appears to be a key reason for societal disregard for the needs of infertile couples, it probably is not the exclusive basis. There may be an element of bias against infertile people on the ground that they could have had children when they were younger and that therefore they are responsible for their predicament.[146] In this view, infertility reflects a person's life choices rather than a medical condition.[147] This would be analogous to the stigma that lung cancer patients face from others who blame the patients for having brought on their disease by smoking cigarettes.[148]

Still while blaming the infertile may be an element of the discrimination against them, it likely is a smaller part than the discrimination from indifference. Many infertile persons cannot conceive because of problems unrelated to their age. As discussed earlier, for example, women may become infertile because of scarring from a ruptured appendix, a pelvic infection, or endometriosis. In addition, IVF is much more common among younger women. More than 40% of IVF cycles occur in women age 35 years or younger, and more than 80% occur in women 40 years of age or younger.[149] If couples are being blamed for their infertility, one would expect such blame to be reserved for couples over age 40. Also, the previously discussed studies of infertile persons did not find that expressions of blame from others are prominent. Finally, if denial of coverage for infertility treatment were driven primarily by bias against couples that have delayed childbearing, then we would expect to see IVF covered until a specific age cutoff (whether 35, 40, or another age), just as Israel covers infertility treatments only until a woman reaches age 45.

CONCLUSION

Medical advances have done much to overcome the barriers to procreation from infertility. More and more couples are able to have genetically related children than in past generations. And in many ways, society supports efforts of the infertile to bear and raise children.

But infertile couples also face a significant societal indifference to their interests in having children. The absence of health insurance coverage may make some treatments, such as IVF, unaffordable, and legal prohibitions may limit access to other options, such as surrogacy. Public policy is much less responsive to the needs of the infertile than it is to the needs of people with other disabilities.

As a general matter, it is important to respect the needs of all persons, and especially so for fundamental interests, such as procreation. Society needs to reform its policies on treatments for infertility to ensure that the needs of the infertile are fairly met.

Acknowledgments

This chapter builds on themes developed in "Discrimination out of Dismissiveness: The Example of Infertility," *Indiana Law Journal* 85 (2010): 143–186, and "Toward Acceptance of Uterus Transplants," *Hastings Center Report* 42 (Nov–Dec 2012): 12–13. I am grateful for the comments of Leslie Francis. I also am grateful for the research assistance of Miriam Murphy.

Notes

1. Brian R. Winters and Thomas J. Walsh, "The Epidemiology of Male Infertility," *Urologic Clinics of North America* 41 (2014): 195–204, 197.
2. Kristin P. Wright and Julia V. Johnson, "Infertility," in *Danforth's Obstetrics and Gynecology*, 10th ed., ed. Ronald S. Gibbs et al. (Philadelphia: Lippincott Williams & Wilkins, 2008), 705. For example, data do not support the claim that environmental or other factors have caused a decline in sperm counts worldwide. Harry Fisch, "Declining Worldwide Sperm Counts: Disproving a Myth," *Urologic Clinics of North America* 35 (2008): 137–146. See also Harry Fisch and Stephen R. Braun, "Trends in Global Semen Parameter Values," *Asian Journal of Andrology* 15 (2013): 169–173, 172 (finding that eight studies "suggest a decline in semen parameters" while twenty-one "show either no change or an increase in semen parameters").
3. Adam H. Balen and Anthony J. Rutherford, "Management of Infertility," *British Medical Journal* 335 (2007): 608–611, 608.
4. Wright and Johnson, "Infertility," 705.
5. Wright and Johnson, "Infertility," 706.
6. Bradley J. Van Voorhis, "In Vitro Fertilization," *New England Journal of Medicine* 356 (2007): 379–386, 380. As with any medical intervention, IVF carries health risks, both for the mothers and their children. Ibid., 382–384.
7. Gianpiero Palermo et al., "Pregnancies After Intracytoplasmic Injection of Single Spermatozoon into an Oocyte," *Lancet* 340 (1992): 17–18. There are some concerns, however, that ICSI may raise the risks of abnormalities in the child. Sacha Lewis and Hillary Klonoff-Cohen, "What Factors Affect Intracytoplasmic Sperm Injection Outcomes," *Obstetrical and Gynecological Survey* 60 (2005): 111–123, 111. Data from Scandinavia suggest

a small increase in risk with ICSI compared to nonassisted reproduction, but similar risks compared to IVF. André Van Steirteghem, "Celebrating ICSI's Twentieth Anniversary and the Birth of More Than 2.5 Million Children—The 'How, Why, When and Where,'" *Human Reproduction* 27 (2012): 1–2, 2.

8. The chances of having a baby in a single cycle are close to 30% in the United States, with younger women having greater chances of success than older women. Older women can improve their odds by using eggs from a younger woman. U.S. C.D.C., *2012 Assisted Reproductive Technology Fertility Clinic Success Rates Report 6*, no. 24 (August 2013), available at http://www.cdc.gov/art/ART2011/PDFs/ART_2011_Clinic_Report-Full.pdf.

9. Most countries put some limits on coverage. There might be a maximum number of cycles covered (e.g., four in France), or couples might age out of coverage (e.g., at age 43 in France). Some countries provide full coverage of costs for a covered cycle, while other countries impose some cost-sharing requirements. Karen Berg Brigham, Benjamin Cadier, and Karine Chevreul, "The Diversity of Regulation and Public Financing of IVF in Europe and Its Impact on Utilization," *Human Reproduction* 28 (2013): 666–675.

10. Peter J. Neumann, "Should Health Insurance Cover IVF? Issues and Options," *Journal of Health Politics, Policy & Law* 22 (1997): 1215–1218, 1215.

11. Tara Siegel Bernard, "Insurance Coverage for Fertility Varies Widely," *New York Times*, July 25, 2014.

12. Mercer Health and Benefits, "Employer Experience With, and Attitudes Toward, Coverage of Infertility Treatment" (May 31, 2006), available at http://familybuilding.resolve.org/site/DocServer/Mercer_-_Resolve_Final_Report.pdf?docID=4361&JServSessionIda004=wp81gwj7l1.app212d (reporting lifetime coverage caps ranging from $1,500 to $50,000).

13. Joseph C. Isaacs, "Infertility Coverage Is Good Business," *Fertility & Sterility* 89 (2008): 1049–1052, 1049.

14. Some of these benefits are now mandated by the Affordable Care Act.

15. *Indiana University PPO High Deductible Health Plan (PPO HDHP) & Health Savings Account* 46, 54 (January 2015), available at http://hr.iu.edu/benefits/2015/pubs/PPO_HDHP-booklet.pdf; IU PPO High Deductible Health Plan (PPO HDHP) & Health Savings Account Benefit Summary 2015, available at http://hr.iu.edu/benefits/2015/pubs/PPO_HDHP-Summary2015.pdf.

16. *Indiana University PPO $500 Deductible Healthcare* Plan 45, 51, available at http://hr.iu.edu/benefits/2014/pubs/PPO500_booklet.pdf.

17. Ann Kurth et al., "Reproductive and Sexual Health Benefits in Private Health Insurance Plans in Washington State," *Family Planning Perspectives* 33 (2001): 153–160 (+179), 157. The percentage of plans offering abortion coverage was even higher—67% or more, depending on the type of plan (e.g., HMO, PPO, etc.). Ibid., 156. A national study found that 87% of insurance plans covered abortion, but some of those plans only covered the procedure when a pregnancy threatened the woman's health. Adam Sonfield et al., "U.S. Insurance Coverage of Contraceptives and the Impact of Contraceptive Coverage Mandates, 2002," *Perspectives on Sexual and Reproductive Health* 36 (2004): 72–79, 76.

18. Sonfield et al., "U.S. Insurance Coverage." Some of the coverage of contraceptive services reflected state mandates for coverage, though other factors were more important. Ibid., 77 (estimating that state mandates were responsible for 30% of the increase in coverage between 1993 and 2002 and that changes in national policy and growing public attention to the issue were responsible for 65% of the increase). See also Danielle N. Atkins and W. David Bradford, "Changes in State Prescription Contraceptive Mandates for Insurers: The

Effect on Women's Contraceptive Use," *Perspectives on Sexual and Reproductive Health* 46 (2014): 23–29 (finding that state mandates increased by 5% the likelihood that women would use a prescription contraceptive).

19. The New York State Task Force on Life and the Law, *Assisted Reproductive Technologies: Analysis and Recommendations for Public Policy* (1998), 96.

20. Ibid.

21. *Indiana University PPO*, 19, 34–35. This is not to say that coverage for medical equipment and devices is optimal. Private health plans may limit the kinds of medical equipment that are covered. On the other hand, when private health insurance is not available, government programs may pick up the slack. Overall, disabled persons or their families pay 40% of the costs of assistive technologies, which include medical equipment and devices, as well as architectural modifications in the home. Dawn Carlson and Nat Ehrlich, "Sources of Payment for Assistive Technology: Findings From a National Survey of Persons With Disabilities," *Assistive Technology* 18 (2006): 77–86 (noting that the federal government spent $845 million on powered wheelchairs in 2002).

22. Elizabeth C. Britt, *Conceiving Normalcy: Rhetoric, Law, and the Double Binds of Infertility* (Tuscaloosa: University of Alabama Press, 2001), 1–2 (observing that state laws were proposed and lobbied for by RESOLVE, a support and advocacy group for infertility treatments). RESOLVE's website is at www.resolve.org. For a discussion of state mandates, see Katie Cushing, "Facing Reality: The Pregnancy Discrimination Act Falls Short for Women Undergoing Infertility Treatment," *Seton Hall Law Review* 40 (2010): 1697–1731, 1726–1728; Jessica L. Hawkins, "Separating Fact From Fiction, Mandated Coverage of Infertility Treatments," *Washington University Journal of Law & Policy* 23 (2007): 203–227, 204.

23. National Conference of State Legislatures, *State Laws Related to Insurance Coverage for Infertility Treatment* (June 2014), available at http://www.ncsl.org/research/health/insurance-coverage-for-infertility-laws.aspx.

24. Cal. Health & Safety Code § 1374.55; Cal. Insurance Code § 10119.6 (1989); Tex. Insurance Code Ann. § 1366.001 et seq.

25. Cal. Health & Safety Code § 1374.55; Cal. Insurance Code § 10119.6 (1989); La. Rev. Stat. Ann. § 22:1036; N.Y. Insurance Law § 3216 (13), 3221 (6), and 4303.

26. Hawaii Rev. Stat. §§ 431:10A-116.5, 432.1–604. In other words, when the cause of a couple's infertility is uncertain, the couple does not qualify for benefits under the mandate.

27. Timothy S. Jost and Mark A. Hall, "The Role of State Regulation in Consumer-Driven Health Care," *American Journal of Law and Medicine* 31 (2005): 395–418, 398.

28. National Conference of State Legislatures, *Insurance Coverage for Contraception Laws* (February 2012), available at http://www.ncsl.org/research/health/insurance-coverage-for-contraception-state-laws.aspx. See also Atkins and Bradford, "Changes," 26. Coverage mandates for mental health services also are much stronger than mandates for fertility services. On multiple occasions, Congress passed legislation to require coverage for mental health treatment that is comparable to coverage for treatment of physical illnesses such as cancer or heart disease. Full coverage parity was finally secured with the enactment of the Affordable Care Act in 2010.

29. Janice G. Raymond, *Women as Wombs: Reproductive Technologies and the Battle Over Women's Freedom* (San Francisco: HarperSanFrancisco, 1993), 9–11 (reporting live birth rates below 10% from IVF).

30. U.S. C.D.C., 2012, 6, 24. "Fresh" embryos are distinguished from cycles in which the embryos have been frozen and thawed before transfer to the woman's uterus. Among

women under age 35, frozen embryos result in a live birth about 39% of the time. Ibid. at 24. For women aged 38–40, the success rates drop to 27% for fresh embryos and 30% for frozen embryos. Ibid. Note that the success rate from an embryo transfer is higher than the success rate from an IVF cycle because not all cycles result in an embryo that can be transferred to the woman's uterus.

31. Martha Griffin and William F. Panak, "The Economic Cost of Infertility-Related Services: An Examination of the Massachusetts Infertility Insurance Mandate," *Fertility & Sterility* 70 (1998): 22–29, 27. While overall costs increase from IVF coverage, there is an important savings. When IVF is covered, couples can use fewer embryos per cycle, and parents are less likely to have twins, triplets, or other multiple births. Multiple births are more expensive per child, and they result in greater health problems for mother and children. Thus, a Canadian study found that economic costs per child decreased after the adoption of coverage for IVF. M.P. Vélez, "Universal Coverage of IVF Pays Off," *Human Reproduction*, 29 (2014): 1313–1319, 1316.

32. Lisa Garceau et al., "Economic Implications of Assisted Reproductive Technologies," *Human Reproduction* 17 (2002): 3090–3109, 3090.

33. Daphna Birenbaum-Carmeli and Martha Dirnfeld, "In Vitro Fertilisation Policy in Israel and Women's Perspectives: The More the Better?" *Reproductive Health Matters* 16 (2008): 181–191, 184. While Israel provides ample financial assistance to women who want children, the national health service does less to help women who do not want children. For contraceptive services or abortion, only partial health coverage is available; abortion also requires a committee's approval. Ibid., 183. For more information about the abortion committee process, see Delila Amir and Orly Biniamin, "Abortion Approval as a Ritual of Symbolic Control, *Women & Criminal Justice* 3(1) (1992): 5–25.

34. In re Baby M, 537 A.2d 1227 (N.J. 1988).

35. Baby M, 1240–1242. With "gestational surrogacy," on the other hand, the surrogates are not the genetic mothers—the eggs come from either the women who have hired the surrogates or from third women who have donated their eggs to the intended mothers—and there is generally less opposition to the surrogate relationship. Sperm and egg donors are more accurately described as sellers rather than donors because they are compensated for their donations.

36. See, for example, Ky. Rev. Stat. § 199.590(4); NY Dom. Rel. Laws §§ 122 (with civil and criminal sanctions in § 123); Mich. Comp. Laws § 722.855 (with criminal sanctions in § 722.859).

37. See, for example, Fla. Stat. § 63.213 (giving the surrogate up to 48 hours after birth to rescind her agreement); R.R. v. M.H., 689 N.E.2d 790 (Mass. 1998) (also rejecting compensation beyond pregnancy-related expenses).

38. See, for example, 750 Ill. Comp. Stat. § 47/15; *Culliton v. Beth Israel Deaconess Medical Center*, 756 N.E.2d 1133 (Mass. 2001); *J.F. v. D.B.*, 879 N.Ed.2d 740 (Ohio 2007). For a helpful discussion of the societal trend in support of gestational surrogacy and the important factors that have influenced the debates over traditional and gestational surrogacy, see Elizabeth S. Scott, "Surrogacy and the Politics of Commodification," *Law & Contemporary Problems* 72 (2009): 109–146.

39. See, for example, Ariz. Rev. Stat. § 25-218 (also prohibiting traditional surrogacy); D.C. Stat. § 16-401-402 (also prohibiting traditional surrogacy).

40. Elizabeth S. Anderson, "Is Women's Labor a Commodity?" *Philosophy & Public Affairs* 19 (1990): 71–92. Anderson discusses traditional surrogacy but criticizes it not only because

it breaks the genetic ties between surrogate and child but also because it breaks their gestational connections.

41. In some cases, women act as surrogates for family members or friends without seeking compensation.

42. Anderson, "Women's Labor," 87.

43. Anderson, "Women's Labor," 91. Martha Field also responds to the desire for surrogate motherhood by observing that alternatives to surrogacy such as adoption would allow infertile couples to have children in ways that are "much more beneficial to society." Martha Field, *Surrogate Motherhood: The Legal and Human Issues* (Cambridge, MA: Harvard University Press, 1988), 55.

44. Anderson, "Women's Labor," 91.

45. Heidi Malm, "Paid Surrogacy: Arguments and Responses," *Public Affairs Quarterly* 3 (1989): 57–66, 63. Judge and former law professor Richard Posner makes the same argument. Richard Posner, "The Ethics and Economics of Enforcing Contracts of Surrogate Motherhood," *Journal of Contemporary Health Law and Policy* 5 (1989): 21–31, 24.

46. Margaret Jane Radin, "Market-Inalienability," *Harvard Law Review* 100 (1987): 1849–1937, 1932 (emphasis added).

47. David Orentlicher, "Cloning and the Preservation of Family Integrity," *Louisiana Law Review* 59 (1999): 1019–1040, 1030.

48. Concerns about the child's interests also are important.

49. Vasanti Jadva et al., "Surrogacy: The Experiences of Surrogate Mothers," *Human Reproduction* 18 (2003): 2196–2204, 2200. See also Olga B.A. van den Akker, "Psychosocial Aspects of Surrogate Motherhood," *Human Reproduction Update* 13 (2007): 53–62, 56 (reporting that relinquishing the baby is usually a happy event for the surrogate).

50. Jadva et al., "Surrogacy," 2198, 2200.

51. Jadva et al., "Surrogacy," 2199; van den Akker, "Psychosocial Aspects," 56.

52. Olga B.A. van den Akker, "Psychological Trait and State Characteristics, Social Support and Attitudes to the Surrogate Pregnancy and Baby," *Human Reproduction* 22 (2007): 2287–2295, 2293.

53. Elly Teman, "The Social Construction of Surrogacy Research: An Anthropological Critique of the Psychosocial Scholarship on Surrogate Motherhood," *Social Science & Medicine* 67 (2008) 1104–1112, 1104; Lina Peng, "Surrogate Mothers: An Exploration of the Empirical and the Normative," *American University Journal of Gender, Social Policy & the Law* 21 (2013): 555–582, 563.

54. Karen Busby and Delaney Vun, "Revisiting *The Handmaid's Tale*: Feminist Theory Meets Empirical Research on Surrogate Mothers," *Canadian Journal of Family Law* 26 (2010): 13–92, 17, 41–42 (describing critiques of surrogacy).

55. Posner, "Ethics and Economics," 25.

56. Busby and Vun, "Revisiting," 43–44, 563–564.

57. Busby and Vun, "Revisiting," 51–52.

58. According to one estimate, 95% of surrogate pregnancies involve gestational surrogacy. Diane Hinson and Maureen McBrien, "Surrogacy Across America," *Family Advocate* (Fall 2011): 32–36, 33. Rather than use the surrogate's eggs, infertile couples can obtain eggs from another woman. Mark A. Hall, Mary Anne Bobinski, and David Orentlicher, *Health Care Law and Ethics*, 8th ed. (New York: Wolters Kluwer Law & Business, 2013), 841.

59. Kavita Shah Arora and Valarie Blake, "Uterus Transplantation: Ethical and Regulatory Challenges," *Journal of Medical Ethics* 40 (2014): 396–400, 397; Giuseppe Del Priore et al.,

"Uterine Transplantation—a Real Possibility? The Indianapolis Consensus," *Human Reproduction* 28 (2013): 288–291.

60. Mats Brännström et al., "Livebirth After Uterus Transplantation," *Lancet* 385 (2015): 607–616.

61. Arora and Blake, "Uterus Transplantation," 396; Shari Rudavsky, "Uterine Transplants: A New Frontier in Science," *Indianapolis Star*, December 18, 2011.

62. Art L. Caplan et al., "Moving the Womb," *Hastings Center Report* 37 (May-June 2007): 18–20.

63. Anjana Nair et al., "Uterus Transplant: Evidence and Ethics," *Annals of the New York Academy of Sciences* 1127 (2008): 83–91, 84.

64. Caplan et al, "Moving the Womb."

65. Nair et al., "Uterus Transplant," 86; Dianne B. McKay and Michelle A. Josephson, "Pregnancy in Recipients of Solid Organs—Effects on Mother and Child," *New England Journal of Medicine* 354 (2006): 1281–1293; Lainie F. Ross, "Ethical Considerations Related to Pregnancy," *New England Journal of Medicine* 354 (2006): 1313–1316.

66. Rudavsky, "Uterine Transplants."

67. Hall et al., *Health Care Law*, 837–841.

68. Arora and Blake, "Uterus Transplantation," 398.

69. Ibid.

70. Noa Ben-Asher, "The Curing Law: On the Evolution of Baby-Making Markets," *Cardozo Law Review* 30 (2009): 1885–1924, 1891–1899; Scott, "Surrogacy," 126.

71. Indeed, it is more likely that employers would prefer an infertile employee than one who may ask for leave to care for a newborn or who may have unexpected absences because of childcare needs.

72. Anita Silvers, David Wasserman, and Mary Mahowald, *Disability, Difference, Discrimination: Perspectives on Justice in Bioethics and Public Policy* (Lanham, MD: Rowman & Littlefield, 1998), 8–9.

73. 45 C.F.R. § 84.3(j)(2)(ii).

74. Silvers et al., *Disability*, 8.

75. Skinner v. Oklahoma, 316 U.S. 535 (1942).

76. Bragdon v. Abbott, 524 U.S. 624 (1998).

77. *Bone Health and Osteoporosis: A Report of the Surgeon General* (2004), 69, available at www.surgeongeneral.gov/library/bonehealth/docs/full_report.pdf. To be sure, insurance coverage also may be limited for some age-related disabilities, such as hearing aids for hearing loss. Michelle Andrews, "Say What? Most Insurance Covers Little of the Cost of Hearing Aids," *Kaiser Health News*, April 9, 2012, available at http://www.kaiserhealthnews.org/features/insuring-your-health/2012/hearing-aids-coverage-skimpy-michelle-andrews-041012.aspx.

78. Most of the arguments in favor of treatment for infertility would apply as well to a postmenopausal woman who wants to gestate a pregnancy with a donor egg. While use of a donor egg does not implicate the postmenopausal woman's interest in a genetically related child, it does implicate her interests in developing gestational ties with her child and in limiting the involvement of other women in her childbearing. Accordingly, coverage for assisted reproduction should be provided in the case of donor eggs for postmenopausal women.

79. Deirdre Madden, "Is There a Right to a Child of One's Own," *Medico-Legal Journal of Ireland* 5 (1999): 8–13, 8; Lori B. Andrews and Lisa Douglass, "Alternative Reproduction,"

Southern California Law Review 65 (1991): 623–682, 629–630; Judith F. Daar, "Accessing Reproductive Technologies: Invisible Barriers, Indelible Harms," *Berkeley Journal of Gender, Law & Justice* 23 (2008): 18–82, 30; Katherine T. Pratt, "Inconceivable? Deducting the Costs of Fertility Treatment," *Cornell Law Review* 89 (2004): 1121–1200, 1126–1130.

80. Ellen W. Freeman et al., "Psychological Evaluation and Support in a Program of In Vitro Fertilization and Embryo Transfer," *Fertility and Sterility* 43 (1985): 48–53, 50. Fewer men described their infertility as the most upsetting experience of their lives—15% overall. Ibid. While the studies find high levels of distress among women regardless of the cause of the infertility, men appear to experience comparable levels of distress only when their infertility is the cause of the couple's infertility. Robert D. Nachtigall et al., "Stigma, Disclosure, and Family Functioning Among Parents of Children Conceived Through Donor Insemination," *Fertility & Sterility* 68 (1997): 83–89, 87–88.

    Because studies of the psychological impact of infertility typically involve couples who seek treatment, they may find higher levels of distress than they would in a random sample of infertile couples. Linda Hammer Burns and Sharon N. Covington, "Psychology of Infertility," in *Infertility Counseling: A Comprehensive Handbook for Clinicians*, ed. Linda Hammer Burns and Sharon N. Covington (Pearl River, NY: Parthenon, 1999), 7.

81. Mimi Meyers et al., "An Infertility Primer for Family Therapists: I. Medical, Social, and Psychological Dimensions," *Family Process* 34 (1995): 219–229, 223.

82. Carrie L. Nieman et al., "Fertility Preservation and Adolescent Cancer Patients: Lessons From Adult Survivors of Childhood Cancer and Their Parents," *Cancer Treatment and Research* 138 (2007): 201–217, 201.

83. "Personal Accounts of Cancer and Infertility," *Cancer Treatment and Research* 138 (2007): 243–248, 243. Whether infertility results in elevated levels of depression or other psychological dysfunction is less clear. On this question, the studies are mixed. Some researchers have found that infertile women are much more likely than fertile women to suffer from depression, Tara M. Cousineau and Alice D. Domar, "Psychological Impact of Infertility," *Best Practice & Research Clinical Obstetrics and Gynaecology* 21 (2007): 293–308, 295, that their depressive symptoms are more severe, Ibid., and that infertile women suffer levels of depression comparable to those of women with cancer, HIV infection, or who were undergoing rehabilitation after a heart attack, Alice D. Domar, Patricia C. Zuttermeister and Richard Friedman, "The Psychological Impact of Infertility: A Comparison With Patients With Other Medical Conditions," *Journal of Psychosomatic Obstetrics & Gynecology* 14 (Suppl.) (1993): 45–52, 47. Other studies have not found an increased level of psychological distress among infertile couples. See, for example, Kevin J. Connolly, "The Impact of Infertility on Psychological Functioning," *Journal of Psychosomatic Research* 36 (1992): 459–468 (finding generally low levels of depression among infertile couples studied). Psychological distress among the infertile may reflect general psychological factors rather than their infertility. Uschi Van den Broeck, "Predictors of Psychological Distress in Patients Starting IVF Treatment: Infertility-Specific Versus General Psychological Characteristics," *Human Reproduction* 25 (2010): 1471–1480, 1477–1478.

84. Britt, *Conceiving Normalcy*, 41.

85. Margarete Sandelowski, *With Child in Mind: Studies of the Personal Encounter With Infertility* (Philadelphia: University of Pennsylvania Press, 1993), 72.

86. Ibid., 12.

87. Arthur L. Greil, *Not Yet Pregnant: Infertile Couples in Contemporary America* (New Brunswick, NJ: Rutgers University Press, 1991), 128.

88. Greil, *Not Yet Pregnant*, 129.
89. Greil, *Not Yet Pregnant*, 130. See also Karey Harwood, *The Infertility Treadmill: Feminist Ethics, Personal Choice, and the Use of Reproductive Technologies* (Chapel Hill: University of North Carolina Press, 2007), at 54 (finding that infertile persons often are told to "Just relax, you'll get pregnant"). Surprisingly, some previously infertile couples who became pregnant adopted the same views. Sandelowski, *With Child*, 66.

    The "just relax" advice is consistent not only with a dismissive view of infertility but also a stigmatizing view of infertility. Charlene E. Miall, "Community Constructs of Involuntary Childlessness," *Canadian Review of Sociology & Anthropology* 31 (1994): 392–421, 405–407 (studying infertility in Canada). Undoubtedly, perceptions of the infertile encompass a range of views, including both dismissiveness and stigma. And infertile women report feelings of alienation and having an outsider status. Sandelowski, *With Child*, 76–78; Anne Woollett, "Having Children: Accounts of Childless Women and Women With Reproductive Problems," in *Motherhood: Meanings, Practices and Ideologies*, ed. Ann Phoenix, Anne Woollett, and Eva Lloyd (London: Sage, 1991), 47, 61. Nevertheless, the weight of evidence indicates that dismissiveness plays a very important role in the response of others to infertility, particularly when compared to earlier periods in history.
90. Greil, *Not Yet Pregnant*, 132. See also Constance N. Scharf and Margot Weinshel, "Infertility and Late-Life Pregnancies," in *Couples on the Fault Line: New Directions for Therapists*, ed. Peggy Papp (New York: Guilford Press, 2000), 108 (observing that the infertile "couple's experience is usually little understood and not valued by their family and friends"). To be sure, some infertile individuals face negative sentiments from others.
91. Greil, *Not Yet Pregnant*, 128.
92. Carl H. Coleman, "Assisted Reproductive Technologies and the Constitution," *Fordham Urban Law Journal* 30 (2002): 57–70, 68–70; Radhika Rao, "Assisted Reproductive Technology and Reproductive Equality," *George Washington Law Review* 76 (2008): 1457–1489, 1478.
93. Coleman, "Assisted Reproductive," 68. I have more to say about the views of Coleman and Rao later in this chapter.
94. Ruth Hubbard, "The Case Against In Vitro Fertilization and Implantation," in *The Custom-Made Child? Women-Centered Perspectives*, ed. Helen B. Holmes, Betty B. Hoskings, and Michael Gross (Clifton, NJ: Humana Press, 1981), 260.
95. Hubbard, "The Case Against," 261. As indicated, Hubbard wrote in the early days of IVF, and part of her concern lay in the uncertain health risks involved. Ibid., 260, 262.
96. Eric Hirsch, "Negotiated Limits: Interviews in South-east England," in *Technologies of Procreation: Kinship in the Age of Assisted Conception*, 2nd ed., ed. Jeanette Edwards, Sarah Franklin, Eric Hirsch, Frances Price, Marilyn Strathern (London: Routledge, 1999), 115.
97. Sandelowski, *With Child*, 72.
98. Ibid., 38 (describing the views of other scholars).
99. Ibid., 38–39.
100. Ibid., 39, 74.
101. Pratt, "Inconceivable?," 1125.
102. Ibid., 1124. Ironically, the same expert argued that expenses for treatment of sexual dysfunction (e.g., costs of Viagra) might qualify for a tax deduction. Ibid., 1124–1125.
103. Elaine Tyler May, *Barren in the Promised Land: Childless Americans and the Pursuit of Happiness* (New York: Basic Books, 1995), 181–182.
104. Ibid., 196.

105. Ibid., 185, 208. Some studies have found that marital happiness is greater both before the arrival of the first child and after the last child leaves for college. Peggy L. Dalgas-Pelish, "The Impact of the First Child on Marital Happiness," *Journal of Advanced Nursing* 18 (1993): 437–441 (finding greater marital happiness in childless couples than in couples with a first pregnancy or first child); Sara M. Gorchoff, Oliver P. John, and Ravenna Helson, "Contextualizing Change in Marital Satisfaction During Middle Age: An 18-Year Longitudinal Study," *Psychological Science* 19 (2008): 1194–1200 (finding increased marital satisfaction for married women when they became "empty nesters"). See also S. Mark Pancer et al., "Thinking Ahead: Complexity of Expectations and the Transition to Parenthood," *Journal of Personality* 68 (2000): 253–279, 257 (discussing studies that find a decline in marital satisfaction with reproduction, but not for all couples).

106. Fiona McAllister and Lynda Clarke, "Voluntary Childlessness: Trends and Implications," in *Infertility in the Modern World: Present and Future Prospects*, ed. Gillian R. Bentley and C.G. Nicholas Mascie-Taylor (Cambridge: Cambridge University Press, 2000), 209, 223–224. See also Jean E. Veevers, *Childless by Choice*, 73–74 (Toronto: Butterworths, 1980) (reporting the importance of spontaneity for couples who choose not to have children).

107. McAllister and Clarke, "Voluntary Childlessness," 222–223. For some personal reflections on not having children, see Meghan Daum, *Selfish, Shallow, and Self-Absorbed: Sixteen Writers on the Decision Not to Have Kids* (New York: Picador, 2015).

108. Germaine Greer, *Sex and Destiny: The Politics of Human Fertility*, 1st ed. (New York: Harper & Row, 1984), 3. See also May, *Barren*, 16 (referring to society's collective hostility toward children); David Orentlicher, "Spanking and Other Corporal Punishment of Children by Parents: Overvaluing Pain, Undervaluing Children," *Houston Law Review* 35 (1998): 147–185, 173–177 (discussing the many ways in which the law withholds fundamental rights from children).

109. Jed Rubenfeld, "The Right of Privacy," *Harvard Law Review* 102 (1989): 737–807, 788.

110. Ibid., 791, 784.

111. Ibid., 796–797.

112. Raymond, *Women as Wombs*, ix. See also Robyn Rowland, "Of Women Born, But for How Long? The Relationship of Women to the New Reproductive Technologies and the Issue of Choice," in *Made to Order: The Myth of Reproductive and Genetic Progress*, ed. Patricia Spallone and Deborah Lynn Steinberg (Oxford: Pergamon Press, 1987), 77–80 (expressing concern over the loss of choice for women from IVF).

Raymond is not the only person to worry about the violence of IVF. In its first "Instruction" on new reproductive technologies, the Catholic Church characterized IVF as a "dynamic of violence and domination," albeit one against the embryos rather than the woman. Congregation for the Doctrine of the Faith, *Instruction on Respect for Human Life in Its Origin and on the Dignity of Procreation: Replies to Certain Questions of the Day* (February 22, 1987), 21. In a 2008 revised Instruction, the Vatican continued to condemn IVF but did not repeat the dynamic of violence and domination language. Congregation for the Doctrine of the Faith, *Instruction* Dignitas Personae *on Certain Bioethical Questions* (September 8, 2008).

113. Raymond, *Women as Wombs*, 86.

114. See, for example, Gayle Letherby, "Challenging Dominant Discourses: Identity and Change and the Experience of 'Infertility' and 'Involuntary Childlessness,'" *Journal of Gender Studies* 11 (2002): 277–288; Charlene E. Miall, "The Stigma of Involuntary Childlessness," *Social Problems* 33 (1986): 268–282, 271–272 (finding that infertile women

regarded their condition as a "discreditable attribute"); Charlene E. Miall, "Perceptions of Informal Sanctioning and the Stigma of Involuntary Childlessness," *Deviant Behavior* 6 (1985): 383–403; Diana C. Parry, "Work, Leisure, and Support Groups: An Examination of the Ways Women With Infertility Respond to Pronatalist Ideology," *Sex Roles* 53 (2005): 337–346 (reporting on infertile women who felt that they were "considered lacking, incomplete, or inadequate").

115. Chloé Diepenbrock, "God Willed It! Gynecology at the Checkout Stand: Reproductive Technology in the Women's Service Magazine, 1977–1996," in *Body Talk: Rhetoric, Technology, Reproduction* (Mary M. Lay et al., eds. Madison: University of Wisconsin Press, 2000), 98; John A. Robertson, *Children of Choice: Freedom and the New Reproductive Technologies* (Princeton, NJ: Princeton University Press, 1994), 29–42.

116. Naomi Cahn and June Carbone, *Red Families v. Blue Families: Legal Polarization and the Creation of Culture* (New York: Oxford University Press, 2010), 2.

117. Cahn and Carbone, *Red Families*, 10.

118. 524 U.S. 624 (1998).

119. Because of her HIV infection, Ms. Abbott's dentist, Randon Bragdon, was willing to fill her cavity only in a hospital, and Ms. Abbott would have been responsible for the costs of using the hospital's facilities. *Bragdon*, 524 U.S. at 628–629.

120. An infertile person might be protected from discrimination by an employer who fires the person for missing time from work while seeking medical treatment for the infertility. See *Hall v. Nalco Co.*, 534 F.3d 644 (7th Cir. 2008); *LaPorta v. Wal-Mart Stores, Inc.*, 163 F.Supp.2d 758 (W.D. Mich. 2001).

121. There have been cases in which an infertile person successfully challenged a denial of coverage for treatment, but those cases involve claims that the insurer has in fact promised to provide coverage. See, for example, *Egert v. Connecticut General Life Ins. Co.*, 900 F.2d 1032 (7th Cir. 1990) (finding that the insurer viewed infertility as an illness, that it had committed to covering necessary treatment for illness, and that IVF was a necessary treatment for the plaintiff's infertility under the terms of the insurance contract).

122. 117 F.Supp.2d 318 (S.D. N.Y. 2000).

123. She also brought claims under Title VII of the Civil Rights Act and under the Pregnancy Discrimination Act but was unsuccessful with those claims as well. Those claims failed, said the Second Circuit, because an insurer's denial of coverage for IVF and other infertility treatments disadvantage both the female and male members of the couple. *Saks v. Franklin Covey Co.*, 316 F.3d 337, 345–349 (2nd Cir. 2003). For a discussion of the current failure of these antidiscrimination statutes to protect infertile persons and observations for how antidiscrimination claims might succeed in the future, see Elizabeth A. Pendo, "The Politics of Infertility: Recognizing Coverage Exclusions as Discrimination," *Connecticut Insurance Law Journal* 11 (2005): 293–344, 317–325; Brietta R. Clark, "Erickson v. Bartell Drug Co.: A Roadmap for Gender Equality in Reproductive Health Care or An Empty Promise?" *Law & Inequality* 23 (2005): 299–362; Katherine E. Abel, "The Pregnancy Discrimination Act and Insurance Coverage for Infertility Treatment: An Inconceivable Union," *Connecticut Law Review* 37 (2005): 819–850.

124. *Saks*, 117 F.Supp.2d at 326–327. However, if insurers cover a type of treatment for some patients who need it but not for others who need the same treatment, they may be in violation of the ADA. See *Henderson v. Bodine Aluminum, Inc.*, 70 F.3d 958, 960 (8th Cir. 1995) (requiring the insurer that provided bone marrow transplants to some cancer patients also to provide the transplants to patients with comparable cancers when

evidence indicates that the transplants provide a significant improvement in outcome over alternative treatments). Under this reasoning, if Franklin Covey covered IVF for women who had a fallopian tube blockage but not for women who were infertile for other reasons, it might be in violation of the ADA. Franklin Covey escaped the *Henderson* principle because it denied coverage for IVF to everyone.

125. 469 U.S. 287, 301 (1985). The 14-day cap disfavored persons with disabilities since they were more likely to require more than 14 days of hospital care in a given year. Ibid. at 289–290.

126. *Saks*, 117 F. Supp. 2d at 320.

127. 42 U.S.C. 12201(c)(3). Under ERISA, private employee benefit plans must satisfy minimum federal standards. The Act also preempts many state benefit plan regulations, including regulation of health care plans. The application of ERISA to health care plans is complicated and beyond the scope of this chapter. Suffice it to say that it has proved controversial—a statute designed to protect the interests of employees has often served to compromise their interests with respect to health care coverage. Linda P. McKenzie, "Eligibility, Treatment, or Something In-Between? Plaintiffs Get Creative to Get Past ERISA Preemption," *Journal of Contemporary Health Law & Policy* 23 (2007): 272–301, 275–276.

128. *Saks*, 117 F.Supp.2d at 327–328.

129. 42 U.S.C. 12201(c)(1).

130. *Saks*, 117 F.Supp.2d at 328. While *Saks* and other courts have held that insurance provisions adopted before the ADA's enactment can never be viewed as a subterfuge to evade the requirements of the Act, the Equal Employment Opportunity Commission and others disagree on that point. Melissa Cole, "In/ensuring Disability," *Tulane Law Review* 77 (2003): 839–884, 876–879.

131. John Hart Ely, *Democracy and Distrust: A Theory of Judicial Review* (Cambridge, MA: Harvard University Press, 1980).

132. Coleman, "Assisted Reproductive Technologies," 68–69; Rao, "Assisted Reproductive Technology," 1478.

133. Rao, "Assisted Reproductive Technology," 1478.

134. Judith Daar, "The Role of Providers in Assisted Reproduction: Potential Conflicts, Professional Conscience and Personal Choice," in *Oxford Handbook of Reproductive Ethics*, ed. Leslie P. Francis (New York: Oxford University Press, 2017), I.B.1; Marcia C. Inhorn and Michael Hassan Fakih, "Arab Americans, African Americans, and Infertility: Barriers to Reproduction and Medical Care," *Fertility & Sterility* 85 (2006): 844–852, 845.

135. Daar, "Accessing Reproductive Technologies," 40, 80–81; Inhorn and Fakih, "Arab Americans," 845; Deborah L. Steinberg, "A Most Selective Practice: The Eugenic Logics of IVF," *Women's Studies International Forum* 20 (1997): 33–48.

136. See, for example, Dorothy E. Roberts, "Punishing Drug Addicts Who Have Babies: Women of Color, Equality, and the Right of Privacy," *Harvard Law Review* 104 (1991): 1419–1482, 1436–1450 (discussing the history of public policies in the United States that devalued Black motherhood).

137. Ben-Asher, "The Curing Law," 1918.

138. Daar, "Accessing Reproductive Technologies," 38–43; Inhorn and Fakih, "Arab Americans," 845–847; Dorothy E. Roberts, "Race and the New Reproduction," *Hastings Law Journal* 47 (1996): 935–949, 937–942.

139. 100 U.S. 303, 304 (1880).
140. Ibid., 308.
141. 347 U.S. 483, 494 (1954).
142. 411 U.S. 677, 686–687 (1973).
143. 133 S. Ct. 2675, 2693 (2013).
144. 42 U.S.C. § 12101(a)(6) (2006).
145. § 12101(a)(7).
146. Greil, *Not Yet Pregnant*, 127. Such views have a long pedigree. In the nineteenth century, physicians often took the view that women were infertile because they had eschewed a life of maternity and chosen instead to postpone childbearing in favor of higher education, work, and other pursuits in the public sphere. Sandelowski, *With Child*, 27–28.
147. Naomi Cahn, *The New Kinship: Constructing Donor-Conceived Families* (New York: NYU Press, 2013), 158.
148. Alison Chapple, Sue Ziebland and Ann McPherson, "Stigma, Shame, and Blame Experienced by Patients With Lung Cancer: Qualitative Study," *British Medical Journal* 318 (June 11, 2004): 1470.
149. U.S. CDC, *2012*, 24.

CHAPTER 17

IS SURROGACY ETHICALLY PROBLEMATIC?

LESLIE FRANCIS

RISKS of exploitation in surrogacy, especially commercial surrogacy, are impressive, as eloquently documented by Donna Dickenson in this volume. Many commentators also have written about potential harms to the child when gestation is achieved through surrogacy—from commodification in apparent baby selling, to unsafe pregnancy conditions, to unfit parents or parents with abusive conceptions of who or what they want their child to be.[1] Concerns have also been raised about the frequency with which apparently voluntary commercial surrogacy is really a form of trafficking, either of the surrogate or of the child. This chapter will assume that exploitation and its extreme form in trafficking, as well as these forms of harm to the child, are wrongs to be avoided in any permissible surrogacy. If a surrogacy practice inevitably incorporates or creates serious risks of these wrongs, the practice would be wrong. But supposing these harms do not actually exist or could be left aside, is surrogacy itself ethically permissible? Are there ethical reasons to question all surrogacy, even noncommercialized, uncoerced, and altruistic arrangements among family members?

This chapter takes up less well-trodden questions[2] about whether a surrogacy arrangement in which one person carries a pregnancy for another is ethically problematic in itself—and if so, why. Pregnancy and delivery are quintessential bodily labor. One set of arguments tests whether carrying a pregnancy is the type of bodily labor one person ethically may perform for another, whether or not for pay. These arguments contend that surrogacy cannot be a permissible service, no matter how well intended or structured. Another set of questions probes the value and identity of the child, asking whether surrogacy is inevitably akin to baby selling or, if not, devalues the child in some other way. A final set of related questions attends to whether surrogacy properly respects the relationship between the pregnant woman and the child-to-be. The general strategy of the argument is to show that we cannot reject all surrogacy on any of these grounds without also rejecting other practices that we find acceptable. The conclusion is that although there are serious ethical issues about surrogacy arrangements, they can be allayed by how these arrangements are structured and are far outweighed by the interests of infertile individuals or couples in becoming parents.

Most surrogacy today is "gestational" surrogacy, in which neither the surrogate nor her partner contributes the gametes to be used in the pregnancy. I address this form of surrogacy primarily[3] but begin with some remarks about "traditional" surrogacy, because it initiated the practice and has to some extent continued to frame the debates.

TRADITIONAL AND GESTATIONAL SURROGACY

Surrogacy exploded onto the legal scene in the 1988 New Jersey case of *Baby M.*[4] In this case, Mary Beth Whitehead was the genetic and gestational mother of the child; William Stern was the child's genetic father; and William and Elizabeth Stern were the child's intended rearing parents. The pregnancy was achieved by artificial insemination using sperm from William Stern. The surrogacy contract provided that Whitehead was to be paid $10,000 for gestation of the child and doing whatever was necessary to terminate her maternal rights so that Elizabeth Stern would be able to adopt the child. Mary Beth Whitehead's husband was also a party to the contract; he agreed to do whatever was necessary to rebut presumptions of paternity under state law. After the baby's birth, Whitehead became emotionally distraught and sought to keep the child; Stern brought suit to enforce the surrogacy contract. The New Jersey Supreme Court ultimately concluded that the surrogacy contract violated the public policy of the state, using instructive reasoning.

Core to the court's reasoning was New Jersey's adoption statute. That statute prohibited money payments in exchange for an adoption and imposed strict requirements on the relinquishment of parental rights, which was not permitted until after the child's birth. The court determined that the surrogacy arrangement employed private contract law to circumvent these restrictions of the adoption statute. In the court's view, the money was being paid to obtain an adoption and not for personal services, despite provisions in the contract reciting that it was for services. Moreover, the contract was necessarily coercive because it created an irrevocable agreement, prior to birth or even conception, for the surrender of any resulting child, also not permitted for private adoptions under New Jersey state law. Adoption is for humanitarian purposes, the court said; in contrast, the surrogacy arrangement between William Stern and the Whiteheads was an economic arrangement "without regard to the interest of the child or the natural mother."[5]

Several themes stand out in the court's critique of contractual surrogacy. The first is that carrying a child for another is not an ordinary service that can be the subject of ordinary contract law. The second is that the woman carrying the child as its genetic and gestational mother is the child's "natural" mother. This relationship can only be terminated under very special conditions of either voluntariness (as with adoption) or malfeasance (as with the termination of parental rights for cause). These themes continue to sound in criticisms of surrogacy arrangements today.

In another early surrogacy case, this time involving gestational surrogacy, the California Supreme Court reasoned quite differently.[6] Mark and Crispina Calvert contracted with Anna Johnson to bear a child created from Mark's sperm and Christina's egg. Anna was to be paid $10,000 and was to relinquish all parental rights to the child in favor of the Calverts. Rejecting adoption as a model,[7] the court turned instead to the Uniform Parentage Act's treatment of the parent–child relationship between natural or adoptive parents and their children. Under that Act, any interested party can bring suit to determine the existence of a mother–child relationship; this includes the genetic mother of the child. Just as fathers can establish paternity by establishing the genetic linkage, so can mothers, reasoned the California court. Cristina's claim to parenthood was genetic, Anna's gestational; in that sense both had claims to a maternal relationship with the child. According to the court, California law provided no basis for choosing between the two; thus, the court examined the terms of the surrogacy agreement to establish intended parenthood. According to the court: "although the Act recognizes both genetic consanguinity and giving birth as means of establishing a mother and child relationship, when the two means do not coincide in one woman, she who intended to procreate the child—that is, she who intended to bring about the birth of a child that she intended to raise as her own—is the natural mother under California law."[8]

Like the New Jersey court, the California court uses the language of "natural" motherhood to describe what is also a legal choice—that is, the identification of the legal mother. Unlike New Jersey, however, California contends that the surrogate would not have been able to conceive the child in question without the intentions of the planned parents. The gestational mother is "agreeing to provide a necessary and profoundly important service without (by definition) any expectation that she will raise the resulting child as her own."[9] The arrangement could be fully voluntary, as at the time of contracting Anna was not expected to "part with her own expected offspring."[10] The court also opined that it is unlikely that prospective parents would choose to procreate in this way without taking the child's interests as central.

Perhaps the difference between the New Jersey and California courts' analyses hinges on the difference between traditional and gestational surrogacy. Gestational surrogacy may involve a biological relationship between the intended mother and the child that traditional surrogacy does not, the genetic tie; with traditional surrogacy, the intended mother bears no biological relationship with her prospective child. Of course, gestational surrogacy also may involve the use of third-party gametes, in which case neither the surrogate nor the intended mother is a source of the child's genetic makeup. Subsequent case law in New Jersey does reflect consideration of such genetic ties, at least to some extent. In a case decided in 2000, a sister carried an embryo created from the sperm of her brother-in-law and the egg of her sister who was unable to carry a pregnancy. The intended parents (with the surrogate's agreement) petitioned for a prebirth order to have the birth certificate list them as the child's parents. Bowing to the postbirth right of the surrogate not to relinquish the child for adoption for 72 hours after birth, the court refused to issue the requested prebirth order. To support this conclusion, the court relied on the emotional ties created by pregnancy: the intended parents' "simplistic comparison to an incubator disregards the fact that there are human emotions and biological changes involved in pregnancy."[11] However, as the window for relinquishment of parental rights opened before the birth certificate needed to be filed at 5 days after birth, the court issued an order permitting the certificate to be changed before filing to list the intended parents as the child's parents, on condition that the gestational mother agree to relinquish her rights to the child. In a later decision, however, the New Jersey courts declined to extend this strategy to a case of gestational surrogacy in which the parties used a donated egg, so that the intended mother bore no biological relationship to the child and the gestational mother bore only a gestational relationship.[12] The intended parents claimed that application of the Uniform Parentage Act—the statute employed in the *Baby M* case—to allow the intended (and genetic) father to claim parentage on the birth certificate but not the intended mother violated equal protection, but the New Jersey court found that it did not as it tracked actual biological differences.[13]

This reasoning of the New Jersey court that biological ties somehow matter—whether gestational or genetic—persists in some criticisms of surrogacy arrangements. Yet it leaves puzzles about which biological ties matter and why. Moreover, in contemporary surrogacy arrangements involving oocyte donation, neither the gestational nor the intended mother has genetic ties to the child (and the intended father might not have such ties as well). Fuller examination of the services and relationships involved in surrogacy is thus critical to understanding its ethical permissibility.

SURROGACY AS SERVICE

Surrogacy is a quintessential act of bodily labor for another. It is physically intrusive, involving pregnancy, birth, and in its gestational form, hormonal stimulation and embryo transfer. Are there reasons for thinking that it is wrongful for one person to perform such invasive bodily labor as a service for another? This section addresses the ethical permissibility of providing gestational services, whether or not in exchange for pay. If it were unethical to perform these services altruistically, it would presumably also be unethical to do so for less compelling economic reasons.

The most sweeping objection to surrogacy doubts the permissibility of one person performing any invasive bodily labor for another. This claim is surely too strong: we permit and even applaud people for donating organs for others or bearing babies in loving relationships where the nongestating partner has the primary desire for the child, both examples of invasive bodily labor performed for the benefit of others. A thought experiment in Judith Jarvis Thomson's famous abortion article (1971) illustrates. Thomson analogized pregnancy to dialysis with a human being providing the kidney: suppose, she asked, you were kidnapped by a society of violin lovers and attached to a great violinist. The plan was to allow the violinist use of your kidneys for 9 months in a manner that would save the violinist's life and that would be inconvenient but not physically risky to you. Thomson's conclusion was that because the violinist had no right to the use of your kidneys, it would be ethically permissible for you to unhook yourself from the arrangement; the analogy was used to show that it does not follow from a claim of the right to life (by the violinist) that there is a right to the means of life. To be sure, a "good Samaritan" might continue to allow the kidney use, and a "minimally decent Samaritan" might do so for a short period of time, Thomson observes; her point is only that allowing the continued kidney use is not morally obligatory. Subsequent commentary on Thomson's thought experiment has been primarily directed to supposed disanalogies between the hypothetical kidnapping and actual pregnancy. I know of no discussions that have attacked Thomson's observation that it is ethically permissible for good—or decent—Samaritans to permit the ongoing use of their kidneys in this way. Yet this is exactly what would be questioned if it were thought impermissible to allow one person to provide such invasive bodily labor for another.

A more limited objection contends that it is wrong for one person to provide particularly risky or burdensome invasive bodily labor for another. For example, in organ donation living donors are assessed and rejected if the risks to them are judged to be too high, even if they are willing to consent to the use of their bodies in this way (e.g., Reichman et al. 2011). Surrogates are also assessed for risk and—at least in programs complying with professional guidelines—rejected for significant physical or psychological risk (ASRM Practice Committee 2015; Daar, this volume). Thus if surrogates are appropriately screened for risk, it would appear that level of risk does not present a principled distinction between this use of the body of another and other uses that are judged ethically permissible. To be sure, kidney or liver transplants from living donors are performed as life-saving measures for their recipients; carrying a child for another is not typically life saving, although it may be deeply meaningful. But to defend this distinction in this way is to rely on contested judgments about whether assisted reproduction is a sufficiently weighty purpose to override the risks it might impose. One such judgment might be that services that carry a risk of death (as organ donation or pregnancy may in very unusual cases) are only permissible if their goal is to save the life of another. But this judgment would prohibit any rescue that risks the life of the rescuer (no matter how small the risk) to save another from serious but nonfatal harm. Another such judgment might be that reproduction is not a sufficiently important service, but this defense devalues reproductive bodily services in a manner that remains to be argued.

Indeed, we regard as ethically permissible other forms of physical labor for others that are quite risky. Nursing is an example. Over a third of nurses suffer debilitating back injuries primarily attributable to repetitive lifting and transferring of patients (Brown 2003). Residential care workers have similarly high rates of injury (Harris 2013). These injury rates are far beyond those associated with normal pregnancy and birth. Although many lifts and transfers are performed to avoid morbidity such as sores, others are for quality of life reasons such as a nursing home patient's ability to have meals with others or go outside. Many family members also perform these tasks in order to enable loved ones to remain at home and in the community; although I know of no data studying familial injury rates, presumably they would be at least similar to those of trained professionals performing the same service, likely with better equipment.

Another more limited way to argue against surrogacy as a service is to argue that it is a special form of bodily labor for another that ought not to be compensated but that might permissibly be performed altruistically. As in the example of the New Jersey case described above, intrafamilial surrogacy arrangements or close-friend arrangements may be desirable for some infertile couples (ESHRE Task Force 2011). Implementing this approach are laws prohibiting commercial surrogacy but allowing uncompensated arrangements.[14] This is only an objection to commercialized forms of surrogacy, however; uncompensated surrogacy would remain permissible (as in many countries of the world), unless it is inevitably tied to commercial surrogacy. However, examining arguments offered against commercial surrogacy presents the opportunity to consider whether they extend to noncommercial surrogacy as well.

COMPENSATED SURROGACY

Many jurisdictions prohibit paid surrogacy while permitting supposedly uncompensated versions of the practice. Although my primary focus is the ethics of unpaid surrogacy, examining issues about paid surrogacy can be revealing about unpaid surrogacy.

A threshold problem with drawing the commercial/noncommercial line is the difficulty in distinguishing commercial from purely uncompensated forms of surrogacy (van Zyl and Walker 2013). Although there no doubt are arrangements in which the surrogate receives no form of payment, many surrogacies—including those in jurisdictions that do not permit paid surrogacy—compensate for expenses the surrogate would not otherwise have incurred but for the gestation. These typically include medical expenses, maternity clothes (and perhaps new clothes post birth), compensation for lost wages, and other expenses associated with the pregnancy. Of note, these pregnancy-related expenses are so significant that it would arguably be unfair to the surrogate to expect her to bear them on her own.[15] Moreover, pregnancies do go awry at times, and it would seem especially unfair not to provide a surrogate with insurance against unexpected medical expenses.

Recognizing these issues in distinguishing commercial from noncommercial surrogacy, van Zyl and Walker (2013) argue that neither fully commercialized models nor fully altruistic models are appropriate for understanding the practice. As another reason for rejecting the purely altruistic paradigm, these authors also contend that it fails to take into account the reciprocal obligations parties in a surrogacy arrangement have to one another; for example, the surrogate has obligations to take care during the pregnancy and the intended parents have obligations to treat the surrogate with respect. Instead, van Zyl and Walker defend surrogacy as analogous to helping professions in which altruistic motivations are important, but fair compensation and the legitimate expectations of the parties also are recognized. An additional advantage of the professional analogy, they observe, is that professionals typically have organizations and rules to protect them from unethical conduct—both their own and those of others. On their view, if surrogacy arrangements were subject to proper oversight, it would be appropriate to enforce contracts on which the surrogate agrees in advance to relinquish the child to the intended parents.

Unfortunately, surrogacy also may be cast in altruistic terms when this is not at all what is taking place. Critics of commercial surrogacy such as Dickinson (this volume) rightly demonstrate how blatantly economic surrogate arrangements may be masked as gifts—and how this mischaracterization may conceal exploitation of surrogates. The point is important that misleadingly characterizing surrogacy as a pure gift may devalue the pressures and burdens on the surrogate. But similar concerns apply to regarding family caregivers as altruistic actors—and the ethical response is that these caregivers should be treated fairly and compensated reasonably, not that they should not engage in the care at all.

In assessing paid surrogacy, it is worth noting that we do allow some intimate activities for others to be compensated, so it cannot be the intimacy alone that explains opposition to compensation. Assistants are paid to wash, bathe, feed, and perform bowel care for people who cannot achieve these functions independently. While families often take primary roles in performing these functions—and desire to perform such caregiving functions out of love—on many views they are neither obligated to do this nor thought less of because they rely on help from others who are paid for their work (e.g., Levine 2005). Wet nursing as a social practice historically was identified with infant abandonment or with aristocratic women handing off tasks they regarded as unpleasant to the poor, but today it has garnered increased interest in light of evidence about the negative health effects of formula feeding (Stevens, Patrick, and Pickler 2009).

On the other hand, there may be intimate functions that only or primarily families can do, especially functions that rely on close personal knowledge. Hilde Lindemann (2009), for example, argues that family members have special responsibilities to construct continuing identities with people with dementia. Or there may be functions that should be reserved only to intimates such as the performance of sexual services for people with disabilities.[16] But that some intimate functions are or should be special to families does not show that all are; reasons would still be required for concluding that gestation is a service that can or should only be performed within the familial or close friend relationships that are likely to be the context for noncommercial surrogacy.

Further reasons offered for viewing surrogacy as special in a way that precludes commercialization rest in accounts of the surrogate's own flourishing, the identity of the child, or the desirability of preserving certain forms of parent–child relationships. Two early and powerful criticisms of surrogacy—by Margaret Jane Radin and by Elizabeth Anderson—both developed arguments that performing this particular kind of intimate bodily labor for another is inconsistent with the pregnant woman's own flourishing. Writing before the transition from traditional to gestational surrogacy, both authors addressed commercial forms of traditional surrogacy primarily, but with arguments that have more general import.

In her seminal article about commodification of intimate activities, Margaret Jane Radin (1987) defended a view of market-inalienability rooted in human flourishing. On her account, the dividing line between permissible and impermissible commodification lies in core aspects of personhood, freedom, and identity, set in context. Freedom is the power to choose for oneself, and identity is the continuing integrity of the self that is necessary for individuation; these interact in the context of environments in which persons seek to constitute themselves. Surrogacy (along with baby selling and prostitution) should not be subject to purchase and sale in an ideal world, Radin concludes, because they alienate important personal attributes and relationships (p. 1904). A complication for a nonideal world is that some forms of at least partial commodification may be tolerated to avoid even worse injustices. Commercialized sex is problematic because sex should be "freely shared," not engaged in only if the parties believe it is economically worthwhile. However, there may be nonideal contexts in which selling sex is the best of very bad options for otherwise impoverished or oppressed women. By contrast, babies are not fungible; to sell them is deny their individual identity (p. 1908) and is never ethically permissible, even in the worst of contexts.

Surrogacy, Radin thinks, is a more difficult case for a nonideal world, but she concludes that reproductive services should be market-inalienable even in contexts in which women have few other choices. Her reasoning is that to sell these services is to alienate a core aspect of identity. Much of her concern lies with commercialization, of both child and gestating mother, but some of what she says applies also to surrogacy in which the gestation is not commercialized. In particular, she deploys her understanding of identity to query whether the gestating woman is regarded as a fungible source of something—the child—produced to satisfy the needs or wants of others. Still worse, Radin says, what the surrogate does is embedded in gender hierarchy, at least in traditional surrogacy, where the goal is the father's but not the intended mother's genetic child: she is expected to give up her own child, and the intended infertile mother is expected to raise someone else's child, all to satisfy the intended father's desire for a genetic heir (pp. 1929-1930). These points—that the surrogate's body is being used to satisfy the wants of another, and that the desire for a surrogate-borne child (that may or may not be genetically related) is ineluctably gendered—apply even to noncommercial forms of the practice, on Radin's view.

Along similar lines, Elizabeth Anderson (1990) contends that surrogacy attributes the wrong sort of value—use value—to gestation. Legal rules that deprive the surrogate of any claims to her child, for example by requiring her to relinquish claims prebirth or even preconception, deprive her of what is "hers both genetically and gestationally" (p. 79). Gestational ties are critical to avoid reducing "the surrogate mothers from persons worthy of respect and consideration to objects of mere use"[17] (p. 80). If these ties are not respected, we fail on Anderson's view to treat the surrogate in accord with principles consistent with her autonomy and her deeply felt emotions (p. 81).

Undoubtedly, surrogacy uses the woman's body and in this respect treats the body as having a use value. The surrogate's body is physically essential for the gestation of the resulting child. It is a significant leap from this biological fact, however, to the conclusion that the surrogacy relationship fails ethically to treat her as a subject of respect and consideration. Surrogacy arrangements that are exploitative would surely be ones in which she is not treated with the respect due persons, but this would be true of any exploitative arrangement. Surrogacy relationships in which the intended parents regard the surrogate only as a vessel for the production of their child and not as a person in her own right would also fail to respect the surrogate as a person. But similar concerns apply to many service relationships in which the servant is devalued. Moreover, while these concerns likely attend some surrogacy arrangements—medical tourism suggests illustrations (Pande 2014)—there is no reason to think they must attend all.

Concerning the surrogate, some have contended that in entering into a surrogacy arrangement she fails to treat herself with appropriate self-respect and thus devalues herself. This view requires an account of self-respect that would explain why gestating a child with the intention that others be its parents cannot demonstrate sufficient respect for oneself. Cecile Fabre (2006) attributes such a view to certain theories of the integrity of the body found in liberalism. On these liberal views, personal services involving the body are radically different from taxation: while it might be permissible (albeit not for libertarians) to require taxation to meet the material needs of others, it is impermissible to command personal services to the same end. Fabre replies that if there are duties in justice to provide the poor with material goods needed for a meaningful life by means of taxation, there are also duties in justice to provide them with necessary personal services—at least, absent some other reason to differentiate personal services from material goods. But what might these reasons be, and can they be applied to surrogacy? I have already set aside arguments that these services are uniquely burdensome or intimate. Drawing once again from Radin and Anderson, other arguments might be that surrogacy services can never be freely chosen, that these services must compromise the surrogate's integrity and thus her ability to lead a flourishing life, or that reproduction must be regarded in a special way that surrogacy does not allow.

Radin holds that market-inalienability should apply when needed to protect individual freedom. Some reasons are prophylactic, if in practice prohibiting any surrogacy is necessary to prevent the emergence of coercive surrogacy. Analogous arguments have been made recently about the Swedish law prohibiting the purchase of sex (but not its sale) that prohibition of voluntary prostitution is necessary to root out human trafficking.[18] Actual likelihoods of coercion are an empirical question, but it might be hypothesized that coercive surrogacy is more likely in trans-border arrangements than in domestic surrogacy contracts and in arrangements where there is a great deal of economic disparity between the parties.[19] At a minimum, it is surely important to have adequate protections against exploitation implemented in all surrogacy arrangements. At present, it is questionable whether voluntary self-regulation on the part of reproductive professionals is sufficient to ensure that these protections are implemented and followed.[20]

Radin also hypothesizes a kind of domino effect, if permitting commercialized versions of a practice undermines keeping noncommercialized versions intact. It would thus be an argument against commercialized surrogacy if its presence undercuts altruistic surrogacy, at least assuming that it is desirable for altruistic surrogacy to continue. I know of no empirical evidence that this is the case, however, although there surely are concerns about unregulated commercial surrogacy in some US states. Moreover, noncommercial surrogacy (including compensation for expenses and lost wages) is permitted in many nations across the globe and continues despite the availability of commercial forms elsewhere.[21] A concern on the other side is that those who favor noncommercialized surrogacy are more likely to engage a traditional surrogate, which is a far riskier endeavor from a family law perspective.[22]

A related reason given by Radin is that a surrogate cannot act freely. But it is unclear why as a general matter decisions to carry a surrogate pregnancy should all be unfree, any more so than other pregnancies. Indeed, surrogate pregnancies have an advantage over as many as half of other pregnancies at least in that they are planned. So it would need to be true that clear, deliberative choices to undergo pregnancy in these circumstances cannot be freely undertaken. Surely with appropriate counseling surrogacy arrangements can be entered into with full information. Appropriate legal protections can give assurances that surrogacy contracts are not adopted as a result of threats or coercive economic need. Categorical views about the types of pregnancies that can be voluntary—such as that only pregnancies within marriage can be voluntary, or that no pregnancies can ever be fully voluntary—would seem to rely on questionable essentialist assumptions about the forms that free reproduction can take.

These points do not take fully into account the possibility that many surrogacy choices arise out of such complex circumstances and emotions that they should be regarded with suspicion. For example, Fabre cites data to the effect that surrogates most frequently enter into the arrangement out of a complexity of emotions, including guilt over prior abortions and other "mistakes" (2006, p. 192). If so, this would provide a reason for concern about whether surrogacy can be seen as evincing appropriate self-respect, or as manifesting problematic self-blame. Other data indicate that the most likely motivation for surrogacy is the altruistic desire to give parenthood to others (Jadva et al. 2003). Here, too, however, there are concerns about whether in intrafamilial arrangements subtle forms of coercion might be operative; for example, a fertile sister might feel guilty about her ability to reproduce when confronted with the pain of a sister who cannot (ESHRE Task Force 2011). Surely these pressures are operative in some surrogacy decisions; whether they are operative in sufficient numbers to say that the practice is unethical is another matter. Moreover, careful counseling can identify many cases of inappropriate pressures, even if some may remain. In assessing the evidence about the likelihood that surrogates are not choosing freely, care must be taken not to assume that reproductive choices must be irrational or subject to emotions so strong as to overwhelm choice.

A related argument made by surrogacy's critics is that the surrogate fails to recognize the inevitable emotional ties resulting from gestation. Some claims about these ties were hypothesized before gestational surrogacy's replacement of traditional surrogacy. But even with gestational surrogacy, surely the biological changes associated with pregnancy and birth will generate emotional reactions. It is an empirical matter what forms these emotions are likely to take, how severe they are likely to be, or whether they are likely to interfere with the surrogate's subsequent life to an extent that suggests that surrogacy is wrong. One recent (albeit small) study indicates that although the immediate postbirth period is difficult, surrogates do not show signs of depression or reduced self-esteem 10 years after birth (Jadva, Imrie, and Golombok 2014). Moreover, surrogates frequently maintain contact with the intended parents and offspring to an extent that they find satisfying. Arguing that the emotional reactions of pregnancy must be so strong or manifested in a parent–child relationship—so that surrogacy is inconsistent with self-respect—would appear at best a risky strategy for feminists who want to avoid essentialist commitments about the nature of women's emotions.

Another freedom-based concern is that surrogacy contracts may be structured to commit the woman to relinquish the child before birth, or even before pregnancy has been achieved. Critics argue that this precommitment does not respect the woman's liberty to change her mind about a very important life event. Some contend that women even when they believe they have completed their own families may not be able to anticipate the emotions they will feel upon being expected to surrender the child they have borne after birth, and so should not be committed to this until after the child's arrival. On this view, no surrogacy contracts could be enforceable unless they provide a window of choice postpartum for the surrogate to decide whether to relinquish her parental rights. These arguments against precommitment were developed when traditional surrogacy was the primary form of the practice; it is understandable that women with genetic ties to the child might feel differently about relinquishment than women without genetic ties as would be the case with gestational surrogacy, as is also illustrated in the case of adoption.

In assessing surrogacy arrangements involving prebirth commitments, it is useful to ask whether surrogacy contracts are unique in the likelihood of subsequent regret, or whether there are other proposed contracts that are judged impermissible because of their unanticipated emotional burdens when the time comes for enforcement. Several doctrines in contract law might be analytically helpful here (see Fabre 2006, pp. 215–216). On a theory of unilateral mistake, contracts are voidable if one party held a mistaken belief at the time the contract was entered, that party does not bear the risk of the mistake under the contract, and either enforcement of the contract would be unconscionable or the other party had reason to know of the mistake at the time of contracting or was at fault for the mistake.[23] Typical cases of unilateral mistake are sales in which the seller was grossly in error about the nature of the item sold and seeks to undo the deal. In surrogacy, the mistake would be the surrogate's belief about her future feelings about relinquishing the child and the judgment that enforcement of the contract would be unconscionable would be based on the surrogate's attachment to the child. Cases in which contracts are voidable for unilateral mistake are very unusual, however, given the aim of contract law to introduce stability into exchange relationships. If surrogacy is different, perhaps the conclusion to be drawn is that surrogate contracts lacking a post-partum window should be unenforceable as unconscionable. This introduces an element of uncertainty into any surrogacy agreement, although in the vast majority of cases the arrangement will conclude as planned. In any event, a determination that freedom requires this limitation on surrogacy contracts is not an argument against surrogacy, but only for structuring surrogacy contracts to give surrogates the liberty to change their minds within a postpartum window.

Yet another reason for rejecting surrogacy is the judgment that surrogacy expresses the wrong sort of regard for one's reproductive capacities. On this view, the surrogate sees her reproductive capacities as something to be used to produce a child for someone else rather than for her own parenting. It would be question begging to argue that surrogacy is wrong because it is wrong to use ones reproductive capacities for another—whether or not this use is wrong is exactly what is at issue. Radin, Anderson, and other writers argue that reproduction is alienated if the child is for another; the idea here is that reproduction must be linked to the intention to parent (even though there are circumstances such as wartime, privation, or disease in which it seems unlikely that the intention will come to fruition). For example, Stuart Oultram writes that "women who donate eggs arguably do so in an alienated way in so much as they donate to assist others rather than because they want to become parents themselves" (2015, p. 472). Christine Overall advances a similar point in arguing that surrogacy demonstrates inadequate levels of care for the child: "it must be acknowledged that the gestating woman creates the baby not because she wants it for its own sake but precisely *in order* to give it away; so her caring certainly has strict limits (2015, p. 354). And Carole Pateman (1988) argues that surrogacy is wrong because it detaches women from their reproductive identities.

Now, powerful reasons for linking reproduction to the intention to parent are protection of the resulting child or the parent–child relationship. It is unclear, however, why the parenting intention or the parent–child relation must lie between the gestating woman and the child she bears, and not between the child and the intended parents (notably even in cases in which they are the genetic parents of the child, having contributed the gametes used in in vitro fertilization, or in which neither the surrogate nor the intended parents are genetically related to the child because conception was achieved with a donated embryo). In any event, subsequent sections will take up regard for the child and regard for the parent–child relationship. Here, the issue is why reproduction would be problematic because it is not linked to the gestating woman's own intention to parent and it is hard to see what an answer would be that is not simply a rejection of surrogacy.

A final possibility is that in becoming a surrogate, a woman compromises her own ability to have a meaningful conception of her good. Conceptual claims to this effect might be that having a child for another cannot be part of a meaningful conception of the good, or that intending to parent a child one bears must be part of a meaningful conception of one's good. But it is hard to see why these claims are not question begging. Empirical versions of this concern would be that surrogacy is such a commitment that it precludes other activities that are critical to a meaningful conception of one's good.

If surrogacy compromised women's later capabilities to form partnerships or families, or reduced the likelihood of surrogates pursuing educations or satisfying careers, this would indeed be a weighty concern. But there are ways of selecting surrogates that blunt this objection. Surrogacy could be limited to women who have already had children or to those whose partners consent—although either of these limits might themselves be regarded as impermissible restrictions on reproductive liberty. Moreover, many women become surrogates because they believe that surrogacy will further their conceptions of their good. With commercial surrogacy, women may engage in the practice to provide more than they would otherwise be able to for their own children, or to stay at home with their children rather than entering the workforce in other ways. Some women become surrogates in order to pay for their educations. To be sure, care must be taken that these arrangements are not exploitative. But in practice there surely are contexts in which surrogacy does not detract from and even furthers the surrogate's well-formed conception of her good.

Surrogacy's critics also argue that the practice is inevitably gendered, as it imposes the male intended parent's preferences on the surrogate or compels his partner to raise another's child. This objection, if it has purchase at all, applies most clearly to situations such as the Baby M case in which the traditional surrogate is artificially inseminated with the intended father's sperm. Many surrogate pregnancies today involve the gametes of the intended parents or gametes from unrelated donors. In such cases, the genetic tie to the child may be as important to the female partner as to the male. Surrogacy is also a reproductive option for same-sex couples wanting to become parents through means other than adoption. Although surely some pregnancies and some surrogate pregnancies involve gendered pressures to have "his" child, it is by no means necessary for all or many surrogate pregnancies to do so. It would seem particularly odd to make this argument in the cases in which a woman's oocyte and donated sperm are used, or gametes from neither intended parent are used, or the intended parents are a same-sex couple. At most, the concerns about gender hierarchy seem applicable to surrogacy using sperm from the male intended parent but donated oocytes, as might be the case for older couples seeking to become parents. But this would yield the odd result: that surrogacy is ethically problematic in just the case in which gametes of the male intended parent are used. A far more reasonable position is to screen and counsel surrogates and intended parents to do the best to assure that the choices of all parties are genuinely made in a manner free from pressure.

SURROGACY: THE CHILD'S INTERESTS AND IDENTITY

Surrogacy is about assisting in the creation of a baby for another. Many objections to surrogacy contend that it is "baby selling." In noncommercial surrogacy, these objections do not hold, but other concerns about the baby may apply. Before turning to these other objections, however, it is important to unpack what might be the subject of sale in commercial surrogacy. Here are some possibilities: the child, rights of the child, rights over the child, or gestational services. It is generally agreed that the sale of a human being by another human being is wrong: it treats the person as a commodity, violates the person's freedom and dignity, and likely subjects the person to oppression or worse. It also treats persons as fungible commodities, exchangeable for other commodities with more desirable characteristics if the price is right. Children are not fungible commodities and must not be treated as such, either by the producing surrogate or by the intended parents. Fabre draws the conclusion that the surrogate must regard the child as more than an object with exchange value, as must the receiving parents. This regard, she thinks, differentiates surrogacy from the case of a celebrity couple having a baby to sell it to the highest bidder, or of parents deciding to put an older child up for bids.

But if we distinguish such sales regarding the person as a fungible commodity—in which there is a paid transfer of all rights and duties over the person as object—from the sale of more particular rights of or over the person (Fabre 2006, p. 190; Hanna 2010), whether these other forms of sale are objectionable is more complex. Parenthetically, it should be noted that there are other cases in which the use value of a child is coupled with respect for the child in his or her own right. Consider the creation of so-called replacement babies for a child who has died (Encyclopedia of Death and Dying 2016) or savior siblings for a child in need of stem cell replacement after high-dose chemotherapy (Sheldon and Wilkinson 2003). Although these practices are ethically controversial, many contend that they are ethically permissible as long as the resulting child will be raised in a loving fashion.

The impermissibility of the sale of rights of the person depends on what those rights are and the process of sale. Many rights of persons—ordinary property rights, for example—are subject to sale at the discretion of the person. Other rights—liberty rights, rights to be a property owner, or rights to nondiscrimination—are judged on many political theories not to be alienable in this way. Commercial surrogacy presses whether the child's right to particular parents could be subject to sale. But a core question about surrogacy is whether the child has a right to be raised by a gestational parent—or instead whether genetic or social ties are the basis for the child's right to be parented by the persons with those ties. From the claim that the child has a right to be parented, or the weaker claim that the child has a right to be assured that his or her needs will be met and that she will be afforded the opportunities requisite for a meaningful life, it does not follow that the child has a right to be parented by her gestational parent. It would, of course, follow that the child's rights to adequate parenting, welfare, or opportunities must be protected in any surrogacy arrangement and that surrogacy arrangements without such protections are impermissible.

An additional complication about the child's rights is that children cannot act for themselves. This complication does not mean that rights of the child cannot be alienated, but it does mean that any alienation must be subject to conditions that protect the interests of the child and that hold open critically important choices for the child to make at a later time to the extent possible (e.g., Davis 1997, Feinberg 1980, Mills 2003). To be permissible, surrogacy arrangements must respect these constraints. In this regard, there is an important dispute about whether children should be told the circumstances of their conception or gestation, including information about the identity of gamete donors or surrogates. This issue is considered by Glenn Cohen's contribution to this volume.

In commercial surrogacy, another possible object of sale is the gestating parent's parental rights over the child. Elizabeth Anderson, for example, has argued that parental rights of genetic parents should not be bought or sold (1990, p. 79). In considering whether selling these rights is objectionable, it is worth noting that some sales of rights over persons may be permissible, depending on the context and the rights in question. Although most political philosophies agree it is wrong for persons to sell themselves into slavery, or to be sold into slavery, it is not so clear that it is wrong for people to buy themselves out of slavery or for others to do so on their behalf, thus extinguishing the rights of slaveholders. (Of course, this would only be an issue in partial compliance theory, as slavery itself is wrong.) Radin contends that it is wrong for parents to sell their rights to a child, because it is in effect selling the child (1987, p. 1904). But this raises the question whether sale of these particular rights over a child treats the child as an object of sale; I have argued earlier that it need not do so if the rights and interests of the child are protected.

Yet another possibility is that it wrongs the gestational parent for her parental rights to be subject to sale. Surely it does when the circumstances of sale are coercive, but it is a different question whether it does so in other cases. The preceding section argued that the sale of gestational services is not a wrong to the surrogate if it occurs in a context in which she is adequately protected. Such sales need not interfere with her liberty, her integrity, or her ability to lead a meaningful life if they are structured in ways that protect her adequately. Leaving for the next section whether commercial surrogacy appropriately respects the parent–child relationship, similar reasoning can be applied to the sale of parental rights.

A further question is whether the gestational surrogate has parental rights to sell or to give away in the first place. Why parental rights should attach exclusively or at all to the gestational parent is itself at issue in surrogacy. Elizabeth Anderson argued about traditional surrogacy that a "consent-intent" conceptualization of parenthood—that the intended parents are the possessors of parental rights—makes parenthood arbitrary. Instead, she argues for recognition of genetic ties as determinative of parenthood: in recognizing these ties, she says, "we help to secure children's interests in having an assured place in the world, which is more firm than the wills of their parents . . . [it] does not make the obligation to care for those whom one has created (intentionally or not) contingent upon an arbitrary desire to do so" (1990, p. 79). This view, however, would vest parental rights in the surrogate only when she is the genetic parent, which she will not be in cases of gestational surrogacy where the genetic parents will either be the intended parents or donors. It would seem implausible to assume that vesting parental rights in this way will be most protective of children. This suggests that the determination of where to locate parental rights is a normative choice, constructed rather than determined by some "natural" feature such as gestation or genetics. For a variety of historical reasons, among them identifying stable sources of parenting for children, legal regimes have identified gestating women and their partners during gestation as the legal parents of the child, but there is nothing inevitable about this location. On the other side of gestational parenting is the argument that the failure to recognize the role of the intended parent devalues the role of persons in initiating reproductive projects (Robertson 1996; see also Oultram 2015).

In addition to stable parenting and protection of the child's interests, another issue that has been raised about surrogacy is the child's identity. Understanding identity is far beyond the scope of this discussion, but it should be noted briefly that there are many different accounts of identity not at all linked to genetics or gestation. Especially important here are views of identity as social (e.g., Appiah 2014, 2005). Such accounts may link identity to nation, culture, race, sex, disability, or religion, among other social constructions. To hold that children's identity is violated if their genetic parents do not raise them is to ignore the complexity of these matters. And it is also, of course, to reject any reproduction in which gamete donation plays a part, as well as adoption. Children need identities, but it is far from clear that these must be identities constructed by their genetic parents.

The Relationship of Gestating

A final set of criticisms of surrogacy claims that it has a mistaken view of the parent–child relationship. The surrogate interacts with the baby in carrying it, these critics argue, and this relationship is not respected if the child is given away. In this respect, pregnancy is a unique form of labor. Overall writes: "The situation of a pregnant woman is radically different from the situation of a factory worker. The factory worker brings only his skill and labor to the factory; he does not provide the materials on which he labors or the environment in which he labors. The pregnant woman, on the other hand, is, herself, the environment in which her reproductive labor is performed. She also provides the materials out of which the child is created" (Overall 2015, p. 357). Earlier sections of this chapter have considered the interests of the surrogate and the child separately; the view to be explored here is that the pregnancy itself creates a relationship that is not properly respected by relinquishment of the child. On this view, there must be overriding reasons—such as the incapacity of gestators—to warrant sundering this relationship, but these reasons do not obtain in surrogacy.

But why should gestation be regarded as ethically weighty in this way? To be sure, 9 months of interaction with a fetus (assuming the pregnancy is carried to term) has effects on the woman's body and emotions that must be taken into account. And the child in utero has experiences, too; there is evidence that after birth children respond in particular ways to prebirth experiences. These facts may be taken to have metaphysical significance, as Hilde Lindemann (this volume) explores. But whether these considerations yield the conclusion that the gestational relationship should have over-riding ethical force is another matter.

Conclusion

This chapter has addressed objections to surrogacy that do not depend on exploitation or commercialization. It has argued that reasons offered for claims that surrogacy wrongs the surrogate, the resulting child, or the parent–child relationship would rule out other practices widely regarded as permissible, devalue the desire of infertile couples to become intended parents, or assume the impermissibility of surrogacy. The examination of these arguments does reveal important cautions about surrogacy, however. Care must be taken to assure that all parties are well informed as to risks. Both surrogates and intended parents must be carefully evaluated. Interests of the child in adequate parenting must be assured. Although payment for surrogacy is not per se problematic, exploitation is a risk of surrogacy; the protections in place today in at least some jurisdictions may not be adequate safeguards, especially when surrogacy is commercialized. Finally, protection of the woman's choice about matters important to identity and relationships is a reason for giving her the option to relinquish any parental claims she might have after birth.

Notes

1. For example, Christine Overall (2014) has recently proposed a system of parental licensing for people using surrogates.
2. A symposium issue of the *Washington Law Review* published in December 2014 does consider whether commercial surrogacy should be more widely available in light of the decision of the US Supreme Court rejecting California's ban on same-sex marriage. The contribution by David Orentlicher to this volume contains an excellent summary of state laws concerning surrogacy, including limits on traditional surrogacy and commercial surrogacy.
3. For an argument that legal preferences for gestational surrogacy mistakenly limit the liberty of surrogates and intended parents, and impose greater risks and costs on all parties, see Shapiro (2014).
4. *In the Matter of Baby M*, 109 N.J. 396, 537 A.2d 1227 (N.J. 1988).
5. 109 N.J. at 425.
6. *Johnson v. Calvert*, 19 Cal. Rptr.2d 494, 851 P. 2d 776 (Cal. 1993) (en banc).
7. 851 P.2d at 784.
8. 851 P.2d at 782.
9. 851 P. 2d at 787.
10. 851 P.2d at 784.
11. *A.W.H & P.W. v. G.H.B.*, 339 N.J.Super. 495, 503 (2000).
12. In re T.J.S., 212 N.J. 334, 54 A.3d 263 (N.J. 2012).

13. Ibid. at 336 (Hoens, J., concurring) (per curiam).
14. Washington is an example, West's RCWA 26.26.101, 26.26.230. By comparison, organ donation is another example of bodily use in service of another that many believe ought not to be commercialized, even leaving aside risks of exploitation; this view is implemented in the prohibition on organ sales in the United States and elsewhere.
15. Shapiro (2014) extends this fairness concern in arguing that compensation isn't the important issue for feminist analysis of surrogacy; instead, power dynamics and exploitation are critical to judgments of forms of surrogacy.
16. Commercialization aside, the therapeutic sex performed with a man with severe physical disabilities in the movie *The Sessions* would be regarded as inappropriate on this basis. The movie is based on the story of Mark O'Brian, "On Seeing a Sex Surrogate," http://noteasybeingred.tumblr.com/post/16646893808/on-seeing-a-sex-surrogate-mark-obrian.
17. For a discussion of the difference between use value and exchange value, see Dickenson, this volume.
18. estonicia!co. "Sweden's Prostitution Solution: Why Hasn't Anyone Tried This Before?" http://prostitutionresearch.com/wp-content/uploads/2014/11/Swedens-Prostitution-Solution.pdf.
19. Jeffrey Kirby (2014) explains why current transnational practices are coercive and how they might be rendered less so.
20. For an excellent discussion of protections for surrogates, see ASRM Ethics Committee 2013. Although ASRM requires its members to subscribe to the standards and principles of the Society, this does not prevent nonmembers from engaging in activities that ASRM would find unethical.
21. The European Society of Human Reproduction and Endocrinology, for example, takes the position that noncommercial surrogacy is the only permissible form of the practice, including payment for medical expenses not otherwise covered, expenses of pregnancy, and lost wages (ESHRE Task Force 2005).
22. I owe this point to Judith Daar.
23. Rest. (2d) Contracts § 153.

BIBLIOGRAPHY

Anderson, E. 1990. Is women's labor a commodity? *Philosophy & Public Affairs* 19, no. 1: 71–92.
Appiah, K. A. 2014. *Lines of descent: W.E.B. du Bois and the emergence of identity*. Cambridge, MA: Harvard University Press.
Appiah, K. A. 2005. *The ethics of identity*. Princeton, NJ: Princeton University Press.
Brown, D. X. 2003. Nurses and preventable back injuries. *American Journal of Critical Care* 12, no. 5: 400–401.
Davis, D. 1997. Genetic dilemmas and the child's right to an open future. *Hastings Center Report* 27, no. 2: 7–15.
Encyclopedia of Death and Dying. 2016. Replacement children, *Encyclopedia of Death and Dying*, http://www.deathreference.com/Py-Se/Replacement-Children.html.
ESHRE Task Force on Ethics and Law. 2011. Intrafamilial medically assisted reproduction. *Human Reproduction* 26, no. 3: 504–509.
ESHRE Task Force on Ethics and Law. 2005. Surrogacy. *Human Reproduction* 20, no. 10: 2705–2707.

Ethics Committee of the American Society for Reproductive Medicine. 2013. Consideration of the gestational carrier: A committee opinion. *Fertility & Sterility* 99: 1838–1841.

Fabre, C. 2006. *Whose body is it anyway?* Oxford, UK: Oxford University Press.

Feinberg, J. 1980. The child's right to an open future. In *Whose child? Children's rights, parental authority, and state power*, ed. W. Aiken and H. LaFollette. Totowa, NJ: Rowman & Littlefield.

Hanna, J. K. M. 2010. Revisiting child-based objections to commercial surrogacy. *Bioethics* 24, no. 7: 341–347.

Harris, S. 2013. Injury, illness rates among nursing, residential care workers triple U.S. Average. http://www.shrm.org/hrdisciplines/safetysecurity/articles/pages/injury-illness-rates-nursing.aspx.

Jadva, V., S. Imrie, and S. Golombok. 2014. Surrogate mothers 10 years on: A longitudinal study of psychological well-being and relationships with the parents and child. *Human Reproduction* 30, no. 2: 373–379.

Jadva, V., C. Murray, E. Lycett, F. MacCallum, and S. Golombok. 2003. Surrogacy: The experiences of surrogate mothers. *Human Reproduction* 18: 2196–2204.

Kirby, J. 2014. Transnational gestational surrogacy: Does it have to be exploitative? *American Journal of Bioethics* 14, no. 5: 24–32.

Levine, C. 2005. Acceptance, avoidance, and ambiguity: Conflicting social values about childhood disability. *Kennedy Institute of Ethics Journal* 15, no. 4: 371–383.

Lindemann, H. 2009. Holding one another (well, wrongly, clumsily) in a time of dementia. *Metaphilosophy* 40, no. 3–4: 416–424.

Mills, C. 2003. The child's right to an open future? *Journal of Social Philosophy* 34, no. 4: 499–509.

Oultram, S. 2015. One mum too few: Maternal status in host surrogate motherhood arrangements. *Journal of Medical Ethics* 41, no. 6: 470-473.

Overall, C. 2015. Reproductive 'surrogacy' and parental licensing. *Bioethics* 29, no. 5: 353–361.

Pande, A. 2014. *Wombs in labor: Transnational commercial surrogacy in India.* New York: Columbia University Press.

Pateman, C. 1988. *The sexual contract.* Cambridge, UK: Polity Press.

Practice Committee of the American Society for Reproductive Medicine and Practice Committee of the Society for Assisted Reproduction Technology [ASRM Practice Committee]. 2015. Recommendations for practices using gestational carriers: A committee opinion. *Fertility & Sterility* 103, no. 1: e1–e8.

Radin, M. J. 1987. Market-inalienability. *Harvard Law Review* 100: 1849–1937.

Reichman, T. W. et al. 2011. Living donor hepatectomy: The importance of the residual liver volume. *Liver Transplantation* 17, no. 12: 1404–1411.

Robertson, J. A. 1996. *Children of choice: Freedom and the new reproductive technologies.* Princeton, NJ: Princeton University Press.

Shapiro, J. 2014. For a feminist considering surrogacy, is compensation really the key question? *Washington Law Review* 89, no. 4: 1345–1373.

Sheldon, S. and S. Wilkinson. 2003. Should selecting savior siblings be banned? *Journal of Medical Ethics* 30, no. 6: 533–537.

Stevens, E. E., T. E. Patrick, and R. Pickler. 2009. A history of infant feeding. *Journal of Perinatal Education* 18, no. 2: 32–39.

Thomson, J. J. 1971. A defense of abortion. *Philosophy & Public Affairs* 1, no. 1: 47–56.

van Zyl, L. and R. Walker. 2013. Beyond altruistic and commercial contract motherhood: The professional model. *Bioethics* 27, no. 7: 373–381.

CHAPTER 18

PARENTS WITH DISABILITIES

ADAM CURETON

HAVING and raising children is widely regarded as one of the most valuable projects a person can undertake.[1] Yet many disabled people like myself find it difficult to share fully in this value because of obstacles that arise from widespread social attitudes about disability.[2] A common assumption is that having a disability tends to make someone less fit to parent than other people, while having a severe disability tends to make someone unfit to parent at all.[3] Parenting a child, some think, is just too burdensome for a disabled person who is already struggling to maintain herself. Disabled people, it is also assumed, are more likely to have disabled children with lives that are often worse than those of other children.[4] And some people with disabilities are discouraged from procreating altogether because they are regarded as asexual and romantically undesirable in virtue of being seen as "sick" or "defective."[5]

These attitudes about people with disabilities played a prominent role in the forced sterilizations of the eugenics movement, but even now the assumptions that disabled people are ill equipped to parent, genetically inferior, or asexual have profound effects on our ability to have and raise children. Many disabled children, particularly those with more severe disabilities, are not taught much about sexuality, reproduction, and parenting; they are not usually encouraged to date, nor are they commonly subject to social expectations and informal inducements to raise a family of their own; and many of us are not seen as potential romantic partners by nondisabled people. Some health care professionals, who regard it as improper for people with certain kinds of disabilities to reproduce or parent, are less likely to screen for sexually transmitted diseases, discuss sexual health, dysfunction, or contraception, or provide access to assistive reproductive technologies; they may also discourage their disabled patients from becoming pregnant and pressure them to have an abortion if they do conceive.[6] If a disabled person decides to have or adopt a child, she is likely to meet with suspicion and scrutiny from adoption agencies, social workers, family court judges, friends, family, and society at large.[7] She may also have difficulty securing the kinds of accommodations she needs to be a good parent. These forms of treatment can send disabled people the message that procreation and parenting are not for them. Many people with disabilities simply acquiesce by choosing not to raise families of their own while others have persevered by, for example, forming mutually supporting communities that help them to be better parents.

The assumption that having a disability tends to make someone an unfit or bad parent may seem especially relevant as a factor in decisions about whether to allow, encourage, and assist disabled people to reproduce and raise children. Yet there are reasons to doubt whether there is such a close connection between having a disability in general and lacking the ability to raise a child well. We may not fully appreciate the potential that many disabled people have to be good parents because of various unconscious biases we have about disability and because we lack adequate information about whether, for example, blind people or quadriplegics can, with the right accommodations, adequately care for a child. Some people have physical and mental impairments that prevent them from taking primary responsibility for an infant, yet other disabled people are fine caregivers who are able to meet the physical, psychological, and emotional needs of their child very well.

Moral questions about allowing, encouraging, and assisting disabled people to reproduce and raise children are likely to be contentious because they often depend on empirical facts that are difficult to know as well as conflicting values that are difficult to interpret and apply. One way to make some progress on these issues is to identify more specific questions to address along with some widely shared values that can guide our deliberations about them.

There are questions about what the law should say regarding disabled people who wish to procreate and parent; there are questions about what socially enforced moral rules a society should affirm regarding such matters; and there are questions about what choices a disabled person should make about procreating. A person with a disability may have the moral and legal right to reproduce, for example, even though it would be morally inadvisable for her to do so because her condition is so unpredictable.[8] Laws may not be fine-grained enough to give adequate guidance in uncommon cases or to fully realize the values that justify having the laws in the first place—the federal 15/22 rule, for example, says that if a child is in foster care for 15 of the last 22 months then states must file a petition to terminate parental rights. Some disabled people, however, may run afoul of the rule through no fault of their own because they were forced to spend time separated from their child in order to adapt their homes, learn new parenting techniques, and otherwise satisfy social workers that they are fit to parent.[9] Professional rules and guidelines that are sensitive to some of the nonstandard but effective ways that many disabled people fulfill their parental responsibilities should guide courts, social workers, adoption agencies, and assistive reproductive providers in their assessments of disabled parents. The law may give parents significant latitude about how they raise their children, but stricter social moral rules and individual judgment may be needed to determine the risks they may impose on their children as well as the circumstances in which others should intervene on behalf of another person's child. Disabilities of various kinds will raise different moral questions about procreation and parenting children of different ages and abilities, and disabled women and female caregivers face pressing issues about body image, gendered roles, sexual vulnerability, exclusion, and oppression.[10] And many of us, disabled and nondisabled alike, have conscientiously asked ourselves whether we would be good parents, and, if we already have children, we wonder whether we are doing enough for them.[11]

The aims of this chapter are, *first*, to identify and clarify some values that are relevant to questions about allowing, encouraging, and assisting disabled people to procreate and raise children; *second*, to give an overview of how these values can help us to address certain legal questions that arise for disabled people who aim to procreate and parent; *third*, to consider the challenge that the rights to procreate and parent are formal and empty for many people with disabilities; *fourth*, to raise concerns about how to properly assess the parenting capacities of people with disabilities; and *fifth*, to suggest some ways in which having a disability can actually make someone a better parent.

REASONABLE VALUES

We can identify several values that are at stake when assessing practical issues that arise for (prospective) parents with disabilities. The values are widely shared when described at a relatively high level of generality, which allows us to set aside, for practical purposes, questions about their foundation and focus instead on how to interpret and apply them as a whole. The values can conflict with one another, and none of them takes absolute priority over the rest. Our task is not simply to weigh and balance the values against one another in order to determine what would bring about the best overall state of affairs. Some of the values are to be respected, honored, and cherished, not just promoted, so moral judgment involves reconciling various presumptions that can override, defeat, and enable one another.

First, many people deeply value reproduction and parenting. Although a life can go perfectly well without children, procreation and parenting usually involve creating a valuable relationship between parent and child that paradigmatically involves mutual love, trust, and intimacy as well as special responsibilities and obligations to care for the child and to help her develop. Such relationships often give shape and meaning to the lives of parents, they tend to become part of their identity, and they often provide a deep source of satisfaction. Those who are unable to become parents but wish to do so tend to experience deep sorrow and despair for their inability to participate in what they see as a very great good.

Second, it is good for people to have the ability to make significant decisions about their own lives without undue influence from others, especially with regard to reproduction, marriage, parenting, religious faith, and so on.[12] Autonomy in this sense may ground a presumptive moral right that imposes duties on others. A right to autonomy would include a right to make one's own choices about when and with whom to reproduce and how many children to have, as well as a right to direct their upbringing. Autonomy rights must be interpreted and qualified, however, to specify what counts as undue influence on our decisions and what counts as a significant life decision; they must also say how potential conflicts among the autonomous choices of different people should be reconciled.

Third, well-being is important as well, but different aspects of it matter in different ways. Basic needs for food, shelter, security, and health may ground presumptive moral rights and duties while other aspects of happiness may be good to promote without generating any moral requirement to do so. The well-being of children, whose basic needs also include education and moral development, may warrant special moral protection because of their vulnerability and dependence. A substantive theory of well-being, or perhaps a set of such theories that are suited to different purposes and contexts, would specify in more detail the ingredients of a good life.

Fourth, it is also important to avoid relying on morally irrelevant distinctions among persons in how we treat or regard them, particularly when such treatment is to their detriment.[13] A fuller account of discrimination in this sense would specify the kinds of distinctions among persons that are legitimate to rely on and in what contexts, but we can agree that, for example, denying university admission to someone simply because she is African American is unjustified discrimination while forbidding a blind person from driving a school bus because of safety concerns is not. Other kinds of potentially unjustified discrimination are more implicit, such as relying on morally irrelevant factors because they correlate with relevant ones or disproportionately disadvantaging people on account of morally irrelevant characteristics as a side effect of an act or policy that was not aimed at doing so.

Finally, the dignity of persons is a great value, which means we have strong reasons not to demean, humiliate, or ridicule others as well as reasons to *express* respect to them. This value needs further elaboration depending on the context in which it is applied, but various kinds of verbal and physical abuse, cruelty, objectification, and neglect are incompatible with having and showing full respect to the dignity of children, while it can be humiliating and degrading, for example, to be forced to justify one's parenting abilities to others.

LEGAL ISSUES

To see how these values can come into conflict in certain contexts and be reconciled for particular purposes, let's consider how the US legal system has addressed questions of disability, procreation, and parenting.

Parental Rights and Child Interests

The legal rights to procreate and raise children are included in human rights documents and recognized by the Supreme Court as falling under the Due Process Clause of the Fourteenth Amendment.[14] The Supreme Court has consistently affirmed that parents have fundamental but limited legal rights to reproductive freedom as well as to nurture, care for, educate, and direct their children as they see fit.[15] These rights are grounded in the values of autonomy, liberty, privacy, and the parent–child relationship. The legal right to reproductive freedom is a right to decide for oneself whether or not to have children and, if so, with whom, when, and how many children to have. It is not recognized in US law as a positive right to assistance from others to reproduce, but only as a negative right that protects us from various kinds of interference from others when making certain reproductive choices.[16] Having the legal right to raise children involves certain authorizations to make decisions for them regarding, for example, food, education, and association; this right also comes with certain parental responsibilities to, for instance, meet the child's basic needs.

Human rights documents and the Supreme Court have also afforded children basic legal rights to security of the person, freedom from cruel or degrading treatment, and basic subsistence.[17] These rights are grounded in their dignity, well-being, and status as future full citizens.[18]

The Supreme Court has held that parental rights must be balanced against the interests of others, especially children and potential children.[19] In one kind of case, a person's parental rights can be terminated if an individualized hearing, which satisfies standards of due process, finds that she is an unfit parent. But there is a strong legal presumption in such proceedings for retaining parental rights, according to the Court, so the government must provide compelling and convincing evidence that the person, for example, abused or neglected her child. Simply showing that someone is not the best parent possible, or only mediocre at parenting, is not legally sufficient to override her parental rights, even if severing them would be good for the child.[20] Others, however, may prefer different legal arrangements that give greater legal priority to the interests of children over the rights of parents by, for instance, allowing courts to abnegate or limit parental rights when there are alternative arrangements that are found to be practicable and significantly better for the child, even if the parents are capable of adequately caring for the child themselves.[21]

Another kind of conflict between the rights of parents and the interests of children can arise when the parents of a child divorce, or when a child is born outside of marriage, or when the parents disagree on fundamental matters about how to raise the child. The law allows significant latitude for parents to decide among themselves how to handle such issues, but when an agreement cannot be reached and courts must step in to resolve a dispute, judges are directed to base their decisions on what is in the best interests of the child.[22] Some may think, however, that courts should play a more active role in scrutinizing even private child custody, visitation, and rearing arrangements among parents in order to ensure that the parents do what is best for the child.

Tensions between the interests of children and the legal rights of *prospective* parents can arise when a person seeks to adopt a child. Prospective parents have the legal right to try to adopt a child, but the government can impose eligibility requirements on adoption that are (perhaps mistakenly) taken to be in the best interests of those children. In practice, states have placed relatively few legal restrictions on who may adopt a child, although some of them forbid adoption by people who have been convicted of a sexual offense, who are under a certain age, or who are gay.[23] Adoption agencies are for the most part legally free to make adoption decisions based on their own extra-legal criteria, which are ostensibly aimed at placing children with parents who will best serve the child's interests. A different legal arrangement, however, would be to recognize a positive legal right to become a parent, perhaps one grounded in the value of the parent–child relationship, and so alter eligibility and placement criteria to allow and encourage adoption by more people who can satisfy the basic needs of children.[24] Or some may favor the current system but insist that the government should play a more active role in ensuring that adoption arrangements are in the best interests of the child.[25]

Finally, legal conflicts can arise between the rights of *prospective* parents and the interests of *potential* children. Although the law does not recognize fetuses as full legal persons, the Supreme Court found in *Roe v. Wade* that the state has reasons to protect the interests of potential legal persons, although it also held that these reasons are not strong enough to override the reproductive rights of women. In some states, for example, a pregnant woman who engages in substance abuse that is likely to substantially harm her fetus can be prosecuted or involuntarily committed to a treatment center, while federal law makes it a crime to commit violent assault against a fetus.[26] Another context in which the interests of prospective parents and potential children can be at odds is when someone seeks to use assistive reproductive technologies, such as in vitro fertilization, to produce a child. The federal government and many states have mostly left unregulated how assistive reproductive technology providers decide who is eligible for their services.[27] This has allowed them to consider the ability of prospective parents to care for a potential child when making those decisions. These various legal arrangements would be substantially different, however, if there were a positive legal right to reproduce or if fetuses were regarded as full legal persons. Some have gone so far as to argue, for instance, that the government should regulate who can reproduce by issuing parenting licenses only to those who can prove that they are likely to secure the best interests of their potential child.[28]

Discrimination and Child Interests

In addition to protecting the rights of parents and prospective parents along with the interests of children and potential children, US law forbids certain kinds of discrimination on the basis of race, sex, religion, or disability. One kind of illegal discrimination would occur if, for example, the parental rights of a disabled person were terminated just because she has a disability, or if a disabled person were not awarded custody of her child or denied access to assistive reproductive technologies or adoption services simply on the grounds that she is disabled. Often, however, disabled people are at a disadvantage in such situations, not merely because we are disabled, but because it is assumed that having a disability tends to make someone an unfit or bad parent, so there is a question of whether such treatment counts as unjustified discrimination.

The Americans with Disabilities Act of 1990 and its subsequent amendments, along with the Rehabilitation Act of 1973, prohibit many kinds of discrimination on the basis of disability.[29] These laws also aim to give disabled people an equal opportunity to participate in and benefit from a variety of public and private programs and services. Someone has a disability, according to US law, if she has as an impairment that substantially limits a major life activity, such as seeing, hearing, or walking, or she has an impairment that substantially limits a major bodily function, such as digestion, respiration, or reproduction.[30] Taken together, the Americans with Disabilities Act and the Rehabilitation Act forbid public entities, such as governments, commercial facilities, and public transportation, from excluding disabled people from their activities solely on the basis of disability.[31] These laws also require public entities to provide reasonable accommodations so that disabled people can participate fully in their programs.

There are several explicit exceptions to these antidiscrimination provisions, however, that are included in the law. Public entities may include disability as a criterion of eligibility and refuse to provide certain reasonable accommodations to disabled people as long as doing otherwise would (1) fundamentally alter the nature of their programs, (2) place an undue burden on them, or (3) pose a *direct threat* to the health and safety of others.[32] When public entities choose to exclude certain people with disabilities from their programs because of the direct threat that including them would supposedly pose to others, they are legally required to conduct individualized assessments that take into account current medical knowledge and objective scientific evidence in order to assess the "nature, duration, and severity of the risk; the probability that the potential injury will actually occur; and whether reasonable modifications of policies, practices, or procedures or the provision of auxiliary aids or services will mitigate the risk."[33] Public entities may not legally rely on stereotypes or mere speculations about disability when making such determinations, and they must take into account reasonable accommodations when making their assessments.[34] Although the law is not always followed in these respects, in order for adoption agencies, assistive reproductive technology clinics, and courts to exclude or disadvantage a disabled person as posing a direct threat to his (potential) children, they must legally show a connection between that specific person's disability and his parenting capacities.

Many states nonetheless use disability in general as one among several factors that can justify terminating a person's parental rights. Family courts often take into account the physical and mental health of parents when deciding what custody arrangements are in the best interests of the child. Jurisdictions vary regarding what sort of connection (if any) must be made between a person's disability and her ability to parent, which leaves room for discrimination by social workers, psychologists, judges, and juries, who can rely to some extent on common stereotypes about the parenting abilities of disabled people. A trial court judge, for example, altered a custody order because, in his judgment, the child's quadriplegic father could not take his son fishing, play baseball with him or otherwise have a "normal" relationship with the child.[35] Another trial judge granted primary custody to a father because the mother had a developmental disability that, he assumed, meant that the woman could not help the child develop normally.[36]

And, in a more recent case, two blind parents were separated from their child because they were deemed to be unfit parents.[37] Subsequent proceedings overturned the rulings in each case on grounds that there was not sufficient evidence to establish that having a disability made these people unable to care for their children.[38]

Adoption agencies and most assistive reproductive technology providers are public entities that fall within the scope of the Americans with Disabilities Act. Many of them, however, deny their services to prospective parents with disabilities altogether or significantly discount disabled applicants as such.[39] They defend such treatment by claiming that, even with reasonable accommodations, people with disabilities are unlikely to be good parents because they are disabled. Assistive reproductive technology providers also tend to assume that pregnancy is too dangerous for many disabled people and that certain people with disabilities are likely to pass on their disability to their child. As they see it, there is no positive right to reproduce; they are not preventing the disabled people from procreating or adopting a child, only refusing to assist them in doing so; and they reasonably think that assisting a disabled person to become pregnant or adopt a child would pose a significant risk to others that could not be mitigated by reasonable accommodations.

Further Legal Issues

There are various other legal questions that arise for disabled people who wish to have and raise children. Perhaps there should be a positive legal right to reproduce or parent, which would require providing greater assistance to disabled people in the form of, for example, surrogacy or home attendants. There are questions of distributive justice about people with certain kinds of disabilities who are less capable of becoming pregnant naturally than other people yet who have fewer resources to devote to hiring expensive adoption agencies and assistive reproductive technology providers. Disabled people who are economically disadvantaged as a result of their conditions may not have the money to secure legal representation in custody proceedings or to hire outside parenting assessments by those who are more familiar with alternative and accessible parenting styles.[40] We can also ask what sorts of accommodations, if any, the government should provide to specifically allow disabled people to fulfill parenting responsibilities. There are issues of respect that may arise when disabled people are disproportionately called upon in formal and informal settings to justify their parenting abilities, particularly when people who can reproduce by natural means are typically not required to explain why they would be good parents. This kind of treatment can intimidate otherwise capable disabled people from becoming parents and lead the ones who have children to avoid associating with others, asking for help, revealing the extent of their disability, or leaving bad marriages for fear that their children will be taken from them. Finally, there are legal questions about whether the government should respond differently to people who have a disability before they become parents as opposed to those who acquire a disability after they have become parents.

WORTH OF LIBERTY

Negative rights to procreate and parent guarantee the liberty to reproduce and raise children free from certain kinds of interference by others. Those who have these rights cannot be prevented from reproducing by natural means, formally excluded from seeking artificial methods of reproduction, formally denied access to adoption services, or prevented from rearing their child as they see fit. As long as someone is not explicitly disqualified from seeking custody of her children or applying for adoption and in vitro fertilization services, however, these rights allow judges, adoption agencies, and reproductive clinics to consider parental ability and other criteria when prioritizing their applicants. Negative rights to procreation and parenting are not absolute because they must be balanced against the rights and interests of children and potential children. When such conflicts arise, a person who is unfit to parent may have her parental rights terminated or she may be formally prevented from adopting a child, from receiving fertility services, or, in extreme cases, from reproducing by natural means.

It may seem that, for some people with disabilities, their negative rights to reproduce and parent are merely formal and empty. A disabled person who cannot reproduce by natural means may have the freedom to submit applications to adoption agencies and fertility clinics, but she may have very little, if any, chance of successfully adopting a child or receiving assistive reproductive technologies because she does not have the resources to pay for these services or to adapt her home so that she fares well against the metrics used to decide where children are placed or who receives fertility treatment. A disabled person who has children may have the freedom to seek to maintain custody of them, but she too may have little, if any, chance of success in such proceedings because she lacks the resources to effectively make her case in court or to hire aides that can help her fulfill her parenting responsibilities. If the negative rights to procreation and parenting are justified in part by the great value of the parent–child relationship then some people with disabilities may worry that they are, in effect, still excluded from one of the main values that those rights are meant to secure and protect. They may think that additional measures are therefore needed, beyond the negative rights to procreate and parent, so that everyone is guaranteed fair, and not just formal, access to parenthood.

One possible response to this problem is to argue for a positive right to procreate and parent that would not only prevent others from interfering in those activities but also require them to assist people who have difficulty reproducing or raising children. This suggestion, however, faces several problems. First, these positive rights must specify what kinds of assistance others are obligated to give. Would the rights require doctors to perform in vitro fertilization procedures if they have a general objection to such measures on religious grounds or require scientists to research new reproductive technologies for those who cannot effectively reproduce with current techniques? The concern is that the obligations associated with positive rights to reproduce and procreate may conflict with the basic rights and liberties of other people. A second concern is that if these positive rights mainly require providing people with sufficient economic resources so that they can procreate and parent, perhaps through taxes and transfers, then enforcing these rights equally for all will likely require significant economic resources. The problem is that basic rights in a just society are commonly thought to take precedence over considerations of economic efficiency and the overall good. To justify positive, and not just negative, rights to procreating and parenting, we must explain why it is more important for people to be able to achieve these particular goods than for others to use their resources to effectively pursue their own aims and projects. Negative rights to procreation and parenting arguably have a justification of the required sort, because they derive in part from the values of autonomy and privacy, so we would need similarly strong arguments for why we should guarantee positive rights to procreation and parenting in light of the significant economic strain this is likely to place on others. Finally, a related concern is that those who do not choose to have or raise children may object that they are being forced to contribute resources to people who choose to do so. They may think that such choices are mostly a matter of individual taste and preference and that basic justice should not be concerned with helping people to achieve the particular aims and aspirations they happen to adopt. Instead, on their view, basic justice should aim to secure everyone with a fair share of means to pursue her own permissible aims and projects, whatever they happen to be.

Perhaps these concerns can be overcome, but an alternative proposal is to maintain the negative character of reproductive and parenting rights but also seek to arrange our economic system fairly so that everyone is provided with a fair share of income and wealth that she can then use to procreate and parent, if she so chooses.[41] Some people may not wish to have and raise children and so may decide to devote their resources to other aims and activities. Those who want to have and raise children may nonetheless decide to spend their money on other activities and pursuits that they value more highly. Others may be willing to sacrifice some of their other aims in order to bear the cost of procreation and parenting. Even in a just economic system, however, some people who deeply want children may not have the resources to pay for reproductive procedures or for assistants to help them with parenting tasks, but such an outcome would not conflict with the requirements of justice, on this view, as long as these people are afforded their fair share of resources.

Whether this kind of account can adequately address the concern that negative rights to procreation and parenting are empty and formal depends on what is meant by a fair economic arrangement. According to John Rawls, fair economic arrangements are those in which the only inequalities in income and wealth that exist are ones that benefit the worst-off members of society by, for example, spurring economic growth that is then partially transferred to the poorest members of society.[42] Some people, on Rawls's view, would have greater economic resources than others, which they could use to hire expensive adoption agents and reproductive specialists, but the worst-off members of society would also have more economic resources than if income and wealth were distributed equally. Suppose a disabled person who is very poor wishes to have children but cannot do so through natural means. She requires resources to adapt her environment for parenting and to secure the services of an adoption agency or reproductive clinic. If there were a positive right to reproduce and parent that ensured everyone had the same ability to exercise these rights then it is likely that she would have fewer resources to exercise her rights as compared to a system in which some people were allowed to have more income and wealth than others as long as such inequalities benefited everyone. Under the latter scheme, she would be afforded a fair share of income and wealth that is greater than what she would have had if income and wealth were distributed equally. Procreation and parenting may be more expensive for her than it is for others, but she is allotted her fair share of economic resources that she may spend as she pleases, so it is up to her to decide whether she is willing to accept the trade-offs that come from having and raising children. If it turns out that she still cannot afford to procreate and raise children, even though she has been afforded a fair share of economic resources that is likely greater than if everyone had positive rights to procreation and parenting, society would not owe her further compensation as a matter of justice.

A view of this sort can respond to the three problems I raised about positive rights to reproduce and raise children. First, a Rawlsian view does not conflict with the basic rights and liberties of others when it requires the more fortunate members of society to pay taxes that improve the position of the worst-off members. Second, this view gives priority to securing negative rights to procreation and parenting while also ensuring that the economic system is more efficient than if everyone had an equal right to the same ability to procreate and reproduce. And third, this view does not require people to help others satisfy their specific personal tastes and aims but instead ensures that everyone has a fair share of means to pursue whatever permissible ends she chooses.

Further assistance for parents with disabilities may be required under another requirement of justice, which is to ensure that children are afforded fair equality of opportunity. Fair equality of opportunity, which is one of Rawls's other principles of justice, holds that if two people have the same natural abilities and the same willingness to put them to use then they should have the same chances over the course of their lives to secure privileged offices and positions in society.[43] One of the factors that significantly influences how well a person can compete and secure offices and positions in later life is her upbringing and early family life, so justice favors instituting programs that assist children from less fortunate social circumstances so that they will eventually be able to compete for jobs on a fair basis with those who come from more privileged backgrounds. If a disabled person has a child then, in some cases, measures should be taken by the government to ensure that she has the resources and accommodations she needs to help her child develop his natural talents and abilities well.

Rather than establishing positive rights to reproduce and parent, a society can ensure that the negative rights people with disabilities have to procreate and raise children are not merely empty and formal by arranging its economic system so that everyone has a fair share of resources that he can use to pursue his various aims and projects. For disabled people who become parents, justice may also require measures designed to ensure that their children enjoy the same fair equality of opportunity as those who come from more privileged backgrounds.

PARENTING ASSESSMENTS

If people with disabilities have negative rights to reproduce and raise children under just economic arrangements in which they can decide whether or not to allocate their fair share of resources to exercising these rights, questions remain about whether a disabled person is an adequate or good parent. Let's now consider how we should go about assessing whether and to what extent a disabled person can and will serve the interests of a child she has or may have. As we have seen, this issue is central for addressing legal questions about parental rights, custody, adoption, and access to assistive reproductive technologies. Within the bounds of the law, a disabled person may also sincerely ask herself, or seek guidance from others about, whether she should have children in light of her condition and her social environment or, if she already has a child, what accommodations she should seek and what decisions she should make in order to be a good parent to her child. Her friends and neighbors may wonder as well what kinds of parenting assistance they should offer her, whether it is appropriate to allow her to babysit their children or drive them in a carpool, under what circumstances they should raise concerns about the welfare of her child, and so on.

When we consider whether a disabled person is able to be a fit and good parent, we must try as best we can to identify and overcome any biases we may have that may prejudice our assessments. There may be connections between a person's disability and her parenting skills, but in making such determinations we should be careful not to assume that an impairment in one area automatically diminishes other abilities, that impairments are permanently disabling even with reasonable accommodations, or that the usual ways of completing parenting tasks are the only ones available. We may initially find ourselves assuming that our own experiences make us good judges of what people with disabilities can and cannot do for children—we may think, for instance, that if we were to become blind then we would certainly be unable to keep track of a child or give her appropriate medicine, which may lead us to conclude that those who are congenitally blind must lack those essential parenting skills as well. Further investigation, however, would have revealed that many blind people have developed adaptive strategies that allow them to fulfill these parental functions. We may also have a tendency to over-ascribe certain behaviors to a person's disability rather than to her choices and luck—we may take the irritation an autistic man shows at a recalcitrant social worker or the difficulty a blind woman has at breastfeeding as confirming evidence that their disabilities make them unfit parents. Yet we would not usually draw the same conclusions if we observed these behaviors in nondisabled people. Shocking news reports, folk wisdom, gut reactions, and social stigma about disability may all lead us to overgeneralize about the parenting abilities of people with disabilities.

There are other biases that those who work for government services such as public health clinics, housing departments, and welfare offices should be particularly careful to avoid. People in these positions are often required by law to report suspicion of child abuse or neglect, yet because disabled people are in general more likely than others to require government services, disabled people tend to come to the attention of government workers more often than those who are more financially secure.[44] This heightened scrutiny can lead to more reports of abuse and neglect by disabled people than by others and to the illicit inference that disabled people are therefore more likely than others to abuse or neglect their children. Yet, because of sampling bias about who is likely to receive such enhanced review, the rates of abuse and neglect among disabled people may be the same as or lower than the population as a whole. Once a report to child protective services is made, there may be a tendency to assume that the accusations contain some truth, which can lead to invasive and overly thorough investigations, especially when combined with other commonly accepted assumptions about the parenting fitness of disabled people. There is some evidence that parents with disabilities are thus disproportionately put into the child welfare system, and once there, they are disproportionately likely to lose their children.[45]

When we attempt to assess a person's fitness as a parent, either formally or informally, we must also be careful to take account of various accommodations that have been or could be made for the person's disability. Observing a disabled person in an environment that has not been modified for her parenting needs may not fully reveal her ability to rear a child effectively. In some cases, parenting assessments are simply made in an unfamiliar office, other times a "home study" may be completed before the person has completed modifications to her home, while in most cases an observer may simply lack the training, rubrics, or data to determine whether an individual with a disability has the potential to be a good parent in an adapted environment.[46]

It is difficult to determine, however, what sorts of accommodations should be taken into account when making such assessments. If someone has the resources and willingness to secure structural modifications to her home and to hire an extensive support staff then such accommodations should be considered, whereas if she has not made such accommodations or cannot to do so given her fair share of economic resources then perhaps her parenting skills can be justifiably assessed at a lower level as compared to others. A further problem is how parenting assessments are to be made if certain accommodations or resources are legally required but are not actually being provided. If, for example, public transportation for the disabled were dependable; if medical offices, parks, and schools were accessible; if teachers provided accessible materials to parents; and if people with disabilities were afforded a fair share of income and wealth then a disabled person might be a fine parent. But, as things stand, these areas of life give her great difficulty and she lacks the resources to accommodate them adequately, so her parenting abilities may be justifiably assessed at a lower level than other parents, even though what this calls for is a more just set of economic, political, and social institutions that could allow her to be a very good parent.

PARENTING WITH A DISABILITY

Some people may have a remaining suspicion that, even after correcting for various biases about disability and taking into account reasonable accommodations for disabled parents, children nonetheless tend to be better off, all else equal, if they are raised by sighted parents rather than blind ones, by people who have full use of their limbs rather than by those who are quadriplegic, and by people who are mentally well adjusted rather than by those who are chronically depressed or cognitively disabled. Perhaps we should do more to support disabled parents and exercise greater caution before severing their parental rights, but we may nonetheless think that some hesitation is appropriate before allowing, encouraging, or helping people with certain kinds of disabilities to become parents or take primary custody of a child.

We must strike an appropriate balance, it may seem, between the interests some disabled people have in procreating and parenting with the interests of their (potential) children, for it may appear obvious that children are usually worse off when their parents are disabled. It is true that some people have disabilities that prevent them from taking primary responsibility for the care of a child while other disabled people are unfit or bad parents for other reasons. But in many cases the interests of disabled parents and the interests of their children are aligned and mutually supporting. Having a disability need not prevent someone from meeting her child's basic needs, while being disabled can actually make someone an even better parent.

One major concern may simply be that people with certain kinds of disabilities cannot provide for the basic physical needs of a child for food, clothing, shelter, and safety. People with disabilities, however, have developed effective and clever ways of caring for their children. Many of us who have children have extended the adaptive strategies that allow us to meet our own physical needs to allow us to fulfill our parental responsibilities. Blind and visually impaired people, for instance, often do our own grocery shopping with ease by navigating public transportation, relying on smell and feel when picking out food, utilizing technology that can read aloud labels and paper money, and relying on contingency plans if we become lost or disoriented. There are also many types of equipment that are specially designed to assist disabled parents. Wheelchair users, for example, can use accessible cribs, changing tables, bathtubs, and highchairs; they can attach child seats to their wheelchairs; and they can use lifting harnesses. People with disabilities have developed adaptations for particular parenting functions. Blind and visually impaired people, for example, can install security alarms on bookcases, cupboards, and doors as well as attach bells to our child's shoes; we can purchase different sized medicine plungers; we can use labeling tape around the house; we can train guide dogs to find changing tables; and we can rely on our other senses to determine if our child is clean and eating properly. Disabled people can train our children in various ways by placing special emphasis on, for instance, teaching them not to run off or to come when called. We can utilize specialty training from occupational therapists to ensure that the physical needs of a child are met. And, like nondisabled people, we can rely on our spouses, family, friends, and wider community to assist us as parents.

Creating an environment in which the basic needs of a child are taken care of requires planning, ingenuity, flexibility, perseverance, patience, and good sense. Disabled parents often must exhibit these qualities to a higher degree than other parents in order to care for our children, however, because we often do not have access to the same kinds of received parenting wisdom that others may rely on. Disabled parents often must work harder than others to decide how we will care for our children given our abilities and social circumstances, which are not widely shared by others. Until an extensive fund of parenting knowledge is available to blind parents, for example, assessing a blind person's parenting skills should sometimes take account of how well she manages her own disability as well as her ability and willingness to develop parenting strategies that allow her to meet the basic needs of her child.

Parents with disabilities can also provide various special benefits to our children that need to be considered when assessing our fitness as parents. Disabled parents can be especially attentive to our children because our parenting strategies often require extensive sensitivity, time, and effort, as well as close proximity to our child, which can lead to a stronger bond between us. Children of disabled parents can learn greater patience, self-reliance, and flexibility when it takes their disabled parent greater time and effort to accomplish various parenting tasks.[47] They can become sensitive to their parent's abilities and needs, which may encourage sensitivity and compassion for others as well. If our child is disabled then we may be in an especially good position to guide the child's development.

Children of disabled people have opportunities to assist their disabled parent. When the assistance that children are expected to provide to their disabled parent or their siblings is age appropriate and tailored to avoid placing undue burdens on them, children can develop independence, problem-solving skills, a sense of responsibility, and self-esteem.[48] These experiences also teach them that people often rely on one another without shame or disgrace. And they learn how to offer and give help in respectful ways.

Disabled people often exhibit virtues that can positively influence our child's character development. Disabled people are often humble because of our limitations but also confident in advocating for our rights. We tend to be independent in securing our own basic needs but also gracious when asking for and accepting help. We usually accept our limitations, hardships, and vulnerabilities, and we are often accepting and tolerant of physical and cultural differences more generally. We have usually suffered prejudice, oppression, and injustice without lapsing into despair or cynicism, but we also tend to appreciate the good will of others who have helped us. Many disabled people have a sense of humor, especially in adversity, and we often take a broader perspective on the world that downplays various kinds of fads and social expectations. Disabled people can also pass down our concern for social justice, compassion, and respect as well as the high value many of us place on family and friends.

Having children can provide great benefits to disabled people as well. People with disabilities sometimes find ourselves somewhat socially isolated because of our condition—we may have difficulty forming close relationships with nondisabled people because we have difficulty communicating with others, engaging in the kinds of activities where people often make new friends, or relating with nondisabled people who are awkward around us. Raising a child can be an opportunity to form and foster deep, loving, and lasting relationships, with our child as well as with other parents, that we may not otherwise have much opportunity to form. Like people who are not disabled, the bonds we form with other adults in our capacity as parents often improve our parenting abilities, give us a sense of community, and give greater structure and meaning to our lives. Raising a nondisabled child can give a disabled person some understanding of how nondisabled people view disability, while raising a disabled child can help us to find more ways to adapt. And having a child is likely to require people with disabilities to exert our own powers to a greater extent than we otherwise would, which tends to improve our self-esteem and sense of accomplishment, and so make us even better parents.

Conclusion

When my wife and I were deciding whether or not to have children, I was concerned that my visual impairment would prevent me from being the kind of parent I aimed to be. What I have found, now that we have two children, is just the opposite. The skills I have developed adapting to new environments, handling adversity, advocating on my own behalf, and seeking necessary assistance, as well as my heightened patience, compassion, and sensitivity, have prepared me to recognize and appreciate the responsibilities and joys of parenthood. Although my children have responded in different ways to my disability, one spontaneously reading movie subtitles for me while the other sends me down wet slides she knows I cannot see, both of them will grow up with an awareness and appreciation of the good that people with disabilities have to offer.

Notes

1. For discussions of the parent–child relationship and the value of having and raising children more generally, see Anderson 1990; Brighouse and Swift 2006; Hursthouse 1987; Overall 2012; Paul 2015; and Robertson 1994. This paper has significantly benefited from discussions with Kimberley Brownlee, Leslie Francis, Anita Silvers, Thomas Hill, and Julie Cureton.
2. NCD 2012. This chapter has especially benefited from this government report, which outlines many of the legal hurdles that disabled people currently face if they decide to reproduce and raise children. Those who want to investigate some of the empirical claims I make should look at this excellent report in detail.
3. Asch 1989; Tankard Reist 2006.
4. Asch and Roussou 1985; Fine and Asch 1981; A. Harris and Wideman 1988.
5. A. Harris and Wideman 1988.
6. Tankard Reist 2006.
7. Bonner 2015.
8. Some people argue, for example, that we are permitted to become parents only if we reasonably believe we can satisfy the basic needs of our prospective children or can ensure that they will live a life of at least average well-being. See Cassidy 2006.
9. 1997 Adoption and Safe Families Act. 42 USC. § 675.

10. See Card 1996; Kittay 1998, 1999, 2000, 2001; Overall 2012; Silvers 1995; Silvers et al. 1998; Silvers 1998; Wendell 1996; and Young 2005.
11. For discussions about who should have children, what sort of children they should aim to have, how far they ought to go in helping them and how difficult it is to know these things in advance, see Cassidy 2006; O'Neill et al. 1979; Overall 2012; Savulescu and Kahane 2009; Steinbock and McClamrock 1994; and Velleman 2005.
12. Dworkin 1993.
13. Boxill 1984; Hill 1991.
14. See, for example, the UN Declaration of Human Rights and the UN Convention on the Rights of Persons With Disabilities.
15. Major cases guaranteeing reproductive freedom include *Griswold v. Connecticut*, 381 US 479 (1965); *Roe v. Wade*, 410 US 113 (1973); and *Planned Parenthood of Southeastern Pennsylvania v. Casey*, 505 US 833 (1992). Major cases guaranteeing parental rights include *Meyer v. Nebraska*, 262 US 390 (1923); *Pierce v. Society of Sisters*, 268 US 510 (1925); *Stanley v. Illinois*, 405 US 645 (1972); *Wisconsin v. Yoder*, 406 US 205 (1972); and *Troxel v. Granville*, 530 US 57 (2000).
16. *Harris v. McRae*, 448 US 297 (1980).
17. See the United Nations Convention on the Rights of the Child as well as the Supreme Court cases, cited earlier.
18. For a discussion of the moral status of children, see Schapiro 1999.
19. *Stanley v. Illinois*, 405 US 645 (1972); *Wisconsin v. Yoder*, 406 US 205 (1972).
20. *Lassiter v. Department of Social Services*, 452 US 18 (1981); and *Santosky v. Kramer*, 455 US 745 (1982).
21. Tittle 2004.
22. NCD 2012, 138.
23. Gateway 2012; James 2013; Press 2009.
24. Daar 2013; J. Harris 1998; Robertson 1994.
25. A further set of considerations that some people think should be considered in such decisions is the interests of the genetic or the gestational parent, such as whether the biological mother should be allowed to choose who may adopt her child.
26. Eckholm 2013; Rights 2000; Unborn Victims of Violence Act of 2004.
27. Some states, such as California, prevent fertility clinics from denying same-sex couples access to their services simply because they are gay. See *North Coast Women's Care Medical Group, Inc. v. Superior Court*, 44 Cal.4th 1145 (2008).
28. Tittle 2004.
29. The Rehabilitation Act applies to any organization that receives federal money while the ADA also covers parts of the private sphere, such as commercial facilities, telecommunications and employment, as well as state and local governments, including public transportation and public schools.
30. See 42 USC. § 12102 and *Bragdon v. Abbott*, 524 US 624 (1998).
31. The Rehabilitation Act, more specifically, covers publicly funded entities; Title II of the Americans with Disabilities Act covers public services; and Title III of that act covers public accommodations.
32. 28 C.F.R. § 36.104, 208.
33. 28 C.F.R. § 36.208.
34. 28 C.F.R. § 35.130(h), 139.
35. *In re Marriage of Carney*, 24 Cal.3d 725 (1979). See Stein 1994.

36. *Holtz v. Holtz* ND 105, 595 N.W.2d 1 (1999).

37. James 2010.

38. For discussion of these and other cases, see NCD 2012.

39. Bartholet 1996; Collier 2008 (both cited in NCD 2012).

40. The Supreme Court held in *Lassiter v. Department of Social Services,* 452 US 18 (1981) that parents do not always have a right to council in proceedings that may terminate their parental rights.

41. This account draws on Rawls's discussion of what he calls the "worth of liberty." See Rawls 1993, 325–331; 1999, 179–180.

42. Rawls 1999, 65–73.

43. Rawls 1999: 73–77.

44. Chand 2000; Shade 1998; Watkins 1995 (all cited in NCD 2012).

45. Swain and Cameron 2003 (cited in NCD 2012).

46. McWey et al. 2006 (cited in NCD 2012).

47. Asch 1989.

48. For discussions of what is called "parentification," see Chase 1999.

BIBLIOGRAPHY

Anderson, E. S. 1990. Is women's labor a commodity? *Philosophy and Public Affairs* 19, no. 1: 71–92.

Asch, A. 1989. Reproductive technology and disability. In *Reproductive laws for the 1990's*, ed. S. Cohen and N. Taub, 69–124. Clifton, NJ: Humana Press.

Asch, A., and H. Roussou. 1985. Therapists with disabilities: Theoretical and clinical issues. *Psychiatry* 48, no. 11: 1–12.

Associated Press. 2009. Most states have not adopted sex offender rules. *NBC News.* http://www.nbcnews.com/id/34226683/ns/us_news-crime_and_courts/t/most-states-have-not-adopted-sex-offender-rules/#.VpQmZJMrJn4.

Bartholet, E. 1996. What's wrong with adoption law? *Journal of Children's Rights* 4: 265–266.

Bonner, H. 2015. How a disabled pregnant woman handles insensitive questions. *Scary mommy.* http://www.scarymommy.com/disabled-pregnant-woman-handles-insensitive-questions/.

Boxill, B. R. 1984. *Blacks and social justice.* Totowa, NJ: Rowman & Allanheld.

Brighouse, H., and A. Swift. 2006. Parents' rights and the value of the family. *Ethics* 117, no. 1: 80–108.

Card, C. 1996. Against marriage and motherhood. *Hypatia* 11, no. 3: 1–23.

Cassidy, L. 2006. That many of us should not parent. *Hypatia* 21, no. 4: 40–57.

Center for Reproductive Rights. 2000. Punishing women for their behavior during pregnancy. http://www.reproductiverights.org/document/punishing-women-for-their-behavior-during-pregnancy-an-approach-that-undermines-womens-heal.

Chand, A. 2000. The over-representation of Black children in the child protection system: Possible causes, consequences and solutions. *Child & Family Social Work* 5, no. 1: 67–77.

Chase, N. D. 1999. *Burdened children: Theory, research and treatment of parentification.* Thousand Oaks, CA: Sage.

Child Welfare Information Gateway. (2012). *Who may adopt, be adopted, or place a child for adoption?* Washington, DC: U.S. Department of Health and Human Services, Children's Bureau. https://www.childwelfare.gov/topics/systemwide/laws-policies/statutes/parties/.

Collier, K. 2008. Love v. love handles: Should obese people be precluded from adopting a child based solely upon their weight? *Texas Wesleyan Law Review* 15, no. 1: 31–60.

Daar, J. 2013. Accessing reproductive technologies: Invisible barriers, indelible harms. *Berkeley Journal of Gender, Law & Justice* 23, no. 1: 18–82.

Dworkin, R. M. 1993. *Life's dominion: An argument about abortion, euthanasia, and individual freedom.* New York: Knopf.

Eckholm, E. 2013. Case explores rights of fetus versus mother. *The New York Times.* A1.

Fine, M., and A. Asch. 1981. Disabled women: Sexism without the pedestal. *Journal of Sociology and Social Welfare* 8, no. 2: 233–248.

Harris, A., and D. Wideman. 1988. The construction of gender and disability in early attachment. In *Women with disabilities*, ed. M. Fine and A. Asch, 115–138. Philadelphia: Temple University Press.

Harris, J. 1998. Rights and reproductive choice. In *The future of human reproduction: Ethics, choice, and regulation*, ed. John Harris and Søren Holm, 5–37. Oxford: Oxford University Press.

Hill, T. E. 1991. The message of affirmative action. *Social Philosophy and Policy* (Spring issue): 108–129.

Hursthouse, R. 1987. *Beginning lives.* Oxford: Blackwell.

James, S. 2010. Baby Sent to Foster Care for 57 Days Because Parents Are Blind. *ABC News.* http://abcnews.go.com/Health/missouri-takes-baby-blind-parents/story?id=11263491.

James, S. 2013. Same-sex adoptions next frontier for LGBT advocates. *ABC News.* http://abcnews.go.com/Health/sex-adoptions-frontier-lgbt-advocates/story?id=20780309.

Kittay, E. F. 1998. On the expressivity and ethics of selective abortion for disability: Conversations with my son. In *Norms and values: Essays on the work of Virginia Held*, ed. V. Held, J. Graf Haber, and M. S. Halfon, 172–203. Lanham, MD: Rowman & Littlefield.

Kittay, E. F. 1999. *Love's labor: Essays on women, equality, and dependency.* New York: Routledge.

Kittay, E. F. 2000. At home with my daughter. In *Americans with disabilities*, ed. L. P. Francis and A. Silvers, 64–80. New York: Routledge.

Kittay, E. F. 2001. A feminist public ethic of care meets the new communitarian family policy. *Ethics* 111, no. 3: 523–547.

McWey, L. M., T. L. Henderson, and S. N. Tice. 2006. Mental health issues and the foster care system: An examination of the impact of the Adoption and Safe Families Act. *Journal of Marital and Family Therapy* 32, no. 2: 195–214.

National Council on Disability (NCD). 2012. *Rocking the cradle: Ensuring the rights of parents with disabilities and their children.* https://www.ncd.gov/publications/2012/Sep272012.

O'Neill, O., W. Ruddick, and Society for Philosophy and Public Affairs. 1979. *Having children: Philosophical and legal reflections on parenthood: Essays.* New York: Oxford University Press.

Overall, C. 2012. *Why have children? The ethical debate.* Cambridge, MA: MIT Press.

Paul, L. A. 2015. What you can't expect when you're expecting. *Res Philosophica* 92, no. 2: 1–23.

Rawls, J. 1993. *Political liberalism.* New York: Columbia University Press.

Rawls, J. 1999. *A theory of justice* (rev. ed). Cambridge, MA: Belknap Press of Harvard University Press.

Robertson, J. A. 1994. *Children of choice: Freedom and the new reproductive technologies.* Princeton, NJ: Princeton University Press.

Savulescu, J., and G. Kahane. 2009. The moral obligation to create children with the best chance of the best life. *Bioethics* 23, no. 5: 274–290.

Schapiro, T. 1999. What is a child? *Ethics* 109, no. 4: 715–738.

Shade, D. 1998. Empowerment for the pursuit of happiness: Parents with disabilities and the Americans with Disabilities Act. *Law and Inequality* 16: 153–218.

Silvers, A. 1995. Reconciling equality to difference: Caring (f)or justice for people with disabilities. *Hypatia* 10, no. 1: 30–55.

Silvers, A. 1998. Women and disability. In *A companion to feminist philosophy*, ed. A. M. Jaggar and I. M. Young, 330–340. Malden, MA: Blackwell.

Silvers, A., D. T. Wasserman, and M. Mahowald. 1998. *Disability, difference, discrimination: Perspectives on justice in bioethics and public policy.* Lanham, MD: Rowman & Littlefield.

Stein, M. 1994. Review of: "Mommy has a blue wheelchair: Recognizing the parental rights of individuals with disabilities." *Brooklyn Law Review* 60: 1069–1099.

Steinbock, B., and R. McClamrock. 1994. When is birth unfair to the child? *Hastings Center Report* 24, no. 6: 15–21.

Swain, P. A., and N. Cameron. 2003. "Good enough parenting": Parental disability and child protection. *Disability & Society* 18, no. 2: 165–177.

Tankard Reist, M. 2006. *Defiant birth: Women who resist medical eugenics.* North Melbourne, Victoria: Spinifex Press.

Tittle, P. 2004. *Should parents be licensed? Debating the issues* (Contemporary issues; Amherst, NY: Prometheus Books.

Velleman, J. D. 2005. Family history. *Philosophical Papers* 34, no. 3: 357–378.

Watkins, C. 1995. Beyond status: The Americans with Disabilities Act and the parental rights of people labeled developmentally disabled or mentally retarded. *California Law Review* 83: 1431–1432.

Wendell, S. 1996. *The rejected body: Feminist philosophical reflections on disability.* New York: Routledge.

Young, I. M. 2005. *On female body experience: "Throwing like a girl" and other essays.* Oxford: Oxford University Press.

CHAPTER 19

··

LATE-IN-LIFE MOTHERHOOD

*Ethico-Legal Perspectives on the Postponement
of Childbearing and Access to Artificial
Reproductive Technologies*

··

IMOGEN GOOLD

WOMEN are regularly confronted with pronouncements on the "right" time to conceive children, which taken together present a confused, unrealistic message. Very young mothers face criticism, as do women who postpone childbearing until their late 30s and 40s. Those who choose to procreate postmenopausally face even greater censure and sometimes ridicule.[1] Women who cannot financially support their children are criticized, yet postponement decisions based on improving earning capacity often butt up against accusations of putting career first or wanting to "have it all," choices that are often regarded negatively. Into this mix of messages come warnings from the medical profession that women are incorrectly assuming that ART will help them conceive if they leave conception until the point when their fertility is on the decline, yet those who seek to address this via egg freezing are often considered to be foolishly relying on an insurance policy that will not pay out. It seems almost as though women are being told that there is some perfect age for conception, yet little account is taken in these messages of women's reasons for conceiving when they do and the rationality of their choices.

This chapter focuses on women who choose to delay reproduction, many of whom will require access to artificial reproductive technologies (ARTs) such as in vitro fertilization (IVF) to conceive. It analyzes the ethics of the choice to delay childbearing and how the state should respond to such a decision. It contextualizes this analysis by drawing on both the messages women receive and data about the reasons for their decisions to delay. Spanning the choices of women who are pre-, peri-, and postmenopausal (that is, from around 40 to 50 years of age), it is informed by data about the success of ARTs in assisting such women to conceive, as well as the risks of their doing so. It also questions whether social age limits, which often translate into legal age limits, should have the power they currently hold.

This analysis centers on one core question: Would it be ethical for the state to deny women suffering from age-related fertility decline access to technology that may enable them to conceive? This chapter could simply barrel into an often polarized debate between the argument that infertility, whatever the cause, is deeply harming and hence demands our aid based on the importance of reproductive autonomy, and the view that those who put off reproduction and then find they cannot procreate have brought the harm (which is not a medical harm) on themselves and should face the consequences of their choice. In these terms, the matter seems irresolvable, or simply based on a difference of opinion about which harms are more important. This chapter avoids pitting arguments for reproductive autonomy directly and simplistically against those objections often raised against late motherhood. Rather than pitting choice against harm, it will provide a way of thinking into these broad questions by raising and then answering some subsidiary questions. In so doing, it offers an approach that avoids the impasse to a degree. There will still be disagreement, but in working through a series of questions and introducing relevant empirical data to answer them where possible, it at least focuses the debate on the key areas of contention, rather than reducing to a battle of harms, or of rights versus consequences.

Postponing Reproduction

There is some dispute over the point at which a woman's fertility seriously declines, but no doubt that for most women, at some point by the time they are in their mid-40s, they will be approaching infertility.[2] The prevalent lay view seems to be that fertility remains stable until a sharp drop in the mid-30s, but this may not be accurate. Some studies suggest instead that fertility declines gradually as women proceed through their 20s and 30s.[3] Very few women will conceive naturally after the age of 45, while cases of women conceiving after the age of 50 are exceptionally rare.[4] This occurs in large part because women are born with their full complement of ova, which declines over time.[5] Those eggs that remain are more likely to be chromosomally abnormal, resulting in higher rates of miscarriage even if a pregnancy is achieved.[6] As women age, their fertility is also more likely to decline as they have had more chances to contract infections or develop conditions that adversely affect fertility, such as endometriosis.[7] Male aging does seem to have some impact on the fertility of a couple, although far less than that of the woman.[8]

Despite this natural decline in fertility, in developed countries, women (and men) are increasingly having children later in life.[9] Across Europe, the average age of mothers at birth is close to or equal to 30 years old.[10] In the United States a similar trend can be observed, with the average age of mothers increasing in the same period from 21.4 years in 1970 to 25 years in 2006.[11] The number of children born to older mothers is also rising. In the United Kingdom, the number of children born to mothers aged 40 years or older has more than quadrupled, rising from 6,519 in 1982 to 29,158 in 2013.[12] The age at which women are bearing their first child is also increasing: Almost a quarter of live births to women over 40 years were firstborn children.[13] In the United States, between 1970 and 2006, the proportion of first births to women aged 35 years or older increased from 1% to 8.5% of all births.[14] In Canada, the rate for births to women over 35 years increased from 4% in 1987 to 11% in 2005.[15]

A consequence of this trend toward delaying is that women are increasingly turning to ARTs, particularly IVF, to help them conceive when they struggle to do so naturally. The availability of such technologies may also be a reason for some women's decision to delay. Some have also begun to have their eggs frozen, so they are ready for use if their fertility later declines. In some countries, they may have access to state-funded treatment (as in the United Kingdom), but in others, ARTs may be available only on a private basis. Age limits on ART are imposed in most jurisdictions, both on access generally (usually up to about 45 years of age) and as recommended limits on access to state-funded treatment.[16] This gives rise to the question: Would it be ethical to deny such women treatment? Relatedly, is it right that such women whose fertility has declined naturally are helped to conceive children they could not otherwise have borne? We might answer that they should be helped, that they should be denied help, or simply that they may seek help, but there is no duty on anyone (or the state) to assist them.

How Can We Decide Whether to Help Women Facing Age-Related Fertility Decline?

To answer the central question, we need to work through a number of subsidiary questions. The first is whether it is right that women who delay reproduction should bear the consequences of their decision. This question encompasses two objections to aiding such women—that their declining fertility is their own fault, and therefore they should bear the responsibility (and consequences) of it; and that it is natural that fertility declines with age, and that therefore they should not be helped when this befalls them. On this basis, a distinction might be made between infertility that is considered in some way unnatural or "medical" (which deserves treatment), and self-induced infertility (which does not). The second question is whether the possible harms that result from delaying reproduction are grounds for denying assistance to women who do so. These include harms to the mother herself, to the resulting child, and to others. The third is whether given that health resources are finite and scarce, they should be offered to women who have brought their infertility upon themselves, and hence diverted away from the treatment of other illnesses and conditions. Each is considered in turn, drawing on both the ethical considerations that bear on them and empirical data that can support the ethical analysis.

CAN WE MAKE MORAL DISTINCTIONS BETWEEN CASES OF INFERTILITY BASED ON CAUSE?

Infertility as a result of illness (such as infections that cause scarring of the fallopian tubes), or treatment for illness (such as chemotherapy), is largely accepted as something that should be treated. The same is true for infertility from which a woman suffers naturally. This includes premature menopause, follicle problems, anovulation and gland malfunctions, and endometriosis.[17] Call this "natural infertility." By contrast, what this chapter will refer to as "age-related infertility" occurs when an otherwise fertile woman delays reproduction, and then struggles to conceive due to the inevitable decrease in her fertility that accompanies aging. There is far less consensus on whether age-related infertility should be treated, whether with state-funded ARTs or at all.[18]

This raises the first subsidiary question: Can we make a moral distinction between cases of infertility based on cause? Put another way, would it be ethical to treat only some cases of infertility, where we distinguish based on the reason the woman cannot conceive? If we believe that only natural infertility should be treated (or be treated via state-funded services), this is the distinction that has been made. Even the most cursory glance of media portrayals of delayed motherhood demonstrates that such a distinction is readily made by many, both in the lay and scholarly literature. A cursory reading of the comments on most press articles about provision of state-funded fertility treatment will yield a slew of vituperative objections. The thrust of many such comments is that delay is a choice and one for which the chooser should bear the consequences, particularly given the shortage of resources for funding medical treatment generally. This view is not confined to the lay person; scholars, too, have made such arguments.[19]

Two main distinctions are usually offered to distinguish cases of infertility that are worthy of treatment and those that are not: choice and "naturalness." The first, choice, is based on the idea that where infertility arises due to the choices a woman has made (specifically the choice to delay reproduction), then that is her own fault and this renders her underserving of treatment. Call this the "she has made her own bed" argument. The second is that age-related infertility is natural. It happens to all women, and therefore to treat it is to "play God" or interfere with nature, which is considered wrong. Call this the "unnaturalness" argument. This argument applies to all cases of age-related infertility, but particularly to peri- and postmenopausal women.

If either position is convincing, it would provide a basis on which to treat natural infertility and age-related infertility differently. This does not necessarily justify refusing to treat the latter, only that differential treatment could be justified. However, as the following sections will demonstrate, neither distinction stands up to scrutiny, leading to the conclusion that there is no relevant moral distinction to be made between types of infertility based on their *cause*. Opponents of treating age-related infertility therefore need an alternative basis for their objection.

Relevance of Choice

To evaluate the "she has made her own bed" argument, we need to consider why a woman's choice might provide a morally relevant distinction between her age-induced infertility, and that of a woman who suffers from natural infertility. It is a complex question, and there is not scope here to do it full justice, but we can consider a number of important aspects of the question: whether women are really making a free choice and the constraints they may face; the relevance of their personal goals; the nature of the risk/benefit calculation they make; and whether choice is a sufficiently good reason to leave people to suffer the consequences of their choices.

Are Women Really Choosing?

The "she has made her own bed" argument rests on the assumption that women who delay childbearing are choosing to do so freely and so (the argument runs) they should bear the consequences of that choice. This argument often accompanies a charge regularly leveled at women who postpone reproduction: that they are selfish and have chosen to delay childbearing for their own reasons regardless of the negative impact on others.[20] Shaw and Giles, in a media framing study of the representation of delayed motherhood, identified multiple instances of such attitudes, with older mothers variously referred to as "self-indulgent and rather vain" (Guardian, Wed), "wrong and selfish" (Sun, Tue), and to modern women as wishing "to have it all" (several sources).[21] Shaw and Giles locate these sentiments toward women within a wider view of the current generation of fertile and recently infertile women as an "indulgent generation."[22]

There are a number of implicit assumptions within such views, first and foremost that delayed childbearing is freely chosen. Claims of selfishness on the part of women also focus on the woman's agency alone, rather than taking account of the role (if any) played by the woman's partner in decisions about procreative timing. In doing so, as in many other areas of reproduction, men are devolved of responsibility for reproductive choices, with this burden (and hence the moral responsibility) resting largely on the woman despite the fact that in most cases two people will be involved in such reproductive decisions. Shaw and Giles's findings support this view; they identified a "general lack of a male perspective in these media portrayals," which they posit "implies their absence from the decision to have children and whether the process of conception progresses in a normalized way."[23]

Whether women *should* bear the consequences of their choice to delay is examined next, but before we do so, we need first to consider why women are postponing procreation (and increasingly doing so). Anna Smajdor makes the very salient point that "If treatment is denied on the basis of poor choices, it becomes supremely important to establish the nature of those choices."[24] An understanding of these women's motivations will cast doubt on just how freely many of them might be said to be choosing.[25] These women's choices need to be contextualized within the socioeconomic forces that drive many women to delay procreation, and numerous studies have tried to divine why women delay and risk childlessness.[26] Women's possible motivations for postponement are many and varied, but they can be divided into two broad groups: lack of knowledge about fertility problems, and the desire to maximize beneficial outcomes.

Lack of Knowledge About Fertility Problems

It is often suggested that women who postpone reproduction do so because they do not fully appreciate the risk of infertility, or they are at least unaware of how early their fertility may decline.[27] Some surveys indicate that this may be true.[28] For example, Nichole Wyndham et al. cite another study from the United Kingdom in which only 75% of women who had not considered the issue of infertility realized that their chances of conceiving would decline between the ages of 30 and 40 years.[29] They comment: "It is only when these women experience infertility themselves and find themselves in the office of a fertility clinic that they begin to understand the reality of their situation."[30] In another study, only just over half of women surveyed realized that age was the strongest risk factor for infertility.[31]

However, there is also considerable research that indicates that women are made very well aware of the risks of putting off childbearing by the media.[32] For example, the Tough survey demonstrated that both men and women are aware of the relationship between age and declining fertility, with over 70% of people of both genders surveyed aware that aging could compromise their chances of conceiving.[33] Another demonstrated that health care professionals underestimate the proportion of their patients that do understand the relationship between aging and fertility decline.[34] All that can be concluded, then, is that some women understand the risks they run, while others do not. Lack of awareness therefore might explain some postponement, but not all.

What does seem to be more widely the case is that women are less cognisant of the relationship between aging and risks to both the mother and fetus. The Tough survey found that less than half those surveyed knew that increased maternal age was associated with higher risks of stillbirth, caesarean delivery, and preterm delivery.[35] Another found that many did not realize that reproducing via intracytoplasmic sperm injection (ICSI) (a form of ART) may result in children with more long-term health problems.[36] Such findings suggest that it may be true that women are making a risk-benefit calculation about postponement without an accurate understanding of the nature of those risks.

Another, related, explanation is that women place undue faith in the capacity of ARTs to alleviate any fertility problems they will face if they attempt reproduction later in life.[37] For example, Daniluk et al. found in a survey of over 3,000 women, that 91% were "unrealistically confident about the ability of [ARTs] to assist most women to have a child using their own eggs until they reach menopause."[38] Benzies et al. found that:

> Women were confident that, if they needed it, reproductive technology would be available to assist with conception whenever they decided to bear a child. Sheila who was older than 30 years without children stated: "Women are having babies later because of technology, fertility technology that allows us to kind of extend our fertility period, where before we couldn't, you know?"[39]

They also found that these women had not considered the risks that attend late-in-life pregnancy, preferring to pursue other personal goals first.

However, there are data that show that women are well aware that IVF is not a "magic bullet" for fertility decline, and often fails.[40] As Khalaf et al. put it, "there is an article on 'my IVF heartbreak' in almost every women's magazine in the newsagents."[41] That said, women appear not to understand *why* their fertility declines with age, with many seeming to believe that if they maintain good health and fitness, their own fertility is less likely to decline.[42] This view is, however, mistaken.

Overall, it seems that while some women fully appreciate the risks they run, others do not, meaning a denial of access amounts to a harsh declaration that they must bear the consequences of their ignorance. If the entire rationale is that people should be responsible for the choices they make, it cannot apply to those who have made choices based without information or understanding: They lack responsibility for the result. Perhaps they should have, or could have, done more to educate themselves, but requiring pursuit of knowledge about a risk of which you had no suspicion (particularly given the examples we see of women conceiving in their 40s, as Wyndham et al. note[43]) is probably too much to ask, and certainly insufficient to justify denying access to ARTs. This is particularly so when we consider, as we will, the harms women (and men) suffer in such situations.

For those women who do appreciate the risks they run, the argument has more bite. But as Khalaf argues:

> Delayed childbearing has social, financial and personal causes. To presume that improving women's education on the biology of their reproduction and the risks of delayed childbearing would solve this complex problem is clear, simple but, as such, may be wrong![44]

And indeed, focusing only on their knowledge of risks as determinative of how we should respond assumes their knowledge of those risks is perfect. This is not and cannot be the case. As women age, the number of eggs in ovaries declines, as does the "quality" of those eggs; that is, their viability decreases and they are also more likely to be chromosomally abnormal. It is possible to determine a woman's ovarian reserve—the quantity of eggs she has left—but not their quality. Therefore, as a woman ages, her ability to reproduce can be evaluated to some degree, but lack of knowledge about her egg quality will prevent a truly accurate evaluation.

Given all this, it is clear that if we focus only on their knowledge of the risks, we have considered only one half of the risk-benefit calculation they have made and one in which they may not even be able to make a perfect calculation. We turn now to the benefits side to consider what might motivate women to take such a risk with their fertility and why, in fact, they may be taking a reasonable and rational approach to decisions about reproduction.

Desire to Maximize Beneficial Outcomes

Assuming, then, that many women are aware of the risks they run, what else might be motivating their decisions? In reality, multiple reasons must motivate these decisions, some of them highly personal. There are numerous studies in which women are asked why they delayed childbearing, and three main reasons emerge.[45]

First, many women report wanting to be in a stable relationship with a person they see as a suitable co-parent who is likely to stay with them. In the Tough survey, 80.2% cited "partner suitability to parent" as reasons for delaying procreation.[46] Similarly, Berrington found that "a lack of a partner is a key variable affecting the chance of starting a family at older ages."[47] Such a rationale is indicative of a desire to ensure any child created is brought into a stable relationship. Women driven by such a motivation are weighing the risk of potentially no children as worth taking if the benefit is bringing any child who does result into the kind of loving, secure environment that is important to raising a happy, well-adjusted person. This seems a very rational and reasonable way of thinking about the decision to reproduce. To respond when the woman has achieved such stability and tries, but fails, to procreate by telling her she must bear the consequences when IVF might offer her a chance to avoid them seems perverse. If the concern is that it is somehow bad to produce children later in life, because of putative harms to that child, these potential harms should at least be weighed against the benefits the child will receive by being brought up in a family environment where that child is secure and wanted. We will return to the weighing of harms and benefits later.

The second reported reason women postpone childbearing is to pursue higher education. Higher rates of childlessness are correlated with the attainment of degree level qualifications,[48] and consequently income.[49] Increased age of first childbirth is correlated with women's increased participation in higher education.[50] One possible reason for this is that both pursuits are time-consuming and hence may not be compatible for some women.[51] Childrearing can severely undermine a woman's capacity to undertake higher study, and so postponement is a rational strategy. This is particularly the case when we take account of the third, and highly related reason for postponement: the impact of childbearing on women's careers and therefore their income. There is substantial data supporting the thesis that women postpone childbearing for career-related reasons.[52] As higher education is often tied to employment in more highly paid careers, the two reasons are often interlinked. For example, women residents have been shown to intentionally postpone childbearing to avoid perceived threats to their career that might result from extending their training. These women were more likely to make this choice than their male counterparts (41% of men were prepared to have a child during residency, whereas only 27% of women were).[53]

It is clearly the case that women who delay childbearing experience economic benefits:

> A year of delayed motherhood is found to increase career earnings by 9%, work experience by 6%, and average wage rates by 3%. The effects are heterogeneous across women; those with college degrees and in professional and managerial occupations receive the greatest career returns to delay. Post-motherhood wages are also shown to vary with motherhood timing.[54]

The timing of a woman's exit from the workforce to have children has been said to account for as much as 12% of the gender wage gap due to its impact on work experience and the consequence depreciation in a woman's skills.[55] From the time they give birth, women experience reduced earnings and their wage profile "flattens," meaning their earnings increases will be smaller, although the impact differs across employment sectors. Women entering more highly skilled workforces are those who gain the most from delaying childbearing.[56] Some explanations for these phenomena offered by Miller are:

> On the supply side, mothers may reduce their hours in the labor market and invest less in skill development. From the demand side, employers may offer mothers fewer training and advancement opportunities.[57]

Wilde et al. suggest that one explanation is that wage growth is dependent on effort and that "if actual effort is hard to monitor, employers may rightly or wrongly perceive mothers as less committed to their jobs."[58]

Miller goes on to point out that the data show that

> Motherhood remains an obstacle to women's economic equality with men (Fuchs 1988); its deferral may constitute an important mechanism for reducing that inequality. On the other hand, if one considers equality the benchmark, the financial rewards to delay represent an effective penalty for early motherhood.[59]

As Wilde et al note, "professional women face sizable career costs and difficult trade-offs in deciding to become a mother."[60]

It might be replied that both men and women face the same choices about opting out of education or career to care for children. Both can be carers, but if women are postponing on this basis, it is their choice (as it is their partner's) to do so. This might suggest that women deserve the characterization that they want (unreasonably) to "have it all."[61] This needs some unpacking. First, this is rarely, if ever, a charge laid at the feet of men who have children yet seek to remain in the workplace. An explanation for this is that women still continue to take on the bulk of child care responsibilities, and if they wish to retain or progress in their careers, they must do so simultaneously. In doing so, they are not necessarily simply pursuing their own career interests (as the characterization goes), but actually seeking to achieve independence and financial stability: a reasonable goal both for themselves and the child they seek to bear. Indeed, as Khalaf comments, many women reported delaying reproduction in the interests of achieving a stable environment in which to raise a child, which encompasses both financial stability and the formation of a lasting relationship.[62] In one Canadian survey of over 1,500 people, 85.5% cited financial security as a reason to delay having children.[63]

Second, in the early days post birth, the woman often *has* to bear a greater share of the carer role if she is breastfeeding (and this is reinforced in jurisdictions where women receive more leave entitlements than men).[64] As Mills et al. argue, the result of this and in general as a response to the birth of a new child is often . . . a crystallization of gender roles, with women increasing time spent in housework and childcare in comparison with men only after the birth of the first child.[65]

Furthermore, as Bewley rightly states

[women's] delays may reflect disincentives to earlier pregnancy or maybe an underlying resistance to childbearing as, despite the advantages brought about by feminism and equal opportunities legislation, women still bear full domestic burdens as well as work and financial responsibilities. The reasons for these difficulties lie not with women but with a distorted and uninformed view from society, employers, and health planners.[66]

Women also report delaying childbearing until they feel they are emotionally ready, or because they wanted to achieve their personal goals before childbearing so that they were fully committed.[67]

As we have seen, opposition to assisting women who are motivated by these reasons for postponement often stigmatizes such women as "selfish"[68] and (unreasonably) wanting to pursue both a career and motherhood (while no such stigma attaches to similarly minded men). But what the data here reveal is that, in many cases, child welfare is the motivation. The woman is in fact weighing the risk of having no children against the risk of bringing children into a situation where she cannot fully provide for them, whether that means emotionally or financially. Far from being a morally unworthy rationale, such a balancing should be regarded as praiseworthy. To respond to such behaviour by refusing to assist her in bearing that child again seems perverse and poorly founded.

Where a woman has chosen to pursue her own personal goals, refusing assistance may be too harsh anyway: It is not unreasonable for people to want to achieve and experience many different things in their lives. Doing so is not morally wrong, and therefore probably does not deserve the severe impact of refusal to aid when that pursuit reduces fertility.

Furthermore, the data suggest that women's choices are often not really "choices" in the fullest sense. They are made against a backdrop of social and economic realities that place women in the role of carer, but restrict her from achieving the same degree of education, career success, and economic independence as men. A woman's choices are constrained by these conditions, as well as her own biological limitations. To say that she has simply chosen to postpone childbearing gives only a very shallow picture of the reality of how she arrived at the point of infertility. It is not surprising, then, that in a qualitative study of 18 women having their first child after the age of 35 or still without children, many reported that the view that the delay was by choice (a popular perception) was incorrect in their case.[69] It is rare that anyone makes a serious life choice in isolation from its context and impact, a fact that must bear on whether to leave them to bear the consequences of that choice.

Therefore, it can be seen that for many women there may not be enough of a choice for us to attribute the resultant infertility solely to their decisions and so attribute blame. Furthermore, given their context, women's motives for delaying childbearing are often rational (in the face of educational or economic penalties they otherwise face) and focused on ensuring a good environment into which to bring a child, namely one that is financially stable and sufficient, and in which the woman is in a secure relationship with a partner who is likely to make a good parent. The notion that such choices are made entirely freely is open to question, given that creating such an environment is affected by factors beyond a woman's control in many cases—she cannot simply procure an appropriate partner, nor can she entirely control the forces that shape her financial position.

Bearing the Consequences of Our Choices

It can be intuitively appealing to say that we should bear the consequences of our choices. We see this in the many epithets summing up the sentiment: "you reap what you sow"; "you have made your bed, now you must lie in it"; "what goes around, comes around"; and so on. This is particularly the case when someone else might be otherwise burdened by those consequences, whether it is the state (and therefore the community) who bears it in terms of cost of treatment, or the child who will bear the (arguable) detriments of being born to an older woman, such as stigma, risk of illness, or the premature death of a parent. These consequences are considered later in this chapter. For now, we must ask how committed we should be to this idea of responsibility.

Let us say, then, that people should bear the consequences of their own choices. If we take this position in response to one choice-induced disorder, to be morally consistent, we should take the same position toward all other choice-induced disorders unless there is a good reason to support differential treatment. So, if choice is relevant to whether someone receives health care resources for age-related fertility, it should be relevant to whether someone receives treatment for other conditions they might have avoided had they made other choices. It follows that the smoker with lung cancer should be denied treatment, as should the obese person who develops diabetes. The horse rider should be denied assistance when she breaks a limb, having known the risks and decided to run them. So, too, the mountaineer who suffers a fall, or the rugby player whose cornea is detached. All should be turned away from the hospital, as they are the authors of their own destiny.

There are many reasons why we should reject such an approach. First, we should distinguish between choosing an outcome and running the risk of an outcome. Like the overeater or the smoker, it is not certain that delaying reproduction will result in infertility. It depends on the duration of that delay, the woman's underlying fertility and that of her partner, and numerous other factors. The longer she delays, the more likely it is that she will face infertility until it becomes almost a certainty in her late 40s or early 50s, but she cannot know exactly when her personal fertility will decline to the point of needing assistance. Delays into the late 30s and early 40s (usually) then only equate to running the risk of infertility; it is not equivalent to choosing it as a certainty and then demanding help, although as the woman ages (and continues to delay), that decision becomes increasingly similar. The extent to which we decide a woman should bear the consequences of her decision to delay should take account of the fact that they equate to the running of a risk, not the pursuit (usually) of a certainty. It should also take account of the reasons for the delay and factors that the woman may not have foreseen (or been able to foresee) when calculating the risk. These range from rejecting a partner (or being rejected herself) to losing employment to facing an illness, any of which might mean at the point at which the woman had intended to begin procreating, she finds the conditions unfavorable and must continue to postpone. It is probably fair to say people should bear the consequences of the risks they take, but we might also think some of those consequences are too harsh if the reasons for running the risk were reasonable (and we have seen earlier that women have many good reasons for delaying procreation), or unknowable, or simply unknown due to ignorance or misinformation. We all take risks in life, and doing so enriches that life. No one has perfect information or the capacity to always make perfect choices based on perfect evaluations of risk and benefit. For these reasons, it is often right to soften the impact of the consequences that result when someone runs a risk, and reproductive decision making always involves risk of some kind of another.[70] Infertility can be devastating for women (and men), and this is not a situation in which facing that consequence will lead them to choose differently next time: There is no next time. This, combined with the terrible impact infertility may have, is a good reason to soften the consequences through the provision of ARTs where we can, just as we treat the smoker or the horse rider when the risks they chose to run play out badly.

Second, and more compelling, is the fact that the choices we make in life are made for complex reasons. We are, after all, human. We may balance risks against benefits, or short-term pleasures against long-term goals. We each have different histories that shape the choices we make, and even how we approach choosing. Our choices are not made in isolation, but within complicated contexts, often with others in mind (whether voluntarily or because of our obligations to them). To respond to this balancing of goals by simply leaving all those whose choices lead to bad consequences to bear them takes no account of the variables involved that we cannot control. It assumes complete control (and hence responsibility), when in most cases this is not the reality. This is particularly true of decisions about reproduction, where women cannot have perfect knowledge of their reproductive capacity and how long it will last. This, taken together with the constraints on the choices before them, undermines the case for leaving them simply to bear the results of their choice to delay.

The complexity of making choices also means that it will be very difficult to determine in most cases whether someone's choice is one for which he or she should bear responsibility. This is particularly true in the context of lifestyle choices that affect health (and fertility) outcomes, because these choices are made up of multiple decisions over a long period of time. Just as the obese person does not instantly become overweight because he or she decides to overeat, so a woman rarely chooses to postpone childbearing until she is 40. Much more likely is that she puts it off for different reasons at different stages in her life. A new job opportunity may mean postponing for a year until she is secure in her employment and eligible for maternity leave. But then at the end of that year, perhaps her father becomes ill and she must take on the burden of his care, or her partner leaves her, or she falls ill. And so on. Just as there are epithets to express the idea that we should bear the consequences of what we choose, so to "the best laid plans of mice and (wo)men often go awry."[71]

Given this, and given the very sensible, reasonable motivations women generally cite for their delaying reproduction, and the fact that many of these are driven by a desire to be in the best position to do well by their child, the idea that these women deserve the consequence of childlessness seems rather hollow. It makes little sense to say someone who makes a constrained choice with the welfare of his or her future child in mind (that is, a constrained but morally well-motivated choice) deserves to suffer, particularly when that suffering could be alleviated without significant harm to others. Desert derives from having done something morally unworthy; women who delay reproduction for good reasons do not fall into this category.

Judging Choices, Calibrating Responses

Probably there are those women who delay for "selfish" reasons, or at least self-regarding reasons. It is very likely they exist, that there are women who wish to pursue their own personal goals before having children, knowing that once they do so, their ability to pursue other things in life that are important to them will be lessened. The arguments made in the previous section would not then apply. In such cases, however, proportionality of response becomes highly relevant. Let us accept that it may be ethical to leave someone to bear the consequences of his or her choices in some cases. We could ground this in arguments from autonomy and responsibility, that we treat people as moral agents by respecting their choices, but this brings with it the need for them to take responsibility for those choices.

But we then need to consider whether the consequences (which could in some cases be avoided by permitting access to ARTs) are proportionate to the responsibility they bear. We need to be clear, then, on what those consequences are. It is demonstrably the case that reproduction is an important aspect of the great majority of people's lives. This is evident from the ubiquity of childbearing: Almost everyone does it, and in fact those who do not face curiosity and sometimes censure precisely because their choice is unusual. There is considerable evidence that unwanted childlessness has deleterious impacts on both men and women's lives. Many women report that, with hindsight, they regret their decision to postpone motherhood (particularly those who then experience unwanted childlessness).[72] Others express feelings of guilt or failure when they discover that they face fertility problems related to age.[73] In one qualitative study, a participant stated she felt she had failed her husband, while another said: "You feel like you're not a woman, that is the worst thing . . . you can't do what you're put on earth to do" (Emma, age 37).[74]

Individuals who wish to have children but fail to do so experience higher levels of clinical depression, as well as feelings of lower self-esteem, guilt, and isolation.[75] It is not simply that they do not get what they want; in many instances the involuntarily childless suffer deeply precisely because they fail to participate in a human experience that so many find so enriching.

This is, in fact, precisely why respecting people's reproductive autonomy is considered so vital. As Anna Smajdor rightly notes: "Having children is important to women. Doing so when they feel ready, and in ways that suit them, is valuable."[76]

There is not the scope here to fully explain why reproductive autonomy is important, but we can point to a few expressions that encapsulate the value of respecting such choices. Nicky Priaulx argues that the value of such autonomy "lies in its instrumentality in fostering basic human needs and one's sense of self."[77] Such decisions operate at a deeply emotional and personal level, she argues, concurring with John Robertson that it is their very intimacy that captures what is so very important about procreative liberty.[78] Decisions about if, when, and how to have children go to the core of what it means to be human. They affect our sense of self, they are part of the core goals we may have in life, and therefore demand our respect. It is far from surprising that when those choices are thwarted, people (men and women) can suffer deep and lasting harms.

Furthermore, if we are to use choice as the basis for judging when someone will receive ARTs, then as Smajdor has argued, we put ourselves in the position of needing to be a perfect judge. To avoid being unfair, we must be sure that we can judge accurately. When we place legal limits, this means further that we must create a system by which such judgments can be made. It is unlikely that anyone can take on such a role and make no errors, and even less likely that the legal system can design mechanisms to ensure this is the case. In using choice as the basis for deciding whom to help, we run the risk of not helping those who actually (on this account) deserve it. Given the harms these people will suffer, it may be preferable to provide support and ARTs to all who want them rather than risk inadvertently denying those who are "deserving."

Finally, if we are to make such judgments about ART access based in choices, we should take account first of why it is important to allow people to make choices and then sometimes assist them if these lead to problematic consequences. We should promote people's capacity to live life according to their own values. Experimentation and making choices about which goals we pursue enrich our lived experience and, as Mill argued, are important in developing as persons.[79] Providing a safety net of care when this pursuit goes awry enables people to lead fulfilling lives: doing otherwise and restraining their choices potentially leads to a life lived less well. Additionally, not providing aid to people who harm themselves through their own choices is likely to create a society in which we are less sympathetic. The cancer-afflicted smoker or the horse rider with a broken leg will be left to suffer, and we as a community will therefore bear witness to that. Such a community would be far from pleasant to inhabit.

There is, of course, much more that could be said on these matters, but this section has demonstrated that the simplistic view that those women delay reproduction because they make selfish choices is far from accurate. Furthermore, it has shown that choice is a flawed basis on which to distinguish who deserves assistance with conception, and also a weak basis on which to leave people to bear the consequences of their own choices.

Naturalness

The second argument that often emerges in response to women seeking ART, particularly postmenopausal women who cannot conceive in any other way, is that it is "unnatural" for them to do so, and so they should not be assisted in their attempts to "fool nature." Older women, particularly those who use ARTs to conceive, are also often perceived as acting "unnaturally." Such women are often reminded of their "ticking biological clocks" and as Shaw and Giles found, referred to as trying to "cheat time" or avoid their "physical destiny," or even "bend nature to their will."[80] They also found examples where the unnaturalness charge itself was absent, but older motherhood (and parenting in general) was constructed as "freakish."[81]

Such constructions become increasingly common and judgmental when the woman involved is postmenopausal. For example, when 62-year-old Patti Farrant gave birth, the *Tuesday Express* ran a feature article on her in which her public breastfeeding was described by one onlooker as "a sight I'll never forget."[82] Older mothers, particularly those who conceive postmenopausally, are also warned of being "mistaken for granny at the school gate" (warned against in a British Medical Association manual),[83] a seemingly problematic consequence of older motherhood. This is asserted to be harmful to the child, who may face teasing. In one article cited by Shaw and Giles, a fertility expert claimed that children would fail to have a good quality of life "if its parents are older than its friend's grandparents."[84]

There are many reasons why such an objection to is untenable as a basis for denying such women access to treatment. First, and most obviously, such a claim in fact applies to all medical treatment. If we genuinely believe that we should simply let nature take its course, then we should reject any medical intervention. It is no more natural to put a pacemaker in someone's chest, or a donor kidney in their abdomen, or an IV drip of antibiotics in their arm, than it is to offer them ART to redress fertility decline. It might be countered that the *reason* these people need treatment is that they have fallen below normal functioning for persons, whereas being infertile is in fact normal for peri- and postmenopausal women. However, this does little to improve the argument. We could easily reply that it is normal for people to develop cancer—it happens every day, and therefore it must be a normal part of human life, even if the sufferer can no longer function *as normal*. If it is normal, and if (as the argument goes) we should leave nature (and normality) well alone, then we have no basis on which to interfere by using medicine. This is not the prevailing view, because treatment alleviates suffering and loss of life. It is driven by a desire to improve quality of life—precisely the same desire of those who seek ART to redress infertility. Their lives will go better if they have it, and they will suffer if they do not, just as the cancer patient will based on whether she receives treatment or not.

Second, say we assume that helping peri- and postmenopausal women to bear children is unnatural. This does not, in and of itself, mean that this action is morally wrong: There is nothing inherently wrong with behaving unnaturally.[85] This is not only because in fact we behave unnaturally all the time in the medical sphere, or because we cannot really even define what is natural. It is because naturalness, if defined, is merely a description of a state, but the fact that something *is* natural does not mean that this thing *ought* to be the case. Perhaps a way to define naturalness is the state of the world unchanged by humans. On that view, when we say something is natural, we are simply saying this is how it is when we do not affect its state: Only the forces of nature (physics, chemistry, perhaps evolution) have made it thus. Those are not forces with moral weight. They do not proceed from any consideration of reasons for acting or other factors that have a bearing on the morality of an action or state. They are amoral. They cannot determine that a state is moral or otherwise. Therefore, to call something unnatural or natural tells us nothing about whether it is immoral or moral. We need to look for another way of determining this, and there are of course many. We might judge an action by its consequences and tendency to increase happiness, good, or utility. We might judge it by what has motivated it. We might wonder if it was what the virtuous person would do. We need not decide which is the most appropriate approach here; we need only realise that naturalness or otherwise cannot determine whether an action, like conceiving peri- or postmenopausally through the use of technology, is moral or not.

Conclusions

The argument from choice is often put forcefully in the media, but the foregoing analysis suggests that this cannot be a basis on which to determine whether those who delay conception should be helped to have children (or prevented from doing so). Similarly, the argument from nature cannot be such a basis. Neither argument can tell us the answer to the question of whether such assisted reproduction is ethical. Therefore, we need to turn to other subsidiary questions to help us to do so, such as the following arguments based on harm.

HARM-BASED OBJECTIONS

An alternative basis on which arguments against assisting older women to conceive are made is that such efforts have harmful consequences: to the woman, to the child, or to others. Each argument is taken in turn.

Harms to the Woman

Women who conceive later in life face significantly higher risks: They are more likely to experience poor health outcomes post birth than younger mothers.[86] Some research suggests that a woman in her 20s faces a miscarriage risk of around 1 in 10, whereas a woman aged 45 faces a risk as potentially as high as 9 in 10.[87] There is some dispute about the accuracy of miscarriage rate data generally,[88] but what is clear is that the miscarriage rate for women who have undergone IVF and had the pregnancy confirmed by ultrasound *does* increase with age. The Centers for Disease Control in the United States data show a rise from a 10% for women aged 25–30 years, to a rate of 30% for woman aged

40 years, 42% for women aged 42 years, and 55% for women aged 44 years.[89] The main reason is the increased incidence of chromosomal abnormalities in the woman's eggs (although, as will be explained, paternal age also plays a role). Around 25% of the eggs of a woman aged 30 years will have chromosomal abnormalities, compared to 40% for women aged 38 years and close to 70% for women aged 44 years.[90]

Women aged over 40 years are also more likely to become hypertensive during pregnancy.[91] They also face a higher likelihood that they will develop gestational diabetes,[92] age increases the likelihood of caesarean delivery,[93] and older women, particularly those aged over 40, also face higher risks of placenta praevia and placental abruption.[94] Those who need to use IVF to conceive face the added risks associated with ovarian stimulation.[95]

Is this a basis on which to deny access to ARTs? Some, such as Art Caplan, would say that the risks are high enough that it would be immoral to allow access to treatment.[96] However, ethically, we can only respect such women's autonomy by allowing them to make free choices about the risks they are prepared to run in relation to their own health. If we see these as self-regarding harms, a Millian perspective would suggest we have no basis on which to constrain their choices. The common law would take a similar approach. For example, the law of England and Wales permits people to refuse treatment even if the decision will result in pain or the end of life.[97] That said, while we do not force treatment, people are not free to *demand* treatment that is not clinically indicated, but as such women are facing infertility, this objection would not apply. As long as women are informed, they should be free to make their own choices about which health care treatments they use.

We should also take account of the *benefits* women who conceive later in life may enjoy as a result of their choice. These include the economic and educational benefits noted earlier but also the fulfilment of their desire for a child and all the enrichment that will bring to their lives. This is particularly true of those who have postponed reproduction for considered reasons, as they will have their child at what they considered the optimal time, with many therefore likely to enjoy pregnancy and childrearing at the point they felt most ready to do so emotional or financially. Only the particular woman can determine whether the risks she runs are worth these benefits. To make that calculation for her would be unduly paternalistic. It is at this point that the reasons we should value and respect reproductive autonomy arise once more, for as Smajdor has pointed out:

> Having children is important to women. Doing so when they feel ready, and in ways that suit them, is valuable . . . risk avoidance is not compatible with reproduction *at all* . . . [and] medical values do not necessarily trump other values that patients may hold. Human wellbeing depends on more than good health.[98]

Finally, the view that all risks to the mother derive from her own advanced age is increasingly open to question. There are some data that suggest that paternal age is also an independent risk factor for miscarriage,[99] a finding that coincides with the fact that increased male age is correlated with higher rates of some fetal abnormalities. Paternal age also appears to be somewhat associated with higher rates of caesarean section delivery, preeclampsia, and placental abruption (but not placenta praevia).[100] Therefore, it is not only the mother's decision to delay that may harm her, but her partner's as well.

Harms to the Child

By contrast, welfare concerns about the health of the child who will result may have more purchase because they revolve around a vulnerable party who cannot have a say, despite the impact on its life. When women conceive later in life, the fetus they create also faces substantially higher risks. Babies born to women over the age of 40 years are also more likely to be low weight at birth or be born preterm (that is, earlier than 37 weeks).[101] Both outcomes are correlated with higher rates of neonatal and childhood morbidity and mortality,[102] and developmental difficulties (both physical and mental). The risk of some congenital abnormalities rises with maternal age: The link with conditions such as Down syndrome, neural tube defects, and abdominal wall defects are well established, and many of these are widely known to the public.[103]

Babies born to older women are more likely to be born as a result of ARTs, which carry their own risks. In some countries, where multiple embryos are implanted, ART use is associated with higher rates of multiple births, which in turn are associated with lower birth weight and preterm delivery. The risk of birth defects is higher where ICSI is used to achieve pregnancy,[104] but the data on IVF are not yet conclusive.[105] Twin pregnancies, which carry risks for both mother and the fetuses, are more likely to occur in older women using ARTs as they may be more inclined to choose to have more embryos implanted at one time to increase their chances of a success. In doing so, their choice to use ARTs potentially increases the risk of harm to the fetuses they hope to carry.[106]

As they go through life, such children are also arguably harmed if they experience stigmatization due to their mother's age (the "grandmother at the school gate" concern). It is also suggested that an older mother is likely to die while the child is still young, increasing the likelihood that the child will experience the grief of losing a parent[107] (and perhaps the problems of a lack of care) than those born to younger mothers. Such children may also face the burden of caring for an aging parent while still young themselves.[108] For example, in a recent Italian case a child born using ARTs was removed from the care of her parents in part because they were regarded as too old to care for her. The original judge commented:

> The couple did not seriously consider the fact that the child will be orphaned at a young age and, before that, she will be constrained to look after her old parents, who could present more or less invalidating pathologies, right at the moment when, as a young adult, she will need her parents' support.[109]

The mother was 57 years old, and the father was 70 years old. Other concerns about parental age and its impact on children include worries that they will lack the stamina to care for a young child, and that they will be unable to understand the child's perspective given the large generational gap.[110] Are any or all of these risks sufficient to deny women ARTs? Three responses are given here.

Balancing Harms

Even if it is true that a child born to an older mother might suffer harms, it is important to remember that he or she may also experience many benefits. Not least, the child will most likely be born to a woman who is committed to having a child (as few people would undergo ARTs without such commitment), and at the point she is best prepared to do so. Numerous studies note the positive aspects of motherhood late in life, such as financial stability, but especially commitment to the parenting experience and women being more prepared for it.[111] There is evidence that childbearing at a later age results in better family functioning and more stable familial structures.[112] One study demonstrated that such stability is correlated with greater self-sufficiency in adulthood,[113] and others show links with better educational and psychosocial outcomes.[114] This stands in contrast to the very many children who are conceived naturally and born into far from optimal conditions because one or both parents is not ready, was not intending to have a child, or does not have the financial or emotional capacity to provide adequate care. It is well established that unstable, stressful childhood environments have a lasting impact, while children who are removed from such contexts into care environments also experience many negative consequences.[115] It has also been suggested that these beneficial aspects might offset the biological disadvantages of late-in-life procreation.[116] Cooke et al. cite a range of studies that show correlations between increased maternal age and increased cognitive ability and intelligence, and lower rates of sudden infant death syndrome.[117]

We can note a range of responses to some of the specific harms listed. Mothers can expect to live until their early 80s based on average life expectancy; therefore, even a child born to a woman of 60 years (with a father of similar age) is unlikely to be rendered an orphan.[118] That said, a potential burden of care from having an older parent is not removed, but this is only a risk, not a certainty. With modern medical care, most people in their 60s and 70s are fit and able, and it should be noted that ill health can strike at any time. A child born to a woman in her 20s who is afflicted with cancer or other illnesses in her 30s may be burdened, too, yet we do not deny her ARTs. Perhaps we might say the risk is higher if the parent is older, but age is not the only determination of health and so cannot alone be the reason to deny access to ARTs on the basis of this risk. Given that care burden is possible but not certain, a much more detailed and case-specific approach than a simple age-focused ban would be needed, one that takes account of other factors that affect ART success such as parental obesity. The same reasoning holds true for arguments about stamina and capacity to understand the child's perspective. A wider age gap alone does not necessarily imply an automatic inability to understand. It is also worth noting that there is little discussion (if any) of a *minimum* age limit for ART use based on parenting capacity, even though arguments might be made that younger adult women may be less well-placed financially to support a child or lack the life experience and maturity to raise it well. Similarly, there is little to no debate on the age at which men should be fathering children, even though we should hope that the male partner will take an equal role in the raising of the child.

Not All Harms Derive from Maternal Age

The harm argument against late-stage conception focuses on the impact of maternal age, but this leaves out the contribution of paternal age to harms. There is some (albeit conflicting) data on associations between paternal age and outcomes for offspring. Some studies suggest that children born to men over 40 years experience shorter life spans, birth defects, and a range of conditions such as various cancers, diabetes, and bipolar disorder. However, as Sartorius et al. point out in the survey of the literature, some of these associations are not well established and should be approached with caution.[119]

Paternal age is also increasingly being identified as a contributing factor to some congenital abnormalities that result in spontaneous abortion, but the impact on abnormalities that do not lead to fetal death is less clear due to a lack of data.[120] One study suggested that children born to fathers aged over 40 years faced a 20% higher risk of suffering an autosomal dominant disease than those born to 20-year-old fathers. As fathers approach 50 years of age, this risk continues to rise.[121] Another review from 2010 found that:

> despite contradictory reports, evidence suggests that increasing [paternal] age is associated with a higher frequency of aneuploidies and point mutations, more breaks in sperm DNA, loss of apoptosis, genetic imprinting and other chromosomal abnormalities.[122]

Harms that come later due to parental age, such as early parental death or a "grandfather at the school gate," should apply equally to older fathers. It is evident that they do not, with older fathers generally not facing the same degree of censure, but this is probably due in part to the assumption that the woman is the primary caregiver and so her age or her loss is more important. The lived experience for the child is probably quite contrary to this assumption, as the loss of either parent is heartbreaking, while it is as much the father's role to provide care as it is the mother's. There is, of course, more to it than this. It is not only that men face little censure when they choose to procreate late in life. In fact, men are positively lauded for this seeming sign of their enduring virility.[123] As Robert Edwards, one of the pioneers of IVF, once commented: "if a man of 60 fathers a baby, then we buy him a drink and toast his health at the pub. But it is totally different with a woman of the same age."[124]

Given this, it seems if we are to be consistent, older men should also not be permitted to conceive children later in life. The problem is that for the most part they cannot be prevented from doing so due to the incursion into their privacy and their bodies this would require. But we could say their contribution is equally morally problematic, and we could restrict them from contributing sperm when ARTs are used.

The Nonidentity Problem

The key reason why the harm argument fails is the nonidentity problem. A child born to an older mother would not have existed had she been prevented from using ARTs or other assistance to conceive in the face of her decreased or absent fertility. When a person is brought into existence who would not otherwise have existed, it arguably cannot be said that creating the person is morally wrong unless existence is worse for the person than never having existed at all. The older mother faces exactly this choice: bring a child into the world, or bring no child into the world. Unless the child she creates will live a life not worth living, her choice to do so cannot be morally wrong (assuming this choice harms no one else, a point we return to later). None of the harms listed earlier seem to be so bad that someone who experiences them would consider one's life not worth having, and so it is difficult to see how absent other harms, the harm-based argument can be a grounds to denying women ARTs.[125]

Harms to Others

Given the implications of the nonidentity problem, the harm argument can bite only if the decision to enable a woman to conceive a child despite her age-related fertility causes harm to others. One major way in which this might be the case is the diversion of resources, which is considered separately later. Other ways in which others might be harmed are the costs if the child is taken into care, or if the mother needs extra support to care for the child as she ages. These arguments are potentially convincing: It may well be unreasonable to conceive a child likely to place burdens on others. But it is mere speculation that such costs will in fact arise, and we should be fine-grained about age here. The age difference between a woman of 30 years and a woman of 40 years is only 10 years, but both can expect to live until their 80s. Therefore, neither is especially likely to die before the child reaches adulthood. Unless that woman has conceived without a partner, there is also likely to be at least the child's father remaining to provide care. It is also true that a child may lose one or both parents for any number of reasons, not solely age, and therefore the concern that the child will be a burden applies across the board and so cannot be a basis on which to deny ARTs to older women.

It has also been suggested that those who are infertile (particularly through their own fault) should adopt. This argument is often joined with claims that the world is overpopulated, and therefore using ARTs to create children who would not otherwise exist contributes to this problem. This view is obviously flawed. Overpopulation affects everyone, and anyone who bears a child by whatever means contributes to the increase in world population. Therefore, any reproductive decision is open to this objection (perhaps rightly). That some need help to conceive which can be withheld from them does not alter the fact that it is not their responsibility alone to tackle the population problem. To use their need for technological assistance to make them take on that responsibility is simply unjustified discrimination.

Furthermore, the adoption argument assumes that adoption is an option available to all such women when in fact it is not. Age may be barrier to adoption, as in some jurisdictions older people are precluded from becoming adoptive parents. It also assumes that adoption is a reasonable substitute for the creation of one's own genetically related child, but this is again not the case for all women. For some, the genetic connection is important. Many parents want to be genetically related to their offspring for the understandable reason that they rejoice in seeing the traits of themselves and their partner in the product of their relationship.[126] Others may wish not to risk what they might see as a lottery in terms of such traits—they may not wish to take the risk of taking on a child who has unknown traits or potential genetically determined health problems of which they are not aware. However, these arguments are not especially strong because the genetic component is only one of the many factors that shape a human being's character, capacities, and future health outcomes. We know that these are affected also by upbringing, environment, diet, and other factors.

But indeed it is this cluster of other factors that mean adoption is not a perfect substitute for creating a genetically related child. Adopters often will not have the choice of obtaining a newborn, but will instead have to adopt an older child, whose background may be troubled. In the United Kingdom, for example, there has been recent discussion of the difficulties adoptive parents experience precisely because those children most likely to need adoption are ones who have come from a difficult background that precipitates behavioral problems.[127] This will not always be the case, but it is certainly not true that adoption is a simple option that provides a woman who wants a child with the perfect substitute for her own offspring. Finally, it should be noted that there are in fact far fewer children available for adoption since the advent of the contraceptive pill, so it is not certain that all who wish to adopt will be able to do so.

For these reasons, adoption is an alternative to the use of technology to offset infertility, but it is not a simple solution nor is it one that everyone would wish to pursue, and their reasons for rejecting it may well be legitimate. Given the importance of reproductive autonomy, and in fact the importance of people creating families to which they are committed, pressing people into adoption when they would prefer to have genetically related offspring may itself create problems. Furthermore, as with the environmental burdens of ARTs, if there are children in need of adoption, anyone who wishes to have a child has an equal responsibility to take them into their care. The fact that some people need technology to reproduce does not mean that the welfare of these children is their responsibility above that of everyone else.

THE RESOURCE ALLOCATION QUESTION

A different kind of objection to providing women who delay reproduction with ARTs is based on concerns about the use of scarce resources. This argument holds that these women should not be allowed to use up resources that might otherwise go to those with "real" illnesses. It is most commonly raised when women seek access to health care that is provided by the state, such as cycles of IVF provided on the British National Health Service (NHS). A woman who paid for IVF for herself in an attempt to conceive late in life articulates the concern well:

> What right did I have to bump an elderly lady with dementia off the waiting list for drugs to ease her suffering because of my maternal longings? Why is a woman's right to motherhood more worthy than a man with prostate cancer ?[128]

Such arguments are often raised in conjunction with overpopulation concerns, and the alternative generally put is that these infertile people should adopt.[129] The question is complex and has many aspects; only some of these are considered here for reasons of scope.

Provision of ARTs to Older Women Diverts Resources Away From Those More in Need

Within any health care budget, only a small proportion is likely to be spent on ARTs for older women, vastly less than that spent on emergency services, cancer treatments, heart disease medications, and so on, but the concern is whether any should be spent at all. We have already seen that the "she has made her bed" argument is not convincing, but we might think that resources can always be better spent on those who are ill rather than those who are merely infertile. This, however, presumes that any illness is worse than age-related infertility. This may not, in fact, be true. This view belittles the negative impact of infertility on those who suffer it. We have seen that men and women suffer greatly in some cases when faced with involuntary childlessness, and it may well be that these impacts are substantially worse than many minor illnesses or health conditions. On this reasoning, funding ARTs for older women might be at least as important as funding treatment for such conditions as both increase quality of life.

However, in the case of more serious illnesses, this argument will not convince. The depression, frustration, and emotional pain associated with childlessness are probably not commensurate with death, permanent disability, or chronic pain in most if not all cases. Perhaps we should always direct funds at these conditions over anything else. Two responses can be made. First, severity of illness is not the only factor that determines how we divide resources. Public funds (at least in the United Kingdom) are distributed based not on the severity of the condition per se, but on the targets likely to produce the most quality-adjusted life years (QALYs). So in funding, we account for length and quality of life. We have seen that childlessness affects quality of life—it may be in many cases that the relatively small spending needed for a few cycles of IVF is good value, in QALY terms, compared to the misery of childlessness. Second, the argument that we should fund only severe conditions works against not just ARTs for older women, but *any* less serious condition. Therefore, on this basis we should divert all funds from less serious illnesses toward only the most serious. And where those minor illnesses to cause less harm than involuntary childlessness, this would place older women *above* those with minor conditions with which someone might be able to tolerate. Perhaps this is what we should do, but we would then have to defend that decision to everyone whose quality of life is decreased by a minor illness who is denied public health care. This approach would also be open to criticism on the grounds that significant numbers of people will have their quality of life depleted for the sake of a few.[130]

Provision of ARTs to Help Older Women Conceive Is a Waste of Resources

It is true that ARTs will not help all older women conceive, and its ability to help them decreases as their age rises: The success of IVF using a woman's own eggs drops from around 50% in her 30s to less than a 5% chance in her early to mid-40s.[131] It may be that these higher rates at later life stages are due to causes other than maternal age, but the size of the decline and the fact that there is a significant difference in the success rates using donor eggs (with a rate fairly constant despite increasing maternal age) and the woman's own eggs (which decreases markedly with age) suggest that maternal aging affects fertility.[132] Women of "very advanced maternal age" (older than 44 years) using their own eggs may succeed with IVF and respond well to ovarian stimulation,[133] although many have insufficient ovarian reserve and more than 90% of women aged over 40 years will not achieve a live birth with IVF.[134] When using donor eggs, IVF success rates remain relatively constant, at around 50%–60%, even for women in their mid-40s.[135] However, once women reach their late 40s, even with donor eggs the success rate begins to decline, markedly once the woman is over 50 years old.[136]

With this in mind, there is a fair point to be made about whether resources used for ARTs in older women are a "good spend." It is for this reason that some, such as Gleicher et al., argue that in women over advanced maternal age (over 42 years), access to IVF should be determined by chance of success as reflected by ovarian reserve and other measures.[137] Similarly, in the United Kingdom, state-funded IVF provision on the NHS is generally limited to women under the age of 40 years (subject to some regional variation).[138] When resources are limited, deploying them in the contexts where they will do the most good is rational. The appropriate cutoff point is difficult to determine, but there is a significant difference between helping a 40-year-old women using her own eggs, who has the same chance as many other "naturally" infertile women, and offering them to a woman of 55 years old, who has almost no chance of success.

We might reply that this should not apply to women who are willing to pay for ARTs themselves. Looked at narrowly, if she wants to spend her money in this way, then she should be free to do so. This takes a very capitalist approach, and in times of declining global resources, there may be valid arguments to be made about the approach generally. Cristina Richie has gone so far as to make the case against ART use on the grounds that it contributes unreasonably to carbon emissions. But even if these arguments are valid, given the small numbers of women who seek to use ARTs to offset natural fertility decline, and the significant benefits they obtain, the impact on resources and carbon emissions is comparatively small. There are many other reductions in consumption that produce much less happiness that we could pursue before asking these women to shoulder the burden of environmental concerns. Furthermore, if we take these concerns seriously (which we should), we should also be directing our energies at encouraging people *generally* to have fewer children; it is unreasonable and misplaced discrimination to suggest that only older women who need ARTs should take it on.

We might also reply by considering what the purpose of publicly funded health care is. If it were simply to cure disease or extend life, then many conditions currently funded would fall outside its remit. But a wider understanding, that it is to promote human flourishing by improving aspects of life that can be improved via medicine (which is probably more accurate) can certainly encompass ART provision for at least women in their 40s with some chance of success given the deleterious impact infertility may otherwise have on their lives. Even though we call it "health care," much of what is performed by medical practitioners, including ART providers, goes well beyond improving health in the narrow sense, and rightly so for, as Smajdor points out, "human well-being depends on more than good health."[139] If that well-being is promoted by treatments provided by health care providers, then that is a strong justification for its provision, regardless of the semantics of whether a problem is one of "health" or otherwise.

SOME FURTHER CONSIDERATIONS

A few further points remain to be made about how we should think about the issue of assisting women to conceive late in life. One is what the overall impact of providing such assistance would be. Will it be a large impact? Probably not, as most women will not face these issues, and many who do choose not to go through the stress and heartache of using ARTs to try to conceive. Assisting those who want help is unlikely to have substantial demographic implications or a huge impact on resources. One possible consequence, however, is a shift in current stereotypes about women's role as primary carer, as providing assistance can enable women to delay reproduction as men do. John A. Robertson goes further when he argues that a technology like egg freezing "may provide some women with reassurance that they can commit themselves to education and work without losing their fertility." It may also remove some of the pressure to find a suitable partner or to ensure they are psychologically and emotionally ready for children. Providing access to ARTs for older women may hence expand female choices and, as such, promotes female empowerment.[140]

I have also argued elsewhere that permitting women to freeze their eggs to postpone motherhood may also have the welcome effect of enabling those women to pursue education and employment such that they attain positions of power and influence. In doing so, there is the hope that they will have greater capacity to push for change to promote workplace conditions more conductive to earlier childbearing (if a woman prefers it), while continuing to break down the traditional male dominance in higher level positions.[141]

There are benefits of providing ARTs to women with age-related fertility issues. There are also problems. While ARTs may help some women, those women will be in the minority, particularly if they must use donor eggs. Many will be disappointed. If women are already unaware that their fertility will drop, and already placing undue hope in ARTs, it could be argued that providing them and offering examples of successful conceptions fuel hopes that are more than likely to be dashed. However, this is not a sufficient reason to refuse access. Rather, it is a reason to offer ARTs in conjunction with increased education to better inform women about the implications of delaying.

As I have also argued elsewhere, we should continue to work to improve the social, employment, and educational conditions that lead women to delay. If we deny women the capacity to delay childbearing in the manner in which they choose, we may see the emergence of unsafe practices such as privately arranged ART use in less regulated juris-dictions. Denying women treatment is unlikely to prevent all from seeking treatment, and some may well take risks with their health to achieve their goal. Given that this chapter has demonstrated the lack of well-established harm stemming from conception later in life, we should try to avoid placing women into the position where their choices are limited to those that prevent achievement of important life goals or harm them. More important, we might well address the challenges that prevent women conceiving at the physically opti-mal time in the future, but this will not help those women who currently face pressures that lead them to delay. If we can help them now, we should, while still working toward a future where fewer women will need to delay unless they truly wish to do so.

Conclusion

At first blush, it appears that there are many strong arguments in support of denying older women access to ARTs. But when we take the time to unpack the reasons why women delay, the conditions in which they do so, and the constraints on their choices, some of these arguments begin to fall away. We may have intuitions about the best time to conceive a child, but life is unpredictable and in most cases women who delay will do so with the best of intentions. In fact, before we criticize, we should notice that a woman who is prepared to take on the burden of having a child late in life and to go through the far from pleasant process of using ARTs to do so is likely to have made a commit-ted, considered decision to be a parent. Many of us are free to simply fall into parent-hood, and then make of it what we can. In the case of those who pursue that goal with commitment and care, whatever the challenges that prevent them, they deserve at least a reasoned consideration of their motivations and some attempt at understanding the impact of missing out of one of life's great experiences, rather than knee-jerk judgment and poorly founded objections.

Notes

1. See, e.g., J. Berryman, "Perspectives on Later Motherhood" in A. Phoenix, A. Woollett, and E. Lloyd (eds.), *Motherhood: Meanings, Practices and Ideologies* (London: Sage, 1991) as cited in R. Shaw and D. Giles, "Motherhood on Ice? A Media Framing Analysis of Older Mothers in the UK News," *Psychology and Health* 24 (2009): 221.
2. See, e.g., J. W. McDonald, A. Rosina, E. Rizzi, and B. Colombo, "Age and Fertility: Can Women Wait Until Their Early Thirties to Try for a First Birth?" *Journal of Biosocial Science* 43 (2011): 685; but compare J. Twenge, "How Long Can You Wait to Have a Baby?" *The Atlantic* (June 19), www.theatlantic.com/magazine/archive/2013/07/how-long-can-you-wait-to-have-a-baby/309374.
3. J. W. McDonald, A. Rosina, E. Rizzi, and B. Colombo, "Age and Fertility: Can Women Wait Until Their Early Thirties to Try for a First Birth?" *Journal of Biosocial Science* 43 (2011): 685.

4. See variously Advanced Fertility Center of Chicago, "Fertility After Age 40—IVF in the 40s," http://www.advancedfertility.com/fertility-after-age-40-ivf.htm; accessed October 14, 2014; D. Dunson, B. Colombo, and D. Baird, "Changes With Age in the Level and Duration of Fertility in the Menstrual Cycle," *Human Reproduction* 17 (2002): 1399; Reproductive Endocrinology and Infertility Committee, Family Physicians Advisory Committee, Maternal-Fetal Medicine Committee, Executive and Council of the Society of Obstetricians, K. Liu, and A. Case, "Advanced Reproductive Age and Fertility," *Journal of Obstetrics and Gynaecology Canada* 33 (2011): 1165; American Society for Reproductive Medicine, *Age and Fertlity: A Guide for Patients* (Birmingham, Alabama, 2012).

5. Faddy, M. J., R. Gosden, A. Gougeon, S. Richardson, and J. Nelson, "Accelerated Disappearance of Ovarian Follicles in Mid-life: Implications for Forecasting Menopause," *Human Reproduction* 7 (1992): 1342.

6. Note that J. Twenge, "How Long Can You Wait to Have a Baby?" *The Atlantic* (June 19), www.theatlantic.com/magazine/archive/2013/07/how-long-can-you-wait-to-have-a-baby/309374 disputes whether the statistics on miscarriage rates rising with age are entirely accurate.

7. S. Bewley, M. Davies, and P. Braude, "Which Career First: The Most Secure Age for Childbearing Remains 20-35," *British Medical Journal* 331 (2005): 588.

8. One extensive review study concluded that the main impact is seen when both partners are older, wherein increased paternal age is associated with fertility decline in couples where the woman is at least 35 and the man older than 40: G. A. Sartorius and E. Nieschlag, "Paternal Age and Reproduction," *Human Reproduction Update* 16 (2010): 65, 71. This appears to be the case even where donor eggs are used, where the average donor age is 25 years, but both male sperm provider and the recipient woman are aged over 39 years: I. Campos, E. Gómez, A. L. Fernández-Valencia, J. Landeras, R. González, P. Coy, and J. Gadea, "Effects of Men and Recipients' Age on the Reproductive Outcome of an Oocyte Donation Program," *Journal of Assisted Human Reproduction* 25 (2008): 445.

9. S. Tough, K. Behzies, N. Fraser-Lee, and C. Newburn-Cook, "Factors Influencing Childbearing Decisions and Knowledge of Perinatal Risks Among Canadian Men and Women," *Maternal and Child Health Journal* 11 (2007): 189; M. Mills, R. R. Rindfuss, P. McDonald, E. Velde, and on behalf of the ESHRE Reproduction and Society Task Force, "Why Do People Postpone Parenthood? Reasons and Social Policy Incentives," *Human Reproduction Update* 17 (2011): 848.

10. Office for National Statistics (UK), *Births in England and Wales, 2013* (2014), 1; T. Mathews and B. E. Hamilton, "Delayed Childbearing: More Women Are Having Their First Child Later in Life," *National Center for Health Statistics* 21 (August 2009): 1, 6.

11. Ibid., 2.

12. Office for National Statistics (UK), *Birth Summary Tables, England and Wales 2013* (2014), table 2a.

13. Office for National Statistics (UK), *Birth Summary Tables: Characteristics of Mother 2012* (2013), table 2a.

14. Ibid., 1.

15. Y. Khalaf, "Cassandra's Prophecy and the Trend of Delaying Childbearing: Is There a Simple Answer to This Complex Problem?" *Reproductive Biomedicine Online* 27 (2013): 17, citing SoOaGo Canada, "Society of Obstetricians and Gynaecologists of Canada: Opinion Committee, Delayed Childbearing," *Journal of Obstetrics and Gynaecology Canada* 34 (2012): 80.

16. See, e.g., National Institute for Health and Care Excellence, *Fertility: Assessment and Treatment for People With Fertility Problems* (Manchester, 2013).

17. R. Cook-Deegan, "What Causes Female Infertility?" (Stanford University, Stanford in Washingtom Seminar and Tutorial), https://web.stanford.edu/class/siw198q/websites/reprotech/New%20Ways%20of%20Making%20Babies/Causefem.htm, accessed September 23, 2014.

18. This is evidenced by the breadth of approaches across jurisdictions. See variously: F. Shenfield, J. Mouzon, G. Pennings, A. Ferraretti, A. Andersen, G. Wert, V. Goossens, and ESHRE Taskforce on Cross Border Reproductive Care, "Cross Border Reproductive Care in Six European Countries," *Human Reproduction* 25 (2010): 1361 (surveys policies across Europe, demonstrating that some limit funding or ban access to certain technologies, such as oocyte donation, or refused treatment based on age); M. P. Connolly, S. Hoorens, and Georgina M. Chambers on behalf of the ESHRE Reproduction and Society Task Force, "The Costs and Consequences of Assisted Reproductive Technology: An Economic Perspective," *Human Reproduction Update* 16 (2010): 603 (on the United States and Australia); M. Peterson, "Assisted Reproductive Technologies and Equity of Access Issues," *Journal of Medical Ethics* 31 (2005): 280.

19. See variously R. Shaw and D. Giles, "Motherhood on Ice? A Media Framing Analysis of Older Mothers in the UK News," *Psychology and Health* 24 (2009): 221: fertility expert Bill Ledger claimed that a child would have poor quality of life if its parents are older than its friends' grandparents; on the "granny at the school gate" argument see discussion in J. Berryman, "Perspectives on Later Motherhood" in A. Phoenix, A. Woollett, and E. Lloyd (eds), *Motherhood: Meanings, Practices and Ideologies* (London: Sage, 1991).

20. R. Shaw and D. Giles, "Motherhood on Ice? A Media Framing Analysis of Older Mothers in the UK News," *Psychology and Health* 24 (2009): 221.

21. Ibid., 226.

22. Ibid., 230.

23. Ibid., 227.

24. A. Smajdor, "The Ethics of IVF Over 40," *Maturitas* 69 (2011): 37, 38.

25. See further Ibid. and also G. Pennings, "Postmenopausal Women and the Right of Access to Oocyte Donation," *Journal of Applied Philosophy* 18 (2001): 171.

26. Men also postpone childbearing, but as they are able to reproduce well into later life (albeit, with some fertility decline), they are not making the same risk/benefit calculation as women in the same position.

27. See discussion in J. C. Daniluk, E. Koert, and A. Cheung, "Childless Women's Knowledge of Fertility and Assisted Human Reproduction: Identifying the Gaps," *Fertility and Sterility* 97 (2012): 420; K. L. Bretherick, N. Fairbrother, L. Avila, S. H. Harbord, and W. P. Robinson, "Fertility and Aging: Do Reproductive-Aged Canadian Women Know What They Need to Know?" *Fertility and Sterility* 93 (2010): 2162. N. Wyndham, P. G. M. Figueira, and P. Patrizio, "A Persistent Misperception: Assisted Reproductive Technology Can Reverse the 'Aged Biological Clock,'" *Fertility and Sterility* 97 (2012): 1044.

28. N. Wyndham, P. G. M. Figueira, and P. Patrizio, "A Persistent Misperception: Assisted Reproductive Technology Can Reverse the 'Aged Biological Clock,'" *Fertility and Sterility* 92 (2012): 1044.

29. Ibid., 1045, citing A. Maheshwari, M. Porter, A. Shetty, and S. Bhattacharya, "Women's Awareness and Perceptions of Delay in Childbearing," *Fertility and Sterility* 90 (2008): 1036.

30. N. Wyndham, P. G. M. Figueira, and P. Patrizio, "A Persistent Misperception: Assisted Reproductive Technology Can Reverse the 'Aged Biological Clock,'" *Fertility and Sterility* 97 (2012): 1044, 1045.

31. K. L. Bretherick, N. Fairbrother, L. Avila, S. H. Harbord, and W. P. Robinson, "Fertility and Aging: Do Reproductive-Aged Canadian Women Know What They Need to Know?" *Fertility and Sterility* 93 (2010): 2162.

32. See, e.g., J Twenge, "How Long Can You Wait to Have a Baby?" *The Atlantic* (June 19), www.theatlantic.com/magazine/archive/2013/07/how-long-can-you-wait-to-have-a-baby/309374; Y. Khalaf, "Cassandra's Prophecy and the Trend of Delaying Childbearing: Is There a Simple Answer to This Complex Problem?" *Reproductive Biomedicine Online* 27 (2013): 17.

33. S. Tough, K. Benzies, N. Fraser-Lee, and C. Newburn-Cook, "Factors Influencing Childbearing Decisions and Knowledge of Perinatal Risks Among Canadian Men and Women," *Maternal and Child Health Journal* 11 (2007): 189. The investigators interviewed 1,006 women and 500 men.

34. Y. Khalaf, "Cassandra's Prophecy and the Trend of Delaying Childbearing: Is There a Simple Answer to This Complex Problem?" *Reproductive Biomedicine Online* 27 (2013): 17.

35. S. Tough, K. Benzies, N. Fraser-Lee, and C. Newburn-Cook, "Factors Influencing Childbearing Decisions and Knowledge of Perinatal Risks Among Canadian Men and Women," *Maternal and Child Health Journal* 11 (2007): 189.

36. J. C. Daniluk, E. Koert, and A. Cheung, "Childless Women's Knowledge of Fertility and Assisted Human Reproduction: Identifying the Gaps," *Fertility and Sterility* 97 (2012): 420, 424 and studies cited therein. See also K. L. Bretherick, N. Fairbrother, L. Avila, S. H. Harbord, and W. P. Robinson, "Fertility and Aging: Do Reproductive-Aged Canadian Women Know What They Need to Know?" *Fertility and Sterility* 93 (2010): 2162; M. J. Davies, V. M. Moore, K. J. Willson, P. V. Essen, K. Priest, H. Scott, E. A. Haan, and A. Chan, "Reproductive Technologies and the Risk of Birth Defects," *New England Journal of Medicine* 366 (2012): 1083.

37. J. C. Daniluk, E. Koert, and A. Cheung, "Childless Women's Knowledge of Fertility and Assisted Human Reproduction: Identifying the Gaps," *Fertility and Sterility* 97 (2012): 420, 424 and studies cited therein. N. Wyndham, P. G. M. Figueira, and P. Patrizio, "A Persistent Misperception: Assisted Reproductive Technology Can Reverse the 'Aged Biological Clock,'" *Fertility and Sterility* 97 (2012): 1044, 1045.

38. J. C. Daniluk, E. Koert, and A. Cheung, "Childless Women's Knowledge of Fertility and Assisted Human Reproduction: Identifying the Gaps" *Fertility and Sterility* 97 (2012): 420, 424. See also A. Cooke, T. A. Mills, and T. Lavender, "Informed and Uninformed Decision Making—Women's Reasoning, Experiences and Perceptions With Regard to Advanced Maternal Age and Delayed Childbearing: A Meta-synthesis," *International Journal of Nursing Studies* 47 (2010): 1317, 1325.

39. K. Benzies, S. Tough, K. Tofflemire, C. Frick, A. Faber, and C. Newburn-Cook, "Factors Influencing Women's Decisions About Timing of Motherhood," *Journal of Obstetric, Gynecologic and Neonatal Nursing* 35 (2006): 625, 628.

40. A. Cooke, T. A. Mills, and T. Lavender, "Advanced Maternal Age: Delayed Childbearing Is Rarely a Conscious Choice. A Qualitative Study of Women's Views and Experiences," *International Journal of Nursing Studies* 49 (2012): 30.

41. Y. Khalaf, "Cassandra's Prophecy and the Trend of Delaying Childbearing: Is There a Simple Answer to This Complex Problem?" *Reproductive Biomedicine Online* 27 (2013): 17.

42. J. C. Daniluk, E. Koert, and A. Cheung, "Childless Women's Knowledge of Fertility and Assisted Human Reproduction: Identifying the Gaps," *Fertility and Sterility* 97 (2012): 420 and various studies referred to therein. See also A. Cooke, T. A. Mills, and T. Lavender, "Informed and Uninformed Decision Making—Women's Reasoning, Experiences and Perceptions With Regard to Advanced Maternal Age and Delayed Childbearing: A Meta-Synthesis," *International Journal of Nursing Studies* 47 (2010): 1317, 1325.

43. N. Wyndham, P. G. M. Figueira, and P. Patrizio, "A Persistent Misperception: Assisted Reproductive Technology Can Reverse the 'Aged Biological Clock,'" *Fertility and Sterility* 97 (2012): 1044, 1045. See also J. C. Daniluk, E. Koert, and A. Cheung, "Childless Women's Knowledge of Fertility and Assisted Human Reproduction: Identifying the Gaps," *Fertility and Sterility* 97 (2012): 420, 421; K. L. Bretherick, N. Fairbrother, L. Avila, S. H. Harbord, and W. P. Robinson, "Fertility and Aging: Do Reproductive-Aged Canadian Women Know What They Need to Know?" *Fertility and Sterility* 93 (2010): 2162.

44. Y. Khalaf, "Cassandra's Prophecy and the Trend of Delaying Childbearing: Is There a Simple Answer to This Complex Problem?" *Reproductive Biomedicine Online* 27 (2013): 17, 18.

45. As Robert Winston has said: "The nature of our society is that women are leaving childbearing until later and later in life, and there are good reasons for it, too": A. Grant, "I'm an 'older' mum whose son was conceived by IVF—so why am I uneasy about the NHS offering more women like me the same chance of motherhood?" *The Telegraph* (May 23, 2012).

46. S. Tough, K. Benzies, N. Fraser-Lee, and C. Newburn-Cook, "Factors Influencing Childbearing Decisions and Knowledge of Perinatal Risks Among Canadian Men and Women," *Maternal and Child Health Journal* 11 (2007): 189.

47. A. Berrington, "Perpetual Postponers? Women's, Men's and Couple's Fertility Intentions and Subsequent Fertility Behaviour," *Population Trends* 117 (2004): 9, 116, and see also as cited therein: F. McAllister and L. Clarke, *Choosing Childlessness: Family & Parenthood, Policy & Practice* (London: Family Policy Studies Centre, 1998); T. Fahey and Z. Spéder, *Fertility and Family Issues in an Enlarged Europe* (Luxembourg, European Foundation for the Improvement of Living and Working Conditions; Office for Official Publications of the European Communities, 2004); R. Schoen, N. M. Astone, Y. J. Kim, and C. A. Nathanson, "Do Fertility Intentions Affect Fertility Behavior?" *Journal of Marriage and the Family* 61 (1999): 790. A. Cooke, T. A. Mills, and T. Lavender, "Advanced Maternal Age: Delayed Childbearing Is Rarely a Conscious Choice: A Qualitative Study of Women's Views and Experiences," *International Journal of Nursing Studies* 49 (2012): 30, 34–35; K. Benzies, S. Tough, K. Tofflemire, C. Frick, A. Faber, and C. Newburn-Cook, "Factors Influencing Women's Decisions About Timing of Motherhood," *Journal of Obstetric, Gynecologic and Neonatal Nursing* 35 (2006): 625, 628.

48. A. Berrington, "Perpetual Postponers? Women's, Men's and Couple's Fertility Intentions and Subsequent Fertility Behaviour," *Population Trends* 117 (2004): 9. See also A. Cooke, T. A. Mills, and T. Lavender, "Informed and Uninformed decision Making—Women's Reasoning, Experiences and Perceptions With Regard to Advanced Maternal Age and Delayed Childbearing: A Meta-Synthesis," *International Journal of Nursing Studies* 47 (2010): 1317, 1323.

49. S. Tough, K. Benzies, N. Fraser-Lee, and C. Newburn-Cook, "Factors Influencing Childbearing Decisions and Knowledge of Perinatal Risks among Canadian Men and Women," *Maternal and Child Health Journal* 11 (2007): 189 and as cited therein: J. Hansen, "Older Maternal Age and Pregnancy Outcome: A Review of the Literature," *Obstetrics

and Gynecology Survey 41 (1986): 726; P. Mansfield and W. McCool, "Toward a Better Understanding of the 'Advanced Maternal Age' Factor," *Health Care Women International* 10 (1989): 395.

50. M. Mills, R. R. Rindfuss, P. McDonald, E. Velde, and on behalf of the ESHRE Reproduction and Society Task Force, "Why Do People Postpone Parenthood? Reasons and Social Policy Incentives," *Human Reproduction Update* 17 (2011): 848, 852.

51. Ibid., 852.

52. N. Wyndham, P. G. M. Figueira, and P. Patrizio, "A Persistent Misperception: Assisted Reproductive Technology Can Reverse the 'Aged Biological Clock,'" *Fertility and Sterility* 97 (2012): 1044 and studies cited therein.

53. L. L. Willett, M. F. Wellons, J. R. Hartig, L. Roenigk, M. Panda, A. T. Dearinger, J. Allison, and T. K. Houston, "Do Women Residents Delay Childbearing Due to Perceived Career Threats?" *Academic Medicine* 85 (2010): 640.

54. A. R. Miller, "The Effects of Motherhood Timing on Career Path," *Journal of Population Economics* 24 (2011): 1071, 1073. Similar results are reported in E. T. Wilde, L. Batchelder, and D. T. Ellwood, "The Mommy Track Divides: The Impact of Childbearing on Wage of Women of Differing Skill Levels," *National Bureau of Economic Research Working Paper Series* 16582 (2010).

55. A. R. Miller, "The Effects of Motherhood Timing on Career Path," *Journal of Population Economics* 24 (2011):1071, 1073–1074.

56. Ibid. See also E. T. Wilde, L. Batchelder, and D. T. Ellwood, "The Mommy Track Divides: The Impact of Childbearing on Wage of Women of Differing Skill Levels," *National Bureau of Economic Research Working Paper Series* 16582 (2010).

57. A. R. Miller, "The Effects of Motherhood Timing on Career Path," *Journal of Population Economics* 24 (2011): 1071, 1097.

58. E. T. Wilde, L. Batchelder, and D. T. Ellwood, "The Mommy Track Divides: The Impact of Childbearing on Wage of Women of Differing Skill Levels," *National Bureau of Economic Research Working Paper Series* 16582 (2010): 8.

59. A. R. Miller, "The Effects of Motherhood Timing on Career Path," *Journal of Population Economics* 24 (2011): 1071, 1098.

60. E. T. Wilde, L. Batchelder, and D. T. Ellwood, "The Mommy Track Divides: The Impact of Childbearing on Wage of Women of Differing Skill Levels," *National Bureau of Economic Research Working Paper Series* 16582 (2010): 5.

61. S. Bewley, M. Davies, and P. Braude, "Which Career First: The Most Secure Age for Childbearing Remains 20-35," *British Medical Journal* 331 (2005): 588, 589; R. Shaw and D. Giles, "Motherhood on Ice? A Media Framing Analysis of Older Mothers in the UK News," *Psychology and Health* 24 (2009): 221, 226 citing several media sources.

62. See Y. Khalaf, "Cassandra's Prophecy and the Trend of Delaying Childbearing: Is There a Simple Answer to This Complex Problem?" *Reproductive Biomedicine Online* 27 (2013): 17.

63. S. Tough, K. Benzies, N. Fraser-Lee, and C. Newburn-Cook, "Factors Influencing Childbearing Decisions and Knowledge of Perinatal Risks among Canadian Men and Women," *Maternal and Child Health Journal* 11 (2007): 189. See also various studies cited in N. Wyndham, P. G. M. Figueira, and P. Patrizio, "A Persistent Misperception: Assisted Reproductive Technology Can Reverse the 'Aged Biological Clock,'" *Fertility and Sterility* 92 (2012): 1044.

64. For example, until 2015, in the United Kingdom men received only two weeks paternity leave entitlement, while women could take up to one year while retaining job security.

65. M. Mills, R. R. Rindfuss, P. McDonald, E. Velde, and on behalf of the ESHRE Reproduction and Society Task Force, "Why Do People Postpone Parenthood? Reasons and Social Policy Incentives," *Human Reproduction Update* 17 (2011): 848, 855 citing S. Bianchi, M. Milkie, L. Sayer, and J. Robinson, "Is Anyone Doing the Housework? Trends in the Gender Division of Household Labor," *Social Forces* 79 (2000): 191; J. Gershuny, *Changing Times: Work and Leisure in Postindustrial Society* (Oxford: Oxford University Press, 2000); J. Hook, "Care in Context: Men's Unpaid Work in 20 Countries, 1965–2003," *American Sociological Review* 71 (2006): 639.

66. S. Bewley, M. Davies, and P. Braude, "Which Career First: The Most Secure Age for Childbearing Remains 20-35," *British Medical Journal* 331 (2005): 588, 589.

67. K. Benzies, S. Tough, K. Tofflemire, C. Frick, A. Faber, and C. Newburn-Cook, "Factors Influencing Women's Decisions About Timing of Motherhood," *Journal of Obstetric, Gynecologic and Neonatal Nursing* 35 (2006): 625, 628.

68. N. Wyndham, P. G. M. Figueira, and P. Patrizio, "A Persistent Misperception: Assisted Reproductive Technology Can Reverse the 'Aged Biological Clock,'" *Fertility and Sterility* 92 (2012): 1044.

69. A. Cooke, T. A. Mills, and T. Lavender, "Advanced Maternal Age: Delayed Childbearing Is Rarely a Conscious Choice. A Qualitative Study of Women's Views and Experiences," *International Journal of Nursing Studies* 49 (2012): 30, 33.

70. A. Smajdor, "The Ethics of IVF Over 40," *Maturitas* 69 (2011): 37, 38.

71. Robert Burns, *To a Mouse, On Turning Her Up in Her Nest With the Plough*.

72. J. C. Daniluk, E. Koert, and A. Cheung, "Childless Women's Knowledge of Fertility and Assisted Human Reproduction: Identifying the Gaps," *Fertility and Sterility* 97 (2012): 420 refs 11, 21–24, 25. See also A. Cooke, T. A. Mills, and T. Lavender, "Informed and Uninformed Decision Making—Women's Reasoning, Experiences and Perceptions With Regard to Advanced Maternal Age and Delayed Childbearing: A Meta-Synthesis," *International Journal of Nursing Studies* 47 (2010): 1317, 1325.

73. A. Cooke, T. A. Mills, and T. Lavender, "Advanced Maternal Age: Delayed Childbearing Is Rarely a Conscious Choice. A Qualitative Study of Women's Views and Experiences," *International Journal of Nursing Studies* 49 (2012): 30, 35.

74. Ibid., 35.

75. M. Mills, R. R. Rindfuss, P. McDonald, E. Velde, and on behalf of the ESHRE Reproduction and Society Task Force, "Why Do People Postpone Parenthood? Reasons and Social Policy Incentives," *Human Reproduction Update* 17 (2011): 848, 849. W. Meller, L. Burns, S. Crow, and P. Grambsch, "Major Depression in Unexplained Infertility," *Journal of Psychosomatic Obstetrics and Gynecology* 23 (2003): 27.

76. A. Smajdor, "The Ethics of IVF Over 40," *Maturitas* 69 (2011): 37, 38.

77. N. Priaulx, "Rethinking Progenitive Conflict: Why Reproductive Autonomy Matters," *Medical Law Review* 16 (2008): 169, 173.

78. Ibid., 174 referencing J. A. Robertson, *Children of Choice: Freedom and the New Reproductive Technologies* (Princeton, NJ: Princeton University Press, 1994), 24.

79. J. S. Mill, *On Liberty* (1869), Ch III.

80. R. Shaw and D. Giles, "Motherhood on Ice? A Media Framing Analysis of Older Mothers in the UK News," *Psychology and Health* 24 (2009): 221, 227.

81. Ibid., 227.

82. Ibid., 227.

83. Ibid.

84. Ibid., 228.

85. Compare the position of the Canadian Royal Commission in opposing postmenopausal IVF: Royal Commission on New Reproductive Technologies, *Proceed with care: final report of the Royal Commission on New Reproductive Technologies* (Ottawa, 1993).

86. J. C. Daniluk, E. Koert, and A. Cheung, "Childless Women's Knowledge of Fertility and Assisted Human Reproduction: Identifying the Gaps," *Fertility and Sterility* 97 (2012): 420 and studies cited therein.

87. S. Tough, K. Benzies, N. Fraser-Lee, and C. Newburn-Cook, "Factors Influencing Childbearing Decisions and Knowledge of Perinatal Risks Among Canadian Men and Women," *Maternal and Child Health Journal* 11 (2007): 189; N. Wyndham, P. G. M. Figueira, and P. Patrizio, "A Persistent Misperception: Assisted Reproductive Technology Can Reverse the 'Aged Biological Clock,'" *Fertility and Sterility* 92 (2012): 1044. See also S. Bewley, M. Davies, and P. Braude, "Which Career First: The Most Secure Age for Childbearing Remains 20-35," *British Medical Journal* 331 (2005): 588, 589.

88. J. Twenge, "How Long Can You Wait to Have a Baby?" *The Atlantic* (June 19), www.the-atlantic.com/magazine/archive/2013/07/how-long-can-you-wait-to-have-a-baby/309374.

89. Centers for Disease Control, "ART National Summary Report Presentations" (2010), http://www.cdc.gov/art/artreports.htm#p5, accessed 13 October 2014, 17.

90. Advanced Fertility Center of Chicago, "IVF and Age—Impact of Female Aging on In Vitro Fertilization Statistics," http://www.advancedfertility.com/ivf-age.htm, accessed July 10, 2012.

91. See studies as cited in S. Tough, K. Benzies, N. Fraser-Lee, and C. Newburn-Cook, "Factors Influencing Childbearing Decisions and Knowledge of Perinatal Risks Among Canadian Men and Women," *Maternal and Child Health Journal* 11 (2007): 189.

92. See studies as cited in Ibid.

93. A. Treacy, M. Robson, and C. O.'Herlihy, "Dystocia Increases with Advancing Maternal Age," *American Journal of Obstetrics and Gynecology* 195 (2006): 760; J. Cleary-Goldman, F. Malone, J. Vidaver, R. Ball, D. Nyberg, C. Comstock, G. Saade, K. Eddleman, S. Klugman, L. Dugoff, I. Timor-Tritsch, S. Craigo, S. Carr, H. Wolfe, D. Bianchi, and M. D'Alton, "Impact of Maternal Age on Obstetric Outcome," *Obstetrics and Gynecology International* 105 (2005): 983; W Gilbert, T. Nesbitt, and B. Danielsen, "Childbearing Beyond Age 40: Pregnancy Outcome in 24,032 cases," *Obstetrics & Gynecology* 93 (1999): 9 as cited in A. Cooke, T. A. Mills and T. Lavender, "Advanced Maternal Age: Delayed Childbearing Is Rarely a Conscious Choice: A Qualitative Study of Women's Views and Experiences," *International Journal of Nursing Studies* 49 (2012): 30.

94. W. Gilbert, T. Nesbitt, and B. Danielsen, "Childbearing Beyond Age 40: Pregnancy Outcome in 24,032 Cases," *Obstetrics & Gynecology* 93 (1999): 9. As cited in A. Cooke, T. A. Mills, and T. Lavender, "Advanced Maternal Age: Delayed Childbearing Is Rarely a Conscious Choice. A Qualitative Study of Women's Views and Experiences" *International Journal of Nursing Studies* 49 (2012): 30; and see S Bewley, M Davies and P Braude, "Which Career First: The Most Secure Age for Childbearing Remains 20-35," *British Medical Journal* 331 (2005): 588, 589 on risks generally.

95. J. S. Cunha-Filho, M. Samama, R. Fanchin, C. Righini, I.-J. Kadoch, and R. F. Olivennes, "Clinical and Laboratory Evaluation of Hospitalized Patients with Severe Ovarian Hyperstimulation Syndrome" *Reproductive BioMedicine Online* 6 (2003): 448.

96. A. Caplan and P. Patrizio, "Are You Ever Too Old to Have a Baby? The Ethical Challeges of Older Women Using Infertility Services," *Seminars in Reproductive Medicine* 28 (2010).

97. See, e.g., *St George's Healthcare NHS Trust v S* [1998] 3 All ER 673.

98. A. Smajdor, "The Ethics of IVF Over 40," *Maturitas* 69 (2011): 37, 38.

99. G.A. Sartorius and E. Nieschlag, "Paternal Age and Reproduction," *Human Reproduction Update* 16 (2010): 65, 71.

100. Ibid., 72–74.

101. See A. Cooke, T. A. Mills, and T. Lavender, "Advanced Maternal Age: Delayed Childbearing Is Rarely a Conscious Choice: A Qualitative Study of Women's Views and Experiences" *International Journal of Nursing Studies* 49 (2012): 30 and multiple studies cited therein.

102. See S. Tough, K. Benzies, N. Fraser-Lee, and C. Newburn-Cook, "Factors Influencing Childbearing Decisions and Knowledge of Perinatal Risks Among Canadian Men and Women" *Maternal and Child Health Journal* 11 (2007): 189 and multiple studies cited therein; M. C. Hoffman, S. Jeffers, J. Carter, L. Duthely, A. Cotter, and V. H. González-Quintero, "Pregnancy at or Beyond Age 40 Years Is Associated With an Increased Risk of Fetal Death and Other Adverse Outcomes," *American Journal of Obstetrics and Gynecology* 196 (2007): e11.

103. J. Rychtarikova, C. Gourbin, A. Sipek, and G. Wunsch, "Impact of Parental Ages and Other Characteristics at Childbearing on Congenital Anomalies: Results for the Czech Republic, 2000–2007" *Demographic Research* 28 (2013): 137, 139. See also A. Cooke, T. A. Mills, and T. Lavender, "Advanced Maternal Age: Delayed Childbearing Is Rarely a Conscious Choice: A Qualitative Study of Women's Views and Experiences," *International Journal of Nursing Studies* 49 (2012): 30.

104. M. J. Davies, V. M. Moore, K. J. Willson, P. V. Essen, K. Priest, H. Scott, E. A. Haan, and A. Chan, "Reproductive Technologies and the Risk of Birth Defects," *New England Journal of Medicine* 366 (2012): 1083.

105. See, e.g., Ibid.,1803.

106. This harm arises only in jurisdictions where it is permissible to implant multiple embryos in one cycle, a practice some jurisdictions have limited due to the risks doing so poses. Where no such regulatory limits are in place, clinics' interests in publishing high success rates may also affect a woman's decision about how many embryos to implant.

107. Numerous studies have demonstrated the negative psychological impact of the loss of a parent in early childhood. Early parental death has been associated with suicide, substance abuse, difficulties with establishing and sustaining intimacy, and anger-management issues (K. Mack, "Childhood Family Disruptions and Adult Well-Being: The Differential Effects of Divorce and Parental Death" *Death Studies* 25 (2001): 419) as well as social withdrawal, anxiety, and low self-esteem in children suffering childhood grief (J. Worden and P. Silverman, "Parental Death and the Adjustment of School-Age Children" *Journal of Death and Dying* 33 (1996): 91). Dowdney suggests that as many as one in five children who lose a parent develop a psychiatric disorder (L. Dowdney, "Annotation: Childhood Bereavement Following Parental Death" *Journal of Child Psychology and Psychiatry* 41 (2000): 819), and other studies show that parental death during childhood is associated with risks of psychological illness in offspring and of later substance abuse, PTSD and health risk behaviours (C. Tennant, P. Bebbington, and J. Hurry, "Parental Death in Childhood and Risk of Adult Depressive Disorders: A Review" *Psychological Medicine* 10 (1980): 289; D. A. Brent, N. M. Melhem, A. S. Masten, G. Porta, and M. W. Payne, "Logitudinal Effects of Parental Bereavement

on Adolescent Developmental Competence" *Journal of Clinical Child & Adolescent Psychology* 41 (2012): 778). However, other studies suggest that parental loss in childhood is not an independent risk factor for adult depression (C. Tennant, "Parental Loss in Childhood: It's Effect in Adult Life," *Archives of General Psychiatry* 45 (1988): 1045).

108. See, e.g., discussion in M. Peterson, "Assisted Reproductive Technologies and Equity of Access Issues" *Journal of Medical Ethics* 31 (2005): 280.

109. Minors' Court of Piemonte and Valle d'Aosta, Sentence n 133, August 16, 2011, 251. It is important to note that there were other bases for the decision, most particularly failures in care of the child unrelated to the parents' age, but the matter is complex and the case was appealed twice. Alice Margaria and Sally Sheldon provide a very useful analysis of the reasoning in all three courts here: A. Margaria and S. Sheldon, "Parenting Post IVF: Is Age Not So Relevant After All?" *Reproductive Biomedicine Online* 29 (2014): 10.

110. See further on these arguments: S. A. Jayson, '"Loving Infertile Couple Seeks Woman Age 18–31 to Help Have Baby. $6,500 plus Expenses and a Gift: Should We Regulate the Use of Assisted Reproductive Technologies by Older Women?' *Albany Law Journal of Science and Technology* 11 (2001): 287.

111. See, e.g., R. Shaw and D. Giles, "Motherhood on Ice? A Media Framing Analysis of Older Mothers in the UK News," *Psychology and Health* 24 (2009): 221.

112. M. Mills, R. R. Rindfuss, P. McDonald, E. Velde, and on behalf of the ESHRE Reproduction and Society Task Force, "Why Do People Postpone Parenthood? Reasons and Social Policy Incentives," *Human Reproduction Update* 17 (2011): 848, 849.

113. Ibid., 849.

114. Ibid., 849.

115. K. Bos, C. Zeanah, N. Fox, S. Drury, K. McLaughlin, and C. Nelson, "Psychiatric Outcomes in Young Children With a History of Institutionalization," *Harvard Review of Psychiatry* 19 (2011): 15; J. Windsor, J. P. Benigno, C. Wing, P. Carroll, S. Koga, C. N. III, N. Fox, and C. Zeanah, "Effect of Foster Care on Young Children's Language Learning," *Child Development* 82 (2011): 1040.

116. F. C. Billari, A. Goisis, A. C. Liefbroer, R. A. Settersten, A. Aassve, G. Hagestad, and Z. Speder, "Social Age Deadlines for Childbearing for Women and Men," *Human Reproduction* 26 (2010): 616, 621.

117. A. Cooke, T. A. Mills, and T. Lavender, "Advanced Maternal Age: Delayed Childbearing Is Rarely a Conscious Choice. A Qualitative Study of Women's Views and Experiences," *International Journal of Nursing Studies* 49 (2012): 30, 31.

118. For example, Banh et al. demonstrate that given the current life expectancy for women, the cutoff for a woman using IVF should be 68 years if the basis on which to restrict access is concerns that the child will not reach adulthood before the mother dies: D. Banh, D. L. Havemann, and J. Y. Phelps, "Reproduction Beyond Menopause: How Old Is Too Old for Assisted Reproductive Technology?" *Journal of Assisted Reproduction and Genetics* 37 (2010): 366. On this basis, they suggest that when IVF is offered to patients over the age of 50, one consideration should be whether the patient has a remaining life expectancy of 18 years or more.

119. G. A. Sartorius and E. Nieschlag, "Paternal Age and Reproduction," *Human Reproduction Update* 16 (2010): 65, 74.

120. J. Rychtarikova, C. Gourbin, A. Sipek, and G. Wunsch, "Impact of Parental Ages and Other Characteristics at Childbearing on Congenital Anomalies: Results for the Czech Republic, 2000–2007," *Demographic Research* 28 (2013): 137, 139, 152. Plas et al. make

the same observation about lack of data: E. Plas, P. Berger, M. Herman, and H. Pfluger, "Effects of Aging on Male Fertility?" *Experimental Gerontology* 35 (2000): 543, 545. Paternal age does not appear to be associated with Down syndrome (p. 151).

121. E. Plas, P. Berger, M. Herman, and H. Pfluger, "Effects of Aging on Male Fertility?" *Experimental Gerontology* 35 (2000): 543.

122. G. A. Sartorius and E. Nieschlag, "Paternal Age and Reproduction," *Human Reproduction Update* 16 (2010): 65, 69.

123. See further on this point: I. Goold and J. Savulescu, "In Favour of Freezing Eggs for Non-Medical Reasons," *Bioethics* 23 (2009): 47, 52.

124. B. Hewitt, "Turning Back the Clock," *People* (January 24, 1994), 36.

125. See further on this point in the context of postmenopausal women's reproduction in particular: J. Harris, "Rights and Reproductive Choice" in ed. J. Harris and S. Holm, *The Future of Human Reproduction: Ethics, Choice, and Regulation* (Oxford: Oxford University Press, 1998), 19–21.

126. Compare Bayles (1984) who argues that this view is irrational; W. Dondorp and G. D. Wert, "Fertility Preservation for Healthy Women: Ethical Aspects," *Human Reproduction* 24 (2009): 1779.

127. See, e.g., M Henderson, "Adoption: Why the System Is Ruining Lives," *Guardian* (October 31, 2012) and references cited therein.

128. A Platell, "I endured the trauma of IVF. Giving it to the over-40s on the NHS isn't just wasteful . . . it's cruel," *Daily Mail* (May 24, 2012).

129. A. S. Daar and Z. Merali, "Infertility and Social Suffering: The Case of ART in Developing Countries" in E. Vayena, P. Rowe, and P. Griffin (eds), *Current Practices and Controversies in Assisted Reproduction* (Geneva, Switzerland: World Health Organization, 2002). The question of adoption also arises frequently in feminist jurisprudence. In E. Bartholet, *Family Bonds* (Boston: Houghton Mifflin, 1993), 24, the argument is made against use of reproductive technologies because they detract from the appeal of adoption, leaving it as a "choice of last resort for infertile . . . women"; R. Colker, "Pregnant Men Revisited or Sperm Is Cheap, Eggs Are Not," *Hastings Law Journal* 47 (1996): 1063, 1080, muses: "I wonder why people engage in IVF at all, because it is such a difficult, painful, expensive, and not very successful procedure. There are always children available to be adopted . . . . Does the use of IVF express a disrespect for the lives of the poor, disabled, and often minority children who are available for adoption?"; and see also M.A. Field, "Surrogacy Contract—Gestational and Traditional: The Argument for Non-enforcement," *Washburn Law Journal* 31 (1991): 6, in which it is suggested that we should restrict access to reproductive technologies to encourage people to adopt hard to place children.

130. For a further discussion of some of these arguments, see W. Dondorp and G. D. Wert, "Fertility Preservation for Healthy Women: Ethical Aspects," *Human Reproduction* 24 (2009): 1779.

131. Centers for Disease Control, "ART National Summary Report Presentations" (2010), http://www.cdc.gov/art/artreports.htm#p5, accessed October 13, 2014, 31.

132. Ibid., 44.

133. S. D. Spandorfer, K. Bendikson, K. Dragisic, G. Schattman, O. K. Davis, and Z. Rosenwaks, "Outcome of In Vitro Fertilization in Women 45 Years and Older Who Use Autologous Oocytes," *Fertility and Sterility* 87 (2007): 74.

134. S. Bewley, M. Davies, and P. Braude, "Which Career First: The Most Secure Age for Childbearing Remains 20-35," *British Medical Journal* 331 (2005): 588, fn 6.

135. Advanced Fertility Center of Chicago, "IVF and Age—Impact of Female Aging on In Vitro Fertilization Statistics" <http://www.advancedfertility.com/ivf-age.htm> accessed July 10, 2012.

136. N. Wyndham, P. G. M. Figueira, and P. Patrizio, "A Persistent Misperception: Assisted Reproductive Technology Can Reverse the 'Aged Biological Clock,' " *Fertility and Sterility* 92 (2012): 1044.

137. N. Gleicher, V. A. Kushnir, A. Weghofer, and D. H. Barad, "The 'Graying' of Infertility Services: An Impending Revolution Nobody Is Ready for," *Reproductive Biology and Endocrinology* 12 (2013): 63.

138. See further National Institute for Health and Care Excellence, *Fertility: Assessment and Treatment for People with Fertility Problems* (Manchester, 2013); NHS Choices, "IVF: Introduction" (National Health Service) <http://www.nhs.uk/conditions/IVF/pages/introduction.aspx> accessed October 15, 2014.

139. A. Smajdor, "The Ethics of IVF Over 40", *Maturitas* 69 (2011): 37, 38.

140. J. A. Robertson, *Children of Choice: Freedom and the New Reproductive Technologies* (Princeton, NJ: Princeton University Press, 1994), 120.

141. I. Goold and J. Savulescu, "In Favour of Freezing Eggs for Non-Medical Reasons," *Bioethics* 23 (2009): 47, 49.

CHAPTER 20

JUSTICE, PROCREATION, AND THE COSTS OF HAVING AND RAISING DISABLED CHILDREN

DAVID WASSERMAN

FOUR types of objection have been raised to the failure of prospective parents to select against, or to their deliberate selection of, (future) children with disabilities.[1] The first is impersonal; it concerns the aggregate good, which is assumed to be reduced by the choice of a disabled rather than nondisabled child. The other three objections concern duties to specific people or groups. The first of these objections concerns the interests or rights of the future child; it claims that avoidably having a child with a disability (i.e., having such a child when one could have another one) wrongs that child. The second claims that failing to select against, or selecting for, disability harms, or poses an unacceptable risk of harming individuals toward whom the prospective parents have personal duties, particularly their other children, aging parents, and other dependents. The third claims that such action is wrong because it violates, or creates an unacceptable risk of violating, duties of justice, duties owed not to specific individuals but to the political community. It does so by voluntarily imposing or threatening to impose substantial costs on that society, in the form of higher medical or personal care expenses, or reduced productivity.

In this chapter, I will explore the last objection, which has seen relatively little discussion in the recent literature. There has been considerable debate about whether having a child with a genetically based disability is wrong when parents could have had a different, nondisabled one (see Boonin 2014 for a comprehensive review). The duties of prospective parents to individual third parties are generally recognized as an appropriate moral constraint on procreation, although those burdens have fare more often been assumed than evidenced (see Asch and Wasserman 2014). Far less has been written about the costs of disability to the wider society.

Some of the reticence about discussing duties of justice, and the social costs of disabilities, undoubtedly comes from the legacy of negative eugenics: no one wants to be accused of evoking the concerns about the genetic fitness of the population raised by US eugenicists like Davenport and Laughlin, let alone of treating people with disabilities as "useless eaters," to use the chilling Nazi phrase (Kevles 1985). But there are other, more philosophical reasons to avoid the issue. Questions about what individuals owe society and vice-versa are central questions in political philosophy, no closer to resolution than they were when Rawls (1971) revived interest in justice as a philosophical topic. And questions about the role of families in theory of justice, or a just society, are particularly contentious (Fishkin 1983). Additionally, those holding widely divergent views about ideal justice agree that all existing societies are far from their ideal, and questions about what duties are owed in nonideal circumstances (Simmons 2010) add another layer of complexity and controversy.

Recently, however, a small number of authors have begun arguing, or suggesting, that the social costs of disability are morally relevant to decisions about prenatal testing for disability. Although I will dissent from their claims, I think they are no less plausible, and in some cases more, than the objections raised on the three other grounds. As Glenn Cohen concludes about related objections concerning what he calls negative reproductive externalities, they are "the best of a not very good lot" (2012, 1220).

The most cautious, qualified argument based on social costs is made by Stephen John (2015). He argues not for restrictions on parental choice, but merely for state financing of prenatal diagnosis (PND) based on expected cost savings. Although he recognizes the force of expressivist concerns about treating people with disabilities as economic burdens, he believes that the public provision of PND could be justified for some disabilities, in societies where its provision would not promote discrimination against existing people with disabilities. He suggests that this cost-savings argument also has implications for the responsibility of prospective parents. Although the moral complexities of decisions concerning pregnancy termination preclude moral blame, they may permit what Scanlon (1998) calls "substantive responsibility" in some circumstances—holding parents responsible for the additional costs of having a child with a disability if state-financed PND gave them a reasonable opportunity to avoid that outcome. John recognizes that as a practical matter, holding parents responsible in this sense would be highly problematic, because in many cases, religious or (other) moral objections to abortion would preclude "reasonable opportunity to avoid" and because the disabled child would usually suffer the consequences of holding its parents substantively responsible.

Other writers, discussing the broader issues of who should bear the costs of raising children, have made claims with harsher implications for the costs of children with disabilities. Serena Olsaretti (2013) suggests in passing that parents should bear the costs of raising disabled children they "deliberately and avoidably" have when they could instead have had nondisabled children. If children with certain disabilities can be expected to cost more than they benefit economically, even in a reasonably inclusive society, they cannot be regarded as either public or "socialized" goods (Olsartetti's term), which would entitle their parents to state subsidy of childrearing costs. Paul Bou-Habib and

Olsaretti (2013) argue in addition that life plans that are unlikely to be chosen by a significant share of the society should not qualify for burden-reducing subsidies. If we adopt a fine-grained specification of life plans, then parenting disabled children certainly would be an even less popular choice than the authors' example of mountaineering, so it clearly would not qualify for subsidies.

Finally, Eve Garrard and Stephen Wilkinson (2006) argue for PND on prioritarian grounds: it is wrong to knowingly create people who are expected to be among the worst off. This is a welfare-based argument, which concludes that the lower the expected well-being of future people we could create, the stronger the reason we have to create better-off people instead. Their argument does not concern political justice, but it might be recast to do so. It could be argued that is would be wrong to impose strong prioritarian claims on one's society by having a badly off child when one could impose no claims, or lesser claims, by having a better-off child.

Arguments claiming injustice in avoidably having a disabled child find a natural home in "luck-egalitarian" theories of justice, which hold individuals responsible for the disadvantages that they choose to risk (the outcome of bad "option luck") but not for the disadvantages they did not choose or risk (the outcome of bad "brute luck"). So although a person's own genetic endowment is, for him or her, a matter of brute luck, genetic technology is making the genetic features of children a matter of option luck (Denier 2010). Eric Rakowski (2002) spelled out one apparent implication for a luck-egalitarian of the increased capacity to choose the genetic features of one's children: "Parents who intentionally bear children entitled to redress, in the form of additional resources, more expensive education, or special educational opportunities, as deaf children are, would be personally liable for the increased costs associated with their choices" (2002, 1398). Specifically addressing the attempt to have a deaf child, Rakowski asserts "the additional expense of providing for the child is not one a parent or parents may justly pass on to others, nor is it one that others are likely to share voluntarily. The increase in the child's educational, medical, and other costs ought to be paid by that child's parents" (2002, 1391–1392).

At the same time, Rakowski's luck egalitarianism does not single-out parents who choose or risk having a child with a disability. On his approach, *all* voluntary parents are liable for the costs of raising their children; parents who voluntarily have or risk having disabled children are merely responsible for any additional costs as well. The arguments on which I want to focus, however, assume or argue that society should share the costs of raising nondisabled children and of children whose disabilities cannot be attributed to parental choice. John explicitly assumes that the state will have default responsibility for children. Olsaretti and Bou-Habib argue that justice requires public support of children and childrearing. All three regard the voluntary creation of children with disabilities as a special case, in which it is warranted to impose a greater share of the costs of childrearing. Parents who can be held responsible for having disabled children should in theory bear all or most of the additional costs, to the extent that they can without impairing the child's welfare.

These arguments cannot be met by invoking "procreative liberty," which John Robertson (1995) describes as liberty from state interference in procreative decisions. As Robertson defends the concept, it requires state restraint, not state subsidy. The only costs the state is required to bear are those necessary to ensure the enforcement of this negative liberty. Individuals or couples must bear the costs of choosing to have children whose gestation, birth, or rearing is expected to be substantially more expensive than average. In such cases, shifting those costs to other people would seriously harm them, and thereby fall beyond the scope of procreative liberty (1995, 251–252). By requiring the additional costs to be substantial, and the harm of shifting them to others to be "serious," however, Robertson does leave room for one of the responses to social justice arguments I will consider later: that the additional costs to society of having disabled children over the costs society routinely bears are *not* substantial, so that it would not seriously harm any third party to have society absorb those additional costs as well.

One reason these arguments appear to be "the best of a not very good lot" is that they appeal to a powerful pretheoretic notion of fairness. In most contexts, few of us care about increasing the total or average well-being in the world except to the extent that it improves the welfare of actual people. And most of us can be made to see (I hope) that in having a disabled child instead of a different, nondisabled child, we are not improving the welfare of any actual child. In contrast, concerns about the social costs of children are widely shared, often plausible, and hardly limited to disabled children. They are expressed by people who worry about the impact of overpopulation on global climate and food supply, people who worry about the urgent needs of existing children in less developed countries, and people who resent paying taxes for education and preschool despite having chosen to be childless.

Although concerns about the social cost of children are not limited to disabilities, however, their application to disability rests on some of the same dubious assumptions as other objections to having children with disabilities. Those concerned with social costs, like those concerned with family impact and the welfare of "the child," often take an exaggerated and oversimplified view of the burdens of raising children with serious disabilities (Asch and Wasserman 2014). In common with other objections—impersonal, child welfare, and family impact—the social cost objections also overlook or understate the potential benefits of raising children with disabilities.

I will offer three responses to objections based on social cost. They draw on and extend arguments Adrienne Asch and I (Asch and Wasserman, 2014) have made to the other objections. The first is that claims about the increased costs and reduced productivity of children with diagnosable disabilities are greatly exaggerated. Moreover, those costs, even if substantial, will only be incurred in a fairly small number of cases, and they may be less overall than the state would incur in a case-by-case determination of whether the costs were avoidably incurred. Finally, much of the cost is attributable to unjustly exclusionary physical structures and social practices. The second response is an appeal to consistency in social policy. Most modern liberal states already subsidize many costs of childrearing, particularly through public education. Although those costs increase with additional children, those states make no attempt to regulate the number of children per family, with one exception: the family caps imposed on welfare recipients in many US jurisdictions. That exception arguably reflects the stigmatization of poverty more than the actual cost of additional welfare payments. The third response is a challenge to the luck-egalitarian accounts that underwrite the imposition of the costs of disabled children on their parents. The rationale on which they do so fails to adequately

respect the institution of the family, and it threatens the state's own interest in its autonomy. But rejecting luck egalitarianism does not require that the state pay *all* the costs of
childrearing, for any parents or children.

The first response can mitigate but not eliminate the social cost claims. However
exaggerated those claims are, and however much the actual costs are attributable to past
injustice, there undeniably will be some additional cost, not attributable to injustice, in
choosing to have children with some disabilities. If that cost is substantial in individual
cases, it raises the question of how it should be fairly distributed, even if the total cost of
such choices is quite small. The second response is a powerful one in policy contexts, but
it does not address the luck-egalitarian claim that all parents should bear all the costs of
choosing to have children of any kind. The third response is intended to meet that claim.

This response emphasizes that the tension between distributive justice and parental autonomy is hardly limited to decisions about what kind or how many children to
have. Those decisions conflict with luck-egalitarian theories of justice no more sharply
than parental autonomy conflicts with the Rawlsian principles of merit and equal life
chances. The latter is the challenging "trilemma" framed by James Fishkin in *Justice,
Equal Opportunity, and the Family* (1983). Fishkin argued that giving parents autonomy
to raise their own children inevitably results in vast disparities in advantage that deny
either equal life chances or the formal equality of merit. I will contend that although the
tension is less acute in the context of procreative decisions than family advantages, it can
only be mitigated, not eliminated. I will conclude, with Fishkin (1983, 193), that justice
in a liberal society can only consist of "a plurality of principles without a unified vision."

THE MAGNITUDE AND CAUSES OF THE ADDITIONAL COSTS OF HAVING A CHILD WITH A DISABILITY

In his skeptical assessment of the "negative reproductive externalities" of having children with disabilities, Cohen suggests that those associated with many disabilities will
fail to rise to the level of significant social harm:

> All things being equal, is it bad if, for example, children have worse rather than bet-
> ter cognitive development, and does that really impose costs on society? In one very
> attenuated sense it does—perhaps there is a probability that children who end up with
> lower IQs will eventually contribute less to the tax base, require more resources in pub-
> lic school, or be more prone to incarceration. But if the Harm principle is to have any
> serious bite as a serious liberal limit on interventions that restrict liberty, such small
> and speculative externalities seem problematic when used as justifications. (2012, 1221)

Because Cohen is primarily concerned with regulation that restricts negative liberty, he
sets a fairly high threshold for harm. A significantly lower one may be appropriate in

determining the limits for public subsidy, and an even lower one in assessing the moral permissibility or the fairness of procreative decisions. Moreover, Cohen's example of mild cognitive impairment may significantly understate the social costs of many or most prenatally diagnosable disabilities.

Setting aside for the moment the issue of reduced productivity, I will focus on increased costs. Consider the following cost estimates: According to Mark Stabile and Sara Allin (2012), the direct and indirect economic costs of raising a child with a disability in the United States average $30,500 per year. This is in addition to general childrearing. According to a 2014 report from the Department of Agriculture, that figure is roughly $264,000 for 18 years. Taking these estimates at face value, a comparison suggests that raising a disabled child to age 18 costs more than three times as much as raising a nondisabled child: $813,000 vs. $264,000. In the domain of health care, Anderson et al. (2011) estimated that over a quarter—26.7%—of national health care spending was attributable to disability-associated health care expenditures.

Several studies have attempted to estimate the additional lifetime costs of specific disabilities or types of disability. A 2002 study of the societal costs of severe to profound hearing loss (Mohr et al. 2002) estimated that with prelingual onset, those costs would exceed $1 million. A 2008 study (Kruse et al. 2009) estimated the lifetime costs associated with cerebral palsy to be 860,000 euros for men and 800,000 euros for women. A 2014 study (Lavelle et al. 2014) found that the additional yearly costs of caring for a child with autism spectrum disorder were greater than $17,000. Despite varying methods, assumptions, and estimates, these are all formidable costs.

There are several reasons, however, for not taking these cost estimates at face value. In some respects, they may be understated; in some, overstated. Concerning the former, many parents of children with disabilities will continue to care for them and face similar or greater costs (because free education and other services end), well beyond their first 18 years. Second, that estimate covers only the quantifiable costs; it does not factor in stress, anxiety, or abandoned or indefinitely postponed projects with no cash value. On the other hand, Stabile and Allin's (2012) estimate for nondisabled children does not include the cost of a college education, or presumably, the cost of the private primary and secondary schools to which a significant proportion of American parents send their children for all or part of their precollege education. Including those costs might well add another $100,000 on average for nondisabled children, somewhat reducing the disparity.

More important, neither cost assessment attempts to assign responsibility for the costs. It would arguably be far less costly to raise a child with a disability in a more inclusive society with a fairer health care system and better child care. Stabile and Allin (2012) provide some indications of the former, noting, for example, that expensive emergency room visits would be less frequent with better primary health care. And for health care in general, Anderson et al. (2011) found that the largest category of disability-associated expenditures was to institutions like nursing homes. They concluded that significant savings could be achieved not only by measures to prevent or delay disability, but measures "to improve the organization and delivery of services to people with disabilities" (2011, 230).

The role of injustice and exclusion may be even greater in other areas. According to the 2000 and 2014 studies, a significant share of the increased cost of specific disabilities is lost productivity. Clearly, productivity could be greatly increased for many or most people with these disabilities by more inclusive workplaces. Similarly, the large share of added cost due to special education might be substantially reduced by more inclusive education. Many disability advocates argue that the costs of separate schools, transit, and so forth exceed those of carefully integrated schools and services: that kind of separate is not only unequal but inefficient. Admittedly, such claims are more plausible, or less controversial, for some disabilities than others; for example, there are strong proponents and opponents of separate education for deaf and autistic children.

The issue of responsibility for incurring costs goes beyond the assessment of the costs of raising children with disabilities or of the cost reductions that could be achieved by greater inclusion. First, there is the issue of how much a just society must pay to make its structures and practice more inclusive. As Linda Barclay (2010) argues, no society can be equally accessible to everyone. Not only is it impossible to achieve "full inclusion," but the attempt to do so would arguably be unjust in a society with other urgent needs and high-priority demands.

There is a further complication. An existing person with a disability can rightly complain if his or her society is far less inclusive than any plausible theory of justice would require. But that complaint would be significantly attenuated if made by prospective parents with elevated odds of having a child with a similar disability. The inadequate provisions for inclusion make it more costly (for someone) to have and raise such a child, and that increased cost may put pressure on their reproductive choices. But they can avoid imposing those costs by carrier screening or PND. If the cost of such "prevention" is minimal, or if it is state subsidized—as John (2015) proposes—the infringement on their procreative liberty will often be slight. It will be substantial only if the prospective parents have a principled objection to, or deep misgivings about, selective implantation or abortion, an issue I will take up later in this chapter.

I cannot hope to resolve the empirical and normative issues underlying these debates about cost. We lack good information on the costs of various services, an accepted way of quantifying intangible "costs," and an accepted theory of justice to determine the entitlements of people with disabilities and their families to various forms of environmental modification, health services, and financial support. For now, then, I will accept the estimates given earlier at face value.

CONSISTENCY IN THE DISTRIBUTION OF SOCIAL COSTS

It is instructive to compare proposals to require or "incentivize" prenatal disability screening and selection with policy, and policy debates, on tax deductions and credits for children, "family caps" for welfare, and state-mandated insurance coverage of IVF. That comparison yields a strong argument from consistency: except in the case of welfare, the government does not reduce benefits, or refuse to share costs, for additional children. Yet those benefits and costs, even for middle-class families, are considerable. Although no US jurisdiction currently offers incentives for carrier screening and PND, or penalties for declining them, the federal government and about half the states impose family caps on welfare recipients, who get no extra payment for children born while they are on welfare. The refusal to pay the relatively small marginal costs of increased welfare benefits seems to reflect the stigmatization of the poor, especially African Americans and single mothers, more than the actual costs of child welfare (Romero and Agénor 2009). Welfare caps were motivated in part by the specter of the "welfare queens" breeding promiscuously to collect lavish benefits—a specter conjured up by demagogic politicians and media.

There is certainly reason to fear that popular support for reduced cost-sharing for parents who did not screen or select against disability would reflect similar biases. This is so for two reasons. First, the same class and racial prejudice would come into play, if as research about current decisions indicates, a disproportionate number of women and couples who decline prenatal testing will be poor Latino or African American. Second, there is no reason to expect that the stigmatization of disability will be limited by class or race. Middle-class white couples who decline prenatal testing may also provoke strong disapproval. That disapproval may be mitigated by the lack of class and racial bias, but exacerbated by the conviction that they declined despite better information and health services.

The example of welfare "reform" should thus give pause to those who would impose a great share of costs on parents who have or risk having disabled children: that the acceptance and implementation of such proposals is likely to reflect prejudice more than fairness or efficiency. Public attitudes toward having a child with a disability may appear more benign than those toward having a child on welfare: parents who make the former choice are sometimes regarded as heroic, while parents making the latter choice are usually regarded as negligent or promiscuous. But that difference may reflect the misleading popular image of raising a disabled child as requiring extraordinary love and devotion. And the difference between attitudes toward having disabled children and having children while on welfare may shrink as the ease of screening and selecting against disability increases.

Few people look askance at a couple who have three or four children, but many would likely disapprove of a couple who failed to screen early and noninvasively for a serious disability for which their single future child was at elevated "risk"—even if the costs of the two reproductive choices were similar. The latter choice may come to be seen as irresponsible or perverse. As Adrienne Asch and I observed (2014), the birth of nondisabled triplets is usually regarded as a joyous occasion; the birth of one disabled child as a trying or traumatic one. If the costs of the two are similar, as suggested by the cost estimates I cited earlier, this once again suggests that social attitudes toward the birth of a child with a disability are not informed by economic judgments.

Between public policy and popular attitudes, infertility clinics, which are unregulated in the United States, impose no limits or liberal ones on the number of pregnancies they are willing to assist (and, until recently, on the number of embryos they were willing to implant at one time). But some require PND to select *against* disability; according to a 2008 survey (Baruch et al. 2008), only 3% permitted clients to select *for* disability.

This difference is particularly hard to justify because the attempt to regulate the number of children parents have is less intrusive than the attempt to regulate the kind of children they have. This is so for several reasons: regulating number does not raise the issues of line drawing and qualitative assessment raised by regulating kind; regulating kind may interfere with family relationships far more than regulating number, and the expressive significance of number regulation is, or can be made, less demeaning that that of kind regulation.

Policies limiting family size, most notoriously, China's 1979 "one-child" policy, have been objectionable mainly for the means they employed—intense social pressure to prevent or terminate additional pregnancies and threats to employment and other services.

But child-limiting policies could be enforced in far less draconian ways, by a mix of financial incentives for having the "right" number of children and disincentives for having too many. The bureaucracy merely needs to count; it does not have to judge the kind or quality of the children. In contrast, regulating the kind of children parents had would have to assess the different costs of their rearing upkeep, and education, and/or job training, and the ease or difficulty with which the parents could have avoided having costlier children. The latter assessment would involve not only the availability and cost of prenatal testing (including PDG), but the greater burden of avoidance facing parents who are more likely to transmit genetic disabilities.

Both size and kind policies would need exceptions for conscientious objection to abortion, but kind policies would have to extend the exemption to "selective objectors"—those who did not object to abortion per se, but only selective abortion. Finally, a kind policy might complicate family relationships in ways a size policy would not. The usual resentment of older siblings at new arrivals might be exacerbated by the financial penalties that accompanied their arrival. But the resentment would likely be far greater if those new arrivals had disabilities that, even apart from financial disincentives, demanded more of their parents' time, attention, energy, and money.

THE TENSION BETWEEN DISTRIBUTIVE JUSTICE AND AUTONOMY IN FAMILY FORMATION

All people choosing to have children make themselves hostages to fortune—even more than they already are. To put it in luck-egalitarian terms, the costs of raising any child one freely chooses to bear are a matter of option luck. The ex ante odds of incurring greater expenses are higher for prospective parents who choose not to test or terminate for disability. But even for prospective parents who make every effort to select a nondisabled child, the odds of their child acquiring a costly disability are hardly negligible. The great majority of disabilities, and of presumably costly ones, are adventitious.

As I argued in the last section, it is intrusive to draw distinctions among choices about which kind of child to have. Indeed, as I noted earlier, luck egalitarians like Rakowski (2002) maintain that all parents are responsible for the costs of raising the children they chose to have, whether or not those children have "bad genes." Although the choice to have a disabled child does not present an exceptional case for a consistent luck egalitarian like Rakowski, it is an exceptionally clear one. That choice is rarely made casually. Indeed, it may typically be made with more reflection than the choice to test and terminate. It is more likely to be voluntary than the latter choice, usually made in the face of social and institutional pressures. And it is more likely to be informed than the decision to terminate, since it would frequently be made with an appreciation of the substantial costs of raising a child with the diagnosed disability, in contrast to a highly exaggerated, stigma-driven expectation of unrelieved trauma and crushing burdens.

I think that Rakowski is right to reject the distinction, but wrong to hold that justice requires that all parents bear all the costs of raising their children. The weakness of luck egalitarianism as a political and moral theory is starkly exposed by its imposition of all the costs of childrearing on voluntary parents. As Elizabeth Anderson (1999) and others have argued, that approach treats all cost-imposing decisions as on a par for the purposes of distributing those costs. But it is only on an assumption of neutrality so strict that it makes no distinction between childrearing and wine collecting that parental choices can be regarded as expensive tastes, for which those making them must bear the costs. Without defending any rival approach, I simply maintain that any adequate theory of justice for a political society requires a thicker conception of the good that includes the flourishing and perpetuation of that society. It must also recognize that the family is a central institution in modern society, although its boundaries are vague and changing. Respecting the autonomy and privacy of the family must therefore be regarded as a political good to the extent necessary for families to fulfill their role in sustaining a society's vitality, strength, and prosperity.

The goal of flourishing and perpetuation for society clearly has the potential to conflict with the constraint on interfering with family autonomy and privacy. Perhaps it does not actually conflict: the best way to ensure a society's flourishing may be to pursue it only indirectly, by supporting family autonomy with both restraint and generosity. But I suspect this conciliatory suggestion is too optimistic. Families may respond in socially more beneficial ways to policies that subtly limit their autonomy than to policies that scrupulously respect it. It may be, for example, that with the advent of comprehensive and noninvasive prenatal testing, states could substantially reduce disability-related health care and educational expenses by making prospective parents liable for those costs, and letting them know they will be, if they fail to test and terminate for positive results. Or, somewhat less intrusively, prospective parents could be made responsible for the additional costs of disabled children if they failed to test but not if they failed to terminate in the face of positive results. That policy would penalize parents who had disabled children negligently but not knowingly. Although that may seem perverse, there is something to be said for such a policy. It would, somewhat cynically, rely on stigma, anxiety, and social expectations to encourage terminations by prospective parents with "positive" results. But at the same time, it would exempt prospective parents who resisted those pressures from state-imposed financial penalties. Nevertheless, the adoption of either policy would be coercive, in making one of the options for prospective parents worse than it is now.

It might be thought that the effect of such pressure on family autonomy would be de minimis, since most prospective parents would be quite willing to test and terminate for major disabilities without any incentives. But that would be taking too narrow a view of the underlying rationale and its implications. The claim that the state has a legitimate interest in the kind of citizens its parents produce could lead to far less popular policies, even in pursuit of goals as reasonable as reducing health care and educational expenses.

Thus, consider a variation on Liao, Sandberg, and Roache's (2012) proposal to mitigate the effects of climate change by human genetic engineering. To avoid the complicated subject of genetic modification, imagine merely that researchers had identified a large number of genetic variants that predicted a smaller "carbon footprint" for the future individual: variants associated with smaller size, slower metabolism, and greater tolerance for heat and cold. Only the last is likely to be the kind of variant prospective parents would favor or select for, but all might play a significant role in the environmental policy of a state committed to doing its part to mitigate climate change. I expect that prospective parents would balk at incentives for selecting future children with those variants, even if the incentives were positive. Selection would either require PGD or selective abortion. Even if the first was fully subsidized and the latter early term, it would significantly complicate and protract the process of having children. And it is not difficult to imagine that as the effects of climate change became more severe, states would be tempted to make the incentives larger and negative as well as positive (a line that would be hard to maintain), especially if the original incentives had few takers. Incentives to have smaller children would likely meet more resistance than even stronger, more effective incentives to have fewer children—and that resistance would likely be fierce.

Some of these examples may be fanciful, but I hope my concern is clear. I believe that there is an unavoidable tension between a society's legitimate interest in its survival and flourishing and its respect for one of its central institutions, the family. As I have argued elsewhere (Wasserman 2009), the best way to reduce this tension is for the state to act in ways that serve its interests without interfering with family autonomy. In the case of disability, one way would be to adopt "universal design" measures for building and education that increased the inclusion of people with a variety of disabilities while reducing the costs of including them. Other ways would include reducing environmental mutagens, introducing more preventative agents into the food supply like folic acid, and improving health care for pregnant woman and their fetuses, and for prospective parents. Although these preventative measures can now be avoided by women, if they so choose, their acceptability does not depend on this. Even if they were almost impossible to avoid—if, say, the government put folic acid in the water as it now puts fluoride—that intrusion would not interfere significantly with the decision making of prospective parents or with family autonomy (Wasserman 2009). Prospective parents would not receive any direct incentives for selecting against spina bifida; they would merely be less likely to have a child with that condition if they declined to screen. (If anything, "folicized" water might make prospective parents less likely to screen, because the odds of having a child with spina bifida would be significantly lower.)

I am not arguing that parents who choose to have or risk having a child with a disability should be exempt from *any* additional costs. No conscientious parent would exempt himself. Those making such a choice should expect to spend significantly more time, money, and energy raising a child with some disabilities than a nondisabled child. Perhaps the best way to respect the privacy of their decisions while demanding minimal responsibility would be to expect *all* parents to pay a fixed share of the costs of rearing their children. That would impose a greater absolute burden on parents who choose to have or risk having a disabled child, but not a punitive one. It would also impose that greater burden on parents regardless of whether the increased costs arose from an "avoidable" disability or the higher cost of living in the area where the parents moved. Or perhaps, if that policy still resulted in overwhelming expenses for parents choosing to have children with disabilities, the share of the costs could decrease as the cost rose. Either scheme would impose a similar burden on parents whose children acquired a similar disability by injury or disease. It may seem unfair to impose the same burden on parents when the costs arose from brute bad luck rather than option luck. But it would avoid intrusive, unreliable, and costly inquires into whether the decision to have or risk having a child with a disability was adequately informed or principled, and whether the costs of prevention (e.g., for an autosomal dominant condition) were unreasonably high.

In conclusion, I want to emphasize that I am not proposing a specific policy. I am merely pointing out that thoughtful policymaking will be necessary to pursue a variety of worthy social goals in ways that preserve parental autonomy and respect the institution of the family. But even the most artful and enlightened policy cannot avoid conflict. There is a fundamental tension between the duties of public officials, responsible for ensuring fiscal solvency, population health, and the survival and flourishing of the society, and the duties and liberties of prospective parents, who need not, and arguably should not, be constrained by those concerns. This tension illustrates, in a different way than Fishkin (1983), the difficulty in encompassing the family within a theory of justice. The tension cannot be eliminated, but it can be mitigated—and more easily mitigated in the case of prenatal selection than postnatal privilege—which is Fishkin's concern. Large differences in family resources for childrearing have a severely adverse impact on the reduction of educational and economic inequality. Although other writers (e.g., Alscott 2004) have struggled valiantly to address Fishkin's concern, none has convincingly argued that the vast inequalities in life chances due to disparities in parental resources, commitment, and skill could be substantially reduced without massively redistributing wealth or restricting parental autonomy. In contrast, the limited uptake of prenatal testing and the failure or refusal to terminate in the face of positive results is unlikely to have, at least in the short term, a significant impact on health care, educational, and personal service costs. (This is so even if it would be "cost-effective" to impose costs on parents on a case-by-case basis.)

Moreover, the tension in the case of prenatal selection can be more readily eased by the kind of policies I suggested earlier which reduce the incidence or cost of genetically based disabilities without interfering with parental decision making. In contrast, the threat to equality of opportunity posed by vast differences in family resources has proven resistant to even the most comprehensive and costly interventions. If we can live with Fishkin's dilemma, we can live with the emerging dilemma I have sketched.

NOTE

1. In this chapter, I will use "disability" roughly as it is defined in the first prong of the Americans With Disabilities Act: a physical or mental impairment that substantially limits one or more major life activities. I will use "impairment" to mean physical or mental atypicalities that reduce function in standard or normal environments. Both these definitions are not only vague but controversial: To what extent do various impairments limit major life activities *because of* social barriers? What does it mean to call a physical or mental feature atypical, and what counts as a standard or normal environment? I will address these issues only as they arise in the context of prenatal testing. As I will argue, the correct understanding of disability and impairment has limited relevance to the permissibility of decisions made in that context.

BIBLIOGRAPHY

Alscott, A. L. 2004. *No exit: What parents owe their children and what society owes parents.* Oxford: Oxford University Press.

Anderson, E. 1999. What is the point of equality? *Ethics* 109, no. 2: 287–337.

Anderson, W. L., J. M. Wiener, E. A. Finkelstein, and B. S. Armour. 2011. Estimates of national health care expenditures associated with disabilities. *Journal of Disability Policy Studies* 21, no. 4: 230–240.

Asch, A., and D. Wasserman. 2014. Reproductive testing for disability. In *Routledge companion to bioethics*, ed. J. D. Arras, E. Fenton, and R. Kukla, 417–432. New York: Routledge.

Barclay, L. 2010. Disability, respect, and justice. *Journal of Applied Philosophy* 27, no. 2: 154–171.

Baruch, S. D., J. Kaufman, and K. L. Hudson. 2008. Genetic testing of embryos: Practices and perspectives of US in vitro fertilization clinics. *Fertility and Sterility* 89, no. 5: 1053–1058.

Boonin, D. 2014. *The non-identity problem and the ethics of future people.* New York: Oxford University Press.

Bou-Habib, P., and S. Olsaretti. 2013. Equality, autonomy, and the price of parenting. *Journal of Social Philosophy* 44, no. 4 (2013): 420–438.

Cohen, I. G. 2012. Beyond best interests. *Minnesota Law Review* 96: 1187–1274.

Denier, Y. 2010. From brute luck to option luck? On genetics, justice, and moral responsibility in reproduction. *Journal of Medicine and Philosophy* 35, no. 2: 101–129.

Fishkin, J. S. 1983. *Justice, equality, opportunity, and the family*. New Haven, CT: Yale University Press.

Garrard, E., and S. Wilkinson. 2006. Selecting disability and the welfare of the child. *The Monist* 89, no. 4: 482–504.

John, S. 2015. Efficiency, responsibility, and disability: Philosophical lessons from the savings argument for pre-natal diagnosis. *Politics, Philosophy & Economics* 14, no. 1: 3–22.

Kevles, Daniel J. 1985. *In the name of eugenics: Genetics and the uses of human heredity*. Cambridge, MA: Harvard University Press.

Kruse, M., S. I. Michelsen, E. M. Flachs, H. Bronnum-Hansen, M. Madsen, and P. Uldall. 2009. Lifetime costs of cerebral palsy. *Developmental Medicine & Child Neurology* 51, no. 8: 622–628.

Lavelle, T. A., Milton, C. Weinstein, J. P. Newhouse, K. Munir, K. A. Kuhlthau, and L. A. Prosser. 2014. Economic burden of childhood autism spectrum disorders. *Pediatrics* 133, no. 3: e520–e529.

Liao, S. M., A. Sandberg, and R. Roache. 2012. Human engineering and climate change. *Ethics, Policy & Environment* 15, no. 2: 206–221.

Mohr, P. E., J. J. Feldman, J. L. Dunbar, A. McConkey-Robbins, J. K. Niparko, R. K. Rittenhouse, and M. W. Skinner. 2002. The societal costs of severe to profound hearing loss in the United States. *International Journal of Technology Assessment in Health Care* 16, no. 4: 1120–1135.

Olsaretti, S. 2013. Children as public goods? *Philosophy & Public Affairs* 41, no. 3: 226–258.

Rakowski, E. 2002. Who should pay for bad genes? *California Law Review* 90, no. 5: 1345–1414.

Rawls, J. 1971. *A theory of justice*. Cambridge, MA: Harvard University Press.

Robertson, J. A. 1995. *Children of choice: Freedom and the new reproductive technologies*. Princeton, NJ: Princeton University Press.

Romero, D., and M. Agénor. 2009. US fertility prevention as poverty prevention: An empirical question and social justice issue. *Women's Health Issues* 19, no. 6: 355–364.

Scanlon, T. M. 1998. *What we owe each other*. Cambridge, MA: Harvard University Press.

Simmons, A. J. 2010. Ideal and non-ideal theories. *Philosophy & Public Affairs* 38, no. 1: 5–36.

Stabile, M., and S. Allin. 2012. The economic costs of childhood disability. *The Future of Children* 22, no. 1: 65–96.

Wasserman, D. 2009. Ethical constraints on allowing or causing the existence of people with disabilities. In *Disability and disadvantage*, ed. K. Brownlee and A. Cureton, 319–351. New York: Oxford University Press.

CHAPTER 21

ETHICAL ISSUES IN THE EVOLVING REALM OF EGG DONATION

LORNA A. MARSHALL

THE concept of one woman donating her eggs to another came about in the early 1980s, and the first donor-egg-conceived child was born just 6 years after Louise Brown, the original "test-tube" baby (Lutjen et al. 1984). Initially, women seeking donated eggs were young women with premature ovarian insufficiency or surgically removed ovaries. Gradually, the number of women interested in receiving donated eggs increased, so that the largest group now is the over-40-year-old woman whose eggs are no longer healthy because of age. Donor egg recipients now also include younger women with inherent egg quality defects or low numbers of eggs, women who have failed to conceive after autologous in vitro fertilization (IVF) cycles, and same-sex couples. Embryos developed using donated eggs are sometimes transferred into a gestational surrogate, as in the case of single or gay men wishing to start a family or older women with health issues precluding pregnancy. In recent years, advances in egg-freezing technology have enabled the development of donor egg banks, which have some similarities to well-established sperm banks.

Donor egg as a reproductive technology is considered to be "third-party," or "collaborative," reproduction, where a child is conceived with others providing essential elements, which are in this case eggs. The genetic mother is the egg donor, who may be known to the intended parents or anonymous. The genetic father is the intended father or sperm donor. In most cases the embryos developed in the laboratory are transferred into the uterus of the intended mother, so the intended mother is also the gestational mother. This strong biological connection to the child provided by gestation has made donor egg an appealing option for infertile women. In some circumstances, however, the intended parent or parents need to contract with a surrogate to carry the pregnancy, either because the uterus is absent or unhealthy, or because the intended mother has health issues.

The term "egg donation" or "donor egg" reflects the initial intent of the procedure, where one woman gifts her eggs to another and generally intends to have no legal relationship to the resulting offspring. The ideal that gametes are beyond commerce and should always be gifted rather than sold has been respected unevenly throughout the world. Acceptable approaches to compensating a donor have varied widely between countries, depending on oversight and regulations in each country. Payment to the egg donor has varied from none at all; to compensating the donor for time, inconvenience, and discomfort; to indirect payment by sharing eggs with a recipient; to frank purchase of eggs with large sums of money. The recent establishment of donor egg banks, where usually a fixed number of eggs are sold by a provider to a user, has led to increased commodification of donor egg services (Quaas et al. 2013b). However inapplicable, the terms "egg donor" and "donor egg cycle" have stuck and will be used whether the eggs have been bought and sold or provided as a gift.

Donating eggs is a much more complex process than is donating sperm, and the evolution of donor egg services has required key clinical and scientific advances in the field of reproductive medicine. Sperm donation has been technically possible for decades, but egg donation required the key development of IVF. A precise understanding of the hormone requirements for endometrial implantation was necessary to allow an embryo developed using a donor egg to successfully implant in the endometrium of another woman. Early IVF cycles employed laparoscopy to access the ovaries and retrieve eggs. Because the first egg donor cycles subjected the donors to the risks of abdominal surgery, eggs were sometimes retrieved for donation when a woman underwent laparoscopic tubal ligation. The development of transvaginal ultrasound and its use to retrieve eggs lowered the risk of egg procurement to a level thought to be acceptable for volunteer egg donors. The most recent medical advance that has changed egg donation is the use of vitrification methods to replace the older and less successful slow-freeze methods. Egg cryopreservation by any method was considered to be experimental by the American Society of Reproductive Medicine, until it lifted the experimental designation of this procedure in 2012 (Practice Committee of the American Society for Reproductive Medicine 2013). Since 2012, when seven egg banks were reported in the United States (Quaas et al. 2013b), there has been an explosion of the number of egg banks and the availability of frozen donor eggs in the United States and the world. This has further separated the egg donor from her recipient couple's treatment cycle and increased the commodification and globalization of this treatment option.

Some of the ethical issues involving egg donation are very similar to those of sperm donation, but the complexities of obtaining eggs from a donor as compared to collecting sperm raise a new set of issues. The egg donor undergoes a prolonged and sometimes painful process of receiving injections and then submits to a surgical procedure to retrieve eggs, usually under an anesthetic.

The most common and serious immediate risk is that of ovarian hyperstimulation syndrome (OHSS), where an exaggerated response to the fertility medications can result in massively enlarged ovaries, fluid shifting into the abdominal space, and dehydration of the vascular space, which can result in distention, discomfort, and sometimes additional procedures, thrombosis, or other serious complications. OHSS and other procedural complications seem to be rare, but most data come from nondonor IVF and not from the egg donor population. Maxwell et al. (2008) found a 0.7% risk of serious complications in 973 donor egg cycles. Bodri and colleagues (2008) reported on complications of 4,052 oocyte donor cycles. Seventeen patients (0.42%) had complications of the retrieval, including hemorrhage and torsion, and 14 required hospitalization with or without surgery. Twenty-two donors had moderate or severe OHSS, and half required hospitalization. In this very large series, the risk of complications was very low, but not zero. Strategies to prevent OHSS in donor patients may further reduce this very low risk of complications. However, the long-term risks of multiple donation procedures to the donor's general health and fertility status have been poorly studied and are largely unknown (Spar 2007). Here, the third party assumes virtually all of the risks of the procedure, and the recipient receives the benefit. The only potential benefits to the egg donor might be the knowledge that she is benefitting an infertile couple or individual, perhaps a discounted IVF cycle, or direct compensation. In contrast, sperm donation requires some effort on the part of the donor, but essentially no short- or long-term risk.

Balancing risks and benefits should be part of the discussion of any medical procedure, but there are so many patients to consider in egg donation that the usual consenting procedures fail to consider many aspects of egg donation. Many patients need to be considered, including the egg donor, the recipient and her partner, and the potential offspring. Minimally, the autonomy of the intended parents needs to be balanced with the duty of nonmaleficence to the donor and offspring, but the autonomy of the donor must also be considered. In addition, the provider must realize that obligations to the various parties can conflict. For example, the provider wants to satisfy the recipient's desire to have many healthy eggs but, in doing so, may hyperstimulate the donor's ovaries and cause her to suffer.

Informed Consent

Informed consent serves to ensure patient autonomy, but whether or not the donor's autonomy is fully respected in the consenting process for egg donation is an area of concern. A prospective egg donor must be able to assess the risks and benefits of the process, and make a voluntary decision to donate, without coercion by any means. The long-term risks are not completely known, and if they were, there is evidence that fertility programs and donor agencies may in general do an inadequate job of describing the risks (Keehn et al. 2012; Alberta et al. 2014).

Some have expressed concerns that young adult women, usually those under 30 years old, are unable to independently assess the risks and benefits of such a complex process and suggest that an advocate should share the consenting process. However, Skillern et al. (2014) have shown that, after an audiovisual information session, prospective donors show adequate subjective and objective comprehension of the process and risks associated with oocyte donation. It seems likely that most young adult women can undergo appropriate informed consent, but that fertility programs must take the appropriate time and care to make sure that prospective donors fully comprehend the process and its risks. Ideally, different providers should obtain consent from both donors and recipients, so that they do not subconsciously entice a donor or minimize the risks for the benefit of a recipient.

Adequate informed consent should begin with the recruitment process of egg donors. In its statement on financial compensation to egg donors, the American Society for Reproductive Medicine (ASRM) Ethics Committee states, "If financial or other benefits are noted in advertisements, the existence of risks and burdens also should be acknowledged" (Ethics Committee of the American Society for Reproductive Medicine 2000). Yet in a survey of 435 ovum donor recruitment advertisements on Craigslist, 97% listed benefits, but 84% of those ads listing benefits did not mention any risks (Alberta 2014). A study of clinics and agencies that recruit egg donors online reported that 44% cite short-term risks, but only 23% mention psychological risk and only 8% acknowledge a possible risk to future fertility (Keehn 2012). This widespread noncompliance with guidelines may encourage prospective donors to enter the consenting process and to discount the risks associated with the procedure.

There is no systematic effort underway to gather information about the short- and long-term risks of these procedures to donors, so it seems unlikely that much additional information to improve informed consent will be available anytime soon. In its practice guidelines, the ASRM has recommended that donors undergo no more than six donation cycles, but that is based on the acute procedural and OHSS risks in the non-donor IVF population (Practice Committee of the American Society for Reproductive Medicine 2014). One study suggested that the ovarian reserve of the donor is not affected by multiple cycles of egg donation (Bukulmez et al. 2010). However, there are no published studies that provide any reassurance that repetitive cycles will not increase a donor's risk of cancer in the future or decrease her eventual fertility. Young women may donate their eggs through several different programs, so an individual program may have inaccurate information about repetitive donors. Moves to establish a nationwide collection center to track all donor cycles have been complicated by concerns for privacy. Until this is realized, it will be very difficult to gather information on the true risks of these procedures.

COMPENSATION TO EGG DONORS

Compensation for the process of egg donation is inevitably linked to the consenting process. This has become a complex issue, with countries diverging in the way they assess the ethical issues of payment to donors. The basic argument against payment is respect for human dignity, which is violated if the human body and its cells and parts are traded or sold. Proponents of donor payment may argue that the donors are being compensated for their time, risk, and inconvenience, and that the recipients are not categorically "buying eggs" but are paying for a treatment cycle that involves donated eggs. Still others believe that both donor and recipient autonomy are most respected if donors are able to sell their eggs for the price the market will bear and recipients are allowed to pay what it takes to secure the donor eggs they want. With the initiation and rapid growth of donor egg banks worldwide, donor egg recipients almost always purchase a set number of eggs, often six, rather than a cycle of treatment. More than ever, buying and selling eggs is becoming an established model for the delivery of donor egg services.

Concerns about selling gametes have been addressed in the legislative bodies of many countries and some US states. Great Britain and Canada have legislated against payment to an egg donor, and they allow only uncompensated friends or family members to donate eggs. In Canada, buying eggs from a donor is a crime, meaning a donor cannot be paid in any way for the donation (Royal Commission on New Reproductive Technologies 2004). Reimbursement for direct expenses is based only on receipts (Royal Commission on New Reproductive Technologies 2004). The Virginia Anatomical Gift Act (Quaas et al. 2013a) specifically legalizes the sale and donation of eggs and sperm. An argument can be made that sperm and eggs are not body parts in the way that a kidney is, for their donation does not diminish the function of the donor. Sperm are a renewable resource, continually developed from the testicular germ cells. Eggs, while they are not renewable, continuously ovulate or die, whether or not they are retrieved for donation.

When payment is allowed, informed consent can be compromised if payment is large enough that the prospective donor might discount the risks of the procedure. An accurate assessment of the risks of single and repetitive donations becomes crucial to this discussion. If the medical and psychological risks of donation are indeed negligible, then there should be few ethical concerns about donors discounting their risks. If the risks are substantial, then large discounts on a donor's own IVF cycle in egg-sharing programs, as well as direct monetary payments to donors, are methods of financial compensation that should be considered carefully.

The amount of money that should raise concerns about donors discounting risks will vary from country to country and between individual cases. Inducements that would ordinarily be acceptable may become undue influences if the subject is especially vulnerable. Ironically, to reduce compensation to egg donors may result in unfair exploitation of the economically disadvantaged. The lower payment will continue to induce the poor to discount risks, while more affluent prospective donors will likely make a donation decision based on other motivating factors like altruism.

In response to published offers of donor compensation as high as $50,000–$100,000 (Levine 2010), the ASRM Ethics Committee tried to quantify reasonable limits on payment in its 2007 statement on "Financial compensation of oocyte donors" (Ethics Committee of the American Society for Reproductive Medicine 2000). This document stated that payments to donors in excess of $5,000 "require justification" and sums above $10,000 "are not appropriate." It also reiterated that compensation is intended for the time, inconvenience, and discomfort associated with the process, and that it should not vary depending on the number of eggs retrieved or the donor's ethnic or other character-istics (Ethics Committee of the American Society for Reproductive Medicine 2000). The recommendations attenuate the discomforting concept that eggs are being bought from donors and sold to recipients. Although many have applauded the guidelines as neces-sary to reduce concerns about exploitation of donors, significant numbers of donor egg agencies and fertility programs have not followed them (Levine 2010).

Confusing the issue of compensation for egg donors in the United States is a class-action lawsuit against ASRM, SART, SART-member fertility clinics, and egg donor agen-cies that agreed to ASRM guidelines for compensation. The suit claims that the Ethics Committee–proposed cap on payment to egg donors is an illegal price-fixing agreement in violation of US antitrust laws, as put forth in the Sherman Act (*Lindsay Kamakahi v. American Society for Reproductive Medicine* 2013). This application of antitrust laws is novel, but if the courts had ruled that the Sherman Act is applicable in the case of egg donors, the landscape of payment to oocyte donors could have changed drastically in the United States (Krawlec 2014). Instead, ASRM settled the lawsuit by removing the dollar amounts, but was able to retain its principles of donor payment in its statement.

ANONYMITY OF DONORS

Balancing the interests of donor, recipient, and offspring is particularly difficult when addressing the issue of anonymity in egg donation cycles. When considering just the egg donor and the recipient couple, anonymity in the arrangement seems generally ben-eficial, for it protects both parties from the emotional complexities and legal complica-tions of an ongoing relationship. It should be mentioned that, even when a donation is designated to be "anonymous," baby pictures make the concept of anonymity provi-sional, since computer-based recognition programs can now be used to search for the linked adult image. Unlike the donor and recipient, the future offspring may prefer an open relationship, for they may have an interest in knowing their genetic parents. In fact, some will argue that offspring have a right to identifying information about the egg donor, as well as the possibility of contact with the donor. The challenge is to find a model that will provide the greatest good for most.

Discussions regarding anonymity are necessarily linked to disclosure to the offspring of the circumstances of their conception, which is discussed in detail in Cohen's chap-ter on anonymity of donors. Many believe that knowing one's genetic origins is a basic human right, and this is violated when children are not informed of their conception by egg donation. However, no country, even the United Kingdom, mandates that parents disclose this information to a child, because such laws are thought to intrude into the privacy of parental decision making. Certainly, if a child is not informed that a donor was used to provide an egg for conception, then the child will not inquire about the identity of the donor. However, a trend toward greater openness with children about circumstances of conception is prompting more discussion about identity disclosure.

In 2011, Washington became the first US state to legislate a modified open identity statute for donors (Washington Rev. Code § 26.26.750). A donor-conceived offspring, after age 18, can request medical and identifying information on her donor, unless the donor has signed an affidavit of nondisclosure at the time of donation. On the other hand, several countries, including Spain and Czechoslovakia, have mandated that all gamete donations must remain anonymous. The law may trump all ethical arguments for and against anonymity in the egg donation process.

Family Members as Egg Donors

Since egg donation was first available, donations by family members, especially sisters, have been common and accepted arrangements (ESHRE 2011). Some couples prefer to use a family member instead of an anonymous egg donor because it preserves the family's genetic connection to the child and may also reduce the cost or waiting time for egg donation. Where there is a shortage of donors, such as in the United Kingdom, or where paid egg donation is illegal, such as in Canada, using a sister to donate eggs may be the only option for a couple. Family oocyte donations are usually intragenerational, such as sister to sister or cousin to cousin, but they may also be intergenerational, such as daughter to mother or niece to aunt.

One of the principal considerations in all family egg donations is to safeguard informed consent. All parties must be able to make autonomous decisions, without undue influence from the intended parents or from other family members. Even though a friend or family member generally accepts no payment to be an egg donor, there can be undue influences on her decision to participate. Special care should be taken to be certain that the donor is adequately informed and that she consents freely to undergo the procedure. Concerns for voluntariness may be greatest in intergenerational egg donation, where a daughter might be still living with her mother or financially dependent on her when asked to donate eggs to her mother (Marshall 1998). Screening and counseling of as many involved family members as possible, including spouses or partners, may be necessary to ensure free and fully informed consent (Ethics Committee of the American Society for Reproductive Medicine 2012).

A second concern is disruption of the family's usual social order and confusion in family relationships. However, in intragenerational family donations, with a sister or sister-in-law as donor, the experiences have been generally positive and donors have maintained their social roles in the family (Jadva et al. 2011). When a sister donates the eggs, she continues to be viewed as an aunt. Intergenerational donations, especially daughter to mother, are more complex, and there are no data that have evaluated the health of the resulting families. Usually a daughter will donate an egg to her mother and stepfather. Although no sexual relations are part of this arrangement, the donor's contribution to her stepfather's child could be perceived as incestuous. This could later be difficult for the child, the donor, or the stepfather (Marshall 1998). Although allowing these arrangements respects the autonomy of the intended parents, great care is necessary to be sure that the interests of all parties are considered and protected.

CONCERNS ABOUT EUGENICS

Except in the case of family donations, most egg donor programs allow recipients to select an egg donor from a menu of qualified candidates, which has aroused concerns about eugenics. According to Wilkinson and Garrard (2013), eugenics can be defined as "the attempt to improve the human gene pool," and it can be either negative, as in avoiding disability, or positive, as in enhancing ability. The term "eugenics" generally evokes negative emotional responses associated with authoritarian coercion to create a superior race, as in the Nazi era. This is very different from individual market-based genetics in egg donation, where prospective parents might choose a donor with greater abilities and capacities over one with less. The concern that recipient couples will aggressively seek a donor whose appearance, intelligence, and talents approach a perceived ideal, in order to create supernormal offspring, has not been realized to the extent predicted. Instead, the experience of fertility clinicians is that the majority of couples seeking an egg donor are most concerned about the likelihood for conception and the health of the offspring. Usually, they also want the offspring to have some physical characteristics of the intended mother, so that the child could appear to be genetically related to her. Reported offers to pay $50,000–100,000 for a donor attending an Ivy League school are rare (Levine 2010). The well-publicized, California-based "Nobel Prize sperm bank," the Repository for Germinal Choice, was initiated in 1980 by Robert K Graham to make smarter, better children. However, it failed to recruit any Nobel Prize winners except William Shockley, and it closed in 1999 soon after the death of its founder (Plotz 2006).

Ethical concerns of large-scale gamete selection include the creation of a society with new types of discrimination. What was average or "normal" would become insufficient, as the population of offspring from donor egg cycles skews the population away from the norm and becomes taller, smarter, or more athletic. However, use of donor eggs to conceive is currently so limited that this future would be unlikely.

Is it really morally wrong for intended parents to choose the egg donor that they believe will give their child a better chance to be successful? When intended parents select an egg donor, they tend to choose young women who are well educated and attractive, to the extent that some fertility programs now offer only egg donors with a college degree. Some specifically choose a donor with a small nose because they always hated their own big one, or they choose a donor who is good at music because they have significant talent themselves and believe musical talent is genetically transmitted. Most parental choices are far from creating the supernormal individuals once envisioned; rather, they reflect the individual preferences of recipient couples. Still, there are some couples that seem to be unable to find a donor "good enough" to provide gametes for the perfect child they envision. Most fertility centers offer or require counseling for recipient couples prior to an egg donation procedure. At this point, counseling may be the best tool to discuss the limits of genetics in determining a child's characteristics and to help recipients see how their careful choices of egg donor characteristics may very well not translate into a perfect child.

The quest for the near-perfect child from a health standpoint seems more defensible and probably more achievable. Genetic screening for carriers of more than 500 severe pediatric diseases is now possible, and the cost of such screening is declining rapidly. Sperm and egg donors are routinely screened for more common genetic disorders like cystic fibrosis, and usually carriers are excluded from donation. To extend this screening to a larger menu of carrier testing will result in a larger percentage of donors being labeled as heterozygote carriers. Here, the interests of the donor need to be considered as well as the interests of the prospective parents and their children. If donors are excluded when they are found to be a carrier of any genetic disease, however rare, this could generate unnecessary anxiety as well as deny them the opportunity to donate. Prospective donors may be chased away if testing might tell them more about themselves than they want to know, especially if testing can be extended to de novo mutations, multifactorial disorders, or even trait selection. At some point, genetic screening may become more harmful to donors than helpful to recipients.

Should There Be Restrictions on the Delivery of Egg Donor Services?

Is parenthood a right, and even if it is, does that extend to the use of donated eggs to conceive? Because no screening is considered appropriate for couples conceiving without assistance, is it appropriate to withhold reproductive assistance from any individual or couple who requests it and can pay? Because a physician and a fertility team are required for assisted reproduction, do they have a greater responsibility if any harm comes to the offspring? In donor egg, do they also have a responsibility to the donor, to ensure that she is taking risks for individuals that will be good parents?

In regard to egg donation, the most extreme assessment is that the well-being of potential offspring is never served when conception is with a donor egg, so this type of collaborative reproduction should never be offered. Velleman (2008) argues that prospects for personhood can only be fully realized when children are raised by their biological parents. To create their own identity and formulate realistic aspirations, children must resemble other family members, he believes. At least in the United States, acceptance of nontraditional family structures is increasing, and this type of argument would generally not be tolerable.

Making the assumption that conception with egg donation is ethically acceptable, decisions about who should and should not be eligible for donor egg services need to consider all parties. Ethical consideration must balance the welfare of the offspring, the interests of the intended parents, the autonomy of the provider, and probably also the interests of the egg donor. The HFEA in the United Kingdom argues that the well-being of the potential offspring is the primary consideration in such discussions, and it explicitly states that treatment services for infertility should not be provided unless the welfare of the child is accounted for (Human Fertilisation and Embryology Authority 1990). The ASRM Ethics Committee argues that providers should be "free to accept persons for treatment as long as they have a reasonable basis for thinking that the child will not suffer significant harm from being raised by these parents" (Ethics Committee of the American Society for Reproductive Medicine 2009). As long as all antidiscrimination laws are followed, providers may or may not choose to treat individuals seeking fertility whom they believe will be inadequate parents.

Even in countries like the United States where young women are compensated for donating eggs, altruism has been shown to be a significant motivating factor in their decision to donate (Marshall et al. 1999). As they enter the process, they need to trust that the clinic will use their eggs wisely. Because providers consider egg donors to be their patients, providers may feel a strong obligation to ensure that the offspring from donor egg cycles will be raised in a healthy environment. For this reason, a provider might extend autologous IVF services to couples that seem to be weak parental candidates but might begin to feel uncomfortable offering donor egg services to the same individuals.

One of the more troubling questions in egg donation is whether or not there should be an age limit on women receiving donated eggs. Since 1997 there have been rare reports of women as old as 63 years conceiving and having successful pregnancies with egg donation (Paulson 1997). Some argue that the usual age of menopause, about age 50, should be the natural limit to reproduction, and that to allow donor egg cycles past that age is not treating a disorder of fertility but responding to a social request. Other concerns include the ability of older couples to parent, the expected life span of older couples, and medical risks to the mother and child when maternal age is over age 45 years. Included in arguments for older women to be egg donor recipients are gender equality and reproductive autonomy. Although requests for egg donation are substantial in the 45–49-year-old age group, they are rare when the female partner is over 50 years old. Several reports suggest that very healthy women can have successful pregnancies over age 50 years. The ASRM Ethics Committee recently concluded that healthy women up to age 55 years could be considered for egg donation cycles, with appropriate medical evaluation and counseling to ensure they are completely prepared for the risks and burdens of pregnancy and parenting in their age group (Ethics Committee of the American Society for Reproductive Medicine, 2013c). It has been proposed that surrogacy can be paired with egg donation when medical issues make pregnancy too unsafe, but others argue that the same issues that make pregnancy risky may also make parenthood too cumbersome.

SAME-SEX COUPLES AND SINGLE PARENTS USING EGG DONORS

Special issues may arise in the use of egg donation by single parents and same-sex couples. In many of these situations, the intended parents are not biologically infertile, but structurally infertile, such as in the case of gay or single men desiring a child but lacking the eggs and uterus to procreate. Although many fertility programs in the United States have refused in the past to treat same-sex or unmarried couples, the ASRM Ethics Committee statement argues that "programs should treat all requests for assisted reproduction equally without regard to marital/partner status or sexual orientation" (Ethics Committee of the American Society for Reproductive Medicine, 2013b). It concludes that the current data do not support restricting access to reproductive technologies in these circumstances. The ESHRE Task Force on Ethics and Law (ESHRE 2014) argues that professionals should use the same standards to predict the welfare of the children in "nonstandard" as well as standard situations. Unlike ASRM, they do support the autonomy of professionals to conscientiously object to offering reproductive care in nonstandard situations, but those professionals have an obligation to provide appropriate referrals.

Legal barriers to building same-sex families are changing rapidly. In its landmark case in June 26, 2015, the United States Supreme Court ruled that state-level bans on same-sex marriage are unconstitutional. At least twenty countries have legalized matrimony and many more legalize civil unions of same-sex couples, but, throughout the world, reproductive access continues to be limited for these groups of individuals. In many countries homosexuality and transsexualism are socially condemned. Those with the financial means often travel to other countries to receive the services they seek, but they still need to consider the difficulties of raising a child in such an environment.

Single women may have unhealthy eggs and be infertile just like married heterosexual women, but then require both donated eggs and donated sperm—or a donated embryo—to conceive. In this event, as with donor insemination alone, the ethical issue is balancing the right of the parent to have the child she wants and the right of the unborn child to have two parents. Single heterosexual mothers who intend to raise a child solo from infancy to adulthood have been shown to have well-adjusted children (Golombok and Badger 2010).

Women in same-sex relationships have conceived using donor sperm and raised children together for decades, but in this arrangement, one partner is the genetic and gestational parent, and the other has only a social relationship with the child. The science of egg donation has increased the reproductive opportunities for lesbian couples. In order for both partners to participate in the creation of a child, one woman may undergo ovarian stimulation and provide eggs, whereas the other partner will bear the child. In this model of "shared biological motherhood," or more simply "shared maternity," one partner is the genetic mother and the other is the gestational mother (Dondorp et al.

2010). Both are also social parents. Marina et al. (2010) have coined the term "ROPA" (reception of oocytes from partner) to refer to the social aspects of this subset of egg donation. Marina argues that this is ethically sound because it respects the autonomy of the intended parents, allows them to have the child they desire, and does not harm the child's development (Marina et al. 2010; Golombok et al. 2010). At least one study has shown that shared maternity has been emotionally advantageous in dual-mother households (Pelka 2009). Still, others question this egg donation arrangement, unless there are medical reasons such as an unhealthy uterus or diminished ovarian reserve in one partner. They argue that physicians are doing good when they treat a medical disorder, but that the cost, complexity, and risk of shared maternity are excessive when donor sperm inseminations are also an option. In individual cases, lesbian couples and providers of fertility care will need to decide if the psychological and childrearing advantages of shared maternity outweigh the potential risks and cost.

In the instance of gay male couples, there is an absolute need for eggs and a uterus, but there is also the same drive as in lesbian couples for the partners to share parenthood equally. Professionals may be presented with many potential arrangements, and they need to evaluate them by considering and balancing the interests of all parties— intended parents, egg donors, surrogates, potential offspring, and family members when appropriate. Often, the couple will plan to have two children who will be half-siblings, using eggs from the same donor, and sperm from each of the male partners. Couples have even requested two surrogates, who will each have one embryo transferred at the same time, so that the half-siblings, if both surrogates conceive, will be social twins. Family donations are also considered, with a sister of one partner donating an egg and the other partner providing the sperm. In this scenario, all offspring will be related to both partners.

Single men have the same issues as gay men, in terms of the need for both eggs and a uterus from a third party. As with single women, the additional consideration is the ability of one parent to raise a child.

Psychological counseling and legal consultation are important early on to clarify all issues and to guide patients to make the best choices to build their family. More social data on the outcomes of these relationships will help professionals balance the interests of all parties in these novel family relationships. However, same-sex couples and single individuals should not be held to a higher standard than heterosexual married couples when reproductive options are offered.

Pennings contends that, even if everyone agrees that the welfare of the children in novel family relationships is of paramount importance, this criterion is difficult to measure (Pennings 2011). Furthermore, the belief structure of many societies is one of the major factors that may compromise the social acceptability and welfare of a child in same-sex families. He concludes that the "well-being of the children would improve considerably were same-sex relationships legally recognized and socially respected, and were same-sex parents treated as adequate parents" (Pennings 2011, p. 1614).

Finally, some prospective egg donors request that their eggs be donated only to married heterosexual couples. This is problematic, because the fertility program or agency may not want to turn away a qualified donor, so it might be willing to act on the donor's preference. Some could argue that the donor assumes the risk in the procedure, and she should be able to limit the use of her eggs if she chooses. In this case, however, the preference is discriminatory against one group of individuals, and many would argue that the woman should not be allowed to donate her eggs with such conditions attached.

DONOR EGG BANKS

Advances in egg-freezing technology have enabled the creation of donor egg banks to provide donor egg reproductive services. Prior to 2012, egg freezing in the United States was designated an experimental procedure by the ASRM, which recommended that this technology be offered only through an Institutional Review Board. Reports by Nagy et al. (2009) and a clinical trial by Cobo et al. (2010) demonstrated the effectiveness of using vitrification methods to freeze donor eggs, allowing the establishment of donor egg banks. Seven egg banks in the United States were in existence by the time the ASRM lifted the experimental designation (Quaas et al. 2013a). Since then, there has been an explosion of egg bank numbers in the United States. Their models vary and have different implications for the delivery of donor egg services. Some egg banks have developed as separate commercial entities, commissioning fertility programs to procure the eggs for their donors and then selling the eggs to patients through their home fertility program. Others have started as a separate offering by a fertility center, to supplement an existing egg donor program using fresh eggs. In addition, sperm banks have diversified to offer eggs as well as sperm, although they still have to partner with a fertility program to monitor donors and retrieve eggs.

This growth of donor egg banks has radically changed donor egg programs in the United States, and it has made it extremely difficult to prevent commodification of the process. If fertility programs follow ASRM Ethics Committee guidelines, they compensate donors for the time, risk, and inconvenience of the process, and they do not increase the payment if the donor has desirable traits or produces more eggs. In the past, recipients were offered a donor egg treatment cycle, often receiving all of the eggs retrieved from the donor, no matter how many were available. The assertion could be made that this arrangement is not a categorical egg sale. For the majority of donor egg banks, however, a fixed number of eggs are sold to a patient, and there may or may not be guarantees that embryos will result from the process. Here, an egg bank explicitly sells eggs to a recipient patient for a price per egg. In this setting, it becomes more difficult to argue that donors who produce more eggs should not be better compensated. If the egg bank is profiting from the sale of the donor's eggs, what is wrong with the donor profiting as well? Should market forces determine the price that egg banks pay a donor for eggs, as well as the price that they can sell them to recipients?

At least one fertility program that initiated one of the first donor egg banks has tried to preserve some semblance of a treatment cycle when using vitrified eggs. There, enough vitrified eggs are warmed and inseminated until two fully expanded blastocysts can be developed and revitrified for the recipient's use (Lamb et al. 2012). Sometimes only four eggs need to be warmed to make two blastocysts, but other times, the blastocyst formation rate is lower and 10–12 eggs need to be warmed for a treatment cycle. This approach minimizes the explicit sale of eggs, which are extremely expensive but worthless by themselves; insemination with sperm can sometimes result in no healthy embryos to transfer. Instead, this cycle approach reassures the patient that she will have embryos to transfer and refocuses attention on the care of the patient.

GLOBALIZATION AND CROSS-BORDER REPRODUCTIVE CARE

For many years, patients have traveled from one country to another to obtain the medical and reproductive services they want. The term "cross-border reproductive care" has recently been applied to this practice, and it refers to "a widespread phenomenom where infertile patients or collaborators (such as egg donors or potential surrogates) cross international borders in order to obtain or provide reproductive treatment outside their home country." (Shenfield et al. 2011, p. 1625.) The major reasons for seeking care in another country are a desire to access broader and higher quality care, a need to lower costs, an effort to circumvent legal restrictions in a departure country, and a desire for privacy or cultural comfort in a destination country (Ethics Committee of the American Society for Reproductive Medicine, 2013a).

Individuals and couples considering cross-border reproductive care are often seeking collaborative reproductive services such as egg donation. Views and approaches toward rights and ethics may differ markedly between Western and non-Western countries but also between neighboring countries. Eighty percent of Canadian women who travel to the United States for assisted reproductive care are seeking anonymous egg donation because Canadian law currently prohibits compensated egg donation (Hughes and DeJean 2010). Shortages of anonymous egg donors in other countries such as the United Kingdom result in long wait times, which prompt some patients to travel to other countries such as Spain for care. The cost of egg donation in the United States has become unacceptably high for many patients, and they may turn to countries like the Czech Republic, where payment to donors and the total cost of a cycle is much less. For various reasons, law or guidelines in many countries, including Turkey, Tunisia, Egypt, Morocco, the Philippines, Germany, China, Norway, and Switzerland, disallow egg donation, so the patients in those countries must travel to receive egg donation. Where egg donation is not allowed or accepted by certain cultures or religions, some couples will seek these services in other countries to maintain confidentiality. Others will travel to the country of their family for a better chance to find a donor matching their own ethnicity. Finally, many countries will not permit certain individuals to use any reproductive services, because they are single, lesbian, gay, or too old. This restricted access forces these groups of patients to seek care in other countries.

With the proliferation of donor egg banks, frozen donor eggs can now be shipped internationally for a program in another country to inseminate and transfer into their patients. Although no patients are traveling, this should also be considered a type of cross-border reproductive care, with donor egg procurement occurring in one country and their use in another. Canadian programs are not allowed to perform compensated donor egg cycles, but they can now receive donor eggs in shipment that have been purchased by a recipient and then develop embryos in their lab that are transferred to the recipient.

Ethical issues for destination countries are different than for departure countries. For destination countries, the major issue is to provide appropriate informed consent for patients that may not be familiar with the language or culture. This may require providing interpretive services for the patients. The same quality of care needs to be provided to all patients, no matter their country of origin or their reasons for seeking care. Destination countries should also be concerned if their reproductive services are diverted to tourists and result in raising prices and limiting access of care for local infertile patients. For departure countries, the physician who has cared for a patient likely has no obligation to inform patients of services in other countries, but he or she should answer questions as accurately as possible if posed (Ethics Committee of the American Society for Reproductive Medicine, 2013a). Even though physicians in the country of departure are likely not directly responsible for providing informed consent for a procedure they do not perform, a general concern for the patient's welfare should encourage frank discussion of the risks of the patient's upcoming procedure. For the health and safety of the patients involved in the arrangement, the ideal model would be to have providers in both the departure and destination countries working jointly to optimize the care of their patients.

Whereas some cross-border care practices raise other ethical concerns, the solutions are not easy for individual physicians or programs to address. In developing countries that recruit international patients for egg donation, payment to the egg donors might be so high compared to average income that it could cause undue pressure on women to donate. Appropriate informed consent may be lacking. If a Canadian woman in her fifties has twins after egg donation in another country, the expenses of her complicated pregnancy will be borne by the Canadian health care system. Globalization of care means that no country can completely control the reproductive practices of its citizens. Taking into account ethnic and religious differences between countries, international professional societies should attempt to establish minimum standards of cross-border reproductive care that can be applied universally (Mainland and Wilson 2010).

COMMODIFICATION OF EGG DONATION

The terms "commodification" or "commercialization" are often applied to the provision of donated eggs for fertility care. The argument against commodification or commercialization is human dignity, which is violated if the human body and its cells and parts are traded or sold. But what do these terms really mean, and are they always bad? Is some commodification of donor egg services appropriate to support the interests of the patients who desire these services?

"Commercial" means "prepared, done or acting with sole or chief emphasis on salability, profit, or success," and "commercialize" and "commodify" both mean to make commercial. There seem to be many opportunities in the provision of fertility services to focus on profitability only. Agencies have been created to recruit donors or surrogates, or even just to match patients with fertility clinics. These charge a separate, often substantial, fee for their services, sometimes as thinly veiled kickback schemes. They are not licensed and have no professional oversight. Some but not all donor egg banks are separate entities that sell eggs to patients to be inseminated and transferred in their fertility clinic.

Are eggs "disrespected" when they are treated as economic commodities? But what does lack of respect mean? How much do we really need to respect eggs, which continually die or ovulate until they are gone?

Laws as well as ethical principles may drive the practice of egg donation. In 30 out of 50 states, the purchase and sale of human tissues and/or organs is explicitly prohibited and considered a felony in the majority of states with such legislation (Quaas et al. 2013a). With the emergence of commercial "egg banks" and the ability to ship vitrified oocytes anywhere, it seems that more attention should be paid to state laws. Although no punitive measures have been taken by states against donor egg banks, egg banks should be aware of the laws that govern the services they provide.

In most circumstances, however, a physician who is ethically compelled to act in his or her patients' interests oversees the care of intended parents. It becomes the burden of the physician to mitigate the commercialism of the many entities that have developed in the delivery of collaborative reproductive services. Physicians need to view themselves as the professionals at the helm of delivery of egg donor services. They need to consider carefully the consequences of any business relationships they develop in an attempt to recruit more patients or egg donors and be willing to deny or terminate relationships that are not acting in the best interests of their patients.

ELECTIVE FERTILITY PRESERVATION AND AUTOLOGOUS EGG DONATION

Elective fertility preservation or "social egg freezing" has increased dramatically in the United States since 2012, when the ASRM lifted its experimental designation from egg freezing (Practice Committee of the American Society for Reproductive Medicine 2013). Fertility preservation is supposed to mean that women freeze their eggs when they are reproductively young so that they can counter future age-related infertility. However, many women who wish to undergo this procedure are now in their late thirties or early forties, when their fertility has already diminished. Unfortunately, fertility clinics and agencies that broker egg freezing have attracted this group of women to freeze their eggs, even holding "egg-freezing parties" to attract patients for this self-pay service. Google and Facebook companies have even begun to offer elective fertility preservation to their female employees. In doing so, they may be deceptively giving hope to women who have already delayed conception and may now benefit little from freezing their eggs (Mertes and Pennings 2011).

Women under 35 years of age will benefit the most from this procedure, because they are reproductively young and will likely have healthy eggs available to achieve a pregnancy years later. Eventually, this may be the largest group to cryopreserve their eggs, and, if so, this may change several aspects of egg donation in the future. Ideally, an increasing number of women in their forties will use autologous eggs that have been frozen for several years, rather than eggs donated from a genetically unrelated younger woman. If a young woman freezes her eggs for later use when young and then conceives spontaneously when older, she may be willing to donate her unused eggs to another woman or couple. Both of these situations may reduce the need to recruit young women to be egg donors, and they may mitigate many of the current concerns about risk and payment involving egg donors.

POSSIBLE FUTURES OF EGG DONATION

Egg donation as part of reproductive care seems likely here to stay, as the population of women seeking childbirth ages, and as acceptance of novel family relationships, such as with same-sex couples or singles, increases in many cultures. Vitrification of eggs and the development of egg banks allow transport of eggs to fertility centers and to countries that do not have egg donor services readily available. However, if these same women should complete their childbearing and do not need their preserved eggs later in life, they may choose to donate unused eggs to others who need them for reproduction. Past practices in many countries have been to inseminate all of the eggs retrieved in an in vitro fertilization cycle and to freeze unused reproductive tissue as embryos. Now, with the success of egg freezing, excess eggs are often frozen instead of embryos. When the female partner is young, her unused eggs can be considered to donate once she has completed her family. An additional, more immediate source of donated eggs may be "freeze-and-share" schemes, which have been championed in the United Kingdom. A woman under 35 years of age seeking elective fertility preservation may agree to multiple treatment cycles and the eggs obtained are split between the donor and an egg bank. In this case, the decision to be an egg donor does not add physical risk to the process. These new sources of donated eggs might increase the availability of eggs for donation (Mertes et al. 2012). If the accepted model for embryo donation is followed, then women who have unused eggs after completing pregnancies generally would not be compensated for their gift and donated eggs may also become more affordable.

Genetic screening options are exploding with the availability of new technology. More genetic screening of donors would risk a strong move toward eugenics. If US law requires that the pressures of a free-market economy drive compensation to donors, more genetic screening with favorable results might translate into increased market value of that donor. New approaches to genetic screening for donor selection are now available, where prospective donors would no longer be labeled as "damaged" because they are a carrier of some rare genetic mutation. One company pairs donors in a bank with the recipient couple's sperm to create "virtual babies" and help them select the healthiest matches (Lim et al. 2014).

Egg donation as part of collaborative reproduction has allowed many individuals and couples to conceive who would otherwise be unable to, but it has raised many questions that still require careful considerations. There is no agreement on how conflicts should be resolved, while respecting the interests of the patients, donors, potential offspring, and surrogates, as well as the autonomy of the providers. The United Kingdom has a centrally regulated model, but its laws are not always specific enough for given situations and they may limit access to care for some groups of individuals. The model in the United States is individualistic and market based with the only legal oversight by the FDA serving to protect the recipient from infectious diseases. There is no formal protection of the donors in the United States, and compensation as an inducement to discount medical and emotional risks of the procedure will continue to be a concern, especially for economically disadvantaged women. Similarly, there is no international consensus or oversight on disclosure and other issues concerning donor egg–conceived children. With the transport of frozen donor eggs as well as patients across borders, ethical concerns must extend beyond the borders of one country and somehow serve the needs of individuals of different ethnicities, religions, and sexual preferences.

Bibliography

Alberta, H. B., R. M. Berry, and A. D. Levine. 2014. Risk disclosure and the recruitment of oocyte donors: Are advertisers telling the full story? *Journal of Law Medicine, and Ethics* 42: 232–243.

Bodri, D., J. José-Guillen, A. Polo, M. Trullenque, C. Esteve, and O. Coll. 2008. Complications related to ovarian stimulation and oocyte retrieval in 4052 oocyte donor cycles. *Reproductive Biomedicine Online* 17: 237–243.

Bukulmez, O., Q. Li, B. R. Carr, B. Leader, K. M. Doody, and K. J. Doody. 2010. Repetitive oocyte donation does not decrease serum anti-Mullerian hormone levels. *Fertility and Sterility* 94, no. 3: 905–912.

Cobo, A., M. Meseguer, J. Remohi, and A. Pellicer. 2010. Use of cryo-banked oocytes in an ovum donation programmed: A prospective, randomized, controlled, clinical trial. *Human Reproduction* 25, no. 9: 2239–2246.

Dondorp, W. J., G. M. DeWert, and P. M. W. Janssens. 2010. Shared lesbian motherhood: A challenge of established concepts and frameworks. *Human Reproduction* 25, no. 4: 812–814.

ESHRE Task Force on Ethics and Law including G. de Wert, W. Dondorp, G. Pennings, F. Shenfield, P. Devroey, B. Tarlatzis, P. Barri, and K. Diedrich. 2011. Intrafamilial medically assisted reproduction. *Human Reproduction* 26, no. 3 (2011): 504–509.

ESHRE Task Force on Ethics and Law, DeWert G, W. Dondorp, F. Shenfield, P. Barri, P. Devroey, K. Diedrich, B. Tarlatzis, V. Provoost, and G. Pennings. 2014. Medically assisted reproduction in singles, lesbian and gay couples, and transsexual people. *Human Reproduction* 29, no. 9: 1859–1865.

Ethics Committee of the American Society for Reproductive Medicine. 2000. Financial incentives in recruitment of oocyte donors. *Fertility and Sterility* 74, no. 2: 216.

Ethics Committee of the American Society for Reproductive Medicine. 2009. Child-rearing ability and the provision of fertility services. *Fertility and Sterility* 92, no. 3: 864–867.

Ethics Committee of the American Society for Reproductive Medicine. 2012. Using family members as gamete donors or surrogates. *Fertility and Sterility* 98, no. 4: 797–803.

Ethics Committee of the American Society for Reproductive Medicine. 2013a. Cross-border reproductive care: A committee opinion. *Fertility and Sterility* 100, no. 3: 645–650.

Ethics Committee of the American Society of Reproductive Medicine. 2013b. Access to fertility treatment by gays, lesbians, and unmarried persons: A committee opinion. *Fertility and Sterility* 100, no. 6: 1524–1527.

Ethics Committee of the American Society for Reproductive Medicine. 2013c. Oocyte or embryo donation to women of advanced age: A committee opinion. *Fertility and Sterility* 100, no. 2: 337–340.

Golombok, S., and S. Badger. 2010. Children raised in mother-head families from infancy: A follow-up of children of lesbian and single heterosexual mothers, at early adulthood. *Human Reproduction* 25, no. 1: 150–157.

Human Fertilisation and Embryology Authority. 1990. Welfare of the child. http://www.hfea.gov.uk/5473.html.

Hughes, E. G., and D. DeJean. 2010. Cross-border fertility services in North America: A survey of Canadian and American providers. *Fertility and Sterility* 94, no. 1: e16–19.

Jadva, V., P. Casey, J. Readings, L. Blake, and S. Golombok. 2011. A longitudinal study of recipients' views and experiences of intra-family egg donation. *Human Reproduction* 26, no. 10: 2777–2782.

Keehn, J., E. Holwell, R. Abdul-Karim, L. J. Chin, C.-S. Leu, M. V. Sauer, and R. Klitzman. 2012. Recruiting egg donors online: An analysis of in vitro fertilization clinic and agency websites' adherence to American Society of Reproductive Medicine guidelines. *Fertility and Sterility* 98, no. 4: 995–1000.

Krawlec, K. D. Egg-donor price fixing and Kamakahi v. American Society for Reproductive Medicine. 2014. *AMA Journal of Ethics* 16: 57–62.

Lamb, J., A. Khabani, C. Khabani, S. Frickleton, L. Shahine, L. Marshall, and L. Hickok. 2012. Donor oocyte vitrification provides an efficient, affordable, and successful option for patients needing egg donation. *Fertility and Sterility* 97, no. 3 (Suppl.): S15–S16.

Levine, A. D. 2010. Self-regulation, compensation, and the ethical recruitment of oocyte donors. *Hastings Center Report* 40, no. 2: 25–36.

Lim, R. M., A. J. Silver, C. Borroto, B. R. Spurrier, R. E. Silver, A. B. Remis, A. S. Cohn, A. Moriss, L. M. Silver. 2014. Autosomosal recessive disease risk in offspring of qualified sperm bank donors and clients: Proof of principle for a novel analysis based on virtual progeny. *Fertility and Sterility* 102, no. 3 (Suppl.): e305–e306.

Lindsay Kamakahi v. American Society for Reproductive Medicine, Society for Assisted Reproductive Technology and Pacific Fertility Center, Civil Action Case No. 11-Cv-1781. (N.D. Cal, filed April 12, 2011).

Lutjen, P., A. Trounsen, J. Leeton, J. Findlay, C. Wood, and P. Renou. 1984. The establishment and maintenance of pregnancy using in vitro fertilization and embryo donation in a patient with primary ovarian failure. *Nature* 307: 174–175.

Mainland, L., and E. Wilson. 2010. Principles of establishment of the First International Forum on Cross-Border Reproductive Care. *Fertility and Sterility* 94, no. 1: e1–e3.

Marina, S., D. Marina, F. Marina, N. Fosas, N. Galiana, and I. Jove. 2010. Sharing motherhood: biological lesbian co-mothers, a new IVF indication. *Human Reproduction* 25, no. 4: 938–941.

Marshall, L. A. 1998. Intergenerational gamete donation: Ethical and societal implications. *American Journal of Obstetrics and Gynecology* 178: 1171–1176.

Marshall, L. A., Emrich, J. R., Hjelm, M., Shandell, A. P., and Letterie, G. S. 1999. What motivates paid egg donors? In *Towards reproductive certainty: Fertility & genetics beyond* 1999, ed. R. Jansen and D. Mortimer, 141–144. New York: The Parthenon Publishing Group.

Maxwell, K. N., I. N. Cholst, and Z. Rosenwaks. 2008. The incidence of both serious and minor complications in young women undergoing oocyte donation. *Fertility and Sterility* 90, no. 6: 2165–2171.

Mertes, H., and G. Pennings. 2011. Social egg freezing: For better, not for worse. *Reproductive BioMedicine Online* 23: 824–829.

Mertes, H., G. Pennings, W. Dondorp, and G. de Wert. 2012. Implications of oocyte cryostorage for the practice of oocyte donation. *Human Reproduction* 27, no. 10: 2886–2893.

Nagy, Z. P., C.-C. Chang, D. B. Shapiro, D. P. Bernal, C. W. Elsner, D. Mitchell-Leef, A A. Toledo, and H. I. Kort. 2009. Clinical evaluation of the efficiency of an oocyte donation program using egg cryo-banking. *Fertility and Sterility* 92, no. 2: 520–526.

Paulson, R. J., M. H. Thornton, M. M. Francis, and H. S. Salvador. 1997. Successful pregnancy in a 63-year old woman. *Fertility and Sterility* 67, no. 5: 949–951.

Pelka, S. 2009. Sharing motherhood: Maternal jealousy among lesbian co-mothers. *Journal of Homosexuality* 56: 195–217.

Pennings, G. 2011. Evaluating the welfare of the child in same-sex families. *Human Reproduction* 26, no. 7: 1609–1615.

Plotz, D. 2006. *The genius factory—The curious history of the Nobel Prize sperm bank.* New York: Random House Trade Paperbacks.

Practice Committee of the American Society for Reproductive Medicine. 2014. Repetitive oocyte donation. *Fertility and Sterility* 102, no. 4: 964–966.

Practice Committees of the American Society for Reproductive Medicine and Society for Reproductive Technology. 2013. Mature oocyte cryopreservation: A guideline. *Fertility and Sterility* 99, no. 1: 37–43.

Quaas, A. M., K. Chung, K. A. Bendikson, and R. J. Paulson. 2013a. Legal implications of commercial "egg banking": Variations in state laws concerning the use of cryopreserved donor oocytes in the USA. *Fertility and Sterility* 99, no. 3 (Suppl.): S5.

Quaas, A. M., A. Melamed, K. Chung, K. A. Bendikson, and R. J. Paulson. 2013b. Egg banking in the United States: Current status of commercially available cryopreserved oocytes. *Fertility and Sterility* 99, no. 3: 827–831.

Richards, M., G. Pennings, and J. B. Appleby, eds. *Reproductive donation: Practice, policy and bioethics*. Cambridge, UK: Cambridge University Press, 2012.

Royal Commission on New Reproductive Technologies. 2004. Assisted Human Reproduction Act of Canada Section 12(2). http://laws-lois.justice.gc.ca/eng/acts/A-13.4/section-12-20120629.html#wb-cont.

Shenfield, F., Pennings G., de Mouzon, J., Ferraretti, A. P., and Goossens, V., on behalf of the ESHRE Task Force 'Cross Border Reproductive Care' (CBRC). 2011. ESHRE's good practice guide for cross-border reproductive care for centers and practitioners. *Human Reproduction* 26, no. 7: 1625–1627.

Skillern, A. A., M. I. Cedars, and H. G. Huddleston. 2014. Oocyte donors' comprehension as assessed by the EDICT (Egg Donor Informed Consent Tool). *Fertility and Sterility* 101, no. 1: 248–251.

Spar, D. 2007. The egg trade-Making sense of the market for human oocytes. *New England Journal of Medicine* 356: 1289–1291.

Velleman, J. D. 2008. Persons in prospect. *Philosophy and Public Affairs* 36, no 3: 221–288.

Washington Rev. Code § 26.26.750 (2011).

Wilkinson, S., and E. Garrard. 2013. *Eugenics and the ethics of selective reproduction*. Keele, UK: Keele University. http://www.keele.ac.uk/media/keeleuniversity/ri/risocsci/eugenics2013/Eugenics%20and%20the%20ethics%20of%20selective%20reproduction%20Low%20Res.pdf.

....

CHAPTER 22

SPERM AND EGG DONOR ANONYMITY

Legal and Ethical Issues

....

I. GLENN COHEN

GAMETE donor anonymity has become an increasingly active area of legislative, bioethical, and empirical interest over the last decade or so. This chapter reviews and discusses these developments. It begins by detailing the very different status of gamete donor anonymity, contrasting the United States (where the law does not prohibit it) with the rest of the world (where it has been largely prohibited by law) and examining the effects of these policies. The next part of this chapter examines the major arguments that have been offered in favor of and against mandating nonanonymous gamete donation.

While I will focus on *sperm* donor anonymity, it is worth emphasizing that most of the legal materials, as well as the ethical arguments, apply equally to *egg* donors. Why do these literatures rarely highlight the egg side? Chauvinism is one possible answer, but another is that the tradition of secrecy is much less firmly rooted on the egg side of the business. Narratives of altruism, motherhood, helping another woman have a child, and other forms of personalization are major tools of recruitment in egg donation. In contrast, recruitment of sperm donors emphasizes work and payment and distances itself from fatherhood (Almeling 2011). There may also be a longer history of the use of known donors on the egg side.

One other caveat is in order. Throughout this chapter I will refer to gamete "donors," which is the most common term in the literature and in common parlance. Nevertheless, as I have suggested elsewhere, the term is largely a misnomer. This is especially true in the United States, where the vast majority of sperm and egg donors are compensated— not only for medical expense or time off work but in a way that is meant to remunerate them (Cahn 2012, 380–381).

This chapter unfolds as follows. The first section describes the widespread adoption of legal prohibitions on sperm donor anonymity in most developed countries other than the United States. It also examines the effects these changes in law have had on supply.

The second section examines the United States, where there is largely no legal prohibition on sperm donor anonymity. As this section shows, though, many donor-conceived children have turned to nonlegal means to try to ascertain the identity of their donor. The third section examines the big ethical debate in this area head on: Should the state legally prohibit sperm donor anonymity and require that all sperm donors put their identifying information into a registry available to donor-conceived children at a specified age? The fourth section considers some peripheral debates.

The Turning Tide: Moves Against Sperm Donor Anonymity Outside the United States

Most sperm donation that occurs in the United States proceeds through anonymous donation (Sauer 2009, 922; Kearney 2011). While some clinics make the identity of the sperm donor available to a donor-conceived child at age 18 as part of "open identification" or "identity release programs" (Cahn 2012, 382–383), no US law requires clinics to do so, and the majority of individuals do not use these programs. There has been litigation in the United States requiring the disclosure of a sperm donor's identity in only a single case of which I am aware (described later). By contrast, in Europe, Australia, and elsewhere there have been significant legislative initiatives requiring that sperm donor identities be made available to children after a certain age (typically when the child turns 18). Swimming somewhat against this tide, the United States has become an outlier. But before I discuss the United States, I will describe the lay of the land in the rest of the world and how it developed.

Sperm Donor Anonymity Outside the United States

In 1985, Sweden became the first country to prohibit anonymous sperm donation by requiring that donor-conceived children be able to receive identifying information about their sperm donor when "sufficiently mature" (Gottlieb, Lalos, and Lindblad 2000, 2052). The law has an interesting intellectual origin, in that the driving force behind it appears to be studies on the welfare of adopted children, which the Swedes extrapolated to donor-conceived children (Dennison 2008, 8; Gottlieb, Lalos, and Lindblad 2000, 2052). The Swedish effort was followed by a number of jurisdictions: Austria, Germany, Switzerland, the Australian States of Victoria and Western Australia, the Netherlands, Norway, the United Kingdom, and New Zealand (De Jonge and Barratt 2006; Dennison 2008, 8–9; Turkmendag, Dingwall, and Murphy 2008, 283–284; Daniels and Douglass 2008, 137).

The United Kingdom gives a good example about how these systems currently operate. The Human Fertilisation and Embryology Authority (HFEA)'s website announces
to prospective egg or sperm donors:

> Those who donated sperm, eggs or embryos after 1 April 2005 are, by law, identifi-
> able. Any person born as a result of donation after this time is entitled to request and
> receive their donor's name and last known address, once they reach the age of 18.
>
> Donors who donated before 1 April 2005 are automatically anonymous. This
> means that donor-conceived people can only access non-identifying information
> provided by the donor at the time of donation.
>
> As a donor, you have no legal rights to contact your donor-conceived offspring;
> the decision to initiate contact is solely that of the donor-conceived child.
> . . .
>
> It is a right of those who donated before 1 April 2005 to choose to remove their
> anonymity—and potentially become identifiable to any children born from their
> donation.
>
> As a consequence of removing your anonymity, your donor-conceived offspring
> may choose to make contact with you once they reach the age of 18. The HFEA will
> try to contact you first using the details held on file to let you know that a request for
> your contact details has been made. Before making this decision, you may wish to
> consider how this could impact on you and your family. If you wish, you can ask to
> speak to a counsellor at the clinic you donated at to talk through the implications of
> re-registering as an identifiable donor.
>
> Bear in mind that you may not be contacted by any donor-conceived offspring.
> This could be for a number of reasons, including the possibility that they do not
> know they are donor-conceived.
>
> If you donate through an HFEA-licensed clinic, you will not be legally responsible
> for any child born as result of your donation. (Human Fertilisation 2013a)

In terms of the information requested and available, the HFEA distinguishes between
identifying and nonidentifying information it makes available to donor offspring at
different ages:

> From 1 April 2005 this is the information the HFEA collected from you at the time of
> donation:
>> your physical description (height, weight, eye and hair colour)
>> the year and country of your birth
>> your ethnicity
>> whether you had any children at the time of donation, how many and their gender
>> your marital status
>> your medical history
>> a goodwill message to any potential children
>> identifying information (your name, date of birth and last known address).
>
> Donor-conceived people conceived after 1 April 2005, when they reach 16 years
> old, are able to apply to the HFEA to receive the non-identifying information that

their donor provided (all information given by the donor except for their name and last-known address).

Donor-conceived people conceived after 1 April 2005, when they reach 18 years old are able to apply to the HFEA to find the information their donor provided, including identifying information. (Human Fertilisation 2009)

To emphasize a point I will raise later, the UK scheme (like most of the donor registries in the world), makes information available *to the resulting child about his or her donor* (not to the donor about the child), *only if the child requests it at the requisite age* (not if the child does not request it), and the child can only know to request the information *if the child's parents inform the child that he or she is donor conceived or the child figures it out on his or her own and inquires*. I have called this a "passive" registry, as opposed to an "active registry," which would call the child at the requisite age or otherwise inform the child that he or she was donor conceived (Cohen 2012b, 445–447). In practice, if an active registry were put in place, the vast majority of parents would likely disclose the information to their children earlier, knowing that otherwise this sword of Damocles would drop.

Effects on Supply

Observational Studies

In general, countries that have prohibited sperm donor anonymity have seen at least a short-term diminution in the pool of willing sperm donors. In 2010, Gaia Bernstein devoted a significant portion of a law review article to determining the effects on supply in various markets (1207–1218). I provide here an adapted version of my previous summary of her work (Cohen and Coan 2014, 718–719):

Sweden adopted sperm donor identification in 1985 and witnessed the number of children born with donor sperm decline from 200 new donors per year just before the law came into effect to 30 new donors per year by 1988. Reports also indicated that half the hospitals that offered artificial insemination by donor closed their programs, both of which commentators attributed to the change in the law (Bygedemen 1991, 266; Daniels and Lalos 1995, 1871–1872; Bernstein 2010, 1207–1208). However, a 1995 study based on data accumulated between 1989 and 1993 indicated a 65% increase in the number of donors, from 69 new donors in 1989 to 106 in 1993, which some commentators took as evidence that the prohibition on sperm donor anonymity only caused an *initial* decline in the number of donors that was later overcome by recruitment measures (Daniels and Lalos 1995, 1872–1873; Bernstein 2010, 1208). Bernstein, however, disputes that reading of the data, noting that no study has looked at the post-1995 data, which are largely unavailable (Bernstein 2010, 1208). She suggests there is good reason to suspect that dwindling donor participation remains a problem in Sweden, pointing to a study showing a steady decline from 900 yearly inseminations in 1985 to 300 yearly inseminations in 2005, shortages causing long waitlists of 6 to 18 months for access to insemination, and that earlier reports of a "rebound" may have been distorted and instead reflected the fact that "demand may have been lower in Sweden than in other countries like the United States because, until 2005, lesbians were not allowed to use donor sperm" (Ekerhovd, Faurskov, and Werner 2008, 311–312; Berstein 2010, 1208–1209). Sweden's rules about compensation have apparently changed over time: Sweden permits compensation to sperm and egg donors, but since 2006 it has "begun prohibiting trading in eggs and sperm for profit," even though "gamete owners who donate their gametes are still compensated" (Genetic Integrity Act 2006; Berstein 2010, 1209).

The Australian state of Victoria enacted laws pertaining to sperm donor identification in two stages. First, in 1984, Victoria created a mandatory donor registry that went into effect in 1988, but under this law no information could be released without the contemporaneous consent of the donor. Then, in 1995, a new law that went into effect in 1998 allowed donor-conceived children to access information about donors once they reach the age of 18 (Infertility Act 1984; Bernstein 2010, 1209). Reviewing the data, Bernstein concludes that they show a "consistent decline in the numbers of newly registered sperm donors" that is coincident in time with the passage of each of the laws (Victorian Assisted Reproductive Treatment Authority 1999, 1209 n. 117; Hickman 1998, 5; Szoke 2004, 358; Turkish Daily News 2005; Bernstein 2010, 1209–1210). The scarcity of sperm donors has been further exacerbated by a 2006 law prohibiting compensation for sperm donation beyond reasonable expenses (Prohibition of Human Cloning 2006; Bernstein 2010, 1211).

Data from the United Kingdom on the effects of sperm donor anonymity are more difficult to interpret. By regulations that went into effect in 2006, all UK sperm donors were required to put identifying information in a registry available to donor-conceived children when they turn 18 (Human Fertilisation 2004). Although the number of newly registered sperm donors has not declined from before the law changed, some contend that this statistic is not particularly probative because there has been an increase in known donors—friends or relatives who donate for one person's exclusive use—such that the amount of sperm from unrelated donors available to most infertile patients for use has significantly declined (Camber 2008; Bernstein 2010, 1211–1212; Human Fertilisation 2013b, 169).[1] Bernstein also finds evidence supporting a decline in the availability of sperm for reproductive use from the fact that "IVF treatment cycles with donated sperm steadily decreased from 939 in 2004 to 711 in 2007 and insemination treatment cycles with donor sperm decreased from 6892 in 2004 to 3878 in 2007" (Bernstein 2010, 1212). However, data from 2009 to 2010 released after her study suggest that these numbers "rebounded" to where they were before the law change, although not for insemination (Human Fertilisation 2012a). As Bernstein documents, reports from the actual British clinics in the years immediately after the passage of the Act also suggested significant shortages and longer wait times for those seeking to use donated sperm (Bernstein 2010, 1212).[2]

Bernstein's read of the data is not shared by all academics working in this area. Naomi Cahn (2012), for example, has written that while

> requiring the release of information may have some initial impact on the number of donors, predictions of drastic long-term effects appear overblown. Moreover, such

legislation may result in the development of new methods to recruit other donors . . . By changing advertising techniques to emphasize helping others rather than the amount of payment, sperm and egg banks may be able to recruit donors who care less about money and more about facilitating the creation of families. . . . But payment, rather than anonymity, does seem to remain a critical component; when Canada outlawed payment for sperm donors, the sperm supply decreased dramatically.

Observational studies such as these are useful, but they can only incompletely inform our understanding of the policy choice that governments face. First, like most observational designs, these studies have difficulty separating coincidence from causation, especially since none of these studies has a comparison state that can be used to evaluate the results. In particular, one might worry about preexisting secular time trends in donor participation in the countries that adopted donor identification laws and also the possibility of reverse causation in that adoption of these laws may be driven by these trends in donation and not vice versa. There may also be omitted variables that affect both the rate of donation and the propensity to pass legislation, such as anticommercialization forces. Second, as Bernstein has noted, during the relevant periods of these observational studies, changes in infertility technology and practices—for example, the introduction of more effective procedures such as IVF and intracytoplasmic sperm injection (ICSI)—make it more difficult to determine whether the data show changes in the supply side alone or also changes in the demand side, which could have reduced the need for sperm donors (Bernstein 2010, 1210).

Furthermore, as Cahn and Bernstein note, because most of these countries also have in place strict prohibition on sperm donor compensation (Sweden being a partial exception), these observational studies are not optimally designed to investigate whether one can "buy" sperm donor nonanonymity through increasing payment to donors.

Interactions Between Compensation and Anonymity

Beyond these observational studies, I have conducted an experimental study with Travis G. Coan to determine whether individuals would be willing to donate sperm nonanonymously in the United States if paid more.

We used an experimental design to assess the effects of donor information on preferences for sperm donation. We conducted the study in March 2012 via an Internet sample of 393 males between the ages of 18 and 60 years who lived in the United States at the time. We sent subjects an invitation to participate in the study, which described the opportunity to "Learn about and share your opinions on the sperm donation process." After reading a short study description, subjects choosing to participate filled out a short questionnaire (15 questions) and earned points that are redeemable for an Amazon gift card. All subjects who chose to participate in the study finished the questionnaire and spent a reasonable amount of time processing it (i.e., between 5 and 10 minutes). Moreover, prior to presenting subjects with the treatment, we asked them: "Would you ever consider donating sperm in the future?" We collected and reported on data for both the full sample of 393 subjects, as well as the subsample of individuals ($n = 332$) who would consider donating sperm.

In our experiment, subjects were randomly assigned into one of two groups: a control group in which respondents received information on donor confidentiality consistent with current US law (i.e., identifying information *is* protected by anonymity) or a treatment group that received information on confidentiality consistent with current UK law (i.e., identifying information *is not* protected in that there is a mandatory registration requirement).

We used a double-bounded contingent valuation study design. Our results showed that subjects in the donor-identified condition needed to be paid significantly more, on average, to donate their sperm than those in the anonymous sperm donor conditions. Anonymous sperm donors are typically paid around $75 per specimen in the United States today (Spar 2006, 39). When examining our full sample of subjects ($N = 393$), we find that individuals in the control (anonymity) condition are willing to accept an average of $83.78 to donate, while individuals in the treatment group are willing to accept an average of $124.21. These estimates suggest that the cost of providing donor information, at least in our sample, is roughly $40, and the results are significant at the 5% level in a two-tailed test. The full sample, however, includes a number of subjects who would never consider donating sperm, based on their answers to a pretreatment questionnaire. When restricting our sample to include only those subjects who would actually consider donating ($n = 332$), we find the cost of providing donor information to be roughly $31, on average, and again these results are significant at the 5% level.

In both cases, the loss of anonymity is associated with a considerable extra estimated cost, although in absolute terms the cost of sperm is still relatively "cheap," even with these increased costs.

This price differential corresponds roughly to that of the one set of published data we have on differential pricing in the United States (based on what donors are paid) for a US sperm bank that operates both anonymous and identity release programs. Gametes, Inc., a major US sperm bank, operates both anonymous and identity release programs. In 2006, the bank paid $65 to anonymous sperm donors per donation and $100 to those who donated as part of the identity release program (Almeling 2011, 121). It is worth emphasizing, though, that participating in an identity release program is different from participating in a mandatory registry of the type we tested in our experiment.

We are currently running a similar experiment on actual sperm donors at a large US sperm bank to help achieve greater ecologic validity; we hope to report that data soon. We also hope at a future point to conduct similar research on egg donation; there are very different gendered narratives propagated around becoming an egg donor, as well as a quite different industrial organization and relationship to the intended parents that is fostered.

Outside of the United States, many of the countries that ban sperm donor anonymity also prohibit or limit compensation for sperm donors, so it is unclear whether increasing payment could lawfully be used to solve any shortfalls in supply.

THE US EXPERIENCE: BREAKING
ANONYMITY THROUGH LEGAL
AND EXTRALEGAL MANEUVERS

As discussed earlier, the United States is an outlier in that neither the federal government nor individual states have imposed a true registry system that forbids anonymous gamete donation. While several sperm banks with identity-release programs exist, prospective rearing parents and prospective donors have to *choose* to use them. This differs from the rest of the world where identification requirements are *imposed* and thus can "benefit" (more on that later) the children born from these sperm donations whether or not the genetic and rearing parents want to use an identified sperm donor. Even in the United States, though, there have been some legal and extralegal chinks in the armor of this regime that I describe in this section.

Legal

In the United States, there are only two instances of which I am aware where the law has in some way compelled disclosure of sperm donor identities.

The first is by common law. *Johnson v. Superior Court* (2000), a decision by the California Court of Appeals, concerned a child born from the sperm of an anonymous sperm donor known as "Donor 276," who supplied sperm for a California-based sperm bank.

Diane and Ronald Johnson used that donor's sperm to conceive their daughter Brittany. Unfortunately, Brittany developed autosomal dominant polycystic kidney disease (ADPKD). The bank assured the Johnsons that the anonymous sperm had been fully tested and genetically screened. Neither parent had ADPKD nor a family history of it, leading them to believe that the donor was the source of the disease. The Johnsons claimed that the bank allegedly knew about the donor's mother and sister's family history of kidney disease, hypertension, and neurological disorders, which were red flags for ADPKD. They sued the bank and its employees for professional negligence, fraud, and breach of contract. The Johnsons sought to take a deposition of Donor 276 to show that the Donor had not misled the bank and thus the bank was at fault, but the bank refused to release his identity. The bank noted that the contract with the sperm donor specified that his identity would be "kept in the strictest confidence unless a court orders disclosure for good cause" and claimed that releasing identifying information about the donor would violate both the contract and the donor's right to privacy (*Johnson v. Superior Court* 2000, 868).

The Court found that the promise of confidentiality in that contract "conflicts with public policy" and was therefore unenforceable. While the court held that the donor had a right to privacy under the California Constitution that included information about his identity, they found that releasing his name for the purpose of allowing a deposition and releasing some of his medical records was nonetheless appropriate. The court held that the donor's "right to privacy is not absolute and must therefore be balanced against other important interests" (*Johnson v. Superior Court* 2000, 877). In this case, it identified three of those interests that it felt won out, namely (1) the state's interest "in making certain that parties comply with properly served subpoenas and discovery orders in order to disclose relevant information to the fullest extent allowable"; (2) the state's "interest in seeking the truth in court proceedings"; and (3) the state's "interest in ensuring that those injured by the actionable conduct of others receive full redress of those injuries" (*Johnson v. Superior Court* 2000, 878). In this case, the donor was the only independent "witness that apparently can reveal the extent of information" he had disclosed to the bank, information that was "not only directly relevant to petitioners' claims, but [wa]s also relevant to Cryobank's affirmative defense" (*Johnson v. Superior Court* 2000, 878).

The court therefore ordered the release of the donor's name and address for the purpose of allowing him to be deposed, as well as the release of some of his medical records. However, the court also indicated that his identity was "to be protected to the fullest extent possible and the identities of [his] family members are not to be disclosed" (*Johnson v. Superior Court* 2000, 879). It left to the lower court to decide how to do this, but suggested that "an order could be fashioned which would allow John Doe's deposition to proceed and documents produced on matters relevant to the issues in the litigation but in a manner which maintains the confidentiality of John Doe's identity and that of his family." For example, the lower court could limit attendance at the deposition to the lawyers and require that the deposition transcript refer to him merely as "John Doe" (*Johnson v. Superior Court* 2000, 879).

While this case is good law in California, whether other courts would follow it in similar situations remains an open question. More important, the case was premised on a credible tort lawsuit against the sperm bank where the identification of the donor was necessary to resolve the claim, which is an unusual setting that will not be present in most cases. Moreover, even in this setting, the court is very careful to protect the identity of the donor and limit the kind of information available about him. Altogether, this case does not seem like a promising root on which to grow a robust doctrine of donor reidentification from judicial order.

If common law has not proven fruitful, what about legislative action? In the adoption context, a practice long shrouded by secrecy, a number of states have mandated openness by legislation. As one author notes: "[S]ix states, including Alabama, Delaware, Maine, New Hampshire, Oregon, and Tennessee, have revised their laws to grant adopted adults 'direct access to their birth records and/or adoption records,'" while Kansas and Alaska never closed their records in the first place (Sharp 2013, 526–527). This post-1970s momentum as to adoption has engendered a similar movement as to sperm donation, but with only one very limited success.

In 2011, the state of Washington passed a law mandating that sperm donors give fertility clinics identifying and medical information that donor-conceived children can access at age 18 (Wash. Rev. Code § 26.26.750). While this appears to mirror the registries in place in other countries, the Washington statute adds a loophole big enough to drive a truck through: Donors can opt-out of providing the information "if the donor has signed an affidavit of nondisclosure with the fertility clinic that provided the gamete for assisted reproduction" (Wash. Rev. Code § 26.26.750 2011).

All in all, the existing US legal landscape has not proven fertile for getting mandated sperm donor identification. Indeed, at least one set of academic writers has suggested that mandating sperm donor identification would violate the constitutional "right to procreate" and "right to raise one's child" (Byrn and Ireland 2012). Others are more skeptical of this kind of constitutionalization of rights related to sperm donation and use of sperm donors.[3] In any event, until a state actually *requires* identification of sperm donors, no court will have an opportunity to pass on this question.

Extralegal

Given the failure to establish legal rights to sperm donor identification in the United States, many individuals have turned to extralegal maneuvers to reconnect donors and build alternative family structures.

The Internet has enabled significant advances in finding one's donor, even when anonymity is enforced by the sperm bank. The initiative that has received the most media attention in the United States is the Donor-Sibling Registry. As Naomi Cahn (2012, 382–387) describes it:

> Thousands of people have begun to "use the Internet to expand their kinship circle" and to create what they often think of as a "unique extended family" in which they are "raising children who are far-flung and yet intimately related." Wendy Kramer and Ryan Kramer, her donor-conceived son, who together started the Donor Sibling Registry (DSR) in 2000, have facilitated contact among more than 8,500 genetically related people, including donors and half-siblings. The sperm banks themselves have recognized this growing interest in connection. For example, California Cryobank has established a "Sibling Registry" that is designed "for clients and their adult children who are interested in extending their 'family circle,' to help in identifying 'potential siblings.';" Moreover, sperm banks are increasingly offering the option of open-identity donation to allow for donor identification once offspring reach the age of eighteen.
>
> Parents and offspring, as well as donors, may all search for one another. While comparatively little research has been done in this area, as the secrecy surrounding use of donor gametes dissolves and as genetic testing becomes more sophisticated, more will become possible. The studies that do exist indicate a variety of reasons that members of donor-conceived families search for donors and for other offspring with the same genetic heritage, and that donors search for their offspring. For example,

one survey of almost 600 people who were members of the Single Mothers by Choice organization found that slightly less than two-thirds wanted their "child to have the possibility of a larger extended family," and half were interested in developing a relationship with other children who shared the donor's genes. Higher levels of searching seem to be associated with households without fathers, perhaps because not only are children in those families more likely to know of their donor-conceived status, but also because of the parents' openness and desire to create larger communities for their children.

Donor offspring may feel that part of their heritage is missing. Donor children may experience a sense of loss for not having information about their biological pasts or being able to establish a relationship with their gamete provider, analogous to the experience of "genetic bewilderment" reported by some adopted children.

. . .

When it comes to relationships with biological half-siblings, the situation is, again, quite complicated, involving the offspring as well as their parents. While the offspring might choose contact, their parents may not. On the other hand, most people feel "'overwhelmingly positive' after some ticklish starts." Contact might be occasional, at the level of sending holiday greetings, or much closer, with the children growing up together and the parents bonding. Indeed, for many donor-conceived offspring and their parents, they want contact, rather than simply written information, and these contacts to lead them to some kind of "family feeling." Many people who have connected feel as though they are starting to create a family, albeit not necessarily a "close" relationship. Wendy Kramer has corresponded with many parents of donor-conceived children who are seeking advice "on how to navigate their new relationships. Some parents in the newly formed donor groups simply want to trade basic information, while others want to form groups that spend holidays together, forming familial-type relationships.

When I checked its current statistics at the time of writing this chapter, the Donor-Sibling Registry claims to have helped connect "11,625 half-siblings (and/or donors) with each other" and that its "total number of registrants, including donors, parents and donor conceived people, is 44,387" (Donor Sibling Registry 2014).

As of now, in the United States, the relationship of anonymous donor to donor-conceived child or donor-conceived child to genetic sibling is largely a nonlegal one in that the anonymous sperm donor is not the legal father of the child born through this process and the genetic half-siblings do not have any legally recognized relationship to one another. Indeed, as I have written elsewhere, there have been a few instances of anonymous *embryo* creation where the same sperm and egg are combined to produce a "batch" of genetically related embryos, with parts of the batch sold to different prospective parents; this would create genetic *full* siblings (Cohen and Adashi 2013). Nevertheless, even such full genetic siblings would ordinarily not have any legal relationship with one another.

All of this is in marked contrast with the world of known donors. There, courts have on occasion held known sperm donors to be the legal fathers of their genetic children. Their reasoning has turned on details as to whether a doctor performed the insemination, whether a contract was in place, whether the genetic father engaged in postbirth contact with the child and in what form, and whether the child would otherwise require public assistance.[4] Often these decisions also turn on peculiarities of state law, including which of the multiple versions of the Uniform Parentage Act the state has put into place.

Legal Relationships and Anonymous Sperm Donation

When it comes to *anonymous* sperm donation and the genetic relations they produce (currently mostly half-siblings but also eventually genetic grandchildren and the like), the call, as we will see, has largely been for *revelation of identity* based on *genetic parenthood*. What we have not seen is a call for *legal* recognition of these genetic relations—that is, for *legal parenthood* (or half-brotherhood, half-sisterhood, etc.).

Perhaps alone among the major writers in this area, Naomi Cahn (2012, 416–417) has floated a tentative balloon in this direction—albeit only briefly in two paragraphs of her major article *The New Kinship*, where she writes:

> Once connections have been made, the newly formed donor-conceived family communities may want more formal respect for their relationship. This does not mean according parental status or providing all of the affirmative legal protections accorded to families under American law. Instead, this might mean, for example, that donor-conceived family communities could opt into a quasi-familial status that would provide them with a weaker form of protection. Their biological connections could give rise to some limited rights that depend on context and on choice. As family law increasingly moves towards privatization, towards customizing the meaning of family through mechanisms ranging from open adoption agreements to cohabitation and premarital contracts, donor-conceived family communities might be able to choose a weak form of legal recognition.
>
> While my goal is not to set out a laundry list of policy prescriptions, this new status could (potentially) provide various privileges and obligations. Members of connected families might, for example, be eligible to take family and medical leave for one another, to inherit, to act as a surrogate decision maker in cases of illness, or to serve as a legal guardian in cases where the parents are incapacitated or have died. It might also involve some form of recognition for sibling associational rights, a step that would have a much broader impact on child welfare. To provide administrative ease, the default rule would remain that these rights are unavailable in the absence of explicit agreements otherwise.

The question of legal status presents an intriguing set of complications and new issues for advocates of mandated openness for sperm and egg donors.

On the one hand, in order to get these kinds of systems of mandated registries passed, it has been important to emphasize that this is only about *information*, and *identity formation*, not the imposition of parenthood. This is how it is emphasized, for example, in the materials of the UK registry (Human Fertilisation 2012b). This is also important in the claim that imposing such a registry will not cause the supply of donor sperm to dry up, which would seem hard to argue in a world where legal parenthood came with the donation. Finally, it would also disrupt the plans of many individuals who want to use donor sperm to create their own families, for which information may be tolerable but the addition of a stranger legal parent would not be.

On the other hand, it is not entirely clear why the reasons that motivate identity revelation should not also motivate something more legal as well. If the claim, as we shall see later, sounds in an understanding of a right of the donor-conceived child or at least an important welfare-promoting interest, why limit the right to information? After all, in many contexts the law has held that parental choices cannot waive rights of support of resulting children (Cohen 2008b, 1128).[5] So why not here as well? That focus on the best interests of donor-conceived children seems in tension with Cahn's suggestion that any potential legal status be voluntarily assumed by the sperm donor who is the genetic father of the donor-conceived child or by the genetic half-sibling. After all, genetic siblings reared together (and indeed even those adopted in) have no say in whether they are recognized by the law as a legal sibling to one another. Why should genetic half or full siblings reared separately due to anonymous sperm or egg donation be treated differently?

One answer is that we have a strong desire not to disrupt the existing legal relationships between the parents rearing the children and the donor-conceived children by allowing the "stranger" anonymous sperm donor to enter or by forcing his entry. But that argument threatens to prove too much in that the revelation of identity information to donor-conceived children also allows the personage of the stranger to enter the existing family unit. Is it possible to argue that this kind of "disruption" is justified while disrupting existing legal statuses (even if it adds new legal status rather than takes away the old ones) is not?

So far, though, most writers in favor of sperm donor identification have not offered such arguments because they have largely ignored the question of legal status or treated it as a nonpossibility. This is in some ways a shame because this is rich terrain worthy of further exploration, even if it may take us to some places that might challenge the underlying raison d'etre for identity revelation to begin with.

THE BIG ETHICAL DEBATE: SHOULD WE LEGALLY PROHIBIT SPERM DONOR ANONYMITY?

As the preceding sections have detailed, the United States has diverged from most of the rest of the world, which has, by force of law, prohibited sperm donor anonymity in favor of a registry-type system. The big question for those interested in reproductive ethics is whether the United States is wrong not to have adopted this approach. To answer that question, I will first try to clear away some underbrush by mentioning two common mistakes that are made in the way people discuss this subject. I will then briefly set out the (now dominant in most of the world) basic argument for adopting a legal prohibition on anonymity based on the welfare interests or rights of donor-conceived children, as well as a less common argument based on the interests of sperm donors and rearing parents themselves. After I set out each argument, I will provide responses to each (full disclosure: the latter is the side of the argument with which my work is most often associated).

Some Incorrect Starting Points

Identification, not Medical Information

Many have written about anonymous sperm donation in terms of a donor-conceived child's right to know his or her medical history (e.g., Ravitsky 2010, 671; Johns 2013, 117–118). This is an important interest of donor-conceived children, but it is not one necessarily connected to the question of whether to prohibit sperm donor anonymity. Sperm banks have endeavored, and government regulation thereof should push, to make available to the parents of donor-conceived children the fullest possible medical histories. Perhaps there should be an obligation to update these records, contractually enforceable by banks against sperm donors, since the bounds of our technological prowess in detecting diseases and dysfunction is constantly evolving.

But this is a good idea that is orthogonal to releasing the name and identifying information about sperm donors, and the relationship is problematic in both directions. On the one hand, it can be done without sharing the identity of the donor. On the other hand, even in countries such as the United Kingdom, where identities are made available to the child at age 18, there is no guarantee that new medical information will be shared beyond what the government already records—the sperm donor may be unwilling to share or may now be deceased.

Therefore, I think discussions of medical information are a red herring in the true debate. The true debate is about access to the name and identifying information about a sperm donor *apart* from his medical history. All that said, one can imagine a future where access to medical information about a donor becomes identifying information. This would require more sophisticated, low-cost, and widely used whole-genome sequencing of the population and large-scale databases where that information can be searched in an identifying way. While possible, I think that future is unlikely for at least the short and middle term. For that time horizon, medical and identifying information will remain quite separate.

Adoption Versus Reproductive Technology

Many people who push for more openness in the gamete donation context point to the data and also the legislative activities of the adoption movement (e.g., Garrison 2000, 900–901; McGee, Brakman, and Gurmankin 2001, 2034–2035; Dennison 2008, 16; Cahn

2012, 8–9). At a rhetorical level this is understandable, but it is not clear we ought to give too much weight to this analogy.

On the data side, we should be cautious about extrapolating data from adoption into the space of reproductive technology; we should instead focus on the data on actual sperm donors and donor-conceived children and not assume that the problems or solutions found in one literature necessarily line up with the other. For example, Brigitte Clark (2012, 646–647) notes that "although research on adopted children indicates that such children need information about their birth as early as possible, no convincing research has found a corresponding benefit in disclosing donor information to donor-conceived children. In fact, research indicates that children who have not been told are well-adjusted and generally stable."

Beyond the data, though, there is an important conceptual point about this discussion related to an argument I will make later pertaining to the nonidentity problem. The failure to mandate the identification of adoptive parents may, if the data back up the claim, harm existing children. Those children would be better off if they were given access to the identities of their genetic parents. The children in question, though, will exist *whether or not* there is a policy of mandated openness. No (or at least very few) parents decide whether to have children (or refrain from having an abortion) or when to have children based on the rules relating to adoption openness for the very simple reason that few if any individuals make the decision to get pregnant (or "decide" to fail to use contraception, the more likely cause) anticipating putting the child up for adoption.[6] By contrast, when one decides whether to become a sperm donor, the rules pertaining to anonymity versus mandated identification are likely to be at the center of one's evaluation in the majority of cases. If, as I will show later, the choice of rules alters when individuals donate sperm, whether individuals donate sperm, or which sperm ends up with which egg, a different child will result. That makes the argument disanalogous to the adoption case in that it will not improve the lives of children (as in adoption), but will instead affect which children come into existence.

For these reasons, all resort to the adoption analogy should be heavily scrutinized.

Arguments from the Interests of Donors Themselves and from Rearing Parents

Though somewhat more peripheral to the larger debate, one of the more interesting arguments that has been made in favor of legally ending sperm donor anonymity draws on an unexpected set of interest holders: sperm donors themselves, as well as the parents who rear donor-conceived children.[7]

As Naomi Cahn (2012) frames it in her landmark work *The New Kinship*:

[A] new paradigm for donor-conceived families considers not just the child, but also the interests of donors, parents, the donor family network, or the larger community. Some parental interests could be furthered through this new paradigm, interests such as making contact with genetically related offspring and even the donor, ensuring the integrity of their own families, and respecting their children's interests. A focus only on regulation, rather than relationships, also overlooks donors' interests in becoming known and possibly establishing connections with their offspring.

The claim would make a powerful argument if persuasive, since it would mean that legally requiring sperm donor identification actually served, rather than set back, the interests of the regulated parties (sperm donors and recipient rearing parents). There is, however, a market-based solution to this concern that is *already* available: Donors who want their donor-conceived children to contact them, or recipients who want the donors to have the option of connecting with their children, can opt for an open-identity donation system, as discussed earlier. It would seem on its face, then, that mandating a one-size-fits-all solution that eliminated an option of anonymous donation and thereby required everyone to be available for contact whether or not they want it, can by definition not serve donors' and recipients' interests; the solution frustrates their ability to choose and thus their ability to maximize their own welfare and carry out their life plans. Therefore, one-size-fits-all regulation cannot be superior.

One potential response to this critique is that the real concern is what goes by the name of affective forecasting or transformative experience or changed-selves problems (Cohen 2008b, 1774–1780). The argument would be that donors or rearing recipient parents (or both) will think they do not want to be identified, but will later in life change their minds and want to connect with the resulting children.

There are several problems with this argument. First, there is the standard concern that such arguments are unduly paternalistic. Second, there is no empirical evidence demonstrating that this hypothesized change in preferences is likely to occur. In fact, it seems equally possible that those who agree to a mandatory identification system later want to undo *that* choice, and it is not clear why their transformative experience should not be given equal weight. Finally, even on its own terms, the argument cannot support the kind of donor registry in place in the United Kingdom and elsewhere that proponents of law change in the United States would like us to adopt. In such a system, donor-conceived *children* can (at the appropriate age) find out whether they were donor conceived and, if they were, determine the name of their donor. This argument would instead only support a different kind of system: one where *recipient parents* can, after a change in preferences, phone the registry and get the name of the donor, or where *donor parents* can phone the registry and get the name of the recipients. If changes in preferences of parental donors or recipients are the concern that motivates this argument, the standard registry does not serve those interests because it relies on the child to initiate contact with the registry, which is *independent* of the donor's or recipient's change in preferences.

Therefore, this whole line of argument strikes me as a nonstarter.

Arguments to Prevent Harm to or Protect the Rights of Donor-Conceived Children

A second and much more common set of arguments that dominates the anti-anonymity discourse is framed in one of two related ways: either (1) donor-conceived children are *harmed* by the anonymity of their sperm donor genetic fathers, and revelation of that identity or no secrecy to begin with would promote their interests; or (2) donor-conceived children have a "right to know" their genetic fathers or at least their identity.[8]

The interrelationship between these two claims depends a lot on your moral theory. In some views, especially that of consequentialists, the difference between the two are direct: Children have a right to know *because* knowing prevents harm or furthers the interest of the donor-conceived children; here the "right" is the conclusion to an argument, not the argument itself. For those with a more deontological bent, the two are more separable: It would be possible, for example, to conclude that it would wrong children to deny them access to their genetic parental information even if doing so does not further the welfare of these donor-conceived children. For those with natural law leanings, the right to know one's genetic parent might be thought to be inherent in our nature, as human beings that live in a particular kind of idealized family structure. Others, such as Vardit Ravitsky (2010, 670), have framed this as a human right (although she does not specify if her conception of human rights comes from natural law or another conception) that would attach even in the absence of any showing of harm to offspring.[9]

My own sense is that the majority of the literature, however framed, really is closer to the consequentialist account in at least the following limited sense: If we became convinced that it *harmed* children to give them access to their genetic father's identity (or, if you prefer, that anonymity regimes, not identification regimes, *furthered* the welfare of donor-conceived children), then few if any would nonetheless push for legal prohibitions on anonymity.

For that reason, it seems fair to say that the harm and benefit to donor-conceived children are the central variables in the analysis, even if for nonconsequentialists it may not be the only thing that matters. That said, in a later section of this chapter I discuss more deontological approaches that argue that children are wronged even when not harmed.

Someone who sought to resist an argument for legally prohibiting sperm donor anonymity based on the welfare of donor-conceived child would have at least three kinds of arguments to offer in response:

1. *Empirical*: Show that there is no evidence that sperm donor anonymity hurts the interests of donor-conceived children.
2. *Counterbalance*: Accept that the interests of donor-conceived children are harmed and that the argument therefore pushes toward legal prohibition, but argue that the interests/rights of recipient parents or sperm donors outweigh the harm to donor-conceived children.[10]

3. *Undermine the premises and entailments*: Show that even if the data substantiate the claim of serious harm and that this harm overcomes the countervailing interest of recipient parents and sperm donors, the argument is nonetheless unpersuasive because it relies on faulty premises or carries with it problematic implications.

In presenting reasons to resist the argument for legally prohibiting sperm donor anonymity, I will focus on this last strategy. That is not to deny that the first two may also be effective argumentative strategies—even proponents of mandated donor identification, such as Ravitsky, candidly admit that data showing harm are currently hard to come by and, because of the nature of the population, hard to study, at least in the short term (Ravitsky 2010, 670–671). But if the third argument I will offer is accepted, it is the most powerful reason for rejecting this push for legally prohibiting donor anonymity, whatever the data show. If the argument does not convince you, then you will have to consider the empirical and counterbalance forms of argument.

Attacking the Underlying Premise: Can Donor-Conceived Children Be Harmed? The Basic Argument

Many people coming from a family law background take as an organizing principle the prevention of harm to existing children or, if you prefer, the protection of children's welfare or best interests. I have argued elsewhere that it is a problem to transpose this principle to justify regulations designed to "protect" children in the reproductive context; if you succeed in altering when, whether, or with whom individuals reproduce, you run afoul of Derek Parfit's nonidentity problem, an idea that has been recognized by courts in less philosophical language in their rejection of wrongful-life tort suits (Cohen 2011a, 437; Cohen 2011b, 13; Cohen 2012a; Cohen 2012b, 435).

Without going too deeply into this other work, I will provide a quick summary: Whenever a proposed intervention will itself determine whether a particular child will come into existence, child-welfare arguments premised on that child's welfare are problematic. As long as the child will *not* be provided a "life not worth living," the child cannot be said to be harmed when its counterfactual was not existing or having a different child (genetically speaking) substituted for it. For that reason, any intervention that will alter whether, with whom, or even when individuals reproduce cannot be justified by concern for protecting the resulting child's welfare unless the child would have a life not worth living absent the intervention. Whatever you think about the harms of sperm donor anonymity, they do not plausibly render a donor-conceived child's life one not worth living or anything close to that line.

Legally prohibiting sperm donor anonymity is likely to alter whether and with whom individuals reproduce. Such regulation may cause some would-be donors not to donate, altering whether and with whom they reproduce. It also changes whether recipients reproduce, in that some intending parents will be unwilling to engage in artificial insemination if donor identification is mandated. Furthermore, regimes that prohibit anonymity usually *ceteris paribus* reduce the number of sperm donors, as has been the experience in countries discussed earlier. If such regulation produced a *true* gamete shortage, then we would end up with a de facto restriction on whether some individuals seeking donors reproduce. But even if this regulation results only in waiting lists (as has been the case in many countries discussed earlier), that too may de facto limit whether individuals reproduce because some women seeking sperm donation will be at the end of their fertility cycle and often multiple attempts are required to successfully inseminate.

But—and I emphasize this point here because some who have responded to my work have ignored it[11]—even if the *quantity* of gametes remained unchanged, that would *not* be enough to avoid the nonidentity problem. As I wrote in 2012:

> To deal with shortages caused by removing sperm-donor anonymity, many countries try to recruit new sperm donors, thereby altering *with whom* individuals reproduce. In Sweden and the Australian province of Victoria, "recruitment efforts have focused increasingly on the older, more altruistically motivated donor as a way of rebounding from the initial dampening effects" of the prohibition on donor anonymity; one clinic in the Australian province of New South Wales even flew "Canadian students to Australia for complimentary vacations" that required sperm donations every second day. Furthermore, even if the same donors provide sperm to the same recipients under either regime, regime choice may alter *when* they donate (earlier in life versus later on) and thus *when* reproduction takes place.
>
> Therefore, a prohibition on sperm-donor anonymity cannot be justified simply by concerns of "harm" to children because the regulation would "protect" these particular children out of existence, and there is no plausible argument that these children would have a life not worth living. (Cohen 2012b, 436–437)

Thus, because they are likely to alter when, whether, or with whom individuals reproduce, bans on sperm donor anonymity cannot be said to improve the welfare of the children that are born through sperm donor anonymity. They instead replace one population of children (those who would have been born had sperm donor anonymity been permitted) with another population (those who would have been born had it been prohibited). They do not make children better off; they bring into existence other, different, substituted children.[12]

That is a very bare-bones reconstruction of the basic argument. Those who want a more sophisticated understanding should consult my other work cited earlier, as well as the work of Parfit and many others who have written about this problem in the context of wrongful life and other areas of reproduction. I will, however, consider a few quick objections and responses to my argument that those who seek to use the child welfare justification for banning sperm donor anonymity could make.

First Attempt to Save the Child Welfare Argument: The "Last Judgment Problem"

Can we reconstruct the argument for informing donor-conceived children as instead an argument for reparation? For example, there is something that can be done *after the fact of birth* to remedy the "injury" to the child, enabling it to access the identity of its donor parent. Axel Gosseries ably presents one such argument as to the application of the nonidentity problem in environmental contexts, which he refers to as the "last judgment" problem (2008, 459–464).

Gosseries imagines a man trying to decide whether to bicycle or drive home from work every day, with attendant effects on the environment experienced by present and future generations. He chooses to drive. Gosseries then imagines that many years later the man's now-17-year-old daughter, who is an environmental activist, lambastes him for making the environment so much worse by not bicycling. The man responds: "[H]ad I done so, *you* would not be here"—because the man would have come home at a different time each day and thus slept with his wife at a different time and produced a different child. The father continues: "Since your life in such a polluted environment is still worth living, why blame me? I certainly did not harm you" (Gosseries 2008, 460).

Gosseries disagrees with the father. He suggests that when there is overlap between generations (to at least some degree), then

> As long as the father's pro-car choice was a necessary condition for his daughter's existence, it remains unobjectionable [such that] his preconception actions are immune to moral criticism when it comes to alleged harms to his daughter.... However, as soon as the daughter is conceived, all the father's subsequent actions no longer fall within the scope of the non-identity context . . . [such that] . . . we should expect the father to *catch up* as soon as his daughter has been conceived in order to be able, at the end of his life, to eventually meet [his obligations to her with regards to the environment]. (Gosseries 2008, 461)

Even if the harm to the environment the father has already inflicted is irreversible, says Gosseries, "he should act in such a way as to compensate for such negative impacts through substitution measures (e.g.[,] replacing an extinguished species with new energy-saving technology)" (Gosseries 2008, 461).

Can we make the same claim here that the recipient parents who have sought to use anonymous sperm donation should "catch up" by revealing the child's identity later on, and that this justifies the legal prohibition on sperm donor anonymity? The argument would suggest that the obligation to reveal to the child his true genetic father—or at least to make sure this parentage information is available in the registry—is like the obligation identified by Gosseries in the environmental context of adopting energy-saving technologies going forward.

I think such an approach fails because of what I call the "anticipation problem." A legal obligation for the sperm donor to place his name in a registry available to the child at age 18 is the very thing likely to alter donor and recipient behavior about when, whether, or with whom they reproduce. Thus, a legally enforceable catch-up obligation feeds back into the conception decision and thus is not immunized from the nonidentity problem. Therefore, even as to sperm donor anonymity, the nonidentity problem cannot be evaded by justifying the regulation in the prevention of harm to the resulting child.

Second Attempt to Save the Child Welfare Argument:
Non-Person-Affecting Principle Approaches

A different attempt to save the argument for harm to donor-conceived children reconfigures it in a subtle but philosophically important way. It concedes that for reasons associated with the nonidentity problem, it would *not* have been better for *these* donor-conceived children had there been a sperm donor anonymity prohibited regime in place (or if you prefer, it concedes these children are not *harmed* by a system that allows anonymous sperm donation). It accepts that if the law changed, these children would not come into existence, and other children would be born in their place instead. It then posits that because these other children would have better lives (knowing their genetic parents), that is a reason to favor adopting this policy.

Philosophers have referred to this as the "non-person-affecting principle" approach (e.g., Parfit 1987, 359–361 and 364–365; Brock 1995, 273). One formulation of this view suggests the world would be better off if instead of person *A*, who will experience serious suffering or limited opportunity, person *B*, who will not experience those things, came into existence—that is, "[a]lthough the person born with the condition in question would not have been harmed by birth, the world is better off if a person without that harm had been substituted in his place" (Robertson 2004, 16). We can also understand this argument to replace the best interests of resulting *children* with the best interests of a resulting *population*, or as an obligation to produce the population of children with the highest welfare possible. It is a claim that the world is better off even though no person is made better off; the world is better in an impersonal sense.

I have critiqued this approach elsewhere as a justification for the regulation of reproduction, including bans on anonymous sperm donation (Cohen 2011a). Among other things, I think the non-person-affecting principle may be limited to cases in which the same number of children will come into existence whichever way we set the regulation, which is unlikely to be true of sperm donor registries.[13] It also faces other problems: If the small population welfare deficits that allegedly result from anonymous sperm donation are enough to justify bans on the practice, we should also endorse much more significant regulation of coital and other reproductive technologies than we currently do. The non-person-affecting principle relies on premises that support the eugenics movements of old, which many find objectionable. Furthermore, it seems to justify equally well regulations requiring parents to have enhanced children, which some would find objectionable. However, perhaps distinctions could be drawn with the old eugenics movements on double-effect kinds of grounds—the old eugenics movements wanted different children to be born, while here we want children who have access to the identity of their genetic fathers to be born, but in so doing we cannot avoid bringing into existence different children. In any event, the approach may have trouble grounding criminal-law-type rules, such as making anonymous sperm donation illegal, depending on one's theory of the moral limits of criminal law (Cohen 2011a).

At base, it is a theory of substitution. It is an argument that banning anonymous sperm donation is justified not to improve the lives of donor-conceived children, but to replace one group of children with another that we think has a higher welfare. At the very least, this is a starkly different justification for banning anonymous sperm donation than most donor-conceived people would identify with—that it would have been better for the world in an impersonal sense that they had not come into existence and had instead been replaced by other children who knew their donor. When properly understood, I am not sure that many donor-conceived children would champion that reason for ending sperm donor anonymity.

Third Attempt to Save the Child Welfare Argument: Wronging While Overall Benefitting

A third way of trying to save the child welfare justification for prohibiting sperm donor anonymity in some senses breaks with the argument and becomes explicitly consequentialist. I call this approach "wronging while overall benefiting." The approach concedes that because of the nonidentity problem, no child is *harmed* by the act of anonymous sperm donation that produces him or her (because the child is not made worse off compared to a counterfactual world in which he or she was not born), but a child is nonetheless *wronged* even while overall benefitted by being brought into existence.

Seana Shiffrin is the most prominent proponent of this view in legal circles, though she applies it to wrongful life cases, not sperm donor anonymity (1999, 119–120). As applied to sperm donor anonymity, this kind of argument would suggest that by depriving a child of access to the identity of his or her genetic father, we have *wronged* the child, even if we have not harmed the child since he or she has a life worth living.

Shiffrin rejects the "comparative model" that treats harm and benefit as two sides of the same scale and its "principle that one may inflict a lesser harm on someone simply to benefit him overall, when he is unavailable to give or deny consent" (Shiffrin 1999, 119–122 and 127). What she endorses is instead an asymmetrical approach in which "harm" is associated with noncomparative, absolutely bad states such as broken limbs, disabilities, death, and significant pain, and "benefit" is associated with goods, such as material advantage, sensual pleasure, and goal fulfillment (Shiffrin 1999, 120–125). Shiffrin then distinguishes between two types of benefits, those that represent the "removals from or preventions of harm" and a residual category she terms "pure benefits" (Shiffrin 1999, 124–125). She argues that it is permissible to inflict a lesser harm to remove or prevent a greater harm, but wrong to inflict that same harm in order to confer a pure benefit, no matter how large that benefit (Shiffrin 1999, 125–127). Shiffrin's next move is to use this idea to explain the right outcome in wrongful-life cases, suggesting that no one is harmed by not being created—being born confers on the child only a pure benefit and not the avoidance of harm (Shiffrin 1999, 119–120).

One could apply the same principle to anonymous sperm donation. The argument would be that by producing a child through anonymous sperm donation, one has harmed the child in order to confer on it a pure benefit, which is wrongful.[14] However, any attempt to apply Shiffrin's approach to anonymous sperm donation seems likely to fail. Shiffrin's argument is rich and complex, and thus my attempts to wrestle with it in other work are quite involved (Cohen 2012a, 1244–1264); for present purposes, I will merely summarize why I think this approach is unlikely to save the argument for banning anonymity.

This approach leads to the conclusion that all acts of reproduction (not just wrongful life or anonymous sperm donation) are prima facie wrongful—a conclusion many will find problematic. To the extent Shiffrin is open to the idea that the wrong caused by the reproduction may be abated by love and support for the resulting child, it is not clear why the recipient rearing parents do not adequately provide that love and support. Furthermore, because the argument relies on a noncomparative conception of harm, it is only as plausible as that account, and others have suggested the account is problematic. The intuition pump Shiffrin uses to generate the rule about harm and pure benefits may not work on its own terms or apply in the reproductive context. Finally, even if this approach can justify tort liability in wrongful life cases, it may run into problems justifying a regulatory regime that seeks to prevent anonymous sperm donation altogether.

In any event, the approach is quite different from the ones put forward by the vast majority of writers who oppose sperm donor anonymity. Therefore, even if it can clear the objections I have raised, adopting this approach would require a dramatic sea change in the reasoning of most proponents of sperm donor registries and may also carry other implications that would make them uncomfortable.[15]

Other Possible Approaches to Save the Child Welfare Argument

There are still other possibilities open to defenders of banning sperm donor anonymity that I think of as even less plausible. Under a virtue-ethics approach, one could argue that the prohibition is needed to ensure that parents act in keeping with the virtues of parenthood (e.g., McDougall 2005, 603). Under a legal-moralist approach, one could argue for the use of criminal law or other regulatory tools to deter acts that neither harm nor offend, but do undermine public morality, all in the name of maintaining traditional family structures (e.g., Feinberg 1988, 3–4). Finally, under a reproductive externalities approach, one can argue that costs to *others* outside of the donor-conceived child, rearing parent, sperm donor triad exist and that it is wrong for members of society not in the triad to bear those costs (e.g., Cohen 2012a, 1216–1244).

Each of these approaches carries with it problems I have detailed elsewhere as frameworks for regulating reproduction more generally (Cohen 2011a; Cohen 2012a). They seem to suffer even greater deficits as theories for requiring sperm donor identification. For example, on the reproductive externalities approach, it seems as though any externalized costs caused by sperm donor anonymity are quite minor and well below the threshold of costs that might make interfering with reproductive decision making even approach a threshold of plausibility. In any event, one seldom sees advocates for prohibiting sperm donor anonymity using these argumentative modes, though the modes may be the last (however unwelcome) refuge if all else fails.

For all of these reasons, I find the argument for legally prohibiting sperm donor anonymity to protect either child or parental welfare unsuccessful on its own terms. Next I turn to a different attack on the argument.[16]

Attacking the Argument by Its Implications:
The Analogy to Sexual Reproduction

Even if one thought that prohibiting sperm donor anonymity was justified by concerns for the harm done to donor-conceived children in not knowing the names of their genetic fathers, the argument runs into a problem of underinclusivity. Why not apply the same rule to sexual reproduction? In my work I have offered a "modest proposal" meant to provoke readers along these lines:

> In particular, why not require every individual who engages in coital sex with a fixed probability of conception to put his or her name and contact information in a registry mirroring the one endorsed [by advocates of sperm donor registries] with the proviso that their names would be erased from the registry if there were no evidence of pregnancy within a few months? This would encompass a "one-night-stand registry" in that never again would a child who results from a temporary relationship suffer the harms which [these advocates find problematic and which thereby call] out for governmental regulation. In fact, my hypothetical registry's beneficiaries are broader still. There is evidence that misattributed paternity—believing like Luke Skywalker that your father is someone other than who he is—is not an insignificant phenomenon, with studies suggesting that it may affect as few as one percent and as many as thirty percent of the population, with most estimates clustering at two to five percent of the population. At age eighteen, these children too could discover that their fathers are not who they thought they were and thus avoid the harms that motivate [the] call for regulation.
>
> To be fair, there are distinctions between my Modest Proposal and [these registries for sperm donors]. Perhaps we have independent worries about the misuse of data on our sexual partners, or we do not trust the government to erase our names from the registry if no child results. There are, though, also ways in which my registry might be thought of as more desirable than [the existing ones]: mine seems less likely to have a chilling effect on the willingness to engage in sex than [the sperm donor] registry's chilling effect on the willingness to engage in donations. To the extent it would increase the use of condoms, my Modest Proposal might be thought to have desirable spillover effects in reducing STD transmission. It would also better enable the state to pursue child support from deadbeat dads.
>
>   . . .
>
> The strongest distinction between [sperm donor registries] and my Modest Proposal is that sperm donors provide sperm with the intention of creating a family while at least some of those affected by my Modest Proposal may not (though there certainly are cases in which individuals seek to produce a child together coitally but down the road the child is reared by a different father and never knows its true genetic origin). Even when this distinction is operative, however, it is not clear that it should make a difference. Courts routinely impose parental status and support obligations upon men who are deceived into believing their partners are using birth control or are incapable of reproducing. A common theme in this case law is that whatever rights the father might have must give way to the best interests of the child, who would otherwise go unsupported; put another way, the right to support belongs to the child and only the child can waive it. If one views information about a

child's genetic parentage as a kind of right of a child or duty that a child is owed—and I think it is fair to characterize [some registry advocates' views as being] along these lines—then, just as in the child support cases, I think there is a strong argument for extending the disclosure right to coital-reproduction cases, even when reproduction happens by accident. (Cohen 2012b, 444–445)

More recently, An Ravelingien and Guido Pennings (2013, 33–41) have made a similar argument that the same rationale that underlies prohibiting anonymity in assisted reproduction should carry over to coital reproduction as well. They argue that

> it would be discriminatory not to extend this right [to know] to naturally conceived children with misattributed paternity. One way to facilitate this would be through routine paternity testing at birth. While this proposal is likely to raise concerns about the conflicting interests and rights of other people involved, we show that similar concerns apply to the context of open-identity gamete donation. Unless one can identify a rational basis for treating the two groups differently, one's stance toward both cases should be the same. (Ravelingien and Pennings 2013, 33)

Others, such as Daniel Sperling (2013, 60–62), have argued against this analogy. In responding to Raveliengen and Pennings, Sperling notes among other things the following distinctions:

> [R]evealing the identity of the gamete donor, with whom the child is in no contact whatsoever, may create very little effect on the relationship between the social parents and the child, and/or between the genetic mother and the social father. This is because disclosure is already made under open and sincere relationship, reflecting also readiness of all parties to cope with familial and emotional hardships, if and when they occur.... On the other hand, a mandatory DNA testing under Misattributed Paternity cases, may, as Ravelingien and Pennings admit, put pressure on the mother to inform the child about his or her genetic father, and affect the sexual and procreative liberties of women more generally. If positive, such testing could create serious tension between the social father and the mother (if, for example the child were born as a result of an unknown affair, or if the child seeks some contact with his genetic father), and/or between the social father and the child, the nature of whose relationship would have changed significantly following the testing. In the case where the child accesses his or her birth certificate and gets in touch with the genetic father who will then refuse to have contact with the child, a serious threat to the child's psychological well-being could be observed.
> ...
> [Moreover,] even if some effects may result following disclosure of donors, one can argue that under systems of open-identity gamete donations, rational people who opt for donation should be presumed to give consent to risks of disclosure as well as to the violation of their privacy, communicational, and familial interests. According to this argument, the choice of the means of procreation (technologically assisted reproduction) entails the acceptance of some limitations on the freedom and well-being of all parties involved. On the other hand, Misattributed Paternity cases do not represent

the exercise of choice pertaining to the means of procreation. At the most, they may reflect some choice as to the circumstances leading to procreation, for example, when nonpaternity is the result of the mother's adultery. Such choice may not necessarily justify imposing detrimental effects on relevant parties. (Sperling 2013, 61)

Attacking the Argument for Settling for Parental Disclosure

One can also find fault with the existing sperm donor registries by showing that they do not go far enough. Unlike my prior point, which really is an attempt to provide a reductio ad absurdum, I am more ambivalent about how to use the point I am about to make. Some will read it and think it too serves as a reductio, while others might view it as a friendly amendment to be championed to the existing registries. Either way, it suggests the existing registries are not optimally designed for their ostensible purpose.

The registries in place in the United Kingdom and elsewhere are what I have called "passive" registries—children have to call the registry at age 18 to learn the identity of their donor—rather than what I have sketched as an "active" registry—one that would itself contact the child at age 18 to let the child know that he or she was donor-conceived and allow (but not force) him or her to receive information about the donor (Cohen 2012b, 446). On the arguments offered in favor of passive registries (especially when framed as a *right* to know one's genetic origins), it is not clear why one should prefer the passive to the active registry. In the shadow of a law mandating active registries, it seems plausible that the vast majority of parents would opt to inform their children of their donor-conceived status rather than wait for a civil servant to do so. Either way, that seems better than the passive registry. With a passive registry, to successfully fulfill its function it requires that children be told by their parents or otherwise find out that they are donor conceived.

Many recipient parents, especially heterosexual parents who can "pass" as the genetic parents, will not disclose to their children that they were donor conceived. Exactly how many is up for debate, although one set of studies suggests that only 5% of recipient parents disclose under anonymous sperm-donation programs, and that 30% of heterosexual recipient parents who have chosen identity-release sperm donations still had not disclosed to their 12- to 17-year-old children that they were donor conceived (Golombok et al. 2002, 966; Scheib et al. 2003, 1120). It thus seems plausible that passive registries will lead to something less than all donor-conceived children being informed that they were the result of sperm donation. Therefore, for some subset of donor-conceived children, possibly the majority, the harms anticipated (or if you prefer, rights violations) will exist even in the face of the passive registry.[17]

The active registry does what the passive registry purports to do, only better. If the arguments for the passive registry hold up, do they not also justify the active registry? Indeed, do they not indicate it is preferable? Moreover, the active registry's benefits go further still: the active registry seems fairer

because donor-conceived children of coupled heterosexual recipient parents would be just as likely to detect their origins as children of same-sex recipient parents and single recipient parents. Moreover, to the extent recipient parents would no longer be able to "pass" as genetic parents to their donor-conceived children, the active registry might decrease the tendency for rearing parents to seek sperm donors who are racial matches for themselves, a practice some have found objectionable. (Cohen 2012b, 447)

And yet many champions of passive registries shy away from supporting active ones. Why? "It is not as though we think that the child who, like Nancy Drew, sleuths out her donor-conceived nature is more deserving of this information than the one who has passively accepted that her father is the man who has reared her" (Cohen 2012b, 447). The best one might do, I think, is to try to develop an intersectionality theory of the harm or the rights violations in which "one demonstrates empirically that the supposed harm to donor-conceived children deprived of their donor's identities is most pronounced for children who already suspect they are donor-conceived" (Cohen 2012b, 447). Another way of framing the idea is that the relevant interest applies only to those who have begun a project of "truth seeking" not those who as yet do not suspect or do not wish to act on their suspicions of their true genetic origin. Doing so would justify supporting a passive registry but not an active one. Unless and until such empirical evidence has been marshaled, though, I tend to think people's discomfort with the active registry is somewhat indicative of some lack of confidence in the premises underlying the argument for the passive registry, though others may read it differently.

I also think the distinction between an active and passive registry nicely sharpens a point on which registry proponents have been somewhat ambiguous. Is the harm (or rights claim) actualized in all or merely some of the following cases: (1) a child who has no suspicion he or she is donor conceived, (2) a child who suspects he or she is donor conceived, wants to verify that fact, but has no interest in finding out who is his or her genetic father, and (3) a child who suspects he or she is donor conceived and wants to find out who is his or her genetic father? The argument typically is framed in terms of the claims of the third kind of child, but what, in particular, of the first? This would take us into some deep philosophical waters relating harm, including whether someone must experience a harm or benefit in order for it to matter morally (Sumner 1996). It would also take us into the question of whether there is a "right not to know" and what are its contours.

I have not played "hide the ball." I have been open in my skepticism as to the arguments that have been offered for mandating by law sperm donor registries, while also pointing out rejoinders to the critique where I see them. Hopefully the reader will get a good sense of the argumentative playing field, even if I cannot claim neutrality.

Additional Issues

While I think the question of whether to legally prohibit sperm donor anonymity is the main issue, I want to close by briefly discussing a few issues that have appeared or should appear at the periphery of the more central debate, and that in many ways deserve more attention from scholars working in this area:

Accidental Incest

Some who have written in this area have worried that sperm donor anonymity carries with it the threat of "accidental incest"—that individuals conceived of sperm donors will meet and have intercourse (Cahn 2009). In other work I have suggested that these worries are interesting because much of the moral horror over incest stems from the fact that children are reared together. To be concerned about accidental incest may depend on premises about best interest of resulting children or forms of legal moralism that I have elsewhere suggested are insufficient to justify legal regulation (Cohen 2011a; Cohen 2012a). Of course, one might say the harm is not to the children but to the adults who would like to avoid incestual sex for their own reasons. The only point I want to make here is that the kinds of steps needed to avoid accidental incest do not require the full-blown revelation of parenthood to donor-conceived children in every case. One could imagine a registry system that would allow donor-conceived individuals to determine if they were genetically related to another individual without directly revealing the identity of the sperm donor. In the case in which one half of the pair knows its genetic origins, I suppose the other will be able to deduce its parenthood. But in cases in which two donor-conceived children meet, they could determine if they were genetically related without requiring identity revelation.

Reciprocity

While registry advocates would give donor-conceived children the right to know the identity of their genetic fathers, there is a curious asymmetry in that they would not allow the genetic fathers to have a right to know the identity of their genetic children. There are distinctions one might offer for this, but it is not clear if they are entirely persuasive.

First, one might argue that children never chose not to know their genetic fathers, while fathers chose to participate in a sperm donation practice that would prima facie hide their genetic child's identity. If one believes in the "changed selves" argument noted earlier, though, one might press on why the donor's Time 1 preference should control his right to know his genetic offspring's identity given changes of feeling now that 18 years have passed. Moreover, if there is a right to know one's genetic *descendants*, it is not clear it should be waiveable in advance any more than a woman's right to have an abortion should be waiveable by contract (Cohen 2008a, 1189–1195).

Second, one might note that the appearance of the genetic father into a family structure of the rearing family might be disruptive to that structure, if he is not wanted. Of course, allowing donor-conceived children to know they are donor conceived and to attempt to contact their genetic fathers is also disruptive of the family structure in which they are reared. The question is whether the difference between the two disruptions is a difference of degree or of kind, or whether one form of disruption is morally problematic while the other is not.

Compensation and Anonymity

As I noted earlier from my own experimental work, it may be possible to use carrots (additional compensation for donors) rather than sticks (legal prohibition) to induce more sperm donors to become identified and thus improve access by donor-conceived children. That assumes, though, that additional sperm donor compensation does not offend anticommodificationist laws. Many of the countries that have prohibited sperm donor anonymity have also prohibited excess compensation. They may have to choose between these policies to some extent in order to maintain their supply of sperm.

Extraterritoriality and Circumvention Tourism

As I have discussed in my other work on medical tourism (Cohen 2014; Cohen 2012c), whatever rules governments adopt on medical services, some will try to circumvent those rules by traveling for services. This is true for anonymous sperm donation as well. Individuals wishing to get sperm without obligations of identification may travel to a place (like the United States) where the law permits anonymity and/or get sperm from that place shipped to their home country. To what extent should countries that prohibit anonymous sperm donation make their law apply extraterritorially to their citizens that travel abroad or create barriers to these shipments?

CONCLUSION

The world is now divided. Most of the world legally mandates that sperm donors must be identifiable and gives children the right to call a registry to find out identifying information about their sperm donor. However, most of those countries do not take the further step of requiring that the children be informed that they are donor conceived; they instead leave that in the realm of family privacy and parental discretion. The United States, on the other hand, is one of the lone holdouts; it does not prohibit sperm donor anonymity. There is a raging debate as to whether donor-conceived children have a right to know their origins or whether the premises and entailments of arguments for that result are problematic. This chapter has introduced the reader to that debate, the underlying law, and some peripheral issues.

Acknowledgments

I am thankful to Jack Balkin, Robert Blecker, Gaia Bernstein, Naomi Cahn, Dov Fox, Axel Gosseries, Holly Fernandez Lynch, Cilla Smith, Jeannie Suk, and Mark Wu, as well as audiences at the Boston College and New York Law School faculty workshops and the Yale Law School Information Society Project workshop for helpful comments on this and related work.

Notes

1. For a lengthier discussion of how to interpret the UK data, see Naomi Cahn's *The New Kinship* (2012). Cahn suggests that in the United Kingdom, "[t]he real problem may not be a decline in the number of donors or donations, but rather an inefficient system of treating women with donor sperm, which can be corrected by improved record-keeping and communication" (Cahn 2012).
2. Bernstein cites several sources to claim that most clinics have a wait of at least 2 years for donor sperm (Camber 2008); that a BBC survey of 78 of the 85 UK fertility clinics indicated over 6-month wait times for clients (Dreaper 2006); that some clinics had long waits and stopped offering donor sperm (Grady 2008); and that other issues exist (Edwards 2005; CBS News 2008). There are also more anecdotal data. For example, Kim Mutcherson (2012) reports that when Canada "made it illegal to pay men for their sperm or women for ova in a 2004 law called the Assisted Human Reproduction Act . . . the number of men in the country willing to sell their sperm dropped precipitously. In short order, all of the agencies that formerly sold sperm closed their doors save for one. One 2010 newspaper article reported that there were only forty sperm sellers available in all of Canada" (Canadian Press 2010). It is also worth noting two reasons why this data may not offer a complete picture. The first is the possibility that there may exist some "underground" exchange of sperm or egg that tries to circumvent the nonanonymity rules, for example through at-home insemination. Second, to anticipate a point I return to at the end of this chapter, medical tourism for reproductive technologies ("fertility tourism" as I have called it elsewhere [Cohen 2014]) may provide parents a way of circumventing these rules through travel. We do not have that much data on the role that anonymity plays in fertility tourism, but here is one pertinent study: In a 2010 study by the European Society of Human Reproduction and Embryology of female patients seeking reproductive technology services through medical tourism at 46 clinics in six popular European destination countries for fertility tourism, Shenfield and colleagues reported that 18.9% of Swedish and 16.4% of Norwegian patients stated they travelled to get anonymous sperm donation unavailable at home (Cohen 2014, discussing Shenfield et al. 2010).
3. In my own work I have stressed that for constitutional purposes it is important to divide an omnibus right to procreate into rights to be a genetic, legal, or gestational parent, and that there are doubts about whether the few constitutional cases on the subject adequately support a right to be a genetic parent through assisted reproductive technology (Cohen 2008a, 1140–1141; Cohen 2011a, 513).
4. See, e.g., *Mintz v. Zoernig*, 145 N.M. 362 (Ct. App. 2008); *Thomas S. v. Robin Y.*, 618 N.Y.S.2d 356 (1st Dep't 1994); *Jhordan C. v. Mary K.*, 179 Cal. App. 3d 386 (1st Dist. 1986); *Ferguson*

v. McKiernan, 940 A.2d 1236 (Pa. 2007); *In re R.C.*, 775 P.2d 27 (Colo. 1989); *Kansas v. W.M.* (unpublished, but a summary of which is available at http://verdict.justia.com/2014/01/27/ craigslist-sperm-donor-owes-child-support).

5. For specific cases, see *S.F. v. State ex rel. T.M.*, 695 So. 2d 1186, 1189 (Ala. Civ. App. 1996); *Faske v. Bonanno*, 357 N.W.2d 860, 861 (Mich. Ct. App. 1984); *Mercer Cnty. Dep't of Soc. Servs. ex. rel. Imogene T. v. Alf M.*, 589 N.Y.S.2d 288, 290 (N.Y. Fam. Ct. 1992).

6. More may make decisions whether to abort based on the rules governing abortion, but I imagine that is true in only a fraction of the cases. Even where it is true, there is still an entity that already exists and the parents are deciding whether to terminate it or not. That too is different from the case of deciding whether to conceive at all.

7. This section and the one that follows are drawn heavily from Cahn (2012) and Cohen (2012b). Direct quotes from either source are cited, but other material from this dialogue is not otherwise demarcated.

8. For examples of those framing this as a "right to know," see Department of Health 1984, 24–25; Chestney 2001, 365; Goodman 2006; Ravitsky 2010, 665.

9. As a matter of positive law, Guido Pennings notes that "a number of international organisations have presented codes of rights which include articles that are relevant for the question of the access to information about genetic origins . . . Especially Article 7 of the United Nations Convention on the Rights of the Child which gives the child the right to know his parents as far as possible and Article 8 of the European Convention for the Protection of Human Rights and Fundamental Freedoms" (Pennings 2001, 2).

10. "The right to privacy of the donor child collides with the right to privacy of the other participants. The weight of the right is partially determined by the importance of the information for the identity of the child" (Pennings 2001, 10).

11. My good friend Naomi Cahn and I continue to "duel" (if that does not sound too violent as to a scholarly disagreement between two friends) on this topic. In her most recent thrust, she conveniently focuses only on the effects of shortages on nonidentity but ignores the point about changing *with whom* we reproduce, in effect confounding the question of whether *any* donor gametes are available with the question of which sperm from which donor meets which egg from which recipient, the relevant question for nonidentity purposes (Cahn 2014, 1114). I think she also makes other mistakes as to abortion and masturbation (Cahn 2014, 1114–1115), but I have already explained those as conceptual mistakes in other work I have written anticipating just these kinds of confusions (Cohen 2011a, 437; Cohen 2012a, 1212).

12. One difference between sperm donor anonymity regulation and, say, the restrictions put in place in some countries that prohibit IVF past a certain age is that the former creates only what I have called an "imperfect" nonidentity problem while the latter creates a "perfect" one. For sperm donor anonymity bans, hypothetically "there may exist at least one child who would have come into existence in both the anonymity-permitted and anonymity-prohibited regimes—one child conceived when the same donated sperm meets the same egg and for whom the rule has no effect on whether, when, and with whom reproduction takes place" (Cohen 2012b, 436, n.23). And "as to that particular potential child (or children), a child-welfare justification will be possible if he or she would be better off with access to the identity of his or her donor genetic parent" (Ibid.). But the number of children for whom this will be true is very small if nonzero, indubitably much smaller than the universe of all donor-conceived children, and elsewhere I have argued in depth that this very small subset of potentially harmed children is not enough to justify this form of regulation (Cohen 2011a, 474–481).

13. The reason is complex and has to do with paradoxes implied by average and total welfarist approaches (Cohen 2011a).

14. I reiterate that Shiffrin herself has largely limited the ambit of her claim to an argument for tort liability for wrongful life, so the argument under consideration is an extension of her claims that she may not endorse.

15. While Shiffrin's account does not exhaust arguments focused on wronging children without harming them, it does seem to me to be the best developed such account in the literature. But while hers is an account of *wronging*, it is one that does depend on a notion of *harming*, just a concept that harm is never outweighed by a pure benefit. Could one imagine a version of the wronging concern related to sperm donor anonymity that does not depend on *any* notion of harm? The claim would not be about the *consequences* to the child of not knowing his or her genetic father's identity—psychological distress and the like—but perhaps a more existential claim of having an "incomplete" identity or lacking the tools needed to form a complete identity. I am grateful to Leslie Francis for suggesting this possibility to me. In the end, though, I am not sure that this reformulation escapes harm, benefit, and the nonidentity problem. If one pressed as to *why* we thought this existential state was something that wronged the child, I think it could only be understood in comparison to a state of being where the child existed without that incomplete identity and a belief that one state was worse than the other. And once we get into comparing one child's state of being against another one, I think we are back in the throes of the nonidentity problem.

16. Several other authors in this handbook also address the nonidentity problem. It would take a whole chapter (or perhaps a book in itself!) to fully wrestle with how our views intersect, conflict and branch out. But for the purposes of some intertextual discussion between the chapters, let me say a few brief words on each:

    DeGrazia's chapter at one point seems to endorse a "wronging without harming" approach similar to Seanna Shiffrin's. My concern with that approach as applied to sperm donor anonymity is telegraphed above and developed in much greater depth in Cohen (2012a, 1244–1264). Later on, though, he specifies that this may not be the way to view true nonidentity problem cases, and instead that in these cases "[t]he parents act wrongly, it seems, without wronging anyone in particular. In my view, the wrongdoing in nonidentity cases such as this must be understood in the impersonal, consequentialist terms of making the world a slightly worse place than it would have been had they acted responsibly." In such case DeGrazia seems to be actually endorsing the non-person-affecting principle approach. I criticize that view's application to sperm donor anonymity earlier and in greater depth elsewhere (Cohen 2011a). For what it is worth I also think that parents who use anonymous sperm donors will not fail the first two of the criteria DeGrazia proposes in his chapter—"Parents owe their children (1) worthwhile lives, (2) in which their basic needs are reasonably expected to be met, and (3) doing more for them if they can without undue sacrifice"; they may, however, run into problems with the third criterion, depending on how we understand "undue sacrifice" in the context of family privacy and procreative liberty.

    Malek's chapter argues that "the interest level at which a life is worth *continuing* to live may not be the same as the interest level at which a life would be worth *conceiving*." I do not think it is plausible to think that the life of an anonymously donor-conceived child without access to the genetic father's identity rises is problematic on either standard and I do not think she believes the contrary, nor that anyone would claim otherwise. Malek's distinction between rigid and nonrigid designators of "this child" deserves a much more thorough discussion and (in my mind refutation) than I can give it in part of a footnote, but my view is closer to Parfit's: that it is linguistically sound but morally unpersuasive. To use a biographical example: My mother was married without children before my father. Imagine in possible world A she had conceived with her first husband and in possible world B she conceived with my father. It is linguistically possible to use the nonrigid designator "her first child" to ask "would it have been better for her first child had she conceived the child with her first husband rather than her second?" But it seems to me to make no moral sense in judging her action to ask whether *I* would have been better off had my mother had a child with her first husband instead of me. And what would we do in the case that she had both of us? In favor of her view Malek argues (among other things) that the nonrigid "designation is more appropriate in the context of conception decision-making" because "it more closely corresponds to the way potential parents normally think about future children." But I venture to say that my mother would think quite differently about a child with one husband as compared to a child with another! Even if her view better adhered with the way potential parents in ordinary language describe their views of producing children, I think that is far from dispositive. Ordinary parents have not thought deeply about the ethics of reproduction and they may just be wrong. It may also be advantageous for them to think about it in these folk ways even if doing so is incorrect. That is, there may be second-order benefits to proceeding as if something false was true (such as, perhaps, belief that posthumous treatment of our body affects our welfare). But we should not confuse these second-order benefits with a belief that the proposition is *actually* true. And the calculus looks quite different when we move from folk beliefs about parenting to what the state is justified in doing in limiting the liberty of would-be reproducers.

I am largely in agreement with the approach in Wasserman's chapter (indeed he quotes me!) that arguments about reproductive externalities turn out to be the best of "the best of a not-very good lot" (2012a, 1220) in justifying the regulation of reproduction. As applied to sperm donor anonymity, the externalized costs for society seem so small and attenuated that I am, if anything, even more skeptical that they can justify legally forbidding anonymous sperm donation. There are also other reasons to be skeptical about reproductive externality approaches I offer elsewhere (Cohen 2012a) and will not rehearse here.

17. The passive registry also leaves open the possibility that children will inadvertently determine they are donor conceived.

BIBLIOGRAPHY

Almeling, Rene. 2011. *Sex cells: The medical market for eggs and sperm.* Berkeley and Los Angeles: University of California Press.

Bernstein, Gaia. 2010. Regulating reproductive technologies: Timing, uncertainty, and donor anonymity. *Boston University Law Review* 90: 1207–1218.

Bernstein, Gaia. 2013. Unintended consequences: Prohibitions on gamete donor anonymity and the fragile practice of surrogacy." *Indiana Health Law Review* 10: 291–324.

Blyth, Eric, and Lucy Frith. 2008. The UK's gamete donor crisis—A critical analysis. *Critical Social Policy* 28: 74–95.

Brock, Dan W. 1995. The non-identity problem and genetic harms—The case of wrongful handicaps. *Bioethics* 9: 269–275.

Bygedemen, M. 1991. The Swedish Insemination Act. *Acta Obstetricia et Gynecologica Scandinavica* 70: 265. Cited in Bernstein, Gaia. 2010. Regulating reproductive technologies: Timing, uncertainty, and donor anonymity. *Boston University Law Review* 90: 1207–1218.

Byrn, Mary Patricia, and Rebecca Ireland. 2012. Anonymously provided sperm and the constitution. *Columbia Journal of Gender and Law* 23(1): 1–28.

Cahn, Naomi. 2009. Accidental incest: Drawing the line—or the curtain?—for reproductive technology. *Harvard Journal of Law & Gender* 32: 59–107.

Cahn, Naomi. 2012. The new kinship. *Georgetown Law Journal* 100: 367–429.

Cahn, Naomi. 2014. Do tell! The rights of donor-conceived offspring. *Hofstra Law Review* 42: 1077–1124.

Camber, Rebecca. 2008. Britain faces fertility crisis as loss of donor anonymity sees sperm and egg donor numbers plummet. *Mail Online*, June 26. http://www.dailymail.co.uk/health/article-1029712/Britain-faces-fertility-crisis-loss-donor-anonymity-sees-sperm-egg-donor-numbers-plummet.htm.

Canadian Press. 2010. Anonymous sperm donation needed fertility experts. October 27. http://www.ctv.ca/CTVNews/Health/20101027/sperm-donation-caanda-101027/.

CBS News. 2008. U.K. facing sperm donor shortage: Experts say scarcity prompted by reversing confidentiality laws. November 13. http://www.cbsnews.com/stories/2008/11/13/health/main4597958.shtml. Cited in Bernstein, Gaia. 2010. Regulating reproductive technologies: Timing, uncertainty, and donor anonymity. *Boston University Law Review* 90: 1207–1218.

Chestney, Elizabeth Siberry. 2001. The right to know one's genetic origin: Can, should, or must a state that extends this right to adoptees extend an analogous right to children conceived with donor gametes? *Texas Law Review* 80: 365–391.

Clark, Brigitte. 2012. A balancing act? The rights of donor-conceived children to know their biological origins. *Georgia Journal of International and Comparative Law* 40: 619–661.

Cohen, I. Glenn. 2008a. The Constitution and the rights not to procreate. *Stanford Law Review* 60: 1135–1196.

Cohen, I. Glenn. 2008b. The right not to be a genetic parent? *Southern California Law Review* 81: 1115–1196.

Cohen, I. Glenn. 2011a. Regulating reproduction: The problem with best interests. *Minnesota Law Review* 96: 423–519.

Cohen, I. Glenn. 2011b. Prohibiting anonymous sperm donation and the child welfare error. *Hasting Center Report* 41(5): 13–14.

Cohen, I. Glenn. 2012a. Beyond best interests. *Minnesota Law Review* 96: 1187–1274.

Cohen, I. Glenn. 2012b. Response: Rethinking sperm-donor anonymity: Of changed selves, nonidentity, and one-night stands. *Georgetown Law Journal* 100: 431–447.

Cohen, I. Glenn. 2012c. Circumvention tourism. *Cornell Law Review* 97(6): 1309–1398.

Cohen, I. Glenn. 2014. *Patients with passports: Medical tourism, law, and ethics.* New York: Oxford University Press.

Cohen, I. Glenn, and Eli Adashi. 2013. Made-to-order embryos for sale—A brave new world? *New England Journal of Medicine* 368: 2517–2519.

Cohen, I. Glenn, and Travis G. Coan. 2014. Can you buy sperm donor identification? An experiment." *Journal of Empirical Legal Studies* 10: 715–740.

Daniels, Ken, and Alison Douglass. 2008. Access to genetic information by donor offspring and donors: Medicine, policy and law in New Zealand. *Medicine and Law* 27: 131–146.

Daniels, Ken, and Othon Lalos. 1995. The Swedish Insemination Act and the availability of donors. *Human Reproduction* 10: 1871–1874. Cited in Bernstein, Gaia. 2010. Regulating reproductive technologies: Timing, uncertainty, and donor anonymity. *Boston University Law Review* 90: 1207–1218.

De Jonge, Christopher, and Christopher L. R. Barratt. 2006. Gamete donation: A question of anonymity. *Fertility and Sterility* 85: 500–501.

Dennison, Michelle. 2008. Revealing your sources: The case for non-anonymous gamete donation. *Journal of Law and Health* 21: 1–27.

Department of Health and Social Security. 1984. Report of the Committee of Inquiry into Human Fertilisation and Embryology. United Kingdom.

The Donor Sibling Registry, 2000–2014. https://www.donorsiblingregistry.com/.

Dreaper, Jane. 2006. IVF donor sperm shortage revealed. *BBC News*, September 13. http://news.bbc.co.uk/2/hi/health/5341982.stm. Cited in Bernstein, Gaia. 2010. Regulating reproductive technologies: Timing, uncertainty, and donor anonymity. *Boston University Law Review* 90: 1207–1218.

Edwards, Gareth. 2005. It's a barren time for city's infertility unit. *Evening News,* March 21, 9. Cited in Bernstein, Gaia. 2010. Regulating reproductive technologies: Timing, uncertainty, and donor anonymity. *Boston University Law Review* 90: 1207–1218.

Ekerhovd, Erling, Anders Faurskov, and Charlotte Werner. 2008. Swedish sperm donors are driven by altruism, but shortages of sperm donors leads to reproductive travelling. *Upsala Journal Medicine Science* 113: 305–313. Cited in Bernstein, Gaia. 2010. Regulating reproductive technologies: Timing, uncertainty, and donor anonymity. *Boston University Law Review* 90: 1207–1218.

Feinberg, Joel. 1988. *The moral limits of the criminal law: Harmless wrongdoing* 4. New York: Oxford University Press.

Garrison, Marsha. 2000. Law making for baby making: An interpretive approach to the determination of legal parentage. *Harvard Law Review* 113: 835–923.

Genetic Integrity Act, The. 2006. 8 ch. 6 §Lag om genetisk integritet. Svensk författningssamling: 351.

Golombok, Susan, Fiona MacCallum, Emma Goodman, and Michael Rutter. 2002. Families with children conceived by donor insemination: A follow-up at age twelve. *Child Development* 73: 952–968. Cited in Cohen, I. Glenn. 2012b. Response: Rethinking sperm-donor anonymity: Of changed selves, nonidentity, and one-night stands. *Georgetown Law Journal* 100: 431–447.

Goodman, Ellen. 2006. Kids' right to know trumps sperm donors' right to anonymity. *Baltimore Sun*, December 22. http://articles.baltimoresun.com/2006-12-22/news/0612220130_1_sperm-donors-sperm-bank-pregnancy.

Gosseries, Axel. 2008. On future generations' future rights. *Journal of Political Philosophy* 16: 446–474.

Gottlieb, Claes, Othon Lalos, and Frank Lindblad. 2000. Disclosure of donor insemination to the child: The impact of Swedish legislation on couples' attitudes. *Human Reproduction* 15: 2052–2056.

Grady, Denise. 2008. Shortage of sperm donors in Britain prompts calls for change. *The New York Times,* November 12, A10. Cited in Bernstein, Gaia. 2010. Regulating reproductive technologies: Timing, uncertainty, and donor anonymity. *Boston University Law Review* 90: 1207–1218.

Hickman, Belinda. 1998. Donors lose interest in sperm bank deposits. *Turkish Daily News*, April 7, 5. Cited in Bernstein, Gaia. 2010. Regulating reproductive technologies: Timing, uncertainty, and donor anonymity. *Boston University Law Review* 90: 1207–1218.

Human Fertilisation and Embryology Authority. 2004. Disclosure of donor information: regulations. No. 1511. United Kingdom. http://www.opsi.gov.uk/SI/si2004/20041511.html.

Human Fertilisation and Embryology Authority. 2009. Conceived After. *Human Fertilsation and Embryology Authority*. http://www.hfea.gov.uk/5554.html.

Human Fertilisation and Embryology Authority. 2012a. Donor conception—Treatments. http://www.hfea.gov.uk/donor-conception-treatments.html.

Human Fertilisation and Embryology Authority. 2012b. Existing donors. http://www.hfea.gov.uk/1972.html.

Human Fertilisation and Embryology Authority. 2013a. Re-register. *Human Fertilsation and Embryology Authority*. http://www.hfea.gov.uk/1973.html.

Human Fertilisation and Embryology Authority. 2013b. New donor registrations. http://www.hfea.gov.uk/3411.html.

Infertility (Medical Procedures) Act, The. 1984. Victoria. Austl No. 10163.

Johns, Rebecca. 2013. Abolishing anonymity: A rights-based approach to evaluating anonymous sperm donations. *UCLA Women's Law Journal* 20: 111–135.

Johnson v. Superior Court, 95 Cal. Rptr. 2d 864 (Cal. App. 2000).

Kearney, Mary Kate. 2011. Identifying sperm and egg donors: Opening Pandora's box. *Journal of Law and Family Studies* 13, no. 2: 215–234.

McDougall, R. 2004. Acting parentally: An argument against sex selection. *Journal of Medical Ethics* 31: 601–605.

McGee, Glenn, Sarah-Vaughan Brakman, and Andrea D. Gurmankin. 2001. Gamete donation and anonymity: Disclosure to children conceived with donor gametes should not be optional. *Human Reproduction* 16: 2034–2038.

Mutcherson, Kimberly M. 2012. Welcome to the Wild West: Protecting access to cross border fertility care in the United States. *Cornell Journal of Law & Public Policy* 22: 349–393.

Parfit, Derek. 1987. *Reasons and persons.* New York: Oxford University Press.

Pennings, Guido. 2001. The right to privacy and access to information about one's genetic origins. *Medicine and Law* 20: 1–15.

Prohibition of Human Cloning for Reproduction and the Regulation of Human Embryo Research Amendment Act. 2006. No. 172. http://www.comlaw.gov.au/ComLaw/Legislation/Act1.nsf/0/71AC9EAE45677788CA2572440012F18A/$file/1722006.pdf.

Ravelingien, An, and Guido Pennings. 2013. The right to know your genetic parents: From open-identity gamete donation to routine paternity testing. *The American Journal of Bioethics* 13, no. 5: 33–41.

Ravitsky, Vardit. 2010. Knowing where you come from: The rights of donor-conceived individuals and the meaning of genetic relatedness. *Minnesota Journal of Law, Science and Technology* 11: 655–684.

Robertson, John A. 2004. Procreative liberty and harm to offspring in assisted reproduction. *American Journal of Law & Medicine* 30: 7–40.

Sauer, Julie L. 2009. Competing interests and gamete donation: The case for anonymity. *Seton Hall Law Review* 39: 919–954.

Scheib, J. E., M. Riordan, and S. Rubin. 2003. Choosing identity-release sperm donors: The parents' perspective 13–18 years later. *Human Reproduction* 18: 1115–1127.

Sharp, Brittney N. 2013. Comparing the rights of adoptees and donor-conceived offspring in states granting access to original birth certificates and adoption records: An equal protection analysis. *Ave Maria Law Review* 11: 515–540.

Shiffrin, Seana Valentine. 1999. Wrongful life, procreative responsibility, and the significance of harm. *Legal Theory* 5: 117–148.

Shenfield, F., de Mouzon, J., Pennings, G., et al. 2010. Cross border reproductive care in six European countries. *Human Reproduction* 25: 1361–1368.

Spar, Debora L. 2006. *The baby business.* Cambridge, MA: Harvard Business Review Press.

Sperling, Daniel. 2013. The right to know one's genetic origin: Are gamete donations and misattributed paternity cases alike? *The American Journal of Bioethics* 13, no. 5: 60–62.

Sumner, L. W. 1996. *Welfare, happiness, and ethics.* Oxford: Clarendon Press.

Szoke, Helen. 2004. The Victorian experience of administering donor birth registers. *International Congress Series* 1271: 357–360. Cited in Bernstein, Gaia. 2010. Regulating reproductive technologies: Timing, uncertainty, and donor anonymity. *Boston University Law Review* 90: 1207–1218.

Turkish Daily News. Clinic asks Australian MPs to donate sperm bank deposits. 2005. January 14. Cited in Bernstein, Gaia. 2010. Regulating reproductive technologies: Timing, uncertainty, and donor anonymity. *Boston University Law Review* 90: 1207–1218.

Turkmendag, Ilke, Robert Dingwall, and Thérèse Murphy. 2008. The removal of donor anonymity in the UK: The silencing of claims by would-be parents. *International Journal of Law Policy and Family* 22: 283–310.

Victorian Assisted Reproductive Treatment Authority. 1999–2009. *Annual Reports.* https://www.varta.org.au/resources/reports. Cited in Bernstein, Gaia. 2010. Regulating reproductive technologies: Timing, uncertainty, and donor anonymity. *Boston University Law Review* 90: 1207–1218.

Wash. Rev. Code § 26.26.750 (2011).

CHAPTER 23

WHO AM I WHEN I'M PREGNANT?

HILDE LINDEMANN

WHO you understand yourself to be when you are pregnant depends to a greater or lesser extent on whether you wanted to be pregnant in the first place. If the pregnancy is unwelcome, you may decide you need to arrange for an abortion in the hope that you can go on as the person you were before. But if there are insurmountable obstacles to abortion, either because you believe it is wrong or because you cannot get access to a provider, then you are forced to reshape your self-conception: you are now going to have to come to terms with the idea that you are a prospective mother to this prospective child, even if you give it up for adoption. If, on the other hand, the pregnancy is wanted, you may step gladly into your new role, happily seeing yourself as a mother-to-be or as already a mother now making room in your life for another child.

No matter how you feel about your future status as a mother to this future child, however, the changes to your body induced by the pregnancy itself can alter your self-conception in a number of different ways. Some women who eagerly look forward to mothering the baby-to-be, for example, do not at all enjoy the experience of being pregnant—they feel invaded by the alien that keeps taking up more room and makes them sick. Other women find the 9-month-long intimacy fascinating and exciting, and they marvel at how their bodies gradually become both their own and another's, making a new someone who has never existed before. Some who have previously had a miscarriage feel guilty, as if they are walking on eggshells, not trusting their bodies to keep the fetus safe and well. And some feel violated, forced to use their bodies in service of a being that has no right to be there. It is possible, of course, to feel all these things at various stages of the pregnancy.

Although I do not have room to argue for it here, I take it that pregnant women's self-conceptions are constituted in part by *master narratives of pregnancy*—stories that circulate widely in one's society—as well as by more personalized stories representing the women's individual circumstances and how they feel about them. But how they see themselves by no means determines who they are. Other peoples' stories also contribute

to the narrative tissue that constitutes their identity. This tissue of stories and story frag-
ments represents the things that matter most about the women, from either their own or
others' point of view. Identities function as guides to our social interactions, in that we
act on the basis of them: my self-conception guides what I do, while others treat me on
the basis of how they understand who I am. Identities, then, are both explanatory and
prescriptive. They are explanatory in that they allow the woman and those around her to
make sense of who she is, and they are prescriptive because they give rise to normative
expectations regarding how the people bearing them are to behave, as well as how they
are to be treated (for a fuller examination of these claims, see Lindemann 2014).

Personal identities are social constructions, not only in the sense that others' narrative understandings contribute to them but also in that many of the stories from both
the first- and third-person perspective are well known socially. But because many people are involved in the construction and what they construct is prescriptive as well as
descriptive, identities are often sites of contestation. In this chapter I will demonstrate
that in the case of pregnant women, master narratives that enter the identity are often
destructive and need to be contested. I will take a close look at three of them, to show
how they go wrong.

THE MASTER NARRATIVE OF
THE FETAL CONTAINER

Master narratives are essential to social life—we wouldn't know how to live together
without drawing on these shared understandings as we navigate our social worlds. The
plot templates and character types they offer help us to understand what we are to do,
and with (or to or for) whom we are to do it. The problem, though, is that power cir-
culates unjustly throughout our social world, and some master narratives arise specifically to conceal this injustice. They do this by purporting to justify the existing social
order, often by depicting the people on the receiving end of the oppressive arrangement
as somehow deserving their oppressive treatment (Lindemann Nelson 2001).

The most prevalent of the narratives contributing to a pregnant woman's identity is
of this kind. It depicts the woman as a container, altogether different from the entity
growing inside her. In the philosophical literature alone, for example, the fetus is said
to be inside the woman "the way a tub of yogurt is inside your refrigerator" (Smith and
Brogaard 2003, 74). Oderberg claims that the embryo is "an organizational entity that
is not a part of its host" (2008, 266), while Howespian asserts that the fetus "could not
merely be a part of some other thing" (2008, 152). Katherine Hawley claims that "no cat
is a proper part of a cat" (2001, 166), implying that either fetal cats are not cats at all or
that pregnant cats contain cats; the analogy to human beings is left unspoken. In keeping
with this containment motif, the bioethics literature is rife with references to the fetus as
an isolated *patient*, imprisoned behind the "maternal abdominal wall" (Phelan 1991; see

also Fletcher 1981; Lenow 1983; Harrison and Adzick 1991; Murray 1996; Chervenak and McCullough 1996). Further emphasizing its ontological distance from the woman gestating it, the fetus is often represented as pitted against its container, particularly in contexts of what is commonly called "maternal–fetal conflict" (Fasouliotis and Schenker 2000; Oduncu et al. 2003; Cummings and Mercurio 2011).

The master narrative of the fetal container is destructive because it degrades the woman. If she is merely a vessel for use, she can be treated like any other piece of equipment. If she is just carrying something, she is to be ignored while the focus is on what she carries. Worse still, if she is pitted against the fetus, she can be treated as hostile and forced to serve the fetus's best interests without regard to the costs to herself (containers do not have selves). All the attention is on the baby-to-be, not on the incubator. Note how this story erases the woman. She exists only as the oven in which the bun is baked.

The fetal container master narrative also erases the profound physical *intimacy* of pregnancy. Far from sitting in its own space on a shelf like the yogurt in the refrigerator, the fetus and the woman gestating it are in the most deeply enmeshed relationship human beings can have. To be pregnant, of course (though it is surprising how many discussions in the abortion literature miss this), is to be occupied by an entity that is both you and not you, and that makes use of your heart, liver, lungs, other organs, blood, hormones, enzymes, and metabolism for its survival. And just as it makes use of your body, so too it makes itself felt in and on that body, changing its contours and the coloration of some of its parts, shifting the organs as it grows to make room for itself, producing nausea, weight gain, euphoria, and varicose veins, and sometimes causing life-threatening diseases such as diabetes, high blood pressure, and preeclampsia. To gestate, as Margaret Olivia Little puts it, is to engage in "a particular, and particularly thoroughgoing, kind of physical intertwinement" (Little 1999, 296). This intertwinement matters. At the very beginning of the pregnancy, the enmeshed fetus constitutes an invitation to a powerful relationship bred of flesh and bone with the potential to last the woman's lifetime. If the woman starts building that relationship, the physical intertwinement with her fetus typically produces an emotional intimacy as well, so that the woman experiences strong feelings of love and protection toward this being she is bringing into independent existence. These feelings usually enter into her self-conception as a mother-to-be, and they are nothing at all like her feelings for the yogurt she had for lunch.

Catriona Mackenzie puts it this way: "In early pregnancy, although the woman's body is undergoing massive changes, the fetus itself is not very physically developed. The fetus' separateness is thus neither physically well established nor is it felt as such by the woman. What happens as pregnancy continues is that, as the fetus develops physically, a triple process occurs. First, from the perspective of the woman, the fetus becomes more and more physically differentiated from her as her own body boundaries alter. Second, this gradual physical differentiation (which becomes very pronounced as soon as the fetus starts moving around . . .) is paralleled by and gives rise to a gradual psychic differentiation, in the experience of the woman, between herself and the fetus. . . . Third, physical and psychic differentiation are usually accompanied by an increasing emotional attachment of the woman to the fetus, an attachment which is based both in her physical connection with the fetus and in anticipation of her future relationship with a separate being who is also intimately related to her" (Mackenzie 1992, 148–149).

The fetal container story captures none of this.

Finally, and perhaps most important, the story also conceptualizes the pregnant woman as passive, being acted upon by biological forces outside her control. In that way it erases the woman's *agency*, concealing the many things she does to bring her child into existence. For one thing, it hides the fact that she may have become pregnant for a reason: she might conceive and carry a fetus because she wants a special relationship that will last over time, or she wants an existing child to have a sibling, or without children she would feel less firmly rooted in the world, or for some other of the myriad reasons why human beings want children.

For another thing, the story erases agency by papering over what the woman must do to sustain the pregnancy. In nonhuman animals, for all we can tell, pregnancy is a process that occurs in the female without any purposive contributions on her part: she passively suffers the fetus to grow in her rather than actively shaping it, so the relationship that ensues is a purely biological one. In human pregnancies, by contrast, what begins as a purely biological relationship is transformed into a recognizably human one because, by what the woman does in imagination, word, and deed, she *calls her fetus into personhood*. It is not until after she starts doing this that the fetus becomes the sort of entity with whom personal relationships are even possible.

I take personhood to consist, not in the possession of certain attributes such as self-awareness or the ability to speak or reason, but in a practice—a practice we engage in as naturally as breathing. As I understand it, the practice rests on four elements: (1) a human being has sufficient mental activity to constitute a personality; (2) aspects of this personality are expressed bodily; (3) other persons recognize it as the expression of a personality; and (4) they respond to what they see. Recognition and response are often a matter of understanding who someone is and treating the person accordingly. Whether these understandings are self-conceptions or others' sense of who we are, they consist of the web of stories that constitutes our personal identities, so who we are plays a crucial role in the practice of personhood.

Although late-term fetuses might be capable of sensing, fearing, and wanting, they cannot yet be said to have a personality, or any way to express it if they did. The communicative repertoire available to the fetus is felt only by the woman, and it is limited to a sharp dig of an elbow, a series of kicks, the fluttering sensation produced by movements of the hands or feet—all of which might mean anything, or nothing. Nevertheless, at some point in the pregnancy the woman beckons to her fetus, calling it into personhood by making physical arrangements for it, giving it a personal identity, creating social space for it, and thinking of it as if it were already the born child she hopes it will become.

William Ruddick has usefully called the forward-looking relationship established in this one-sided way a *proleptic* relationship (Ruddick 2000, 97). Prolepsis, as a literary device, is the treating of a future state of affairs as if it already existed. It is achieved by means of an anticipatory adjective, as in the poetic "While yon slow oxen turn the furrowed plain," where the plain will not actually be furrowed until later, after the oxen have finished turning it. Proleptic *pregnancies* also anticipate the future in this way, because the mother-to-be treats the fetus as if it had already attained personhood. In doing so, she sets the conditions for the born child to be a person. The calling is not just imaginative—it is material. All sorts of activities, from furnishing a nursery to starting a college fund, are apt to take place in the months before the child is actually born. Note how, in accepting the pregnancy and beginning the process of calling to her fetus, the woman adds an important set of stories to her own self-conception. She now not only bears the identity of a pregnant woman but becomes a particular *kind* of pregnant woman: she is a (fittingly proleptic) expectant mother.

It is not just the woman herself who engages her baby-to-be proleptically. Her family, friends, coworkers, health care providers, and strangers on the street all do it, too: "Is it a boy or a girl?" "How's it going, Mama?" "I've brought you some clothes for the baby." Nor is it just individuals who call to the fetus in this way. The entire society mobilizes to help the gestating woman turn her fetus into a person. The pregnancy triggers an elaborate set of formal and informal social mechanisms whose sole purpose is, in one way or another, to call the fetus into personhood.

The fetal container master narrative fails most resoundingly, then, in that it diverts attention away from the woman's role in initiating a new human being into personhood. It does not acknowledge the importance of what she is doing, and it certainly does not honor her for it. In short, it shows a disrespect for her agency and belittles her work.

The Master Narrative of the Good Mother

All stories are selective. Their tellers pick and choose the acts, characters, and circumstances they want to depict, while ignoring or concealing other, sometimes crucial details. The master narrative of the fetal container certainly does this, but at the same time it also displays another feature common to all stories: it is connective. It not only connects one element of the story to another and the teller to the receiver, it also connects itself to other stories. Master narratives tend to be highly interconnected—that is one reason why damaging ones are so tenacious and difficult to uproot. In particular, the master narrative of the fetal container is connected to the narrative of the good mother, which has its grip on women in the United States as never before.

The good-mother story is to some extent a middle-class construct, dating back to the early decades of the nineteenth century. By around 1830 or so, the Industrial Revolution effected a profound change in bourgeois family life. Rather than observing the gendered divisions of labor such families used to observe while working together on the farm or in the shop, men now worked in offices or on assembly lines in factories outside the home, while the rise in middle-class income made it possible for men to assert a prerogative that had until then been reserved for the gentry: their wives and daughters were to tend to the hearth and home rather than joining the paid workforce (Mintz and Kellogg 1989).

According to the good-mother narrative, mothers must always do what is best for their children. This means they must not live in substandard housing. They must arrange domestic life so that it centers solely on the children. They must, of course, be married to the children's father, or at least make it appear as if the family has the appropriate, two-heterosexual-parent makeup. They, not the father, are responsible for providing decent child care when they cannot be at home. They must be kind and patient at all times and willingly make any sacrifice for their child's well-being. They must breastfeed (although never in public), so they must not ingest anything that might adulterate their milk with substances babies should not have. They must be involved in their children's schooling and supervise their studying, sleeping, computer, and eating habits, as well as knowing who their children's friends are. They must never let their children be out of doors unattended. And so on.

Matters are more complicated for women of color. Patricia Hill Collins neatly demonstrates how the stories of the Mammy, the Matriarch, and the Welfare Mother have been used to justify racist and sexist treatment of Black mothers. The Mammy, historically a slave and now a caregiver for more affluent White families, is a character created to justify the economic exploitation of domestic servants—she cares for her White children as "one of the family," so she works for love and she need not be paid much (Collins 1991, 71). She is a good mother so long as she stays in her place, but the Matriarch and the Welfare Mother are bad mothers. The Matriarch is the strong single mother who supports the household she heads by working outside the home, thereby emasculating her husband and failing to supervise her children adequately (Collins 1991, 74). It is these bad Black mothers who cause, in Daniel Patrick Moynihan's infamous words, "The disintegration of the Negro family" (Moynihan 1965). The Welfare Mother, who only became racialized in the 1930s, is "an updated version of the breeder woman image created during slavery [who] provides an ideological justification for efforts to harness black women's fertility to the needs of a changing political economy" (Collins 1991, 76). While the Breeder Woman was valued for her ability to produce children who could be sold, the Welfare Mother's children "no longer represent cheap labor but instead signify a costly threat to political and economic stability . . . [she is] content to sit around and collect welfare, shunning work and passing on her bad values to her offspring" (Collins 1991, 76–77).

These bad mothers are mirror images of what good mothers are supposed to be, and in that way they flesh out the master narrative of the good mother. Because many of that story's norms also establish how the pregnant woman herself is to behave, the good-mother narrative has a great deal in common with the (proleptic) expectant mother identity. The difficulty with it, of course, is that it unfairly constricts pregnant women's agency. Women who disobey its strict prescriptions can find themselves severely punished. Let's look first at what can happen to women who do not conform to the norms in the good-mother narrative, and then see how those norms carry over into the treatment of pregnant women.

In 1991, Denise Maupin went to her first day of work at a fast-food restaurant, leaving her 2-year-old son Michael and his sibling in the care of her boyfriend, Thomas Hale. While she was at work, and apparently acting out of rage *because* she was at work rather than looking after her children, Hale beat Michael nearly unconscious for wetting his pants. The boy was taken to a hospital, where he died that night. A Tennessee jury convicted her of aiding and abetting Michael's murder, apparently because she "failed" to protect him. She was sentenced to life imprisonment (Roberts 1999, 39).

When Casey Campbell got home after work on June 27, 1995, her live-in boyfriend, Floid Boyer, told her that her 4-year-old daughter had burned herself when he tripped and spilled coffee on her. She could see the burns were bad but did not want to get medical help because she was afraid to provoke Boyer, who had viciously abused her in the past. Around 2:00 in the morning, though, she took her daughter to the hospital, where the physician treating the burns called the police. Boyer was convicted of a misdemeanor, while Campbell herself was convicted of the far more serious crime of felony child endangerment (Fugate 2001, 272–273).

And according to Adam Banner, a criminal defense attorney who blogs for the *Huffington Post*,

> In 2006, Robert Braxton, Jr., pled guilty to abusing his girlfriend's three-month-old daughter by breaking her ribs and femur. He was sentenced to two years in prison. The infant's mother, Tondalo Hall, was found guilty of failing to protect her daughter and given a sentence of 30 years in prison. Even though there was no evidence that Hall ever hurt her daughter, and even though there was significant evidence that Hall was abused by Braxton and feared him, her sentence was 15 times greater than his. (Banner 2014)

On September 23, 2015, the Oklahoma Pardon and Parole Board refused to commute that sentence.

Defendants charged with failure to protect are almost always mothers. As one attorney observed, "In the 16 years I've worked in the courts, I have never seen a father charged with failure to protect when the mom is the abuser. Yet, in virtually every case where Dad is the abuser, we charge Mom with failure to protect" (Fugate 2001, 274).

In 2012 Kim Brooks left her 4-year-old son in her locked car for about 5 minutes while she ran into a shop to buy a set of headphones for him to use on a plane trip later that day. A bystander took a photo of the incident and called the police, who arrested her and charged her with "contributing to the delinquency of a minor." Her lawyer persuaded the prosecuting attorney to issue a continuance of the case and to drop the charge if Brooks agreed to perform 100 hours of community service and to undergo parenting education (Brooks 2014).

Other mothers are mocked, shamed, or scolded for allowing their children to walk home from school, ride the subway unattended, or play unsupervised in a nearby playground. They receive harsh criticism for not breastfeeding, for breastfeeding too long, for "letting" young children have meltdowns in public places, for being helicopter mothers, for being too strict or not strict enough. And, of course, mothers blame themselves for all these supposed failings as well.

The same norms of protection and care at any cost enter the expectant mother identity as well. Although the master narratives of pregnancy shown in the movies, on TV, in magazines, and on social media purport only to *represent* women engaging in various practices having to do with their pregnancies, many of them are in fact highly normative, shot through with "oughts," "shoulds," and "mustn'ts." If a woman does not do the things they prescribe, she is lazy, or neglectful, or selfish, or dangerous—in short, she is a morally bad mother, open to others' censure and sometimes to legal sanctions. The stories tell her to refrain from ingesting alcoholic and other adult beverages. They tell her to stop taking antihistamines and other over-the-counter drugs and start taking vitamins and folic acid. They tell her to get enough rest and exercise and to monitor her weight. They tell her to "avoid an array of foods from soft cheese to sushi, to sleep in a specified position (currently, avoiding stomach and back, with left side preferred to right), to avoid paint (including those with low volatile compounds), to avoid changing the cat litter, not to sit in the bathtub longer than 10 minutes, not to sample the cookie dough, to avoid loud music, and even to keep a laptop computer several inches from [her] pregnant bell[y], just in case" (Lyerly et al. 2009, 38).

Here too, failure to abide by the norms of the good-mother narrative can have disastrous consequences for the pregnant woman. For example, in 2014, when she was 12 weeks pregnant, Casey Gloria Allen was charged with criminal endangerment of a child—a felony—because she tested positive for narcotics (Marty 2014). It is not clear how the police knew she was pregnant, although there has been a sorry history, dating back at least as far as the Medical University of South Carolina's policy in the 1980s and 90s, of doctors secretly drug testing pregnant patients and reporting those who tested positive to law enforcement authorities. The National Advocates for Pregnant Women has documented hundreds of cases over the last 10 years in which pregnant women—a disproportionate number of them low income or women of color—were detained, arrested, or forced to accept treatment in the name of fetal protection. According to the *New York Times,* the most extreme example is Alabama, which, using a 2006 chemical endangerment law to prosecute about 100 women whose newborns tested positive for drugs, has sent several new mothers to prison (Eckholm 2013). What goes unreported, of course, is how few drug rehabilitation centers accept pregnant women.

The master narrative of the good mother, then, subjects pregnant women to vast amounts of social policing, treating them as potential criminals who cannot be trusted to carry their fetuses safely to term.

THE MASTER NARRATIVE OF THE PUBLIC BODY

Much of the power of identity-constituting master narratives lies in their masquerading as mere descriptions that make no evaluative demands on us. They operate subliminally, below the faculty of reason, so that they often remain entrenched even in the face of countervailing evidence. They do not have to make sense. And, in fact, they can flatly contradict one another and still remain interconnected. The master narratives of the public body and the fetal container are two such stories.

Whereas the narrative of the fetal container portrays the pregnant woman as merely a flowerpot, an inert object devoid of agency, the master narrative of the public body depicts her as all too agentic, constantly doing things. But, like a hyperactive 3-year-old, there is always a danger that what she does will get her into trouble, which is why she must be monitored. Whereas the story of the fetal container papers over the woman's activity of calling her fetus into personhood, the story of the public body shows the wider society doing just that—it treats the fetus proleptically, as if it were already a born child. But in this version of the story, it calls to the child by supervising the potentially unruly pregnant woman, so that the child can come to no harm from its mother's actions. We have already had a taste of this supervision in the punishment meted out to addicted pregnant women—the public body story is an offshoot of the narrative of the good mother—but it is not only the courts who treat the pregnant body as public. Ordinary citizens do it, too.

According to this story, it is fine for total strangers to pat a visibly pregnant woman's belly, because the pat is an affectionate expression of the society's role as the woman's minder. I once witnessed a man in a bar who was obviously acting on the story as he took a glass of wine away from a visibly pregnant woman, to approving glares from some of the bar's other patrons. The story also adds clout to the list of don'ts depicted by the story of the good mother, because it represents the society as the enforcer with the authority to manage the woman if she misbehaves.

Physicians and hospital administrators are just as eager to build pregnant women's identities around the public body narrative as laypeople are. According to *The New York Times*, for instance, a Florida woman, Samantha Burton, showed signs of miscarrying when 25 weeks pregnant. Her doctor advised her to go on bed rest, for perhaps as long as 15 weeks, but she told him she could not do that—she had two toddlers to care for and a job to keep. Before she could get a second opinion, the doctor alerted the authorities, who asked the Circuit Court of Leon County to intervene. The judge ordered her to stay in bed at Tallahassee Memorial Hospital and to undergo "any and all" medical treatments her doctor deemed necessary. Burton asked to be transferred to another hospital, only to be told that "such a change is not in the child's best interests at this time." Three days later she had to undergo an emergency cesarean section and the fetus was found to be dead (Belkin 2010).

Jennifer Goodall, who was 39 weeks pregnant and already had three children, received a letter dated July 10, 2014 from the Chief Financial Officer of a Florida hospital (why is it always Florida?), informing her that because she intended to undergo a trial labor before she would consent to a cesarean section, her doctors were going to report her to the Department of Children and Family Services, seek a court order to perform a cesarean, and do the surgery "with or without consent." Goodall's three previous deliveries had been by C-section, and based on those experiences and careful research, she had hoped to avoid one this time. There are minuscule risks attached to vaginal birth after cesarean section (VBAC), but undergoing cesarean section for the fourth time is also risky: it carries a 1 in 8 chance of major complications. When the National Advocates for Pregnant Women sought a restraining order to keep the hospital from following through on its threats, the Federal District Judge denied the request, stating that Goodall had no "right to compel a physician or medical facility to perform a medical procedure in the manner she wishes against their best medical judgment" (NAPW 2014). Rulings like this are consistently overturned on appeal, on the grounds that pregnant women retain their constitutional rights to refuse medical treatment and to bodily integrity, but by then the damage is usually already done.

COUNTERSTORIES

The master narratives of the public body, the good mother, and the fetal container each, in their own warped way, arise from the social world's practices of calling fetuses into personhood. The narratives all proleptically depict the fetus as the born child it will become, and they open up social space for it. But they are terrible stories, because in calling to the fetus, they degrade the gestating woman. They treat her as morally subpar and therefore not to be trusted with the baby in her care. This unfairly restricts the woman's moral agency—sometimes even to the point of immobilizing her in bed or in jail and taking the born child away from her.

So, what is to be done? First, even though these identity-damaging stories operate subliminally, so that pregnant women themselves can come to see themselves in the terms the stories reserve for them, it can, perhaps, be helpful if they and everyone else recognized the stories for what they are: sexist and racist mechanisms for keeping women in their place. Second, to counter the master narratives that damage pregnant women's identities, better stories need to be constructed and socially circulated, stories that more accurately represent the women and depict them as worthy of respect. Counterstories such as the one I have been telling about pregnant women calling their fetuses into personhood, are specifically designed to resist oppressive master narratives, and if they circulate widely enough alongside the ones that damage pregnant women's identities, they may eventually uproot the ones that do the damage.

Stories are not enough, of course. Pregnant women also need better material conditions—institutions, policies, and practices—if their work of pregnancy is to be properly valued and supported. Yet it seems to me that social progress requires the insight that is achieved not only by debunking existing oppressive identities, but finding morally better, more accurate ways of understanding who some of us are. This essay is meant to be one small contribution to that work of repair.

BIBLIOGRAPHY

Banner, Adam. 2014. "Failure to protect" laws punish victims of domestic violence. *Huffington Post.* http://www.huffingtonpost.com/adam-banner/do-failure-to-protect-law_b_6237346.html.

Belkin, Lisa. 2010. Is refusing bed rest a crime? *New York Times,* January 12.

Brooks, Kim. 2014. The day I left my son in the car. *Salon,* June 3. http://www.salon.com/2014/06/03/the_day_i_left_my_son_in_the_car/.

Chervenak, Frank A., and Laurence B. McCullough. 1996. The fetus as patient: An essential ethical concept for maternal-fetal medicine. *Journal of Maternal-Fetal and Neonatal Medicine* 5, no. 3: 115–119.

Collins, Patricia Hill. 1991. *Black feminist thought: Knowledge, consciousness, and the politics of empowerment.* New York: Routledge.

Cummings, Christy L., and Mark R. Mercurio. 2011. Maternal–fetal conflicts. In *Clinical ethics in pediatrics: A case-based textbook,* ed. Douglas S. Diekema, Mark R. Mercurio and Mary B. Adam. New York: Cambridge University Press.

Eckholm, Erik. 2013. Case explores rights of fetus versus mother. *New York Times,* October 23.

Fasouliotis, S. J., and J. G. Schenker. 2000. Maternal–fetal conflict. *European Journal of Obstetrics & Gynecology and Reproductive Biology* 89, no. 1: 101–107.

Fletcher, John C. 1981. The fetus as patient: Ethical issues. *Journal of the American Medical Association* 246, no. 7: 772–773.

Fugate, Jeanne A. 2001. Who's failing whom? A critical look at failure-to-protect laws. *New York University Law Review* 76 (April): 272–308.

Harrison, Michael R., and N. Scott Adzick. 1991. The fetus as a patient: Surgical considerations. *Annals of Surgery* 213, no. 4: 279.

Hawley, Katherine. 2001. *How things persist.* New York: Oxford University Press.

Howespian, A. A. 2008. Four queries concerning the metaphysics of embryogenesis. *Journal of Medicine and Philosophy* 33: 140–157.

Lenow, Jeffrey L. 1983. The fetus as a patient: Emerging rights as a person. *American Journal of Literature & Medicine* 9: 1.

Lindemann, Hilde. 2014. *Holding and letting go: The social practice of personal identities.* New York: Oxford University Press.

Lindemann Nelson, Hilde. 2001. *Damaged identities, narrative repair.* Ithaca, NY: Cornell University Press.

Little, Margaret Olivia. 1999. Abortion, intimacy, and the duty to gestate. *Ethical Theory and Moral Practice* 2: 295–312.

Lyerly, Anne Drapkin, Lisa M. Mitchell, Elizabeth Mitchell Armstrong, Lisa H. Harris, Rebecca Kukla, Miriam Kuppermann, and Margaret Olivia Little. 2009. Risk and the pregnant body. *Hastings Center Report* 39, no. 6: 34–42.

Mackenzie, Catriona. 1992. Abortion and embodiment. *Australasian Journal of Philosophy* 70, no. 2: 136–155.

Marty, Robin. 2014. Montana charges woman with "criminal child endangerment" at just 12 weeks' pregnant. *Care* 2. http://www.care2.com/causes/montana-charges-woman-with-criminal-endangerment-at-just-12-weeks-pregnant.html.

Mellor, Hugh. 2008. Microcomposition. *Royal Institute of Philosophy Supplement* 62: 65–80.

Mintz, Steven, and Susan Kellogg. 1989. *Domestic revolutions: A social history of American family life.* New York: Free Press.

Moynihan, Daniel Patrick. 1965. *The Negro Family: The Case for National Action.* Office of Policy Planning and Research, United States Department of Labor (March). https://www.dol.gov/oasam/programs/history/webid-meynihan.htm. Last visited August 16, 2016.

Murray, Thomas H. 1996. Moral obligations to the not-yet-born: The fetus as patient. In *The worth of a child, 96–114.* Berkeley: University of California Press.

NAPW. 2014. Florida hospital says it will force pregnant woman to have cesarean surgery. *Press release.* http://advocatesforpregnantwomen.org/blog/2014/07/press_release_florida_hospital.php

Oderberg, David S. 2008. The metaphysical status of the embryo: Some arguments revisited. *Journal of Applied Philosophy* 25: 263–276.

Oduncu, F. S., R. Kimmig, H. Hepp, and B. Emmerich. 2003. Cancer in pregnancy: Maternal-fetal conflict. *Journal of Cancer Research and Clinical Oncology* 129, no. 3: 133–146.

Phelan, J. 1991. The maternal abdominal wall: A fortress against fetal health care? *Southern Californian Law Review* 65, no. 1: 461–490.

Roberts, Dorothy. 1999. Mothers who fail to protect their children. In Julia Hanigsberg and Sara Ruddick, eds., *Mother troubles: Rethinking contemporary maternal dilemmas, 31–49.* Boston: Beacon Press.

Ruddick, William. 2000. Ways to limit prenatal resting. In ed. Adrienne Asch and Erik Parens, *Prenatal testing and disability rights, 95–107.* Washington, DC: Georgetown University Press.

Smith, Barry, and Berit Brogaard. 2003. Sixteen days. *Journal of Medicine and Philosophy* 28: 45–78.

Young, Iris Marion. 1984. Pregnant embodiment: Subjectivity and alienation. *Journal of Medicine and Philosophy* 9: 45–62.

PART IV

LAST BUT NOT LEAST: ZYGOTE, BLASTOCYST, EMBRYO, FETUS, NEWBORN

CHAPTER 24

···

CONTEMPLATING THE START OF SOMEONE

···

ADAM KADLAC

In the latter stages of *Reasons and Persons*, Derek Parfit introduces the following example:

> *The 14-Year-Old Girl.* This girl chooses to have a child. Because she is so young, she gives her child a bad start in life. Though this will have bad effects throughout this child's life, his life will, predictably, be worth living. If this girl had waited for several years, she would have had a different child, to whom she would have given a better start in life. (1984, 358)

This feature of the 14-year-old girl's predicament creates tension in our assessment of her situation once the child has been born. Though we may still think that it was a mistake for her to have a child, we will generally be unwilling to say that it would have been better if the resulting child did not exist.[1]

Remarking on this example, David Velleman thus writes:

> We think that the birth of a child to a fourteen-year-old mother will be unfortunate, even tragic, and hence that she should not decide to have one. But after the birth, we are loath to say that the child should not have been born. Indeed, we now think that the birth is something to celebrate—once a year, on the child's birthday. (2008, 267)

The girl may later note that having a child at the age of 14 made her life difficult in ways that could have been avoided had she made different choices. But she may be unwilling to trade the life she has now for the life she would have had without her child. In other words, she may fully acknowledge the burdens that her choice has placed on her, and the various ways she has disadvantaged her child, but she may nevertheless be unable to fully regret her decision.

Various attempts have been made to explain how we can adopt these conflicting views of the past without straightforward contradiction. While I am sympathetic to many of these approaches, my aim in the present work is to offer my own account, one which appeals centrally to the notion of our identity as the particular persons we are. My central thesis is that the valence of this identity shifts over time as it becomes more cemented by historical events and our entwinement with those around us. As a result, the reason-giving force of one's status as a particular individual also varies over time in ways that explain the normative and experiential tensions surrounding these sorts of cases. Once this feature of personal identity is in view, the ambiguities in our assessments of the past are not problematic; they are instead largely expected features of our experience.

My discussion proceeds as follows. In the first section, I canvass some of the more recent attempts to understand our ambivalence regarding various events in the past, especially those incidents that have led to our existence. While there are potential problems with these accounts, I think that all of the leading views on offer have something to recommend them. In the second and third sections, I show how a focus on our identity as particular persons helps make sense of what is worth preserving in these accounts. I then conclude in the final section by suggesting some implications of my view for our reflections about what it means to become a parent.

PROBING RETROSPECTIVE AMBIVALENCE

In his own analysis of the case of the 14-year-old girl, Parfit primarily draws a lesson about the impersonal value of various states of affairs. According to Parfit, to say that the girl should not have a child is to say that the overall state of affairs in which she does not have a child is better than a state of affairs in which she does. Thus, if the girl retrospectively concludes that she should not have become a mother at 14, she is committed to the claim that the world would have been a better place without her child. Such a conclusion may be unsettling, but "if we claimed earlier that it would be better if this girl waits, this is what we must claim. We cannot consistently make a claim and deny this same claim later" (1984, 360).

Despite this assessment, Parfit denies that the girl has reason to regret her decision to have a child, all things considered. She may have a basis for some *moral* regret, presumably in light of her failure to bring about the best state of affairs possible. However, the fact that she loves the child, and thinks that his life has genuine value "is enough to block the claim that she is irrational if she does not have such regret" (1984, 306–301). On Parfit's view, the girl's ambivalence arises as a tension between a distinctively moral form of reflection—one which takes a global view of alternative states of affairs and considers which one is best—and a reflective stance which focuses solely on the value of the resulting child. Adopting the former perspective leads to a particularly moral kind of regret, while her justified appreciation of her son keeps her from experiencing what R. Jay Wallace calls all-in regret: "a stable reaction of sorrow or pain about a past action or circumstance, taking into account the totality of subsequent events that [one is] aware of having been set in motion by it" (2008, 51). In other words, the girl may regret her decision morally, but she does not wish that she would have made a different one.

Jeff McMahan ties his discussion of this issue more specifically to reflection on having children with disabilities. As a result, he is concerned with how we can make sense of the fact that many prospective parents would prefer to have children who are not disabled, even as they "confidently anticipate, from their prospective point of view, that if they were to have a disabled child, they too would come to believe that their life with a disabled child was better than life without a child would have been" (2005, 154). Thus, on McMahan's view, there is ambiguity even as one contemplates the possibility of having a disabled child, an ambiguity that is often confirmed in the ways people experience being the parent of a child with disabilities. Individuals may consistently express a preference to have children who are not disabled, but once those children are on the scene, parents are often glad to have had them.[2] Moreover, they often believe that this is how they will feel, despite consistently expressing a preference for nondisabled children.

According to McMahan, what accounts for these differing judgments is a shift of values, one that is common among many parents, not just those who have disabled children. He writes:

> In general, when people have their first child the priorities among their values tend to alter, often quite rapidly. The child becomes their primary focus of concern and their principal source of gratification. Their work, hobbies, and recreations, and even their relations with their spouse and friends, all begin to matter less. This process occurs in parents of disabled children in much the same way that it does in other parents. (2005, 156)

Thus, the prospective judgment about whether it is better to have a child with disabilities or no child at all is made with respect to one's values at the time of the judgment—in this case, the time before one has any children. The retrospective judgment, on the other hand, is made with respect to the values one has after becoming the parent to a particular child.

What is crucial for McMahan's overall view is not simply the contention that our values often change in the ways he suggests. That much seems largely uncontroversial. The key claim is that both the prospective and retrospective judgments can be true. To buttress this idea, McMahan appeals to a pluralism according to which there may be a variety of different values that we can use to organize and direct our lives, all of which are more or less on a par.[3] If, then, "the different personal values of *different people* may be on a par, so may the different personal values that the *same person* may have at *different times*" (2005, 163, emphasis his). For example, if one person can live a good life while choosing not to have any children (because, say, having children will inhibit her from achieving certain other goals that she takes to be important), at the same time as another person lives a good life in choosing to have a child she knows will be disabled, why cannot the same person adopt each of those viewpoints at different times in her life? As

McMahan puts it, "[o]ne's preferences will rationally be dictated by the defensible values that are operative within one's life at the time" (2005, 164). And since those values can change, different preferences can be equally well justified at different times.

Velleman's take on the girl's retrospective ambivalence is to suggest that we can all view her child in two different ways. On the one hand, we can approach her descriptively—under the generic heading of "child of a 14-year-old girl." On the other hand, we can think of her demonstratively as the particular child she is: "this baby" or "her" (2008, 269). The former, descriptive, approach will yield an unfavorable judgment regarding the girl's decision to become a mother (since, we might think to ourselves, 14-year-olds should not be parents) at the same time as we wholeheartedly embrace the existence of the particular child in front of us. As Velleman puts it, the reason our judgments that the girl made a mistake in having the child "withstand our favorable judgment about the baby is that, whereas they rely on descriptions, the favorable judgment is about the baby considered demonstratively" (2008, 269). Given that we can view others through either of these different lenses, we can, therefore, move back and forth between various evaluative judgments about the child and the mother's decision without contradiction.

In his recent meditation on regret, Wallace considers all of these accounts and finds them wanting. To begin with, he argues that Parfit's separation of moral regret and all-things-considered regret is inconsistent. According to Wallace, if it really is the case that the existence of the child is not for the best, then "there is nothing in their evaluative outlook that would render it rational for them not to experience all-in regret about the fact that [the child] was born" (2013, 82). For Parfit, the all-things-considered perspective and the moral perspective are conflated—since they both compare total world states of affairs—and so Wallace thinks there is no way for Parfit to maintain the distinction he wants to maintain (at least in the way he wants to maintain it).

Wallace's criticism of McMahan rests on the seeming arbitrariness of adopting a given set of values at one point in time only to adopt a different set at some later time. On Wallace's view, McMahan's pluralist account gives us "no rational basis for choosing between the values that inform judgments of the prospective and the actual parents of the disabled children" (2013, 84). It may very well be the case that individuals adopt different sets of values at different points in their lives. However, without some explanation of how these different values are *appropriate* responses to one's changing circumstances, any shift of this sort is rationally arbitrary—a peculiar and contingent fact about the psychology of many people who have children rather than "something that is called for by [their] situation, as a correct response to the fact of [a] child's involvement in [one's] life" (2013, 85).

Finally, Wallace criticizes Velleman's approach on the grounds that it attempts to cleanly separate modes of thinking about the 14-year-old's child that are too often run together. Thus, while we may be able to think of the child either demonstratively or descriptively, we can also think of her "through hybrid modes of presentation, such as 'this child, who is the daughter of a fourteen-year-old girl,'" and it is not clear to Wallace what sort of evaluative response is appropriate to this mode of thought (2013, 88). He writes:

> Insofar as it is demonstrative, one would expect it to give rise to the kind of all-things-considered affirmation that is characteristic of love. Yet insofar as it applies to

the child the offending description, it should also express the attitude of all-things-considered rejection that is characteristic of regret. But there is no way of combining complete affirmation and rejection in this way, which is to say that there is no stable set of differently valenced attitudes toward the child that is channeled through demonstrative and descriptive modes of presentation. (2013, 88)

Differing approaches to the child seem to yield totalizing and unambiguous responses that cannot coexist in any stable way when a descriptive approach is combined with a demonstrative one.

Wallace's own solution to the puzzle is to appeal to the ways in which the 14-year-old's normative predicament changes upon the birth of her child. Prior to her decision to get pregnant, she has very good reasons to refrain from so doing—reasons grounded in the strain that having a child will put on her life as well as the limitations she is likely to have as a child trying to parent another child. These reasons combine to justify the conclusion that she should not decide to have a child of her own. But Wallace suggests that the normative landscape changes once the child is on the scene, because the attachment she now has to the child will furnish reasons for her to care for the child that she does not have to care for mere strangers. He thus concludes that "[r]esponding appropriately to the reasons of this kind that her new situation brings in its train, the young girl will naturally affirm and celebrate her child, cherishing her daughter and her daughter's role in her own life" (2013, 90). The girl's values might change over time in a way that justifies a different assessment of her decision to have the child after she is born. However, that change is grounded in her circumstances such that it is neither contingent nor arbitrary but is instead responsive to the value of the child who now exists.

Despite his criticisms of McMahan's account, I think that Wallace's view is best seen as a supplement to McMahan's emphasis on the ways our values might change over time. Wallace's objection seems not to be focused on McMahan's contention that our values change, nor even that our values have an important role to play in shaping the reasons we have to respond to our circumstances in one way rather than another. His primary concern is instead with the seeming arbitrariness of the values that McMahan's position officially allows. Wallace's appeal to the value of the resulting child—and the value of the relationships that various individuals are able to develop with that child—thus provide justification for the change that takes place in the 14-year-old's evaluative outlook as well as the evaluative outlooks of those who may be less directly invested in the situation. In this way, Wallace thinks he has an explanation for what, on McMahan's view, is arbitrary.

What thus distinguishes Parfit and Velleman from Wallace and McMahan is their commitment to see greater ambivalence in our judgments at a single time as opposed to looking at the ways in which those judgments change over time. For Parfit, the 14-year-old girl can experience moral regret about her decision to have a child at the same time she is unable to experience all-things-considered regret about that decision. And Velleman likewise contends that we are able to simultaneously approach others in both a descriptive and demonstrative manner. As I have noted, the simultaneity of these assessments is what Wallace largely objects to in their views, but the contrast between changing judgments over time and ambivalent judgments at a single time may be a helpful way to group the accounts on offer.

My aim in the next section is to more or less adopt the Wallace/McMahan framework and examine in more detail precisely why it is that the present existence of an individual person—as opposed to their merely possible or future existence—can have the kind of effect on us that is so central to their views. What is it, exactly, about the presence of a particular person that justifies the change in the normative landscape to which Wallace and McMahan appeal? While they are correct, in my view, to highlight this change, I think that more could be said about the process by which it occurs and whether that process is itself justified.

My central contention, then, is that an appreciation for the ways in which our identities as particular persons unfold over time—that is, the ways in which we are constituted as the individuals we are as we interact and develop a shared history with others—both explains changes in our normative landscape and provides reasons for us to think that those changes should occur. Importantly, when this account is fully in view, I think that it also lends support to the ways in which Parfit and Velleman maintain the possibility of simultaneously embracing two different (and seemingly contradictory) judgments about one's past decisions. Thus, if what I say is compelling, then distinctions of the sort they advocate are important tools for reflecting on our past choices, our present circumstances, and our relationships to people who are deeply implicated in both.

OUR UNFOLDING IDENTITIES

In invoking the notion of identity, I have in mind what Marya Schechtman has connected to the notion of an "identity crisis" rather than the sense of identity that people have in mind when they are concerned to identify those properties that make an individual at t1 the same person as an individual at t2. She thus writes that, in this context, "identity" refers "to the set of characteristics each person has that make her the person she is. In an identity crisis, a person is unsure about what those defining features are, and so is unsure of his identity" (1996, 74). Most of us, at some point or other, struggle to understand who we are as individuals because we recognize that such an understanding locates us in the natural and social worlds in which we find ourselves. As Charles Taylor has put it, an identity "is the background against which our tastes and desires and opinions and aspirations make sense" (1991, 34).

Various features of these identities are, then, fixed upon our entrance into the world. To begin with, we are all constrained by the truism that we could not have been different people than we are. To paraphrase Bishop Butler: "Everyone is who they are, and not another person." More particularly, our biological parentage seems necessary to our identity as the particular persons we are even to the point that, as David DeGrazia puts it, "none of us could have derived from a different set of gametes than those from which he or she did derive" (2005, 270). Thus, it seems that each possible combination of sperm and egg, to say nothing of each possible combination of parents, would yield a different person.

One might be inclined to deny that these historical contingencies are necessary to our identity, perhaps on the grounds that human beings are not identical to their bodies and so might have had different bodies than they, in fact, have. These views face serious metaphysical difficulties.[4] But even if these difficulties can be overcome, and we conclude that human beings are immaterial minds or souls, or composite entities made up of both material and immaterial parts, rejecting the necessity of origins runs into two significant problems. First, it straightforwardly violates our sense that there is an important connection between who we are as individuals and the historical circumstances that led up to our birth. As Parfit poses the challenge, "how many of us could truly claim, 'Even if railways and motor cars had never been invented, I would still have been born?' " (1984, 361). Perhaps there are some who would grant that they might have existed even if their biological parents had never met, but that seems a significant bullet to bite—one that makes utterly mysterious any connection between our genetic makeup, our parentage, and numerous physical and psychological characteristics we happen to have.

Perhaps more important, in the present context, denying the necessity of origins would change the metric that produces our ambivalence in cases like those of the 14-year-old girl. If each of us could have been the product of gametes other than those which, in fact, produced us, then she could have had *the very same child* at a later time when she was better equipped to satisfy the demands of parenting. She might not know that she would have had the same child. Nevertheless, believing that she might have enjoyed the benefits of having that very child without saddling her child with the burdens of being raised by a young mother would likely temper the degree to which she appreciates her present circumstances. Whatever reticence she has about regretting her decision is tied up with her belief that the positive features of her current predicament could only have come about through that very decision. Getting rid of that commitment would thereby undermine that reticence.

If, then, being the child of our parents is a feature of our identity that is fixed from conception, other aspects of our identity are likewise determined at that time. The genetic contributions of our parents combine to give us the physical appearance we have throughout our lives: hair color, eye color, nose shape, hand size, and so on. Some of these characteristics may change down the line. We can choose to dye our hair or have plastic surgery to alter the shape of our noses; we might break bones growing up and so change the look of various appendages; and numerous environmental factors will no doubt influence what we look like at any given point in time. But regardless of what happens in the future, we come into the world with physical characteristics that are not of our own making and which constitute the first exposure that others have to us.

Moreover, to the degree that there is a genetic basis for our personality traits and intellectual and physical abilities, these are also set from birth. Again, our environment undoubtedly has an important role to play in how these various abilities are developed. But it was probably set from my conception that I was not going to be an NBA point guard. While I may have possessed minimal skill in dribbling and shooting that could have been developed somewhat further through hours and hours of practice, I have no trouble admitting that my talent probably took me as far as it could: getting cut from my eighth-grade team. My basketball ability was simply not enough to allow me to overcome my unimposing 5′ 10′ frame. The rhetoric that we can accomplish whatever we set our minds to accomplish may be inspiring, but it belies the fact that some possible futures are closed to us even before our birth.

While characteristics of this sort clearly play a significant role in determining the person we will become over the course of our lives, our identities remain a predominantly open question at these early stages. We may have brown hair and brown eyes, and we may lack the genetic makeup required to develop an effective crossover dribble or consistent jump shot. As a result, all of the high school girls who are attracted to boys with blond hair and blue eyes are unlikely to be our prom dates, and any future in basketball is unlikely to extend much past the schoolyard. Nevertheless, innumerable possibilities remain open to us: relationships, intellectual interests, athletic pursuits, careers, hobbies, and so on. We may be able to rule out ahead of time certain courses our lives might take, but we will not be able to say with any confidence who we will be in ten, twenty, or fifty years or what route we will take to arrive at that point. Our lives are yet to unfold, and all the experiences, relationships, and accomplishments that will further constitute us as the particular persons we are have yet to occur.

For my purposes, what is significant about the ongoing development of our identities is that we can say comparatively little about precisely who someone is early in that person's life. A newborn girl may be the brown-eyed, brown-haired daughter of a particular man and woman. And she may have a genetic makeup that equips her for some successful years on the high school cross-country team and a career down the line as a biomedical engineer. But whether she will take those paths remains to be seen, as do all the facts about what friends she will make and lose, what hearts she will break and who will break her heart, what subjects she will find interesting in school, or whether she will prefer the arts to athletics. As a result, any attachment we might form to her as the particular person she is will lack a great deal of content in the early stages of her life, since the precise nature of that attachment's object is only very partially determined.

To point out the comparative lack of content in our attachments to very young children is not to deny that these attachments might nevertheless be formed quite strongly. Indeed, given the necessity of origins, I am inclined to see the attachments that parents often form to their newborn children as attachments to those children as the particular individuals they are. Parents might have had similar attachments to any of their possible children; they would, in all likelihood, have loved any child they might have had whether it was a boy instead of a girl or had come out with different hair color and different eye color. However, because any parent who loves his or her child loves an individual who is essentially his or her offspring, parental love seems to focus on individuals whose identity is constituted by having the parents they have. In other words, parental love is a unique case of love for individuals precisely as the individuals they are.

Nevertheless, despite the strength of these sorts of attachments, they are not grounded in much knowledge of who, precisely, the child is. If asked why he loves his newborn daughter, a father might claim that he loves her simply because she is his daughter, and in so doing, he might be expressing an attachment to her as the particular person she is. But that is nearly all he can say about his love. He does not love her because of her appearance; presumably, he would have loved any of his children no matter what they looked like. And he does not love her because of any other aspect of her identity because so much of her identity is yet to be determined. Thus, his attachment to her as the particular person she is may be exceedingly strong, but there is almost nothing he can say at this stage to give others any more information regarding the object of his attachment. That attachment may be exceedingly powerful, but its contours are not well defined; it lacks a measure of depth and nuance because the full nature of its object is yet to be determined.

Moreover, few others will have sufficient reason to love the girl as the particular person she is. Perhaps close friends and loved ones will love her simply because she is the daughter of someone they know and care about. However, the circle of that specific type of concern is unlikely to extend much further. To be sure, strangers and mere acquaintances will celebrate the child's birth and regard her as worthy of moral esteem. But they would respond similarly to strangers they have never met and to whom they have no personal connection. We may celebrate the birth of a coworker's child, and yet, unless we are exceptionally close friends with that coworker, it would be odd for us to announce that, upon that child's entrance into the world, we loved that child as the particular individual she is.

However, the possibility of adding depth and nuance to our attachments increases over time as our lives unfold and our identities take on more content. We not only develop more clearly defined personality traits that heavily influence the ways in which others relate to us. We also develop a track record of accomplishment and relational interactions with others. We are no longer merely the children of our parents who have a particular color of hair and eyes but instead become individuals who roll over at 6 months of age, crawl at 9 months, and walk at 1 year, all while giving our parents memories of sleepless nights, walks in the park, and the occasional anxious trip to the pediatrician's office.

As our personal histories become more detailed, so do the attachments that others might form to us. Viewed as individuals, more can be said of us over time because there is more that is true of us. We develop from infants into toddlers, toddlers into children with increasingly defined personalities, from children into adolescents, and so on. And at each step along the way, we add more to our personal profile as individuals who have done and experienced particular things at particular times and places. We get game-winning hits (or game losing strikeouts) in little league; we get our driver's licenses and go to the prom; we choose colleges (or not) and graduate (or not); we get married (or not), have children (or not), and face all of the unique challenges that every individual life has to offer.

Importantly, even as the various incidents in our lives constitute us as the particular persons we are, they also serve as formative contexts for our relationships with others. We do not typically go through life alone. We far more often experience it together with others, and the shared histories that result from our interactions with those others become essential components of the relationships we regard as most important. It is one thing to have a conversation with a person you like well enough and with whom you share a number of interests. It is another thing to converse with someone you have known for 25 years—someone with whom you share memories of numerous life events. The ability to jointly remember the past enables an intimacy in our present interactions because those who have known us for a long time know where we have been and what we have done. They have, in many cases, been there with us and helped us achieve our goals—they have laughed and cried with us through good times and bad—and as a result, they know most fully who we are.

Nowhere is this dynamic more on display than in the relationships that often develop between parents and children. Not only are parents frequently present for a greater percentage of their children's lives than most any other individual throughout a child's early years; parents are also uniquely responsible for a child's well-being during what is arguably the most vulnerable time of life. As a result, parents are able to watch a child's life unfold from the very beginning and actively participate in the course that life takes. In feeding their children—in changing, bathing, and rocking them to sleep—parents not only provide life-sustaining care; they become part of their children's histories. Whatever else we accomplish in the future—wherever else we go and whatever else we do—we will always be individuals who had our diapers changed by particular individuals at particular times and places. And quite often, those individuals are our parents.

Even at this early stage, then, crucial differences begin to emerge between the attachment that a parent might form with any prospective child and the unfolding nature of that attachment as it relates to an existing child. Parents may know that they will love any child they might have as the particular child she is, and to the degree that our identities are constituted by our parentage, there will be some minimal content to this attachment. But that content pales in comparison to the record of shared experiences that is accumulated once the child is born and parents begin to care for her. One's sense of the child as the particular child she is becomes linked to the particular scenes of interaction with that child in ways that are wholly unique to each child and cannot be predicted ahead of time.

All prospective parents know they will change diapers and feed their children. But they cannot know the particularities of those interactions or the effect on those interactions of historical circumstances, each child's personality, and myriad other influences. As a result, they cannot know exactly what it will mean to be attached to any particular child as the particular child she is until after that child's identity begins to take shape in the context of various contingent historical circumstances. We may know before the child is born that she will take on some identity or other because her life will begin to unfold through some set of circumstances or other. However, without knowing exactly what those circumstances will be, the attachment is largely hypothetical.

This relationship between our attachment to particular individuals and the developing of a shared history with those individuals may explain why some parents report having difficulties in developing (what they regard as) appropriate feelings of attachment to their children. Michael Lewis thus writes that after the birth of his son, Walker, his time was largely occupied with work and caring for his two daughters. As a result, he spent comparatively little time with his son until a bout with respiratory syncytial virus landed Walker in the hospital. Working to minimize the various intrusions of hospital personnel into Walker's room, Lewis writes that he finally devoted significant time to his son's care and, in so doing, came to feel about Walker as he already felt about his daughters.

He thus writes of the experience:

> I change his diapers and feed him and suction the mucus from his nose. I notice for the first time that he has my hands and feet. I study the little heart-shaped birthmark on the back of his head. I discover that if I hold him to my chest and hum against the back of his neck, he falls right to sleep. Tabitha [Lewis's wife] comes and offers to take over, but the truth is I don't want to leave: He feels like my jurisdiction. After every new child, I learn the same lesson, grudgingly: If you want to feel the way you're meant to feel about the new baby, you need to do the grunt work. It's only in caring for a thing that you become attached to it. (2010, 162–163)

There is no reason to doubt that Lewis loved his son prior to this stay in the hospital. Nevertheless, more direct and sustained interaction with Walker enabled him to develop a more intimately shared history with his son which thereby gave more content to his love for Walker as the particular person he is. What started merely as a comparatively generic attachment to "my son" ended as an attachment to "my son whose blood oxygen level I assiduously monitored and out of whose nose I suctioned life-threatening mucus over the course of several nights in the hospital." Lewis's resulting attachment to his son was thus shaped by the emotional resonances of Walker's ordeal as well as their respective identities as the individuals who endured it.[5]

Wallace is, therefore, correct to highlight the role that existing attachments play in altering our normative landscape. Before a child is born, our attachments to particular others cannot play a substantive role in our deliberations because they do not yet exist—the objects of such attachments are simply not around to play that kind of role. However, as it stands, Wallace's account leaves the nature of this shift somewhat underdescribed. After all, most of us can predict with overwhelming accuracy that we will love our children as the particular children they are. Indeed, many people might offer the possibility of such love as a reason for having children in the first place, and they may be entirely right to do so.[6] Thus, the 14-year-old girl in all likelihood believes that she will love any child she might have in this way, and to the degree she is correct, there would seem to be some reason for her to have a child, even at such a young age.

What the 14-year-old girl does not have, and cannot have, prior to that child's existence is any shared history with that child—a shared history that constitutes both of them as the particular individuals they are. She may believe (and perhaps even know) that she will love any child she might have. But she cannot know who, precisely, that child will be, and thus any prospective attachment to that child will lack the detail of her ongoing attachment to the child once it is born. She may know that she will share experiences and participate in activities together with that child. And while she may not know exactly what it will be like to create such memories and have her life progressively intertwined with her son or daughter, she may justifiably believe that these things will occur. However, she cannot know precisely what form that intertwinement will take or what the scenes of interaction with the child will be since those matters await to be determined.

As a result, there are reasons she can give for her attachment as it unfolds that are unavailable to her (or anyone else, for that matter) before the child exists. She no doubt loves the child simply because he is her son. But as time goes on, her attachment also includes the track record of joint experiences that they build up together. She becomes attached to him as the one whom she nursed through a difficult illness and who spit up on her dress at a friend's wedding. The attachments we have to individuals because of the histories we, in fact, share with them are qualitatively different from the attachments we might have to those with whom we are more tangentially acquainted. And they certainly exercise a different influence on our lives than any hypothetical attachment we might form to individuals who do not yet exist.

I want to suggest, then, that it is not enough to say that the shift that interests Wallace and McMahan is occasioned merely by the brute presence of a child to whom the girl happens to have a particularly strong attachment. Rather, what is most crucially at issue is the unique and particular history that she develops with her child—a history that cannot be predicted in advance and which gives that attachment its particular character because it constitutes both individuals as the particular individuals they are.

I think invoking the significance of individual identity at this point provides a more illuminating way to think about the change of values to which McMahan appeals and for which Wallace seeks justification. The emergence of a child for whom one has some responsibility no doubt leads one to reconsider one's priorities. But it is more specifically the track record that one develops with that person that makes it increasingly difficult to imagine one's life without him or her and, as a result, to shift one's goals and aspirations in ways that account for that person's future. In shaping the identity of another human being—and in having one's own identity shaped in return—one begins to view the prospect of a life without that other as the life of someone else. And to the degree that we find our own lives satisfying and rewarding—and to the degree that we regard those other individuals as importantly contributing to that satisfaction—we will regard it as unthinkable to exchange the life we have for the life of someone else.

It is at this point that our existing attachments exercise their normative pull on us. To contemplate a life without certain particular others is not only to consider a life without individuals in whose formation we have been instrumental; it is also to contemplate the rejection of oneself as the particular individual one has become. As Wallace notes, the attachments we have to our own lives run exceedingly deep. It may be theoretically possible to reject our identities as the particular individuals we are, but for most of us, "[t]he same vital forces that lead us to cling to life as we are living also give rise to an unconditional preference to have lived—a preference, looking backward to have lived our actual lives, as against the alternative that we should not have lived at all" (2013, 255). Thus, to the degree that we affirm our own lives, and our own identities as the particular individuals we are, we should be correspondingly reluctant to regret the existence of those who have shaped our identities.

TROUBLING IDENTITIES: MORALITY AND THE DESCRIPTION/ DEMONSTRATION DISTINCTION

Assessments of cases like the 14-year-old girl tend to assume that things work out fairly well for both the girl and her child. In other words, whatever resistance we have to regret in this scenario arises largely because the 14-year-old's life is enriched in numerous ways by the presence of a child whose own life is, on the whole, a good one. However, any clear-eyed discussion of such cases must acknowledge that not everyone has a similar experience. For some, decisions to have children inflict considerable burdens on others—not just the resulting child, but family, friends, and members of the wider community. In other cases, the individuals who result from such choices do not seem to add value to one's life, and as a result, they do not lead one to be particularly attached to one's own life or the particular person one has become. Having argued that the unfolding nature of our identities supports the Wallace/McMahan analysis of these sorts of cases, I turn now to the distinctions invoked by Parfit and Velleman because I think that, suitably refined, they provide some useful resources for thinking about the darker side of this issue.

As I have noted, Parfit argues that there is an important difference between moral regret and all-things-considered regret—that the 14-year-old girl has moral reason to regret her decision to have a child on the grounds that she did not produce the best possible outcome from her circumstances, even though the love she has for her child entails that she cannot fully regret her decision to become a mother. This distinction strikes me as an important one and tracks a distinction that others have drawn between regret and remorse.[7] But whereas Parfit wants to explicate the distinctly moral dimensions of the girl's choice in terms of the contribution she has (or has not) made to the overall happiness in the world, I think it is better to view the moral features of her predicament in terms of how it might be possible to wrong any of the parties involved—for example, her parents, the child's father, and any child who might result from her actions. In other words, distinctively moral consideration of her actions—the sort of reflection that might occasion remorse on her part—should view her actions in relation to particular others rather than the world as a whole.[8]

Taking this perspective, it is possible to see ways in which the 14-year-old girl might experience remorse about her decision. She might, perhaps, think that she has wronged her parents by failing to heed their wishes and advice about whether to become a mother. Seeing in retrospect that they had her best interest at heart, she may regard her past stubbornness as an unfortunate sign of disrespect, and she may experience moral regret as a result of that assessment. Or she may think that the father of her child has been unfairly saddled with responsibilities that he would be better off not having. To be sure, his actions played a part in the resulting circumstances, and had they both made different choices, the challenges they now face could have been avoided. But the thought that she did not fully consider how the decision to have a child would affect him might also lead to some appropriately moral regret on her part.

When her thoughts turn to her child, the relationship between moral regret and other sorts of regret becomes more complicated. Leaving aside the vexed question of whether it was possible to wrong someone who did not exist at the time she made the decision to become a mother, she might experience distinctively moral regret for failing to care for the child to the best of her ability once the child was born. And it is possible that this mode of reflection would lead her to think that she has wronged the child by deciding to raise her. Despite her attachment to the child, and the ways in which the history she shares with her daughter has shaped her own identity, she may think that the child would have been better off raised by someone else and that she has wronged the child by attempting to do what she was not well equipped to do. These feelings may sensibly conflict with the emotional and normative pull of her attachment to the child. Nevertheless, having made the decision to raise the child, the girl cannot now contemplate her life without her daughter and thus may not experience all-in regret about the decision. Put differently, she may experience some remorse about her decision without being able to wish that she had done otherwise.[9]

I do not mean to imply that in every instance in which a 14-year-old girl decides to raise her child, she thereby wrongs that child. It may very well be that some girls in such a predicament do well by their children in raising them, or at least do well enough such that the children are better off than they would be raised by someone else. Nor do I mean to ignore the fact that having chosen to raise the child, new possibilities for wronging the child arise as a result of the shared history they begin to develop. For example, the choice to have someone else raise the child after 4 years of caring for him may wrong the child in ways that giving him up for adoption at birth would not.[10]

What I do mean to highlight, however, is that in all of these cases, the specifically moral assessment can coexist with a different all-things-considered assessment of both the girl's circumstances and the choices that led to them. We can agree that the girl wronged her parents by choosing to have a child even as we appreciate the ways in which her life has been enhanced by the presence of the particular child she has raised. Morality is but one aspect of a life well lived, and while it may be the case that the best sorts of lives contain little to no immorality, the fact that we have sometimes wronged others does not mean that we cannot also appreciate the presence of other goods in our lives.

Morality can take on a different significance when the shared history that one develops with an individual forcefully calls into question whether one made the right decision in having a child. While we may be reluctant to acknowledge them, the experiences that some parents have with their children lead them to question whether they would do it all over again, if they had the chance. And at the extreme end of this spectrum are those whose dissatisfaction with the lives they share with their children leads them to end those lives: the lives of their children, their own, or both.

An example of this phenomenon is the troublingly high rate of filicide among parents of autistic children. As Andrew Solomon has written,

> having a child who does not express love in a comprehensible way is devastating, and having a child who is awake all night, who requires constant supervision, and who screams and tantrums but cannot communicate the reasons for or the nature of his upset—these experiences are confusing, overwhelming, exhausting, and unrewarding. (2012, 290)

Some parents who find themselves in this predicament thus resort to violent measures as a way of ending their struggles. Such incidents may not be common in any absolute sense, but the fact that they occur at all is a stark illustration of the fact that some parents have an exceedingly difficult time with the particular children they have. While all parents likely struggle to love their children as well as they can, and probably endure days when they do not particularly like their children, Solomon directs our attention to those who find their children unbearable. The shared history they have developed with those children is not one they value; they do not value who they have become as a result of this history; and they would be more than willing to exchange their lives for the lives of others. They would, in short, be happy to have different children and be themselves different people as a result.

In this context, perhaps moral considerations do not call into question the value of one's present circumstances so much as provide reasons for one to persevere through circumstances that one does not especially value. Whereas the particular identity of one's child can sometimes neutralize the regret one feels about past moral failings, the demands of morality can sometimes prevent us from wronging those whose particular identities may lead us into darker places. The parent of the severely autistic child may be unable to regard that child's identity as a reason to remain attached to him. Indeed, the pain and suffering caused by the child may seem to provide good reasons to sever any relationship to him by ending his life. But the fact that adopting this course of action would severely wrong the child should be enough to keep despondent parents from going down that road and to instead pursue other means to dealing with their struggles. If morality is but one part of a life well lived, it can sometimes be a crucially important part. The significance of some moral failings may fade in the light of one's present circumstances. The significance of others should not.[11]

If these sorts of considerations support Parfit's distinction between moral regret and all-things-considered regret, albeit in a somewhat different form than he suggests, I think they also lend plausibility to Velleman's contention that we can approach individuals both descriptively and demonstratively. When the parent of the autistic child contemplates her predicament, she may very well regard the child in two different ways. She may think of him as the particular person he is: the child with whom she shares a history that she does not regard as especially valuable. And she may also think of him simply as a human being—a person who, as such, should be treated in certain ways.[12]

As Velleman suggests, the fact that we can adopt these differing approaches is another factor that contributes to the ambiguous nature of our response to various individuals. When the 14-year-old girl considers her child merely as a person who did not have to exist, she might regret her decision to become a mother. But when she focuses more directly on the particular person her child has become in light of their shared history together, she may feel very differently. By the same token, the parent of a severely autistic child may approach that child merely as a person and, in so doing, regard him as one who (in one way of putting it) should be treated as an end in himself. She may also approach him as the particular child he is and thereby think of him in terms of the pain he has inflicted on her—the struggle of getting through each day with numerous violent tantrums—and the apparent lack of quality in her son's own life. Moving back and forth between these approaches, sometimes on a moment-by-moment basis, the mother can experience a variety of different emotions and responses to her child.

More mundane examples likewise illustrate this dynamic. We may not, in general, be overly fond of children in general even as we are utterly smitten with our own. And we may struggle with the trappings of modern childrearing in ways that lead us to bemoan our status as parents, even though we do not at all regret the decision to have children because we deeply love the particular children we have. We may know full well that we cannot have one without the other, but thinking about our experience under broad descriptions nevertheless yields one kind of emotional response, while approaching it more demonstratively will yield a different result.

I noted earlier that Wallace rejects this sort of bifurcated response as implausible on the grounds that "there is no way of combining complete affirmation and rejection in this way, which is to say that there is no stable set of differently valenced attitudes toward the child that is channeled through demonstrative and descriptive modes of presentation" (2013, 88). And he may be right that a totalizing response to any given individual cannot stably maintain competing responses. However, what I think these sorts of examples illustrate is that very often our responses to particular others are neither totalizing nor stable. We may, perhaps, want them to be one or the other, or both. But the ways in which our relationships are shot through with anxiety, desire, self-recrimination, and idealization—if not all at the same time, then very often in rapid succession—belie any thought that stability is a plausible norm in this arena.

Conclusion:
Contemplating Parenthood

If the foregoing discussion has been compelling, then the decision to have a child is the decision whether or not to bring an entity into existence whose identity is, at the time that decision is made, radically undetermined—who may come into the world as the biological child of two particular human beings with a fixed genetic makeup, but whose future is otherwise open, subject to all the vicissitudes life has to offer. Given the role that our relationships with others play in shaping our own identities, it is also the decision to subject one's own identity not only to the uncertainties inherent in our own lives, but to the various ways in which the identities of others will shape the course of our lives. It is, in other words, the decision to subject one's own identity to the identity of another.

To be sure, this dynamic is implicit in all of our relationships. To encounter another person is to be affected by that person, and so all our friendships and acquaintances will exercise some influence on our identities. But when, as adults, we attach ourselves to other adults, we typically attach ourselves to individuals whose identities are more fully established. Not only do our personality traits tend to become more defined as we get older, but there is simply more to our personal histories and, thus, more we can say about precisely to whom we are attaching ourselves. Thus, while there is a measure of uncertainty in all of our attachments, the degree of such uncertainty is markedly higher when it comes to individuals who do not yet exist. Knowing that they will be our biological offspring is pretty much all we have to go on.

Very often, the contribution that our children make to our identities is positive, to the point that we cannot contemplate our lives without them. We affirm the individuals we have become and we thereby affirm those who have played such an important role in constituting us as those individuals. As most discussions of the case of the 14-year-old girl illustrate, this fact is what makes it difficult for many people to regret decisions to become parents that are otherwise questionable. The person who results from those decisions becomes someone whose absence would greatly impoverish the lives of any number of individuals.

However, I hope that I have drawn attention to the fact that there is a potentially darker side to parenthood. The decision to start a life is inherently risky, and things do not always unfold as we hope they will. In this way, the particular course that each life takes not only colors our past decisions—tingeing them with various hues of regret and affirmation; it also determines how burdensome the moral demands of parenting will be for any given child. It seems that anyone who thoughtfully takes on those demands should, therefore, be correspondingly aware of these sorts of uncertainties.[13]

If we then turn our attention back to the 14-year-old girl, it seems that her decision is likely characterized by a failure to engage in precisely this sort of reflection. Whether or not she has wronged her son by choosing to become a parent at such a young age, she has, almost certainly, failed to appreciate the moral stakes involved in that decision. Indeed, as an adolescent, she is, in all likelihood, unable to think through the various future contingencies that will determine the person she ultimately becomes. This inability thus serves as another ground of criticism for her choice. Things may turn out such that she is glad to have made the decision she did, but they might not. And if she is, perhaps, unprepared to handle the demands of raising a child who will contribute positively to her identity, she is almost certainly unprepared to deal with a child whose existence she may come to regret. We can leave as an open question how many other prospective parents can be characterized in a similar manner.[14]

Notes

1. Parfit labels this conundrum "the nonidentity problem" on the grounds that comparing alternative possible outcomes of the 14-year-old girl's decision involves comparing the lives of two different children rather that two possible lives of the same child. As Parfit puts it, no plausible interpretation of this case entails that that the girl's decision was worse *for the child*:

   > If she had waited, this particular child would never have existed. And, despite its bad start, his life is worth living. Suppose first that we do *not* believe that causing to exist can benefit. We should ask, 'If someone lives a life that is worth living, is this worse for this person than if he had never existed?' Our answer must be No. Suppose next that we believe that causing to exist *can* benefit. On this view, this girl's decision benefits her child. (1984, 359)

   The challenge is thus to articulate a way in which the resulting child has been harmed or wronged, given that her life is one worth living (and a world in which the 14-year-old delays motherhood is a world in which the child does not exist). For an overview of the nonidentity problem and various proposed solutions, see Roberts (2013). As will become clear, my concerns are not with the nonidentity problem per se but rather with our retrospective assessments of decisions like those made by the 14-year-old girl.
2. It is worth noting at this point that while many parents of disabled children are glad to have had them, and would do so again given the choice, some have a decidedly different outlook on their predicament. I discuss the significance of this point in more detail later.
3. McMahan clearly notes that accepting this view does not imply that *all* values are on a par across the board. Rather, it implies the much less ambitious thesis that there is more than one way to live a good life (and, therefore, more than one value around which we can legitimately organize such a life) (2005, 162–166).
4. DeGrazia (2005, chap. 2) gives a helpful overview of the metaphysical debate surrounding these issues as well as a defense of the view that human beings are essentially biological organisms.
5. In her recent book on modern parenting, Jennifer Senior echoes a similar line of thought when she notes that love "can be difficult to muster too, contrary to what so many cheerful books about new parenthood contend. It does not come instantaneously to all parents the moment they are handed a new baby in the nursery" (2014, 112). For some, the kind of attachment that characterizes parental love comes only after sustained interaction with their children. As Alison Gopnik puts it, "It's not so much that we care for children because we love them as that we love them because we care for them" (2009, 243. Quoted in Senior, 2014, 112).
6. Harry Frankfurt writes compellingly about this issue in Frankfurt (2004).
7. See, for example, Williams (1981) and chapter 4 of Gaita (2004). The relationship between regret and remorse also runs throughout Wallace (2013).
8. To press this difference is, therefore, to press the significance to morality of bipolar as opposed to monadic forms of normativity. I discuss the relationship between monadic and bipolar normativity in Kadlac (2015).
9. This conclusion differs from Wallace's tentative suggestion that there is "an on-balance wish to have acted otherwise in the cases in which we would most confidently apply the term 'remorse' to characterize a person's retrospective attitudes toward something they have done" (2014, 116).

10. Of course, one can imagine scenarios where this choice would be appropriate. Thus, a drug-addicted mother may recognize that she is incapable of caring for her 4-year-old child and do right by the child in allowing someone else to raise her. But even here, the drug addiction itself may wrong the child in a way that it would not had the child been raised by someone else from birth.

11. It is worth emphasizing here the severity of the cases that Solomon has in view. While autism in all its forms presents parents and children with challenges, a great many families with autistic children are able to find balance and satisfaction with their lives. The cases that Solomon considers are those in which it is a struggle simply to get through each day and where the basic health, safety, and mental well-being of all members of the family are severely imperiled.

12. Rahul Kumar endorses a similar view when he suggests that we distinguish reasons for treating others in a certain way because they are members of a certain type and reasons that are generated on the basis of their particular identity. See Kumar (2003), 110 ff.

13. I am, therefore, sympathetic to David Benatar's (2006) assessment that most people choose to have children with very little consideration of whether they should do so and that things might be better if more people approached that decision with a modicum of reflection. However, his arguments that the conclusion of this reflection should always be a decision not to procreate are not convincing. For compelling criticisms of Benatar, see Harman (2009) and DeGrazia (2010).

14. I am indebted to Emily Austin, Ralph Kennedy, and Christian Miller for their very helpful comments on this paper.

BIBLIOGRAPHY

Benatar, David. 2006. *Better to have never been.* Oxford: Oxford University Press.

DeGrazia, David. 2005. *Human identity and bioethics.* Cambridge: Cambridge University Press.

DeGrazia, David. 2010. Is it wrong to impose the harms of human life? A reply to Benatar. *Theoretical Medicine and Bioethics* 31: 317–331.

Frankfurt, Harry. 2004. *The reasons of love.* Princeton, NJ: Princeton University Press.

Gaita, Raimond. 2004. *Good and evil: An absolute conception,* second edition. London, Routledge.

Gopnik, Alison. 2009. *The philosophical baby: What children's minds tell us about truth, love, and the meaning of life.* New York: Farrar, Straus, and Giroux.

Harman, Elizabeth. 2009. Critical study of David Benatar, Better to have never been. *Nous* 43: 776–785.

Kadlac, Adam. 2015. Does it matter whether we do wrong? *Philosophical Studies* 172: 2279–2298.

Kumar, Rahul. 2003. Who can be wronged? *Philosophy and Public Affairs* 31: 99–118.

Lewis, Michael. 2010. *Home game: An accidental guide to fatherhood.* New York: W. W. Norton and Company.

McMahan, Jeff. 2005. Preventing the existence of people with disabilities. In *Quality of life and human difference,* ed. David Wasserman, Jerome Bickenbach, and Robert Wachbroit, 142–171. New York: Cambridge University Press.

Parfit, Derek. 1984. *Reasons and persons.* Oxford: Oxford University Press.

Roberts, M. A. 2013. The nonidentity problem, *The Stanford Encyclopedia of Philosophy,* Edward N. Zalta (ed.), http://plato.stanford.edu/archives/fall2013/entries/nonidentity-problem/.

Schechtman, Marya. 1996. *The constitution of selves*. Ithaca, NY: Cornell University Press.

Senior, Jennifer. 2014. *All joy and no fun: The paradox of modern parenthood*. New York: Harper Collins.

Solomon, Andrew. 2012. *Far from the tree: Parents, children, and the search for identity*. New York: Scribner.

Taylor, Charles. 1991. *The ethics of authenticity*. Cambridge, MA: Harvard University Press.

Velleman, David. 2008. Persons in prospect. *Philosophy and Public Affairs* 36: 221–288.

Wallace, R. Jay. 2013. *The view from here*. Oxford: Oxford University Press.

Williams, Bernard. 1981. Moral luck. In *Moral Luck*. Cambridge: Cambridge University Press.

CHAPTER 25

THE POSSIBILITY OF BEING HARMED BY ONE'S OWN CONCEPTION

JANET MALEK

THE philosophical debate about whether a person can be harmed by his or her own conception is ongoing. Scholars have held a wide range of views on this question. A persuasive case has been put forward that it is impossible for an individual to be harmed by a decision that results in his being conceived as long as that individual has a life that is worth living. On the opposite end of the spectrum, arguments have been crafted with the aim of demonstrating that life has no ethical advantage over non-existence and that conception is therefore always a harm. Neither of these arguments aligns well with the intuitively appealing view that people are not routinely harmed by their own conception, but that such harm is possible under certain circumstances. This last view, in fact, suffers from a lack of coherent philosophical support. As a result, a consensus position on the possibility of being harmed by one's own conception has not been achieved.

The implications of this debate are significant. If an individual can be harmed by his own conception, that possibility must be factored into the ethical analysis of conception decisions. Potential parents would have at least prima facie duties to avoid harming their future children when making choices about bringing them into the world. Practice guidelines for health care providers who work in areas affecting human reproduction would need to take this possible harm into account. Even policymakers would need to consider whether the regulations and programs that they support could harm future generations. Evaluating whether an individual can be harmed by being conceived is therefore not simply an academic exercise, but is a project with practical importance.

In the following pages, arguments that have shaped this debate will be analyzed and problems with them will be identified. Alternative arguments will be presented that offer coherent support for intuitively appealing views. These resolutions will be found to share defining characteristics, and the implications of these commonalities for work in reproductive ethics will be discussed in the final section. Before addressing these arguments, however, it may be helpful to offer some clarification about the concept of harm.

The Concept of Harm

One author has claimed that "the notion of harm is a Frankensteinian jumble. Thus it is unsuitable for use in serious moral theorizing. It should be replaced by other more well-behaved concepts."[1] There may be some truth in this evaluation; the use of the term "harm" is often imprecise and inconsistent. Even so, jettisoning the concept entirely seems premature. The concept of harm is widely applied in ethics literature, professional education, legal analysis, and clinical practice. The value of avoiding harm has been used to frame guidance in all of these areas. It captures something fundamental to common-sense morality and is strongly intuitive. Perhaps, then, being more specific about what is meant by "harm" is preferable to throwing the concept out.

The concept of harm has been most comprehensively analyzed by Joel Feinberg.[2] Feinberg argues that there are two necessary elements of harm in the morally relevant sense. For an act to cause harm, "(1) it must lead to some kind of adverse effect, or create the danger of such an effect, on its victim's interests; and (2) it must be inflicted wrongly in violation of the victim's rights."[3] In other words, harm only takes place when an individual is made worse off by a wrongful act. This sense of harm is distinguished from a "harmed condition" in which a person experiences an adverse outcome that is not the result of another's action (e.g., getting cancer). It is also different from acts that compromise a person's well-being but that are not wrongful (e.g., losing a fair competition). Although an individual may be made worse off in these types of cases, that individual has not been harmed by another in a sense that would justify the attribution of moral blame.

Feinberg introduces the idea of interest baselines to assess the effect that an act has on one's well-being. Interests are "all those things in which one has a stake."[4] Together, one's interests comprise his well-being. The position of one's interest baseline represents the state of one's interests; the higher it is, the better off the individual is. In Feinberg's terms, then, one individual makes another worse off by compromising the other's interests. That is, an individual who suffers harm has her interests set back, impeded, thwarted, or defeated in a way that negatively affects her interest baseline.

The metaphor of the interest baseline makes clear that it is the *relative* condition of an individual's interests that determines the effect that a particular act has on his or her level of well-being. The judgment that harm has occurred requires a comparison between two states of being. Harm, therefore, is not simply a negative evaluation of an individual's current interest level, but rather the claim that that interest level is relatively lower than it would have been under other circumstances.[5] Which "other circumstances" is the correct point of comparison for assessing harms is a point of some debate. Feinberg advocates the "otherwise condition," claiming that an interest has been compromised when "that interest is in a worse condition than it would otherwise have been in."[6] This approach is probably the most widely accepted, but it is not without its problems, as will become apparent in the following pages.

Finally, it is worth noting that harm is generally thought to be "person affecting." That is, when harm occurs, there is a particular person who is made worse off as a result of that harm; and if an act does not compromise the interests of any individual, that act did not cause harm.[7] As will be discussed in later sections, some work in reproductive ethics has challenged this axiom because it generates unintuitive conclusions in certain cases. For the purposes of this inquiry into the possibility of being harmed by one's own conception, however, it is the traditional, person-affecting understanding of harm that is of interest. The question at hand—whether it can coherently be said that a person, once conceived, has been harmed by decisions that resulted in his or her own conception—concerns person-affecting harm. This sense of harm is of moral importance and has the potential to generate ethical duties.[8]

At least three different claims regarding the possibility of being harmed by one's own conception deserve consideration:

1. That people are *sometimes* harmed by *the fact that* they are brought into existence
2. That people are *sometimes* harmed by *the way that* they are brought into existence
3. That people are *always* harmed by being brought into existence

The philosophical puzzles raised by these three claims are remarkably different. The three following sections address each in turn. The chapter's final section looks for common themes among these analyses and arrives at some conclusions about the use of the concept of harm in the context of reproductive ethics.

That People Are Sometimes Harmed by the *Fact That* They Are Brought Into Existence

Decisions about whether to conceive have been called "different number choices."[9] Choices of this type determine how many people are brought into existence. They are to be distinguished from decisions about when or how to conceive a child (called "same-number choices"). Can a person be harmed by her own conception when the only alternative is that no one is brought into being? We can imagine a number of cases in which this question would be relevant: potential parents choosing whether to have a child during wartime or famine or a couple with a family history of a debilitating genetic disorder who are unable to use genetic testing. There is a high likelihood that the children who could be born into situations like these would lead difficult lives containing much suffering. Their interests would be seriously compromised by the circumstances of their birth. Many people share the intuition that in such cases it would be better for those possible children to not be brought into being. The claim that such children have been harmed by their conception, however, has been a matter of much philosophical debate.

It is relatively uncontroversial to claim that an individual is harmed by her own conception if she is brought into a life that is foreseeably not worth living. These are cases in which a future person's interests are be defeated by the circumstances of her birth to the point that she would be better off dead. Clear examples of this type of harm are cases involving significant suffering and early death with little or no good to balance against that suffering. In such cases, an individual's interest baseline is at such a low level that it compares unfavorably with non-existence.[10] By knowingly and intentionally conceiving a child who is likely to live such a devastated existence, potential parents act in a way that fulfills Feinberg's first criterion of harm; they cause an adverse effect on the child's interest baseline. Their act also fulfills Feinberg's second criterion under any reasonable account of the obligations of parenthood. Parental obligations require that parents ensure that the interests of their children are protected to a reasonable minimum,[11] and creating a life that is not worth living would constitute a violation of that obligation. A child brought into existence in this type of situation has therefore clearly been harmed by his own conception.

More challenging cases involve the creation of people who are likely to have lives that are worth living, but barely so. We might call these lives "marginally worth living." Such people's interest baselines may be thwarted or seriously compromised, but not to the point that death is a preferable alternative.[12] Many people share the intuition that knowingly and intentionally conceiving a child who will live such a life is morally problematic. Furthermore, the source of the moral concern in this case seems to be the pain and suffering experienced by that child. It therefore seems that an individual whose life is marginally worth living could be harmed by his own conception under the same argument used to show harm to those with lives *not* worth living.

However, scholars[13] have claimed that people with lives worth living cannot have been made worse off by the choices that resulted in their conception. If their lives are worth living, the argument goes, these children are not worse off than they otherwise would have been because otherwise they would not have existed. As a result, even if such children have a low level of well-being, their parents cannot have made these children worse off by conceiving them. This argument requires two premises:

> *Life Worth Living Premise:* A child's interest level cannot have been lowered by his own conception if his life is worth living.

> *Worse-Off Condition:* A child is worse off as a result of his parent's conception decisions only if his interest level is lower than it otherwise would have been.

If both of these premises are true, they demonstrate that a parent who brings a child into existence cannot make that child worse off by conceiving him as long as his life is worth living. However, there are good reasons to believe that both of these premises are false.

Life Worth Living Premise

It may appear that the Life Worth Living Premise is obviously true; that if one's life is worth living, his interest level cannot be lower than it would have been had he not been brought into existence. However, David Benatar explains that support for this idea is based on "a crucial ambiguity in the expression 'a life worth living.' This expression could be understood as 'a life worth continuing' or as 'a life worth bringing about.'"[14] This distinction implies that the interest level at which a life is worth *continuing* to live may not be the same as the interest level at which a life would be worth *conceiving*.

Which is the more stringent standard? Benatar holds that the threshold at which a life is deemed worth conceiving is higher than the threshold at which a life is deemed worth living, based on the fact that good reasons are typically required for ending a life, but few if any reasons are needed not to create one.[15] Other scholars have noted an asymmetry in how most people think about non-existence, finding preconception nonexistence to be of little moral concern while death is clearly of great moral concern.[16] This asymmetry supports the idea that the threshold interest level for continuing a life is lower than the threshold interest level for creating a life, since life has to be very, very bad to justify ending it. In contrast, the interest level at which a life would foreseeably be worth conceiving is relatively high because non-existence is a morally acceptable alternative in most cases.

Due to the difference in interest level between a life worth continuing and a life worth conceiving, there are some cases in which a child whose life is worth continuing is worse off than if he had never existed (because he does not have a life that was worth conceiving). Therefore, if the phrase "a life worth living" means "a life worth continuing," the Life Worth Living Premise is false.[17]

As articulated earlier, the Life Worth Living Premise refers to an existing child, equating a life worth living with a life worth *continuing*. Given that conception decisions are made prior to a future child's existence, however, understanding a life worth living to mean a life worth *conceiving* would be the more appropriate interpretation. And using this latter interpretation makes the Life Worth Living Premise false due to cases in which the child is likely to have a life that is worth continuing but not worth conceiving.

If the Life Worth Living Premise is false, it is possible to show that parents can harm their children by conceiving them, even if their lives are worth continuing once they have been conceived. It is nearly tautological to claim that being conceived compromises the interest level of a person whose life was not worth conceiving. Similarly, a parent surely violates his parental obligations by conceiving a child who will live a life that was not worth conceiving and so acts wrongly in doing so. People whose lives are marginally worth continuing may therefore have been harmed by their own conception if their state of well-being was foreseeable.

Worse-Off Condition

According to the Worse-Off Condition, a child is made worse off by a conception decision if and only if her interest level is lower than it otherwise would have been. To explain why this premise is false, it is necessary to look first at the relationship between interest baselines and obligations.

It may initially seem that an individual who does not fulfill his obligations may *fail to benefit* another but does not *compromise* her interests. However, Feinberg's interest baseline can be used to demonstrate that this kind of failure can, in fact, make a person

No Obligation to repay   **Obligation to repay**

Baseline   Failure to pay   Baseline   Failure to pay

                                       L ——

              ↓O   ↓O
L ——   L ——   L ——

FIGURE 25.1 Effect of an obligation and the failure to fulfill it on an interest baseline

worse off. Feinberg claims that "when there is no duty to aid, we use a different baseline to measure benefits and harms [than when there is a duty to aid]."[18] In other words, a person's interest baseline reflects the obligations that others have to her. This means that, all other things being equal, a person to whom another has an obligation is better off than one to whom no one has such an obligation. Consider the following two cases, the first in which Linda *gave* Owen $100 and the second in which Linda *lent* Owen the same amount (see Figure 25.1).

In the case in which Owen has *no* duty to repay Linda, Owen's choice not to pay Linda results in her interest level remaining the same. In the No Obligation case, then, Owen's decision to not give Linda $100 would merely constitute a failure to benefit Linda. In contrast, in the case in which Owen owes money to Linda, her interest baseline is at a higher point (relative to the No Obligation case), and Owen's failure to pay her would lower Linda's interest level by $100, setting back her interests. This explains why Owen merely forgoes benefiting Linda when he fails to act in a case in which he has no obligation, but sets back her interests by doing so when does have one. The failure to fulfill an obligation, then, compromises an individual's interests.

These arguments can be used to show that the Worse-Off Condition is false. A parent takes on an obligation to ensure that her future child's interests are protected to a minimal degree when she chooses to conceive that child. That obligation is reflected in the future child's interest baseline. If the parent chooses to conceive knowing that she will be unable (or unwilling) to fulfill the obligations generated by that choice, she compromises the interests of that future child. As illustrated in Figure 25.2, this is the case even if the child's interest level is not lower than it otherwise would have been. Even though the future child's interest baseline before conception is unknown, upon conception that future child's baseline reflects the parental obligation and is compromised by the parent's anticipated failure to fulfill it. As a result, the child is made worse off even though his interest level is not lower than it otherwise would have been (because he otherwise would not have existed).

One could object to this conclusion about the Worse-Off Condition by claiming that despite the compromise to interests a parent causes by conceiving a child whose interests she knows she will be unable to protect to a minimal degree, the parent's choice does not make the child worse off *overall* if the child's life is worth living. The objector could grant that the compromise to interests occurs, but claim that the benefit of having a life worth living outweighs that negative effect so that the child is still better off overall. There are at least three possible ways to respond to this objection.

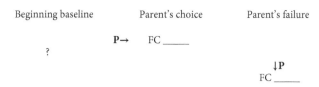

FIGURE 25.2 Effect of a parent's failure to fulfill parental obligations on a future child's interest baseline

First, one could deny that a life worth living, in and of itself, is a good, thus eliminating the benefit that purportedly outweighs the identified compromise. If having a life worth living were a benefit, there would be at least some moral impetus for individuals considering procreation to create lives worth living. However, most people do not have the intuition that they should benefit future children by conceiving them. This reductio ad absurdum suggests that life, in and of itself, is not a benefit to a future child.[19] If life itself is not a benefit, the objection fails because conception does not generate the good needed to outweigh the compromise to interests done by a parent when she conceives a child whose interests she knows she will be unable or unwilling to protect to a minimal degree.

Second, another possible response to the aforementioned objection could be to take an agnostic position on the value of life itself. Acknowledging uncertainty about the benefit of life makes that possible benefit a less compelling moral justification for creating life. In contrast, there is a high level of certainty that an individual is harmed when her parents fail to fulfill their obligations. It seems plausible to claim that a judgment about whether or not the child is better off for being conceived should be based on ethical considerations that can be soundly supported rather than on ethical considerations that are speculative.

Third, a final possible response would be to concede that the child is benefitted by being brought into existence, but to deny that the choice to conceive therefore offsets the compromise to interests that occurs. An action can have distinct effects, some bad and some good. Even if the good effects are significant, they are not necessarily commensurate with the negative effects and therefore they may not negate the existence of the bad effects. As a result, the choice to conceive may be morally problematic even if it brings about significant benefit.

Determining which of these responses is most defensible would require a detailed analysis of the value of life itself that I am unable offer here. Cumulatively, however, they provide a rebuttal to the objection that the child who has such a life is no worse off overall for being conceived.

If the Worse-Off Condition is false, it is possible to show that parents can harm their future children by conceiving them, even if their lives are worth living. This happens in cases in which a parent can foresee (or should foresee) that she will be unable or unwilling to protect the future child's interest to a minimal degree but chooses to conceive (and take on the obligations of parenthood) nonetheless. A parent who takes on obligations to her child knowing that she will be unable or unwilling to fulfill them wrongly compromises a child's interests because the future child's interest baseline reflects that obligation.

I have argued that both the Life Worth Living Premise and the Worse-Off Condition are false and have shown how a future child can be harmed by the fact she is brought into existence, even if no other person would otherwise be conceived. It is worth noting that both of these premises rely on incorrect assumptions about the possible worlds and interest baselines that are used as points of comparison. The Life Worth Living Premise is based on the comparison between a possible world in which an individual already exists and a possible world in which that person no longer exists, where a more appropriate comparison is the difference between a world in which an individual will exist and one in which she never does. Similarly, the Worse-Off Condition neglects to incorporate the relative effect that obligations have on an individual's interest baseline and so incorrectly compares the state of the individual's interests after being conceived with non-existence. While it is difficult to characterize the state of a person's interests when he does not exist, we are able to know that they reflect parental obligations. As we will see in the following sections, similar erroneous assumptions underlie other puzzles about conception and harm.

That People Are Sometimes Harmed by the Way They Are Brought Into Existence

So-called same-number choices do not determine the number of people brought into being but do affect the *genetic identities* of those people. Decisions about *how or when* to conceive a child are same-number choices. Same-number choices that raise the question of harm include those in which potential parents seek to have a child with a disability such as deafness or achondroplasia, fail to use genetic technology to avoid passing on a debilitating genetic condition, or have a child under adverse conditions when it would have been possible to wait to have a child in a better situation. In such cases, the intuition that the parents have harmed their future children is widely held. It seems that the decision is morally blameworthy because of the effect that that decision has on the well-being of the child. It is worth noting that these may not be cases in which the person's interests are defeated or thwarted. The person may, in fact, have a life that is well worth conceiving. It is a life, however, that includes pain and suffering that could have been avoided if a different decision had been made.

As with different-number problems, however, it has been argued that potential parents cannot harm their future children by making same-number conception decisions as long as the children conceived have lives worth living. This is because a person's genetic identity is dependent upon the exact circumstances of his conception.[20] That is, if his parents had conceived at a different time or in a different way than they actually did, a different egg and sperm would have been united and a genetically different individual would have been brought into being. According to this argument, the genetic differences between possible future children mean that same-number conception choices change the identity of the person who is brought into existence, and, as a result, cannot make any one person worse off. Derek Parfit illustrates the consequences of this observation with an example of a 14-year-old girl who chooses to conceive a child. There are only two possibilities for this child: (a) to be conceived when the girl is 14 years old and (b) not to be conceived at all. Parfit argues that "if [the girl] had waited, this particular child would never have existed. And, despite its bad start, his life is worth living . . . We should ask, 'If someone lives a life that is worth living, is this worse for this person than if he had never existed?' Our answer must be No."[21] Because having a life worth living, even if that life faces serious challenges, is not worse than having no life at all, the parent of such a child does not make that child worse off by conceiving him. The fact that another child would have lived a better life is irrelevant from the perspective of the child actually born. Consequently, the child in this case is not made worse off as a result of the young mother's decision. This philosophical puzzle is known as the "non-identity problem."

In this section I will demonstrate that the non-identity problem relies upon an indefensible assumption and that parents *can* make their future children worse off by same-number conception decisions. The argument can be broken down into three premises, the latter two of which were discussed in the previous section:

> *Non-identity Premise:* If a parent had conceived under different circumstances than she actually did, a different child would have been brought into being and this child never would have existed.

> *Life Worth Living Premise:* A child's interest level cannot have been lowered by his own conception if his life is worth living.

> *Worse-Off Condition:* A child is worse off as a result of his parent's conception decisions only if his interest level is lower than it otherwise would have been.

The Non-identity Premise

Whether the Nonidentity Premise is true turns on what, exactly, the phrase "this child" refers to. There are a number of different ways of understanding the referent of this phrase; which is most appropriate depends on the context in which it is used. To refute the Nonidentity Premise, I show that it relies on an understanding of this phrase that is inappropriate for use in the context of reproductive decision making and that the argument is unsound if it is understood in the correct way.

Saul Kripke distinguishes between two types of labels for things in the world. Kripke proposes to "call something a *rigid designator* if in every possible world it designates the same object, a *nonrigid* or *accidental designator* if that is not the case."[22] A rigid designator has the same extension in every possible world. That is, when a term refers to an object rigidly, it picks out the same object no matter what else is true in each world. In contrast, a nonrigid designator can have different extensions in different possible worlds, meaning that it could refer to different objects depending on what is true in each world. For example, "Sean Connery" is a rigid designator because it refers to that particular individual regardless of whether he is playing James Bond or managing a fast food restaurant. On the other hand, "the actor playing James Bond" is a nonrigid designator because different people fill that role in different possible worlds. Both types of designation can be used in everyday conversation. For example, it is equally sensible to state that "Rio de Janeiro, which will host the 31st Summer Olympiad, will need to take adequate security measures for the event" and to claim that "The city that hosts the 31st Summer Olympiad will need to take adequate security measures for the event." The context in which the claim is made determines which type of designation is appropriate.

Both rigid and nonrigid designators can identify objects of moral obligations. A secret service agent assigned to the presidential squad may be directed to protect Barack Obama from threats to his safety and from scandal-hungry journalists. In this case, the individual he is responsible for protecting is referred to in a rigidly designated way. Alternatively, the agent may be directed to protect the President of the United States from those same dangers. The obligation is formulated in a nonrigid way under this directive. Although the agent may be protecting Barack Obama, his exact identity is incidental to the obligation. Both formulations of the directive are equally coherent. On most days, these two assignments would require the same set of duties on the part of the agent. However, on inauguration day, they would entail a different set of responsibilities. These examples demonstrate that moral claims can be sensibly formulated using rigid or nonrigid designation. Which kind of designation is appropriate depends upon the context in which the moral claim is made.

How should the phrase "this child" be understood in the context of reproduction? That is, when parents are making conception decisions, how should the idea of the child who will be created as a result of those decisions be understood? The method used to identify the future child will affect which moral claims can coherently be made about such choices. If the future child is *rigidly* designated, each possible child is considered to be a different moral entity. The concept "this child" picks out a child with a particular combination of genes. Each possible child must be separately identified in moral discourse. Claims made before conception that concern a child who could exist would have to be phrased, "I will teach whichever child I conceive how to cook Sauerbraten" or "No matter which children come into being, I will make sure they learn to play Euchre." Such claims must differentiate among genetically distinct possible future children.

In contrast, designating the future child *nonrigidly* places emphasis on the role the child will have in the world, regardless of the genetic identity of the individual who is conceived. If "this child" were understood as a nonrigid designator, it would refer to any of the possible children who could fill that role and would therefore eliminate the distinction between them. Moral claims about the future child, nonrigidly designated, allow uncertainty about the extension of the object of those claims. Under this conception a parent's claim that "I plan to take my future child to Disneyland," refers to a placeholder for the role that the entity plays in the world. The fact that different individuals may fill that role is morally irrelevant.

The Non-Identity Premise uses rigid designation to refer to a future child. The non-identity problem requires that each possible child be thought of as a separate moral entity. It is only possible to say that a "different child" would have existed instead of "this child" if these entities are referred to rigidly. Its soundness therefore depends upon a rigid understanding of future children. But should future children be referred to rigidly? Or would it be more appropriate to use nonrigid designation in the analysis of conception decisions? Conception decisions (obviously) must take place *before* the child is conceived. There are several reasons to believe that a future child should be referred to nonrigidly rather than rigidly in moral claims made before the child's conception.

The most compelling argument for a nonrigid understanding of the future child is that in most cases it would be nonsensical to use the concept rigidly prior to conception. At the time at which a conception decision is made, the identity of the child has not yet been determined and so "the future child," rigidly designated, has no referent.[23] In contrast, when used nonrigidly, claims about the future child make sense in the relevant contexts. Relatedly, nonrigid designation makes it possible to refer to a child consistently before and after her conception. This means that the claim "I will save money to send my first child (nonrigidly designated) to college" can mean the same thing before and after she is brought into being. Nonrigid designation therefore allows moral claims to maintain continuity in a way that is impossible using rigid designation.

Another reason why nonrigid designation is more appropriate in the context of conception decision making is that it more closely corresponds to the way potential parents normally think about future children. If the fact that possible children are technically distinct entities were morally relevant to potential parents, those parents' thoughts would be likely to reflect that distinction in the way illustrated earlier. Such consciousness does not, however, seem to be reflected in most people's moral thinking about conceiving a child. That is, we do not differentiate morally between possible combinations of genes when considering a future child. Rather, before a child is conceived, it is the place that the child will occupy in the world that is of moral relevance. We are indifferent to which particular child ends up taking that place. Nonrigid designation therefore seems more consistent with the way that potential parents think about possible children than does rigid designation.[24]

Parfit acknowledges the possibility of using this kind of approach when thinking about a future child. Referring to his example of the 14-year-old girl, he admits that "in trying to persuade this girl not to have a child now, we can use the phrase 'her child' and the pronoun 'he' to cover *any* child that she might have . . . By using these words in this way we can explain why it would be better if this girl waits."[25] Parfit rejects this approach as a solution to the non-identity problem, however, maintaining that it does not provide a foundation for a person-affecting moral claim. He argues that "This becomes clear after she has had her child. The phrase 'her child' now naturally refers to this particular child. And this girl's decision was *not* worse for *this* child."[26] These statements demonstrate Parfit's commitment to using rigid designation when applying person-affecting principles. He formulates his argument within the postconception context, after the child's genetic identity is determined, emphasizing the particularity of the child in that context.

The earlier arguments in favor of nonrigid designation of the future child, however, do not use semantic equivocation, as Parfit suggests. Instead, the claim is that he understands the phrase "this child" in a way that is less appropriate for use in the context of reproductive decision making. The Non-identity Premise states that if a parent *had* conceived under different circumstances than she actually *did*, a different child *would have been* brought into being and this child *never would have* existed. This premise looks retrospectively upon the decision to conceive *after* the conception takes place. Furthermore, Parfit explicitly states that his argument "becomes clear after [the mother] has had her child."[27] He approaches conception decisions from the context of hindsight, reflecting upon the parent's choice after the child is conceived. However, actual conception decisions must be made *prospectively* and so moral claims concerning conception decisions should be made within that context, where nonrigid designation is more appropriate. The Non-identity Premise therefore chooses the wrong context from which to analyze the morality of conception decisions. As a result, it invokes the inferior method of designating the future child in Parfit's arguments. The argument about the appropriate type of designation is therefore more than a game of semantics—it represents a morally relevant disagreement with the way the Non-identity Premise portrays the concept of the future child in the context of conception decision making.

This critique of the nonidentity problem takes issue with the implied theory of personal identity and whether it fully captures what must be taken into account in moral decision making about human reproduction. The philosophical debate about what we are, who we are, and what makes us "us" is ongoing. The question of which is the most defensible theory of personal identity is far from settled. The available theories are even more confounded in contexts that involve the *creation* of persons. It is not possible here to fully explore this debate or to lay out and defend a particular theory of personal identity. However, a few comments are in order.

While it is true that a person comes from a unique egg and sperm, it is less clear that this fact is the only, or even the most important, determinant of that person's identity. Her identity is also a function of the family into which she is born, the environment in which she lives, and the culture that surrounds her.[28] These facets of a person's existence affect who she is just as her genetic makeup does. When parents make same-number conception decisions, these determinants of identity remain constant. There is therefore a very real sense in which the identity of a future child does not change as a result of a same-number conception decision.[29]

This latter sense of identity captures what matters morally in decision making better than a genetically based approach. Furthermore, it is particularly appropriate for use in reproductive contexts. When we think about the morally relevant features of existing or future persons, it is not their genetic codes that come to mind, but the other facets of their being that define them. There are therefore good reasons to believe that genetic identity is not the whole story of identity and that this complimentary view of identity captures something important and morally relevant.

If the future child is referred to nonrigidly in the context of decision making about conception, the phrase "this child" in the Non-identity Premise refers to the future child regardless of the genetic identity he may have, making the premise false. Nonrigid designation of the future child creates *continuity of identity* among genetically distinct possible future children, making it possible to compare the interest levels of that future child in different possible worlds. The No-Worse-Off Premise and the Worse-Off Condition were also shown to be problematic in the previous section. Together, these conclusions open the door for the possibility that a person's interests can be compromised by decisions in the way she is conceived.

Recall the assumption that parents have an obligation to promote the interests of their future children when they can do so at a reasonable cost. Their future children's interest baselines reflect that obligation. As a result, if the parents conceive in a way that fails to fulfill that obligation, the future children's interests are compromised, fulfilling one of Feinberg's two individually necessary and jointly sufficient conditions for the occurrence of harm. Because potential parents also act wrongly by failing to fulfill an obligation, Feinberg's second criterion is also met. As a result, potential parents can wrongfully compromise their future children's interests by the manner in which they conceive them. Therefore, people are sometimes harmed by the way they were brought into existence.

It is the realization that identity may be conceived differently in a preconception context than in a postconception context that opens the door for this solution. Assumptions that have served us well in the latter context may fail us in the former. In this case, many different possible worlds are possible and, before conception, all are morally relevant. A potential parent must therefore consider a range of possible worlds when making conception decisions, not just one. The use of nonrigid designation in creating our moral claims about conception enables the proper comparison among the various relevant possible worlds, creating conceptual space for the possibility of harm.

That People Are Always Harmed by Being Brought Into Existence

David Benatar[30] has taken a more extreme position about the possibility of being harmed by one's own conception. He has argued that people are always harmed by coming into existence. On his account, existence has no advantages over non-existence and, as a result, it would have been better for each of us never to have been. This unintuitive conclusion is supported by an intriguing philosophical argument that merits serious consideration. Whether one is ultimately persuaded by Benatar's account, the argument offers important insight into the question at hand.

Benatar's argument is built on the observation that there is an asymmetry in the way that the presence and absence of pleasures and pains are evaluated. He states that it is uncontroversial to claim that:

1. The presence of pain is bad, and
2. The presence of pleasure is good

However, when thinking about the lack of pain and pleasure:

3. The absence of pain is good, even if that good is not enjoyed by anyone, and
4. The absence of pleasure is not bad unless there is somebody for whom this absence is a deprivation

Benatar claims that the evaluation of pain and pleasure in the context of non-existence is not simply the inverse of their evaluation in the context of existence. In the context of non-existence, the avoidance of pain has positive moral value, as might be expected. A symmetrical assessment of pleasures would assign negative value to the lack of pleasure associated with non-existence. However, the absence of pleasure that would otherwise have been experienced does not generate moral concern. In other words, when pains and pleasures are experienced, they are bad and good, respectively. But when those pains and pleasures are *not* experienced because the person who could have been brought into being does not exist, the absence of pain is good and the absence of pleasure is not bad.

Benatar does not offer a direct argument in support of the asymmetry. He instead defends his claims by showing that they explain some commonly held beliefs, including:

(i)   The asymmetry of procreational duties
    While we have a duty to avoid bringing into existence people who would lead miserable lives, we have no duty to bring into existence those who would lead happy lives.
(ii) The prospective beneficence asymmetry
    It is strange to cite as a reason for having a child that that child will thereby be benefited. It is not similarly strange to cite as a reason for not having a child that that child will suffer.
(iii) The retrospective beneficence asymmetry
    When one has brought a suffering child into existence, it makes sense to regret having brought that child into existence—and to regret it for the sake of that child. By contrast, when one fails to bring a happy child into existence, one cannot regret that failure for the sake of the person.[31]

The explanatory power of Benatar's asymmetry provides good reason to believe that it points to something important. However, the asymmetry as he describes it also entails some deeply unintuitive conclusions. The matrix Benatar uses to help show the results of this asymmetry is re-created in Figure 25.3.

The essence of Benatar's argument is that existence has no advantage over non-existence. With respect to pain, box (1) is compared with box (3), making it obvious that never existing is better than existence because it is good to avoid the experience of pain. With respect to pleasure, box (2) is compared with box (4). Because the absence of pleasure is not bad if there is no one to experience that lack of pleasure, existence holds no advantage over non-existence on this measure. As a result, Benatar argues, non-existence is always better than existence and therefore that being brought into existence is always a harm.

X exists	X never exists
(1) Presence of Pain (Bad)	(3) Absence of Pain (Good)
(2) Presence of Pleasure (Good)	(4) Absence of Pleasure (Not Bad)

FIGURE 25.3 David Benatar's view of the asymmetry of benefits and burdens in existence and nonexistence

If sound, this argument has profound implications for the possibility of being harmed by one's own conception. Under this view, it is not only possible to be harmed by one's own conception, but any individual who experiences any pain at all has been harmed by being conceived. It is not surprising that many philosophers have offered criticisms of Benatar's argument in an attempt to show how this conclusion can be avoided. It is not possible to engage all of these critiques and Benatar's rebuttals here.[32] Rather than rejecting Benatar's asymmetry or the conclusions it entails outright, the following paragraphs will explore a modification of the asymmetry that preserves its explanatory power but avoids its extreme implications.

When non-existence is compared with a life of extreme suffering, Benatar's asymmetry captures common intuitions accurately. It is clearly bad for a person who exists to experience significant pain, giving non-existence the relative advantage of avoiding that pain. As Benatar claims, we find that absence of pain to be good even when no one exists to experience that absence. With respect to pleasure, even a life of significant suffering most likely includes at least a few pleasures. Even so, non-existence seems to have no real disadvantage when compared to existence on this measure because no one suffers from the lack of pleasure. This is, then, the paradigm case that serves as the basis for Benatar's formulation of the asymmetry.

Does the asymmetry work as well when non-existence is compared with an ordinary life? Most human lives are filled with a mix of pleasure and pain, where one does not overwhelm the other. When a person exists and has a life of ordinary quality, the pain she experiences is bad for her. But would the avoidance of pain be of positive moral value in this case if she did not exist? The idea that avoiding pain is good by preventing a person's existence is less compelling in this case. When an ordinary couple decides not to have an(other) ordinary child, they are not typically perceived to have done something morally praiseworthy by avoiding the pain that that child would have experienced. Choosing not to bring an ordinary child into the world is generally a matter of moral indifference, not a moral duty. The asymmetry's treatment of pleasures seems appropriate in this second type of case. Just as we do not rejoice in the avoidance of pain for that could-have-been ordinary child, we do not bemoan the absence of pleasure.

Finally, how does the asymmetry fare when considering a life that is on the opposite extreme: one that contains overwhelming pleasure and minimal pain? As in the ordinary case, avoiding a small amount of pain by choosing not to bring into being a person who would lead a very pleasurable life does not seem to be good in the same way that avoiding extreme pain is. In terms of pleasure, is the foregone pleasure of moral concern in this extreme case? Most people would say that it is not; as the asymmetry captures, the lack of pleasure is not bad unless someone experiences that lack, even when the could-have-been person would have had a very pleasurable life.

In crafting his argument that coming into existence is always a harm, Benatar describes an asymmetry that holds in an extreme case and then applies it to other cases. In those other cases, however, the asymmetry does not seem to reflect our intuitions as well. When lives are anticipated to be ordinary or extremely pleasurable, the absence of the pain and pleasure caused by non-existence does not seem to be of great moral importance. It is only when contemplating a life of overwhelming pain that our intuitions support the asymmetry. In the face of this puzzle, should we maintain the asymmetry and claim that it demonstrates our intuitions are wrong? Or should we reject the asymmetry in ordinary cases, claiming that there is a morally relevant difference between extreme and ordinary cases that justifies this approach?

It could be argued that pain is pain and pleasure is pleasure; that they should be treated consistently regardless of the quantities of each a life contains. However, it seems plausible to respond that there is a morally relevant difference between a life that contains significantly more pain than pleasure and one that contains significantly more pleasure than pain. The place at which the pain of life outweighs its pleasure seems to be a breaking point that can be used to differentiate among cases.[33] The asymmetry should therefore be revised as follows so that it applies only to the appropriate type of cases:

1. The absence of overwhelming pain is good, even if that good is not enjoyed by anyone, and
2. The absence of overwhelming pleasure is not bad unless there is somebody for whom this absence is a deprivation

The term "overwhelming" indicates pain or pleasure that clearly outweighs the other aspects of existence. It offers a way to differentiate extreme cases from ordinary ones in which there is a reasonable balance of pain and pleasure. This revised version does not apply to the latter types of cases; as noted earlier, the absent pain and pleasure of non-existence in such cases are not treated asymmetrically. Both are matters of moral indifference.

It is important to emphasize that this revised version of the asymmetry is no less effective than the original at explaining the commonly held beliefs cited by Benatar to support his view. In fact, this version leads more precisely to those conclusions. The beliefs discussed by Benatar refer to "miserable lives" and the "suffering child,"[34] suggesting that the cases under consideration are more likely extreme cases than ordinary ones.

The revised asymmetry has the additional advantage that it does not entail the unde-sirable conclusion that it is good to avoid bringing into existence anyone who would experience any iota of pain. It recognizes that pains and pleasures can be balanced, rather than taking the view that the experience of pain is a trump card that outweighs any possible benefit. As a result, it recognizes that although being brought into existence *can* be a harm, people are not *always* harmed by being conceived.

Benatar's key observation about the asymmetrical treatment of the absence of pains and pleasures in the context of non-existence is correct and important. It offers help-ful insight into some fundamental puzzles in reproductive ethics. The original asym-metry holds when a possible world in which no one exists is compared with a possible world in which an individual exists and lives a life of extreme suffering. However, when non-existence is compared with a different type of possible world—one in which an individual exists and lives an ordinary life—the asymmetry dissolves. This observation illustrates the importance of selecting the appropriate alternative possible world when considering questions involving non-existence.

The conclusion of this section, then, is that Benatar goes too far in claiming that exis-tence is always a harm. This does not mean, however, that one is never harmed by his own conception. Benatar's framework and the revised asymmetry show that in cases where pain clearly outweighs pleasure, there is positive moral value associated with non-existence and that it may therefore be relatively harmful.

Conclusion

The concept of harm in the context of human reproduction raises fascinating paradoxes and philosophical puzzles. Compelling arguments leading to strongly unintuitive con-clusions have been made concerning the possibility of being harmed by one's own con-ception. Scholars have claimed that a person can never be harmed by the fact that she is brought into being or by the way that she was conceived. Others have claimed that people are always harmed by their own conception. Neither of these approaches fits well with the sensible middle ground on which conception is sometimes a harm, depending on the circumstances under which one is conceived.

The discussion thus far has aimed to show that there are problems with each of these arguments. These problems take different forms, but all deal with the way that the interests that exist in life are compared with the lack of interests associated with non-existence. Because non-existence is not a state of being, it cannot be evaluated intrinsi-cally. It would be nonsensical to claim that non-existence is either good or bad in and of itself, because it *is not*. As a result, the value of non-existence must, therefore, be assessed relatively—that is, with reference to another possible world in which the possible person *could* exist.

The trouble seems to be in figuring out which possible worlds are the appropriate points of comparison for evaluating non-existence. If the wrong possible world is used, the relative value of non-existence is incorrectly described and the wrong conclusions are drawn. In posing the non-identity problem, Parfit suggests that non-existence cannot be compared with existence, neglecting to recognize the relative value that can be assessed by reference to another possible world. Furthermore, the idea that one's genetic makeup determines her identity ties our moral reasoning to one possible world rather than acknowledging that before conception many different worlds are possible. Finally, Benatar uses an extreme possible world in evaluating the relative value of non-existence, but fails to see that non-existence may have different value depending on the possible world it is compared with.

Using appropriate possible worlds for comparison, it is possible to draw intuitive, plausible conclusions that offer guidance for reproductive decision making. If a choice causes harm, there are typically good moral reasons to avoid making that choice. A parent who chooses to have a child knowing that she will be unable to protect his interests to a minimal degree harms that child because he will be worse off than he would be in a possible world where the parent fulfills her parental obligations. That parent therefore has at least one important moral reason not to have a child under those circumstances. A clinician who fails to inform his patients about a test for a serious genetic condition could cause harm by bringing into being a possible world in which that child has that condition when a possible world in which the child (nonrigidly designated) did not have that condition was available. That clinician should therefore help to avoid that possible harm by informing the patients about the test. Finally, there is no need for policymakers to create disincentives to procreation if reproduction under normal circumstances does not routinely cause harm—an intuition supported by an accurate understanding of the relative value of a possible world in which an ordinary person does not exist.

There is much more to be said about how the value of non-existence should be understood and how this affects the possibility of being harmed by one's own conception. The preliminary conclusion offered here is limited to several observations: (1) Non-existence must be evaluated relatively, that is, with reference to other possible worlds; (2) The correct possible worlds must be used as a point of comparison to arrive at correct evaluations of non-existence; and (3) When the value of non-existence is appropriately compared with the value of existence, it is possible to make a coherent argument that one may be, but is not always, harmed by her own conception.

NOTES

1. Ben Bradley, "Doing Away With Harm," *Philosophy and Phenomenological Research* 85 (2012): 391.
2. Joel Feinberg, *Harm to Others* (New York: Oxford University Press, 1984) and Joel Feinberg, "Wrongful Life and the Counterfactual Element in Harming," in *Freedom and Fulfillment: Philosophical Essays*, ed. Joel Feinberg (Princeton, NJ: Princeton University Press, 1992). Feinberg's account was developed with the intention of explicating the harm principle, a legal concept used to justify limitations on individuals' liberty. Even so, the account can equally be used to identify cases involving harm of the morally worrisome kind that is relevant to ethics; see note 3.

THE POSSIBILITY OF BEING HARMED BY ONE'S OWN CONCEPTION

3. Feinberg, "Wrongful Life and the Counterfactual Element in Harming," 3–4. The first condition, that there be an adverse effect on a person's interests, applies straightforwardly in the moral (as opposed to legal) context. The second, that the act causing the adverse effect was wrong or a violation of a person's rights, is easier to evaluate in the legal context when the act can be compared with a written set of laws and regulations. Although the moral assessment of an act's wrongness may be difficult in morally controversial cases, Feinberg's more detailed description of his second condition seems helpful in a moral (as well as legal) sense: "acting in a manner that is indefensible, that is, neither excusable nor justifiable . . . is the case of an adverse effect . . . [and] is also a violation of [the individual's] right."

4. Feinberg, *Harm to Others*, 34.

5. David DeGrazia discusses this point in "Procreative Responsibility in View of What Parents Owe Their Children" in this volume. He suggests that a noncomparative understanding of harm might be more appropriate for some questions in reproductive ethics.

6. Feinberg, *Harm to Others*, 34.

7. Derek Parfit, *Reasons and Persons* (New York, Oxford University Press, 1984), 394–400.

8. Jan Narveson, "Utilitarianism and New Generations," *Mind* 70 (1967): 62–72.

9. Parfit, *Reasons and Persons*, 355–356.

10. One could object that it is nonsensical to claim that a child is worse off than he would have been if he had not been conceived because it is impossible to compare the level of well-being associated with nonexistence with that associated with existence. This is the argument made by Justice Proctor of the New Jersey Supreme Court in *Gleitman v. Cosgrove* in 1967: "The infant plaintiff would have us measure the difference between his life with defects against the utter void of nonexistence, but it is impossible to make such a determination." If this were true, however, there would be no kind of life, no matter how bad, that could be accurately described as worse than nonexistence. Most people would not want to accept this extreme conclusion. Even Parfit implies that a child who has a life that is not worth living was made worse off by being conceived (Parfit, *Reasons and Persons*, 358). To avoid this extreme conclusion, it must be acknowledged that there is some way, however imprecise, to compare existence with nonexistence, undermining the objection.

11. A full discussion of parental obligations is not appropriate here, but it should not be controversial to claim that parents have a duty to protect the interests of their future children to a minimal level and to promote their interests when it is possible for them to do so at reasonable cost. This suggestion obviously raises the questions of what constitutes a "minimal level" and what costs are "reasonable" for a parent to bear. It is my view that the requisite minimal level is fairly high and that even significant costs may be reasonable for parents to bear, making parental obligations substantial.

12. It would be tangential to consider in detail the specific characteristics of such lives or how far apart these two thresholds are. One might argue that almost any life worth continuing would also be worth conceiving, but I believe that there are substantive differences between the thresholds. The presence of truly horrific conditions (such as Tay-Sachs disease) would clearly make lives not worth continuing; the presence of significantly painful or seriously disabling conditions (such as autosomal dominant polycystic kidney disease) could make lives not worth conceiving, and the presence of conditions that cause only challenges (such as phenylketonuria) do neither. David Wasserman's paper in this volume, "Justice, Procreation, and the Costs of Having and Raising Disabled Children," addresses questions related to this issue.

13. Derek Parfit, "On Doing the Best for Our Children," in *Ethics and Population*, ed. Michael Bayles (Cambridge, MA: Schenkman, 1976), 100–102; Parfit, *Reasons and Persons*, 351–377; Robert M. Adams, "Existence, Self-Interest, and the Problem of Evil," *Nous* 13 (1979): 53–64.

14. David Benatar, *Better Never to Have Been: The Harm of Coming Into Existence* (New York: Oxford University Press, 2006), and David Benatar, "The Wrong of Wrongful Life," *American Philosophical Quarterly* 37 (2000): 175–183.

15. Benatar, "The Wrong of Wrongful Life," 176–177.

16. Frances M. Kamm, *Morality, Mortality: Volume I—Death and Whom to Save From It* (New York: Oxford University Press, 1993), 25, and Cynthia B. Cohen, "The Morality of Knowingly Conceiving Children With Serious Conditions: An Expanded 'Wrongful Life' Standard," in ed. Nick Fotion and Jan C Heller, *Contingent Future Persons: On the Ethics of Deciding Who Will Live, or Not, in the Future* (Dordrecht: Kluwer Academic Publishers, 1997), 27–40.

17. The premise is clearly true for lives that are worth conceiving and does not apply to lives that are not worth living in either sense. A more precise understanding of the lives this area encompasses would require an exact definition of what it is to have a life worth continuing and what it is to have a life worth conceiving. I will propose without argument that a life worth conceiving is one in which the future child's interests will be protected to some minimal level at which the child can successfully pursue a reasonable range of human activities.

18. Feinberg, *Harm to Others*, 138–143.

19. Stuart Rachels addresses this issue in "Is It Good to Make Happy People?" *Bioethics* 12 (1998): 93–110.

20. Parfit, *Reasons and Persons*, 351–352.

21. Parfit, *Reasons and Persons*, 358.

22. Saul Kripke, *Naming and Necessity* (Cambridge, MA: Harvard University Press, 1972), 48.

23. A possible exception could be a case in which a sperm and egg have been selected and will be united at some point, so that the genetic material will be the same. Even in such a (very unusual) case, however, it is likely that the delay or change of environment could cause different genetic translocations, inversions, deletions, or insertions so that the future child's genetic identity would be altered.

24. The question of when and how the transition from nonrigid designation to rigid designation should take place is an interesting one. Certainly a full-term infant is generally thought of rigidly; perhaps the transition to that way of thinking occurs gradually throughout fetal development or varies depending on the beliefs of the parents. A socalled chemical pregnancy might not reach the point at which that possible child would be rigidly designated in his parents' minds, but a late miscarriage likely would.

25. Parfit, *Reasons and Persons*, 359.

26. Parfit, *Reasons and Persons*, 359.

27. Parfit, *Reasons and Persons*, 359.

28. David DeGrazia introduces a helpful distinction between numerical identity and narrative identity. He concludes that numerical identity depends on one's biological makeup (73) and narrative identity comes out of one's "self-stories" (81–83). DeGrazia's discussion has to do with identity over time rather than identity across possible worlds, and so does not apply directly to the issue at hand. However, his idea that identity is multifaceted is similar to what I am arguing here. David DeGrazia, *Human Identity and Bioethics* (New York: Cambridge University Press, 2006).

29. The scope of the continuity of identity proposed here may be a matter of debate. Potential parents could be indifferent to the genetic makeup of a future child, but only within a certain time frame or with a certain characteristic. For example, parents could distinguish between "our first girl" and "our first boy" or between "the child I could have conceived before beginning graduate school" and "the child I could have conceived after completing graduate school." Such thinking would reflect a nonrigid understanding of the future child with a more specified description of that child's role. Whether continuity of identity among such specialized roles is possible merits consideration.

30. Benatar, *Better Never to Have Been* and David Benatar, "Still Better Never to Have Been: A Reply to My Critics," *Journal of Ethics* 17 (2013): 121–151.

31. Benatar, "Still Better Never to Have Been," 123.

32. Benatar summarizes and responds to these critiques in detail in "Still Better Never to Have Been."

33. This point is obviously not one that can be clearly and simply defined. It would have to include a margin of error that would create a gray area in which there is uncertainty.

34. Benatar, "Still Better Never to Have Been," 123.

CHAPTER 26

UNDERSTANDING PROCREATIVE BENEFICENCE

JULIAN SAVULESCU AND GUY KAHANE

THE MEDICAL CONSULTATION I

IMAGINE that you and your partner are thinking about starting a family. You wonder what you should do. Abstain from drinking? Take vitamins? Yoga? You go to your doctor. She says, "The virus causing German measles has mutated. The vaccine against this is no longer effective. Everyone who was vaccinated, including you, is now vulnerable. There is currently a virulent epidemic. If you become pregnant now and contract German measles, you will be fine but your child is likely to be deaf, blind, or severely intellectually disabled, or some combination of these. This is called congenital rubella syndrome. If you wait 6 months to try to start a family, there will be a new vaccine available and you won't pass on German measles to your baby."

"What do you think we should do, doctor?" you ask.

"Well, that is entirely up to you. I have given you the facts—it is up to you to choose whether you have a disabled or a nondisabled baby. I can't say which is better. I can't say whether you should try now or wait 6 months."[1]

This would be a bizarre medical consultation. Yet it is precisely what the current standard around nondirective genetic counseling prescribes. It is also what some disability activists would advise. It is also what liberal eugenics prescribes. According to liberal eugenics, people ought to be given the choice to have nondisabled rather than disabled children, but it is entirely up to them what they choose.

What the doctor ought to say in this situation is, "You should wait 6 months until vaccination controls the epidemic. It is better for a large variety of reasons to have a healthy, normal baby rather than one who is blind, deaf, and/or intellectually disabled. Unless you have very good reasons to attempt to have a baby now, you ought to wait."

Now if this couple waits 6 months, it will be a different sperm and a different egg that produce the nondisabled baby. The choice they face is between two different potential children: disabled Danny now or nondisabled Nancy in 6 months.

Structurally, their choice is the same as a couple who has preimplantation diagnosis during in vitro fertilization (IVF), which reveals one embryo will be deaf and the other hearing. They *should* select the hearing embryo, unless there is a *very* good reason to do otherwise (we shall discuss such countervailing reasons later).[2]

This is precisely what procreative beneficence (PB) prescribes. According to the principle of procreative beneficence, "couples (or single reproducers) should select the child, of the possible children they could have, who is expected to have the best life, or at least as good a life as the others, based on the relevant, available information" (Savulescu 2002, 415).

This claim can sound surprising. It certainly has many critics. But as we shall show, much of this criticism is based on misunderstanding. In this chapter, we will clarify what PB amounts to exactly, and we will address common criticisms. We shall argue that, despite appearances, it is PB, not complete freedom of reproductive choice or nondirective counseling (Savulescu and Kahane 2009), that is most consistent with ordinary practices and common moral thinking about reproduction.

THE MEDICAL CONSULTATION II

Many accept that we should select a healthy child rather than one affected by disease or disorder. We will return to the moral significance of the health/disease distinction. However, for the present, note that this commitment is not all-embracing. It is not only the prevention of disease that people care about when they consider having a child. To see this, consider the Medical Consultation II.

A couple is intending to conceive a child. They attend the doctor for preconception counseling. The doctor tells the woman, "If you take these pills for 1 month, the child you conceive may be more intelligent. The pills contain vitamins and fatty acids that are completely safe. You should take them for the full month. You should also abstain from drinking alcohol for 1 month because drinking alcohol results in a child with a slightly lower IQ, even if taken in normal levels."

If these factual statements were true, the advice would be sound: you should take the vitamins and abstain from alcohol for 1 month, unless you have a good reason not to. Of course, as the probability that the course of action will result in the valuable result falls, the strength of the normative prescription likewise falls. If the pills are certain to produce a child who is more intelligent (and there are no reasons to believe there are other downsides), the prescription is strong. If there is a 1/1,000,000 chance, it is very weak and easily overridden.

One might object that the caveat "there are no other downsides" is one which it is difficult itself to be confident in. We simply do not know about genetics, the effect of epigenetics, genetic interaction, environment, and so on to be confident that there will not be downsides.

This may (or may not) be true. The strength of the prescription to take the pills will reduce according to the confidence that there is some downside. Once all the relevant available information is at hand, one can only make a decision (and rate confidence) according to the facts at hand. The wheel of fortune analogy (Savulescu 2002) shows that even when there is massive uncertainty about outcome, information slightly favoring one option provides a reason (albeit weak) to choose that option.

A related objection is that this makes reproductive decision making incredibly complex, time consuming, and rationalistic. There is no doubt information relevant to the decision available somewhere, buried in some scientific study. Are parents really meant to spend weeks or even years researching the relevant information for selecting a child?

The cost, including opportunity cost, of searching for and digesting information is a real cost. It is a standard problem in decision theory that one must weigh the value of further information against the cost of getting it. At some point, one has to decide. What that point is depends on the particular decision and context. The more important the decision, the more important it is to obtain relevant information. If you are about to dive into a pool, you should ascertain how deep the water is before you jump. If you are putting a paper boat in, you do not have to worry.[3]

As in Medical Consultation I, the child who would be conceived in 1 month is a different child to the one who would be conceived now if you ignore the doctor's advice. In effect, this is advice to select the more intelligent child. This is a practical instantiation of the advice PB affords.

A Moral Obligation?

PB is a moral principle that should guide our procreative choices. We see it as stating a moral obligation, but it is important to clarify what we mean by this. By moral obligation, we mean "prima facie moral obligation." It would be absurd to hold that PB is an all-things-considered overriding obligation. Perhaps such absolute obligations exist (e.g., never to torture an innocent child), but there is certainly not one to select the best child.[4] To claim that one *must* select the best child, whatever the cost, the risk, and the implications to society, would be as absurd as to suggest we should save someone's life regardless of the cost, risk, and implications for others (as in the movie *Saving Private Ryan*). We do not subscribe to "Let the best child be selected and the Heavens fall." But that is true of many familiar moral obligations (we have an obligation to tell the truth, but this does not mean we should tell the truth in absolutely all circumstances).

"You should select the best child" is similar in force of moral obligation (though perhaps weaker—as we will see in the final section on impersonal reasons) to "You should give your child the best education."

Nonetheless, many people have mistakenly interpreted PB to mean that all couples must always undergo IVF and PGD (preimplantation genetic diagnosis) to select the best embryo (de Melo-Martín 2004; Sparrow 2007; Overall 2012). Clearly the risks and costs of IVF to the mother need to be weighed against the reasons to select a better child. But in many cases, the information is costlessly available and the risks already taken on.

Yet the law and professional guidelines forbid the release of information relating to non-disease-related genotypic traits (such as sex) to prospective parents in Australia and the United Kingdom when making decisions about which embryos to implant.

A related worry is that there is no moral obligation at all, only a reason to select (see Hotke 2014; and Overall 2012) the best child. This can give the impression that PB states some negligible optional consideration. But that is wrong. We take the approach of Derek Parfit (1984, 2011) that what we ought morally to do is simply what there is most reason to do. Because PB states a significant moral reason (Savulescu and Kahane 2009), and because in plenty of cases this reason will not be outweighed by any competing reasons, often enough PB will state what we morally ought to do.

Some have objected that this is an overextension of "moral obligation" (Sparrow 2014a). We do not think so. It is the same sense of prima facie (or pro tanto) moral obligation that exists when we say parents have a moral obligation to give their children nutritious food. This is sometimes easily defeated, but nonetheless it is real and carries considerable weight. We would say it is wrong if parents did not give their children nutritious food.

Sparrow has argued that this interpretation renders PB vacuous (Sparrow 2014b). But this is false (Savulescu 2014). Soon, whole-genome analysis employed during genetic diagnosis will reveal all the genetic information available on an embryo. Couples having IVF for infertility or genetic risk where PGD is already being performed could gain all this information almost costlessly once PGD is undertaken for other reasons. PB implies such couples should obtain this information, and they should use it to select the embryos, or from the range of embryos, expected to have the best chance of the best life. PB also implies that existing laws in the United Kingdom, Australia, and many parts of Europe preventing access to this information are wrong. People *ought* to have access to this important information.

PB, as we have said, is one reason among many. The health of the parents and justice in society are other potentially competing reasons. Building on PB, Douglas and Devolder (2013) and Elster (2011) have argued that there are such general obligations to others, a form of "procreative altruism." One of us previously said, "personal commitment to equality, personal interests and procreative autonomy" could conflict with PB (Savulescu 2002). What we ought to do will depend on weighing all these reasons. But we are not likely to arrive at the correct overall conclusion if we do not take into account all of the relevant reasons, including those given by PB.

Practical ethics in this way is a bit like physics. Reasons exist that push in a certain direction and are of a certain strength. They are like vectors of force. What we have most reason to do involves summing all of these vectors. Practical ethics ought to follow the vector of reasons. The strength of these vectors will vary according to the facts of a given context, a point to which we will return.

We should add one qualifying note. The strength of the vector is the confidence we have in the reason. We have discussed empirical uncertainty as a factor that reduces our confidence in our reasons to act. Another relevant factor is "normative uncertainty"—uncertainty about the reason or value itself. How good is it to be intelligent or empathetic in a given circumstance? Part of the answer to this will be determined by the effects of being intelligent or empathetic. But part depends on the normative framework or theory to which one subscribes. Because of uncertainty at this level, one may also be uncertain, fundamentally, about the value of intelligence or empathy. For Kant, empathy might be a bad quality; for Christians, a good one.

This kind of fundamental normative uncertainty ought to be factored in to the confidence one has about reasons, in addition to empirical uncertainty. Nonetheless, some progress can be made. Some "all-purpose goods," like sufficient self-control, seem good whatever one's plausible higher order commitments. But such normative uncertainty is something we face with very many moral decisions, and it should not be exaggerated. As we will argue later, there are ways of arriving at reasonable conclusions about the factors that promote or reduce well-being.

Social/Legal Sanction and Distributive Justice

Many have argued that PB involves or invites coercion (Bennett 2009; Sparrow 2011). This is wrong. In the Medical Consultations, it is completely consistent with the doctor giving advice saying the couple should wait that the couple should still be free to go off and procreate whenever they want. PB is perfectly compatible with what is often known as procreative autonomy or liberty.

We have been at pains to point out that people should be free to reproduce even when that involves foreseeably and avoidably having less than the best child (see Savulescu 2002; Savulescu and Kahane 2009). Indeed, one of us has even defended the legal right of deaf people to deliberately select a deaf child on the principle of procreative liberty (Savulescu 2002) This view runs counter to the Human Fertilisation and Embryology Act in 2008 in the United Kingdom that explicitly prevents selection in favor of disability (section 14(4)). It is a familiar point that moral obligation, especially prima facie moral obligation, does not necessarily imply any legal obligation. We may have a moral obligation to get our children to clean their teeth. But failing to do so should not be a crime, nor should we be coerced to do it.

The point at which wrongdoing becomes the object of the social or legal sanction is an interesting but separate question to what our moral obligations are. There are a variety of social responses to wrongdoing, such as discouragement, persuasion, blame, social ostracism, incentives for better behavior, and legal responses such as fines and imprisonment, and, in some extreme cases, even surgical or biological intervention (e.g., the castration of pedophiles). The degree of social and legal response depends, among other things, on the degree of harm to others and on considerations of distributive justice. Because reproduction is a private matter, and parents primarily bear the brunt of its costs, and also because the reasons PB generates are impersonal in character and failing to follow them cannot harm the resulting child (see final section), we believe that the social response ought to be limited to prospective advice and encouragement, by making testing cheap and easily accessible, making the relevant information (scientific and ethical) accessible—and removing legal or other barriers. We do not believe stronger moral responses, even overt blame, may be appropriate in this context. But there is nothing remarkable about this. We often judge that other people's parenting decisions are mistaken or even seriously wrong without thinking that it is appropriate to overtly criticize, let alone coerce them[5]—except, of course, when these decisions involve risk of significant harm. While decisions to create one child rather than another cannot be said to harm the resulting child, overt blame and criticism may be appropriate here when parents thoughtlessly decide to create a child who is extremely likely to have a bad life when better alternatives are clearly available. And, as we have argued, decisions to create children whose lives will not be worth living should be made illegal (Savulescu and Kahane 2009).

In practice, it ought only be when there are significant issues of public interest (Savulescu 2002) such as distributive justice at stake, or direct harm to others involved (e.g., selecting an embryo with genes disposing to psychopathy), that stronger responses are warranted.

For example, imagine that a couple were having state-funded IVF. A test is developed to determine whether an embryo will develop into a fetus with anencephaly. This is a condition where the forebrain is missing; such babies will never be conscious and will die within weeks to months of life. In some cases, it is due to either chromosomal or genetic abnormality.[6] In such cases, IVF specialists should use such chromosomal or genetic information to discard embryos that will develop anencephaly. (This practice in general already occurs when embryologists discard embryos based on morphological characteristics predictive of viability.)

This is consistent with letting couples decide to give birth to babies with lethal abnormalities such as Trisomy 18 or anencephaly who have been conceived naturally (Wilkinson 2010).[7] However, if a couple wished to deliberately select an embryo with anencephaly during IVF, this should not be supported with state resources—the benefit does not compare with the cost. This is different from selecting for deafness. Although in our view deafness is a disability (Kahane and Savulescu 2009) because it tends to reduce or limit a person's options, it goes without saying that deafness is consistent with a rich and fulfilling life.

The relationship between social/legal sanction and distributive justice, and moral reasons is thus a complicated one. PB is concerned with what we have moral reason and obligation to do. It is about what should guide the decision making of prospective parents, not about what the state, or others, should try to enforce or prevent.

COMMON SENSE

Although PB is often presented as a radical view, it is really just an extension of widely accepted existing practices and an application of common-sense ethical ideas. Reproductive medicine specialists already routinely pick embryos during IVF. If someone asked for a principle for selection, common sense would suggest "pick the one with the best chance of the best life." Platitudinous as this may sound, the 2001 article that first introduced PB has generated great anger and objection. There are now 343 articles referring to it (and counting), nearly all of them critical.

To pick the embryo that will have the best chance of the best life is simply common sense. Imagine that a couple having IVF produce two embryos. Genetic testing provides evidence that A has a 50% chance of being dead by 65, and B has a 50% chance of being dead by 75. According to PB, they should choose B—it has a better chance of a better life (in this case a longer life), based on information available.

Of course, we would need a lot more information to make a comprehensive determination of the expected overall well-being of each of these embryos. Perhaps A will have a much better quality of life than B, and this offsets the gain in expected length of life. A shorter life can be better if it is extremely good.

But if there is no further information available, there is a reason to choose B rather than A. Absent other considerations, the couple ought to choose B. After all, what could possibly support choosing A or simply ignoring this information?

People might accept that it is common sense to prefer a longer life to a shorter life. But they balk at comparisons of quality of life and estimates of well-being. *Those* sorts of comparisons, they claim, cannot be made. There are two strong objections to PB worth considering. The first is that without an account of well-being, PB is impotent in practice. The second is that because selection does not benefit anyone—it is just a decision to bring into existence one possible person rather than another—the kind of reason it generates is mysterious. Considerations of well-being are irrelevant because violations of PB only constitute harmless wrongdoing. We will spend most of the rest of this chapter considering these two objections.

Well-Being

A whole raft of objections has to do with the very idea that lives could differ in value. In thinking about these objections, it is vital to keep in mind the difference between the value *within* a life—that is to say, how much *well-being* that life contains—and the value *of* a life. There are at least seven different considerations that are often raised in this connection.

Skepticism about Value

The most basic form of this objection is that it is not possible to make value judgments about lives (apart from judgments relating to health and disease). This is either because one is skeptical about making value judgments at all or about human lives or well-being in particular.

All Lives are of Equal Value

A related but different objection is that all lives are equally valuable overall and to say that one life is better than another is discrimination and failure to respect human dignity.

Both of these views should be differentiated from the prescriptive ideal of equality: that people should all be treated with equal concern and respect, regardless of their quality of life or degree of well-being. Call this prescriptive equality (cf. Dworkin 1977; Singer 2011). Prescriptive equality is often thought to arise from the value or dignity that all persons possess. But to say that all persons possess equal value is not at all the same as to say that they all lead lives that are equally good. The latter claim is absurd. If nothing we did and nothing that happened to us could affect the quality of our life, then most action—including most morally and politically motivated action—would be pointless.

PB might be thought to violate prescriptive equality because it involves discarding some human embryos in preference for others. However, embryos are not people. If embryos were persons, PB would involve discrimination. But then the whole process of IVF and PGD with genetic selection, even against disease, would be unjustifiable. For those who believe that embryos are not persons, PB is similar to selecting gametes, or partners, as a way of having a child with a better prospect of a better life. PB is a principle relating to whom to bring into existence, not how to treat people once they are in existence.

When disability activists claim that genetic selection discriminates against the disabled, they may be assuming that embryos or fetuses are disabled people. However, this view of moral status is inconsistent with contraception, abortion, and IVF, which involves the destruction of embryos. This view of the status of embryos is generally only held by religious extremists.

(A related argument is that selection expresses a negative view of disability, that by selecting a nondisabled embryo we are expressing the view that disabled people should not have been born. This objection, however, only has force against *conservative* views that allow us only to select against disability or disease. It makes no sense when leveled against PB. According to PB, *anything* that increases or reduces the chances of a good life is a potential target of selection, not merely deafness, blindness, intellectual disability, and paralysis. Thus, asthma ought to be selected against while, arguably, cheerfulness or greater intelligence ought to be selected for. Such a principle is not specific to conventional disabilities; it expresses a view about the value of all states correlated in some way with well-being.)

Nonetheless, if we cannot evaluate the lives of persons, PB would be an impotent principle because it would have no application. To be action guiding, it requires that some lives differ in value by containing more or less well-being. But you do not need an explicit theory of well-being to make such assessments. Many everyday judgments we make already implicitly involve such assessments of well-being. One way of bringing these assessments to light is the Preservation Test (Savulescu 2007). According to this test, if we should preserve Property X to level Y, then we should also enhance Property X to level Y. In the context of procreation, it would mean that we should select embryos with Property X at level Y, rather than X at some lower level, Z.

Imagine that John's life expectancy is 80. A condition affects him so that it is now reduced to 60. If Juice is given, the condition will be corrected and he will again live to 80. Juice should be given because it is better to live to 80 than 60 (assuming the life is good quality).

Now imagine Jane is born with a life expectancy of 60. If Elixir is given, she will live to 80. Again, Elixir should be given because it is better to live to 80 rather than 60.

This approach can be extended beyond length of life to qualities in life.

Imagine a child, Anna, who is highly empathetic. If event B happens, Anna will become low on empathy. B could be some social event, like the introduction of violent computer games, or it could involve giving, or not giving, some biologically active substance. We can ask, from the point of view of Anna's well-being, should B happen?

If we believe B should not happen (from the point of view of Anna's well-being), it is because it is better to have more rather than less empathy. If we believe B should happen, it is because it is better to have less rather than more empathy. Indeed, studies have suggested that levels of empathy in the United States are in decline (Konrath et al. 2011), and we should ask whether this is good or bad or indifferent.

Now consider child Charlie. Charlie is already low on empathy. If D happens, Charlie will become more empathetic. If we believe that B should not happen, then we should also believe that D should happen. D might be some educational intervention or reading a novel by Tolstoy. Or it might be some biological intervention or neurointervention.

The first case involving Anna is one of preservation of some valuable property. The second involving Charlie is one of enhancement. Such thought experiments can tell us what makes lives better or worse, or at least bring to light our implicit views about this question.

Here are some other examples. Consider IQ. You need an IQ of more than 90 to complete a tax return and 120 to go to university. There are numerous advantages to having a high IQ and numerous disadvantages to having a low IQ (Savulescu et al. 2011).

Assume a child George has an IQ of 120, but H will reduce it to 90. H could be a tumor, lead in the water, lack of some vitamin or education, abuse, and so on. H should not happen because it is better to have an IQ of 120 rather than 90.

Now imagine that a child Isabelle has an IQ of 90. If J happens, Isabelle's IQ will rise to 120.

Of course, there can be other reasons why H or J should happen—perhaps they are necessary to treat some lethal disease. For example, G might have a brain tumor that requires radiotherapy that will reduce George's IQ from 120 to 90. But without the radiotherapy George will die. The radiotherapy should be given, even though the bad side effect is a reduction in IQ.

Using the Preservation Test, we can try to identify what is of value, provided we are not under the status quo bias (see Bostrom and Ord 2006 for a test of this).[8]

PB says we should select those things which the Preservation Test evaluates as valuable.

This approach does not imply that the valuable property is itself genetic or biological in origin. Property X may be mainly socially determined—but to the extent that our genetic endowment has some influence on it, PB tells us to choose genes associated with X, even if they are only weakly connected to the valuable disposition or trait.[9]

Many people accept that disease reduces well-being. Thus, those with absent empathy, such as psychopaths, could be said to have a psychiatric disorder and to have worse lives. But, the argument goes, within the normal range, variation does not matter. Nicholas Agar has articulated such a view in relation to moral capacities and described a state of moral "normalcy" (Agar 2014).

We have elsewhere examined the normative implications of normal human variation (Kahane and Savulescu 2015). It is important to remember that "normal" is an arbitrary statistical term. It implies variation within 2 standard deviations from the mean. Around 4% of any population falls outside this. Thus, intellectual disability is defined as an IQ 2 standard deviations below the mean of 100, that is, less than 70. But there is now good evidence that low-normal IQ (which is between 1 and 2 standard deviations, between 70 and 85) is associated with significantly reduced opportunities in today's world (see Dunlop and Savulescu 2014 for a review).

There are some properties, like empathy, where there may be an optimal amount in the likely range of environments a person today is likely to inhabit. There may be too much or too little. But it is very unlikely that evolution "selected" the right amount of any property for the range of environments we are now likely to inhabit (Kahane and Savulescu 2015). Evolution selected properties that were conducive to small group survival and cooperation in the African savannah. That is utterly different to a technologically advanced, globalized world where, for example, large-scale cooperation is necessary to avoid existential risk (Persson and Savulescu 2012).

Subjectivity/Relativity of Value

Another objection to valuing lives in a way that PB requires is that one's life is good to the extent one judges it good. In this sense, "beauty is in the eye of the beholder." The quality of a life is relative to that individual's own valuation. Because we cannot know in advance how much a person will value his or her own life, we cannot make a prediction about its value, or so the objection runs.

This is a very simple subjective account of well-being (or the value within a life).[10] This is the kind of view that is put forward by some disability activists. They claim that the disabled are as satisfied with the quality of their lives as the nondisabled. Hence, the quality of their lives is just as good.

It is important to recognize that even within such a simple subjectivist framework, a person can be mistaken about what is of value. People can be wrong about the facts, for example believing that they are receiving medical care that is beneficial to them. Or people could be wrong about whether a particular state of affairs instantiates what they value (Savulescu and Momeyer 1997). For example, suppose someone values empathy but mistakenly applies the value of empathy to support a "tough love" approach. People can be "satisfied" with their lives when they are making these kinds of mistakes—as theorists of false consciousness point out.[11]

Disability activists can point to this kind of error in folk judgments about the value of the lives of the disabled: nondisabled people systematically misjudge the quality of life of people with disabilities. Such judgments may be based on mistakes about the facts about what people with disabilities actually can do, mistakes that have been fostered by institutions that place barriers to the development or exercise of capacities.

One implication of such a view is that a person who desires to live must have a life worth living while a person who desires to die must have a life not worth living. Yet we are not incorrigible about the value of our life. People can desire to die, even when their life is very much worth living. Anorexia involves a similar evaluative error about body image and shape.

A standard response to such objections is to qualify the kind of desire or preference that "counts" as tracking or expressing value. Often it is put as an informed "rational preference" (see, e.g., Brandt 1979; Railton 1986; Smith 1994)—that is, when one knows all the relevant facts and is thinking clearly, rationally, or in some other suitably qualified way.

The problem with subjectivist theories of well-being, even highly qualified ones, is that they do not track value (Savulescu 1999). Peter who has 6 months to live may desire to live with 100 units of preference strength. Paul who has 60 years to live may desire to live with 100 units. On a subjective account, their lives appear to be equally good.

John Harris bites this bullet and states that the value of a life is determined by the preference to live. He claims that each rational person wants at least three things from health care: (1) the maximum possible life expectancy *for him or her*; (2) the best quality of life *for him or her*; and (3) the best opportunity or chance *for him or her* of getting both (1) and (2) (Harris 1996, 270).

However, such an approach is inconsistent with the whole of health economics and the attitudes to what is right among lay people. It would imply that life of 70 good years is equivalent to a life of 5 years of miserable pain, blind and deaf, provided people in each condition desire to live to the same degree. As one of us has pointed out elsewhere, people differ in the degree to which they "happen to fear death or even want to live, which is a feature of their individual psychology" (Savulescu 1999, 407).

The problem with subjectivist accounts of well-being—and more generally of value or reasons—is that such accounts are, at base, unfettered: one can literally desire anything. Hume was one of the few people to confront this aspect of his own theory. He admitted that, on his view, "'tis not contrary to reason to prefer the destruction of the whole world to the scratching of my little finger" (Hume 1978, 416).

To provide a real-life instance of this problem, recently, the family of a brain-dead patient, Jahi McMath, has managed to keep her alive for nearly 2 years because they do not accept the brain death definition of death. Even though Jahi is undoubtedly unconscious, on a desire-based view of reasons, they ought to keep her "alive" in this state because they judge her life to be of value (Pope 2015). (In fact, the family are suing her hospital for damages claiming she is alive but suffered negligent care.)[12]

Another account of wellbeing is hedonism. According to this view, what matters is happiness, or as Sidgwick put it, "desirable consciousness" (Sidgwick 1907).

Peter Singer now subscribes to this version of hedonism (de LazariRadek and Singer 2014). One might say that if two lives have equal happiness, then they are equally valuable. A life of 5 years of total happiness is less valuable than a life of 50 years of total happiness. Because Jahi's life in a brain-dead state is devoid of happiness, it has zero quality of life and value.

Such views are again liable to a reduction. Jeremy Bentham accepted it when he famously stated that the pleasures of playing pushpin were of equal value to those of reading poetry (1830, 206). Nozick's Experience Machine (Nozick 1974) provides another powerful refutation of pure hedonistic theories.

Mill tried to avoid this kind of conclusion by distinguishing between higher and lower pleasures, arguing that the pleasure from poetry is higher than the pleasure of playing pinball (or pushpin as it was then called).

But once one has accepted the move to higher and lower pleasures, one has accepted that certain kinds of pleasures are more objectively valuable than others. But if one accepts this kind of objective evaluation, why limit this to pleasure? Why not say that certain states and activities are more objectively valuable than others? Why not say that caring for others, such as one's children, is valuable even if it does not provide pleasure?

Objectivity about Value

Derek Parfit and James Griffin both describe three theories of well-being: hedonistic, desire fulfilment, and objective list theories. Parfit explains objective list theories in the following way: "[C]ertain things are good or bad for people, whether or not these people want to have the good things or avoid the bad things. The good things might include moral goodness, rational activity, the development of one's abilities, having children and being a good parent, knowledge and the awareness of true beauty. The bad things might include being betrayed, manipulated, slandered, deceived, being deprived of liberty and dignity, and enjoying either sadistic pleasure, or aesthetic pleasure in what is in fact ugly" (Parfit 1984, 499).[13]

Objective list theorists, sometimes also called perfectionists, include Aristotle, Plato, Aquinas, Leibniz, Adam Smith, Hegel, Marx, and Nietzsche.

According to Aristotle, what is good for a human is determined by the function of that organism or its nature. For example, humans are social animals who derive meaning, pleasure, and fulfillment through social relationships. Humans are also curious and inventive, and knowledge, creativity, and inventiveness characterize the human organism.

There are good reasons to include at least an objective element within an account of well-being. In a well-cited study, becoming a paraplegic has very negative effects on a person in the short-term—it causes a significant decrement in subjective life satisfaction. However, over time, quality of life returns to nearly normal. Many paraplegics adapt to their state (Kahneman and Varey 1991, 144). If they are less happy than normal people, the difference is not great (Brickman, Coates, and Janoff-Bulman 1978).

This is because of the phenomenon of adaptation, and such studies measure subjective quality of life (Brickman, Coates, and Janoff-Bulman 1978). Yet the loss of independence and mobility are serious disadvantages (though clearly ones whose badness depends on the built environment). Similarly, the loss of a loved one is bad, but people adapt subjectively—they get over their grief surprisingly quickly (see Moller 2007). Nonetheless, the loss of a loved one, such as a spouse or child, makes one's life go worse in objective terms, no matter how well or quickly one subjectively adapts.

There are also objections to purely objective list theories of well-being, but the most plausible account of well-being arguably includes both subjective and objective elements.

Each of the three accounts of well-being—hedonistic, desire-fulfilment, and objective list theories—has some plausibility. Parfit concludes that an adequate account of well-being must accord weight to all of valuable mental states, desire satisfaction, and objectively valuable activity (Parfit 1984, 502). It may be best not only to engage in activities that possess objective value but to also *want* to engage in such activities and to derive pleasure from them.

So while the subjectivist critique of PB has some merit in that we cannot exactly predict how much a person will value his or her own life, it fails in two regards:

1. We can predict to a significant extent what will satisfy people or give them pleasure (Diener 2000; Argyle 2001).
2. We can predict what is more likely to be conducive to possessing the objective goods of life.

Thus, if life has both subjective and objective value, PB can still have valid predictive value insofar as certain features of our genetics or biology are more conducive to possessing, and enjoying, the things that are objectively good for us and insofar as we can predict people's desires. A life of severe autism or psychopathy is deficient at least because of the lack of social value in that life. Moreover, even if, at the subjective level, our psychologies are resilient and adaptive so that even severe disability might not, in the long run, change our natural level of subjective well-being (or what is known as our "hedonic set point"), it remains the case that some people's mood is naturally brighter than others—and that is one more thing that is significantly shaped by our genetic endowment.

We have criticized purely subjective accounts of well-being—whether desire based or hedonist—and argued that well-being also has an important objective component. Although the arguments we provide here are fairly brief, they illustrate how progress can be made in identifying the elements of well-being. These arguments also converge with the Preservation Test we outlined earlier. The features and capacities of people we should try to preserve and protect, for their own sake, include features and capacities that relate to objective goods—for example, the capacity to form deep personal relationships.

Context Relativity of Value

A related objection, sometimes marshalled in support of diversity, is that we cannot predict the future environment and so cannot predict what set of biological dispositions will be maximally advantageous. In terms of disease, genetic diversity is said to protect against a variety of unforeseen infectious insults. Put broadly, one cannot say what a good genome is without considering the environment in which that organism is living.

There is a deep truth that instrumental value claims are highly context sensitive. For this reason, we have defined capability and disability as stable biological or psychological traits that either tend to increase or reduce well-being in a given set of social and natural circumstances (see Kahane and Savulescu 2009; Savulescu et al. 2011).

However, context sensitivity is not value relativity. Insofar as one can predict the likely environment, one can predict which biological and psychological traits are likely to be conducive to a better life. Dyslexia may not have been of significance in the African savannah, or it may have been associated with positive traits of advantage in that environment, but today it is a significant disadvantage. Interestingly, it may be less of a disadvantage in Asian cultures with language involving symbolic representation. (And it may be associated with other mental capacities that outweigh its badness but in itself, the inability to read is a disadvantage.)

Impulse control and IQ are both traits that are of advantage in the contemporary environment. We have made the point that deafness could be of advantage in certain environments, but in the range of environments a person is likely to encounter in the actual world, it is likely to be a disadvantage (Kahane and Savulescu 2009; 2016).

Some disability activists claim that conditions like deafness are only disadvantageous because of social injustice. We have argued that while prejudice and injustice do play an important role in making such conditions disadvantageous, this is not the whole story. Even if prejudice and injustice were removed, deafness would be associated with residual disadvantage, in the way the world is likely to be. This is, at least in part, because of deafness reducing access to the options and goods derived from music and sound. Of course, the residual disadvantage might be quite small compared to the current disadvantage, but it would still likely exist, making selection for genes for hearing likely to be associated with a (perhaps only slightly) better life. Stronger claims can be made about more severe forms of disability.

A related objection appeals to the plurality of goods. Suppose there are other goods— for example, of family and community relationships—that one can still enjoy if one is deaf. A life can still be very good even if it does not contain auditory goods because it contains other significant goods.[14] Although this point is correct, the mistake in this objection is that from the perspective of selecting embryos, a future hearing child can have *both* music and relationships, while a deaf child cannot have music. Having hearing is associated with the same and additional options. It is Pareto superior (Kahane and Savulescu 2009).[15]

Intersubjectivity about Value

As social beings, a large part of how well our lives go is dependent on others. Social constructivists about disability, or some disability activists, claim that the badness of disability is entirely socially constructed. We have denied this. We have argued that there are both social and nonsocial components to the badness of disability, and not all disadvantage associated with disability is due to prejudice and injustice. Indeed, we gave a welfarist definition of disability which refers to a biological or psychological state that is likely to lead to a reduction in well-being in a given set of social and natural circumstances, subtracting the effects of prejudice and injustice (Kahane and Savulescu 2009).

PB seems insensitive to such considerations of injustice. Indeed, a standard objection to PB is that it requires selecting a lighter skinned embryo to a darker skinned embryo from a mixed-race couple in a racist society. Or it requires selecting a male embryo in a sexist society. In both cases, the lighter skinned child or male child will experience less discrimination.

It is correct that according to PB, there may sometimes be a reason to choose the lighter skinned or male child. The reason is that, in some real-world environments, such a child can be expected to have a better life. Imagine some extremely sexist society where women become sex slaves in a harem to some powerful despot (see Savulescu 2002 for this kind of response). Young girls are taken away from their families to be indoctrinated into servitude. A couple is having IVF. According to PB, they should select a male embryo because a male child will have a better life in this society.

However, as we have repeatedly emphasized (Savulescu 2002; Savulescu and Kahane 2009), PB is only one reason among others. There are also reasons of justice. A mixed-race couple might choose deliberately to have a darker skinned child to make a statement about equality. This is a valid reason that could counterbalance PB-related reasons. What kind of child a couple should have will depend on weighing all these reasons.

As we have said, reasons are like vectors. They have a direction and a strength. What we have most reason to do is the result of summing all these vectors. PB represents only one reason, and its strength may be weak, compared to competing reasons. In the case of the sex slavery case, its strength is significant.

Importantly, however, not all socially constructed disadvantage is unjust. Consider attractiveness (full references to this section on the value of attractiveness can be found in Savulescu 2016. See also Minerva forthcoming). There is a science to what people find beautiful in faces—the so-called golden triangle. People find similar faces attractive across different cultures. Facial attractiveness equates to significant social advantage.

In the job market, being attractive is advantageous. An attractive man can earn, on average over a lifetime, $230,000 more than an unattractive one. Attractive solicitors raise more money for charities. Very attractive individuals are less likely to engage in criminal activities, whereas unattractive ones have a higher propensity for crime. Attractive criminals are punished less severely than unattractive ones.

Both children and adults judge attractive people to be more helpful, more intelligent, and friendlier than their unattractive counterparts. Cute infants elicit stronger motivation for caretaking than less cute ones. Moreover, cute infants are rated as most adoptable.

Adults have higher expectations of attractive kids compared to nonattractive ones, and mothers of attractive infants tend to be more affectionate, playful, and attentive when interacting with their children than mothers of less attractive infants. Teachers expect better performances from attractive students. Transgressions of unattractive children are judged more negatively than transgressions of attractive ones.

Being attractive is also an advantage in romantic relationships because there is a positive correlation between physical attractiveness and dating.

Some of these advantages are unjust. It may be unjust that beautiful people earn more or are less likely to be found to be guilty of a crime. But it is surely not a requirement of justice that people mate and pair with people who are less attractive. What people find attractive and like is in part a brute fact of our biology and psychology, as well as social acculturation. To take another example, consider having an affable disposition. It may be that such a person does better in life, but this is not an issue of justice. If one embryo is more likely to be affable, other things being equal, we should select the more affable embryo or the embryo more likely to be affable as a future person.

We can see this as a kind of intersubjectivity in the realization of value: the component of our well-being that depends on the society and people we interact with, and the social relationships derived from them.

Another common objection is that this point renders PB likely to reinforce, be complicit with, or a victim of social fads. Say, for example, that people start to value blond hair and blue eyes. PB instructs couples to have a blond-haired, blue-eyed child, the objection goes.

We should ask two questions. First, is this what PB necessarily instructs? Second, if it does, is it wrong?

First, it is not clear that this is what PB instructs. One needs to predict what people in the future will value or care about. Rarity can become a value. Thus, as the numbers of blond-haired, blue-eyed children increase, it may be more valuable to have a dark-haired, dark-eyed child.

Secondly, there is nothing morally wrong about social fads, provided they do not result in injustice. If red-haired people start to be discriminated against, this creates reasons of justice (not PB reasons) not to select against them. As before, we are left weighing reasons.

As a general rule, however, social stereotypes will have a small or modest influence over the ethics of selection decisions. Consider, for example, height in men.

Height does confer a socioeconomic advantage. But this is not related to height absolutely but rather relatively—being tall is only of advantage if one is taller than relevant others. Height is said to be a positional good (Buchanan et al. 2001) Sometimes this is said to cancel out if everyone becomes taller. "No one sees any better if everyone stands on tippy toes."

Height nicely illustrates some of the simplicity of thinking around selection and enhancement. Even height is not a purely positional good. Height has nonpositional value. For example, being taller is better if you want to be a basketball player or rower. Being shorter is an advantage for gymnasts, slalom skiers, and skateboarders.

The overall value of having a given height will be difficult to predict. It is not, straightforwardly, that taller is better. And if any height has a disadvantage, it is likely to be outside of the normal distribution—that is, very tall or very short. So within a range, it may not matter to well-being whether a man is 170, 175, or 185 cm.

Many of the intersubjective goods are likely to be in this category. Their positional value is likely to be weak and easily outweighed by other considerations. Moreover, the effect of intersubjectivity in our lives means that many objectively disvaluable traits may not turn out to be disvaluable after all.

To take another example, dwarfism would be associated with some residual objective disadvantage even in a just world. But if dwarves were highly valued (say as artistic models, religious leaders or as stars in a new Hollywood movie series), this intersubjective value could mean they have the best of lives (Savulescu 2015a).

Does this intersubjective element mean there is no point in attempting selection? No, all we can do is take account of uncertainty and make the best decisions we can. We need to predict likely intersubjective effects, but this will be difficult, and we cannot be confident the embryo which is expected to have the best chance of the best life will in fact have the best chance of the best life.

Imprecision

Another misconception about PB is that it is committed to a precise cardinal ordering of all genomes, from very best to very worst. An extreme version of this objection is mounted by Sparrow. He claims that PB is committed to reproduction from a single cloned embryo: "it is also clearly possible that one embryo might have a genome that was clearly superior over all others in a given environment" (Sparrow 2015, 4).

Of course, that is *logically possible*, but vanishingly unlikely, given the way the world is. As one of us has claimed, in the way the world is and would be under conditions of justice, there will be many "equally good genomes" (Savulescu 2014, 2016). Sparrow thinks this significantly weakens PB. However, it would be absurd to believe there is a single genome which is best.[16]

This concept of "equally good" is similar to Derek Parfit's recent concept of imprecision about goodness. Indeed, he sees imprecision as blocking the so-called repugnant conclusion, an important challenge in population ethics (Parfit 1984). What does Parfit mean by "imprecision"? He illustrates this with an example from Ruth Chang—Who is a greater genius, or achieved more, Einstein or Bach? Parfit argues that "the truth could be only that one of these people was imprecisely greater than the other, or more plausibly that they were imprecisely equally as great" (Parfit unpublished).

Now Bach and Einstein also clearly had different genomes. Perhaps one of these genomes was better. But it is more likely that their genomes cannot be compared precisely.

To put the point another way, classes of genomes may fall into three broad categories: black, white, and gray. The existence of a gray zone, which may be substantial, does not preclude there being black and white. Perhaps we cannot compare the genome of Bach and Einstein, or their achievements, or perhaps we want to say, with Parfit and Chang, that they are imprecisely equally good (or "on a par"), but their achievements are obviously greater than those of a human being with anencephaly, or, for that matter with very profound intellectual disability and an IQ of under 15.

In many cases, it may not be possible to tell which embryo has a better genome. Is it better to be gifted at music, chess, or sports? Is it better to be creative but disposed to mental illness, or uncreative but happy? There may be no precise answers to these questions, but this should not preclude us from saying that the genome of Bach is likely to be better than many ordinary, normal genomes.

This point applies to many of the cases we have discussed. Even if there are no precise answers to questions about whether enjoying music is better than reading novels, or whether having more friendships is better than knowing deep truths about the universe, this hardly means that we can never compare and rank the prospects of possible future people. As we have argued, it is generally better to be hearing than to be deaf in the sense that while the deaf can enjoy very many goods, and lead good lives, the hearing have (or potentially) have access to the very same goods as well as to the goods uniquely associated with hearing. Of course, a particular deaf individual may have a better life than a particular hearing individual. But deafness reduces access to some objective goods, and there is nothing objectively good about deafness considered in itself (Kahane and Savulescu 2009).

The complex character of questions about well-being thus does not render PB impotent or radically subjective or relative. However, the kind of precise ordering of best to worst, with embryos falling neatly in a line, will not be possible. This is not surprising. However, some embryos will still be better than others. "Best" will indicate a range. This is different to satisficing, which we previously rejected (Savulescu and Kahane 2009): it is not the claim that we should satisfice, only aiming to select an embryo that will have a good enough life. That claim is rather simply that there will be multiple embryos that are among the best.

Consider an analogy. Can you remember the best day of your life? If you are like us, you will remember many days that are candidates. It may not be possible to say which was the very best. But certainly some were very good or excellent or even ecstatic. And some were terrible, and others ordinary. If a genie appeared willing to grant you to relive the best day of your life, you would choose from a range of excellent days you have already experienced without having to say that the day you selected is better than other very good days.

IMPERSONAL REASONS

Let us return now to the Medical Consultations. It is important to bear in mind that in the first consultation, it is not for their future child's benefit that the couple should wait.

It does not benefit disabled Danny if nondisabled Nancy is conceived. And it will not harm Danny to be selected either if the life he will go on to have would be worth living. Danny would only be harmed by being brought into existence if he has a life which is so bad that it would have been better not to have even been conceived.[17]

So PB is *not* concerned with benefits or harms to the child produced. It is a claim about it being better to bring into existence a child without disability as opposed to a severely disabled child—because this would make for a better world, in an impersonal sense. This has been called an impersonal reason.[18]

Some deny that such reasons exist (Bennett 2009). Famously, philosophers such as Narveson (1973) and Heyd (1994) argue that there are only person-affecting reasons— that is to say, only reasons to act in ways that benefit or harm particular people. But eschewing impersonal reasons in this way would mean that in the Medical Consultation I, the doctor could not say, "You should wait 6 months until there is a vaccine available" if the parents wanted to procreate during the epidemic.[19] Even the most conservative thinkers on genetic selection such as Michael Sandel (2007) and Jurgen Habermas (2003) believe that there are reasons to select healthy embryos rather than embryos afflicted by disease. But as we have just seen, with respect to the child, this can only be grounded in impersonal reasons—because health is better than disease.

Moreover, nearly all decisions affecting future generations, especially distant ones, involve impersonal reasons rather than person-affecting reasons. Consider reduction in carbon emissions to reduce climate warming in the longer term. This is said to be done for the benefit of future generations. But at least in the case of those who are not yet born, such large-scale policies would affect who procreates and when, meaning that completely different people would come to exist over time. For example, consider a person who rides a bike rather than drives home from work. As a result of this exercise, he may be tired, or for other reasons have intercourse at a different time to when he had driven home. So the identity of the child whom he would conceive under such a policy will be changed. The child he would have had had the policy not been implemented thus does not in any way benefit from it—that child simply never comes to exist.

When it comes to the next generation, virtually anything said to benefit "them" therefore does not really benefit any specific person. The long-term good done by policies mitigating climate change will be almost entirely impersonal in nature.

We should reject the claim that impersonal reasons do not exist. But how much weight should be given to such reasons? How strong are impersonal reasons compared to person-affecting reasons? Perhaps if they are very weak, they only play a role in tiebreaker cases, such as if parents are unsure what to do.

Derek Parfit has famously argued that such reasons are as strong as person-affecting reasons. He gives the following example:

> The Medical Programmes. There are two rare conditions, J and K, which cannot be detected without special tests. If a pregnant woman has Condition J, this will cause the child she is carrying to have a certain handicap. A simple treatment would prevent this effect. If a woman has Condition K when she conceives a child, this will

cause the child to have the same particular handicap. Condition K cannot be treated, but always disappears within two months. Suppose next that we have planned two medical programmes, [to prevent the effect of condition J and to prevent pregnancies in women who are in condition K] but there are funds for only one; so one must be cancelled. (Parfit 1984, 367)

In other words, implementing either of the two medical programs would mean that healthy children would be born instead of disabled ones. But the first program would achieve that by curing disability before birth, while the second would do so by preventing embryos with the disability from being conceived in the first place.

Parfit supports the No Difference View: he believes that each program is right and there are equal reasons to support them.[20] Let's call the treatment of J, modification, and the identification of K and waiting, selection. K involves selection because a different sperm and egg will create a different embryo 2 months later.

Modification is person affecting; selection involves impersonal reasons. We believe we have a strong reason to fund selection but an even stronger reason to fund modification. Consider the outcome of modification—there will be a child and later adult who has straightforwardly been benefited who could be grateful for the modification. In the case of selection, there does not seem to be any case for gratitude—the person would not have existed were it not for selection.

Let's assume that both individuals have the same quality of life—say level 80 out of 100. One could object that both individuals have been provided with the same thing—a life of quality 80. So, it might be argued, there is the same reason to modify or select. This would support Parfit's view. This can seem plausible. On such a view as Parfit's, PB-related reasons are as strong as reasons to prevent person-affecting harm.

But now consider two ways a deaf couple could deliberately have a deaf child like themselves—something that many deaf couples apparently desire (see Savulescu and Kahane 2009). The first is by having IVF and deliberately selecting a deaf embryo. Say this individual, Doris, has a life of overall quality 80.

The second is for them to take one of their hearing embryos and genetically modify it, by some gene-editing technique like CRISPR, to create exactly the same mutation that was present in the case of Doris. This causes David to exist, and he has a life of quality 80.

Can Doris complain about the act of selection? Given her life is very good, there are no grounds for complaining that she was selected rather than some other hearing embryo.[21] What about David? He could complain that, even though his life has been very good, it could have been potentially even better, say quality 85, if the deafening manipulation had not been performed. This suggests that even though the effects of selection and manipulation can be the same, manipulation can still be worse because it denies an individual an even better alternative life. The reverse would also seem to apply—when manipulation provides a person with a better alternative life than she would have had, this provides an additional reason and cause for gratitude, even if the effects or states are the same impersonally considered.[22]

This suggests to us that person-affecting reasons are stronger and that we should prefer manipulation to selection.

This has important implications. It implies that PB generates real reasons with force, but these are weaker than competing person-affecting reasons. What might such reasons be? Welfare of the parents or siblings or others might compete with the reasons PB generates. The standard case is one where there are risks involved for the woman in having IVF. This analysis shows that not only should these reasons be weighed against the PB reasons, but they may have greater weight. Our understanding of PB thus easily accommodates the point that it is specifically women that carry the burdens and risks of IVF (cf. Overall 2012). Still, in those cases in which there are no competing person-affecting reasons, then PB should decide the day. And such cases are common enough—such as when IVF and PGD are being done for other reasons, such as infertility or risk of genetic or chromosomal disorder.

This point also has important implications about the level of sacrifice that should be made for the sake of future generations. Impersonal PB-like reasons suggest some sacrifice should be made to bring about future generations that have better lives, for example, by reducing carbon emissions. But this analysis suggests that significant person-affecting considerations have greater strength than impersonal considerations. That is, the interests of the present generation have greater priority over those of future generations.

Impersonal reasons then could be relatively weaker when pitted against strong personal reasons. Requirements of PB and to preserve and protect the environment are reasons, but they should not require very significant person-affecting harms. But this does not mean that reasons of PB do not have considerable force, just as the earlier considerations do not show that the present generation should not make any sacrifices to prevent significant impersonal loss of well-being in future generations.

Serious invasion of personal liberty is a harm. According to Mill, it is only justified when that person threatens to directly and seriously harm another. We would add— when that harm is personal in nature.

If our reasons to have the best children (and best future environment) are relatively weak, they may be often overridden by person-affecting reasons. Not only does interfering in procreative liberty constitute a harm, but there are other harms involved in forcing or compelling people to have certain kinds of children. These are psychological and involve loss of dreams, plans, aspirations, and so on.

The view that person-affecting considerations are stronger than impersonal ones also seems to be reflected in law. It would not only be wrong for a parent to fail to treat her child's intellectual disability or pain or disability, a court would order treatment on behalf of the child. There is both a moral and a legal obligation.

Such a legal obligation does not exist in the case of genetic selection. According to Mill's harm principle, the sole ground for interference in the liberty of another is because that person's actions harm or risk harming another person. Although often wrong, procreative decisions to deliberately select a disabled or disadvantaged embryo do not harm anyone, provided the child's life is worth living.[23] From an impersonal standpoint, such decisions are highly problematic, but there is no person-affecting harm.

For this reason, deaf people and dwarfs should be free to deliberately select offspring with genetic forms of deafness or dwarfism using natural reproduction. Even though such choices may be wrong, in a range of common cases, they should be legally permitted. Laws, such as the Human Fertilisation and Embryology Act, which prevent selection for disability, should be repealed, unless significant distributive justice arguments can be mounted to support them.

A further reason to believe that procreative liberty should be respected in genetic selection decisions is that the harm to the couple of not respecting their choices would be a person-affecting harm. If we prevent a deaf couple from selecting a deaf embryo, there is a direct personal harm to them for merely an impersonal benefit of bringing into the world a hearing child.

Giftedness and Reverence
for the Natural

Having discussed well-being and impersonal reasons, it is worth returning to what is probably the most common popular objection to PB, though we consider it less philosophically compelling as the previous two objections related to well-being and impersonal reasons. Even arch conservatives about reproduction like Michael Sandel, Leon Kass, Jurgen Habermas, and others accept selection against major diseases. What they object to is selection of nondisease traits. They believe we should accept natural human variation. Children should be seen as "gifts" and accepted for who they are. Sandel, quoting theologian William May, claims we should be "open to the unbidden."

As with nearly all attractive positions, there is some truth in these claims. Nearly all of us are far from perfect. Prescriptive equality requires that everyone be treated with equal respect regardless of manifest descriptive inequality. And when it comes to our children, we should surely accept them for who they are, their abilities and disabilities.

But this very reasonable principle of the equal treatment and acceptance of people is bizarre when applied to embryos. We have no more reason to treat all embryos equally as we do all sperm or eggs, unless you hold that the embryo is already a person, which many of these bioconservative writers may hold.

It is completely consistent with PB that if your child is rendered severely disabled by an accident, you should continue to love him or her in the same way, accept his life and do whatever you can to make it go as well as possible. In short, to accept that child as a gift.

However, it is one thing to say that we should accept what we cannot change and quite another to say that we must accept what we *can* change. The former is just a basic feature of a mature outlook on life. The latter is a rather dubious idea (see Kahane 2011). If your child is struggling at school and you could do something to help, should you simply accept the situation?

Few would deny that we should change things for the better when we can, rather than simply accept things as they are. The latter attitude is not virtuous. It expresses indifference and lack of concern, or plain stupidity.

But the same unremarkable point also applies in the less familiar context of reproductive decisions. Letting nature decide, when we can intervene, is foolish. Why should we simply accept natural selection, the natural lottery, or "God's will"? As we have pointed out, evolution does not aim at value or human well-being, only inclusive fitness. We are the result of random mutations in particular environments. We have evolved only to live long enough to reproduce, not to be happy, moral, or good.

There is much natural variation, between species and within species, and, in consequence, significant descriptive inequality between individuals. Lives differ vastly in any property leading to some having very good lives and some very bad. Genetic selection would allow this natural inequality to be reduced. Science and ethics enable us to rise above these constraints. We have earlier discussed reasons of justice to override PB. But justice also provides strong reasons to select children with the best prospects as a way of reducing genetic inequality in talent and ability.

Technology gives power to avoid the arbitrary results of the natural. If the expected utility of choice is greater than natural, we should choose according to values/ethics and science. Genetic selection becomes an issue of moral responsibility—once knowledge and technology give us power to change the natural state of affairs, this generates moral responsibility for the choice to remain with the status quo and its effects.

Nearly everyone now accepts genetic selection for avoiding disease. Sandel, Kass, and Habermas are examples of such bioconservative thinkers who accept eugenics about health. But medicine is also routinely used for nonmedical or enhancement purposes: contraception, abortion, sterilization, cosmetic surgery, Ritalin, and circumcision are used for enhancement purposes, not necessarily for the treatment of disease. What matters to people is not merely health, but well-being and making choices about our own lives. Sterilization and contraception are examples of where natural processes are subjugated to improve human well-being.

"Disease" in the naturalistic sense defined by Boorse (1975) is statistically significant species-typical subfunctioning. Such judgments do not track value but just statistical distribution and contribution to survival and reproduction. Understood in this standard way, disease and health do not intrinsically matter ethically.

What matters is human well-being, and disease and health matter only insofar as they affect our well-being. But similar considerations apply in contexts that do not involve disease. Insofar as genes contribute to valuable traits, like self-control or general intelligence, we ought to select the ones which are more likely to lead to a better life. But once a person exists, we should accept that person as a moral equal whatever the talents or disabilities, health or disease, genetic advantage or disadvantage of that individual.

SELECTION AND THE WILL OF ANOTHER

One dominant strand of objection to PB has been that a new life should not be the product of the will or choice of another. The mere act of selection, these critics claim, undermines the capacity for autonomous agency and the right to an open future (Davis 1997).

Objecting to genetic selection and cloning, Leon Kass writes:

> A third objection, centered around issues of freedom and coercion … comes closer to the mark. … [T]here are always dangers of despotism within families, as parents already work their wills on their children with insufficient regard to a child's independence or real needs. Even partial control over genotype—say, to take a relatively innocent example, musician parents selecting a child with genes for perfect pitch—would add to existing social instruments of parental control and its risks of despotic rule. This is indeed one of the central arguments against human cloning: the charge of genetic despotism of one generation over the next. (Kass 2003, 16)

This objection from "coercion" is the objection that Michael Sandel gives to genetic selection which he calls "hyperparenting" (Sandel 2007, 50–57). In a similar vein, Jurgen Habermas argues that germline enhancements would represent a threat to the enhanced child's freedom because the parents' choice of enhancements would not only imply their endorsement of particular goods but also communicate to their child that they expect her to pursue those goods (Habermas 2003, 51). These expectations, Habermas suggests, may serve to hinder the child's freedom to do what she wants, when her desires do not align with her parents' expectations (Habermas 2013, 61–63).

The paradigm case of coercion could be said to be when a robber stops you and says, "Your money or your life." Coercion involves the restriction of freedom (reduction of options), which causes that person to do what she does not want to do. Coercion is wrong when it harms a person or fails to respect that person's autonomy. This is just what the concept of coercion means.

Embryos cannot be coerced because they are not persons and lack freedom of the will (Savulescu 2015b; material in this section is drawn from this article). But more important, future people also cannot be coerced by the act of genetic selection or cloning. Imagine IVF produces two embryos, Roger and Tony. The parents choose Roger because that embryo has a genetic disposition to being a sprinter (or is a clone). Later in life, can Roger complain that his parents coerced or limited his freedom by selecting him on the basis of having sprinting ability (or being a clone)? No—he owes his very existence (all his options and freedom) to their act of selection. Without assisted reproduction and selection (or cloning), he would not have existed. It is metaphysical fact that those who owe their existence to a reproductive act cannot be coerced by that act. Even more broadly, as we saw earlier, they cannot be harmed by that act unless it makes their existence so bad that their lives are not worth living.

Concerns about coercion fail for another reason that also applies to many acts of germline genetic enhancement. Selecting or engineering sprinting ability or increasing intelligence or giving a child a talent *increases* options and freedom. Coercion in such cases only exists if parents choose to then limit options. But how parents choose to react to their child's abilities or disabilities is entirely independent from what those abilities or disabilities are. Genetic selection or enhancement is neither necessary nor sufficient for hyperparenting. Indeed, selection and parenting are independent acts.

In fact, if we greatly value the autonomy of the created child—and such autonomy may be an important component of well-being—then we could try to use genetic selection to select an embryo that is more likely to have the basic capacities and abilities to function as an autonomous person rather than as a mere extension of his parents' will (Schaefer, Kahane, and Savulescu 2014). It is even harder to see how the bioconservative worry about being subject to one's parents' will could even begin to apply in such a case.

What would coerce Roger? It would indeed reduce Roger's freedom (and open future—cf. Davis 1997) to force him as a child to go to Little Athletics for 6 hours a day when he wants to play with his friends. That would be coercion and bad parenting. But couples who select (or clone) can be great parents, and couples who leave selection to nature can be hyperparents. These are conceptually and morally distinct issues.

It might be objected that they might nevertheless be empirically linked: by being given an option to select the traits of their future child, parents are likely to be encouraged to hyperparent. But this gets things the wrong way round. Some prospective parents would be motivated to select *because* they are already inclined to hyperparent. As everyday life without selection shows, such parents are just as likely to flog their children, even without talent. Indeed, it would likely be more harmful to be a flogged untalented child than a flogged gifted child. At any rate, the disease is the parental psychology; the symptom is, among many, an attraction to selection. It is worth remembering that genius pianist Lang Lang was told by his father to commit suicide at the age of 10 because a teacher told Lang Lang that he had no talent and would never pass the entrance exam to the Beijing Conservatory. Lang Lang was not genetically selected.

A similarly contestable objection to cloning is that clones would live in the shadow of their preexisting clone, burdened by the expectations of those around to live a certain way (Holm 1998), or a clone would be discriminated against in various ways. This is true today—Prince Charles must live in the shadow of the expectation that he could become king. Nonetheless, no one sees this as a reason against giving birth to heirs to the throne. Children who are born to sports stars, say, are burdened with such expectations—but they do not have as great a chance as clones to live up to them.

To say that discrimination against children whose genes were selected for certain reasons (including clones) is a reason not to bring them into existence is like saying having an African American child in racist nineteenth-century America would be wrong because such a child would be a slave or victim of discrimination. What is clearly most wrong is the racism, or discrimination, and not the fact of being black or being selected for an advantageous trait.

It is certainly possible that human beings would have discriminatory attitudes to selected children, or clones, or to children produced artificially by IVF, or by mitochondrial transfer, or just because they look different. But the problem is not the manner of procreation, but the primitive, prejudiced attitudes people have. Discriminating against people because of their mode of creation is a new form of discrimination akin to racism and sexism—in the case of clones, "clonism."

If one is worried about selection being at the will of another, this worry equally applies to selection against disease. Whether one was selected because one did not have cystic fibrosis, or because one did have better self-control, one's existence in both cases is determined by the choice of the parents. One's very existence is the result of choice, not chance.

What is plausible about this objection, which surfaces explicitly in Michael Sandel's complaints about "hyperparenting" (Sandel 2007), is the subsequent limiting of choice and freedom by parents based on earlier selection decisions. What they (rightly) worry about is a child selected for exceptional musical talent will be locked in a room for 4 hours a day and forced to practice violin.

This is, indeed, bad parenting. As we have said, it can also easily occur without genetic selection. The best predictor of future talent is present talent. A child who early on displays real talent might equally, or more likely, be subjected to such parental tyranny.

And the same applies to selection for health. Now that parents have a fine healthy specimen, not a child sick with cystic fibrosis, they might choose to flog the child in Little Athletics to produce a running superstar.

What is problematic in all these cases is not selection, or identification of talent, but *parenting*. This is related to but separate from selection. How we treat our children once they are in existence is an important question, and many of us can surely do better. But this is very different to whether we should let nature decide what kind of children we have.

Choosing a gifted child is, in a sense, to give that child a gift—one which should be used for the good of the child, and, ultimately, how that person sees fit. There is nothing wrong with being exceptional at music or math or running. Indeed, it is a capacity that is worth having. It is wrong to be singled out and mistreated on the basis of that feature, just as it is wrong to be discriminated against because you are a woman or a part of racial or religious minority.

One of us has given a similar response to the living in the shadow objection to reproductive cloning, which could be called "clonism." The discrimination against children on the basis of a gift could be called "giftism." Children may well have a right to an open future, but that does not preclude genetic selection and PB is not in tension with it. Indeed, we have elsewhere argued that it can *increase* the openness of one's future (Schaefer, Kahane, and Savulescu 2014).

CONCLUSION

The two best objections to PB are that it requires a conception of human well-being and that it is committed to the existence of impersonal reasons. We have argued that the most plausible account of well-being has subjective and objective elements, is not culturally relative, but is context sensitive, and includes intersubjective elements. Importantly there is much imprecision about evaluations of well-being.

PB is committed to the existence of impersonal reasons, but this is less metaphysically queer than initially appears—many commitments to future generations involve impersonal considerations. We have argued that person-affecting reasons are stronger than impersonal reasons, and this lessens some of the force of several objections to PB, such as it involves significant sacrifices of procreators.

PB, we believe, articulates a prima facie reason or obligation rooted in common sense. It is a reason that has real implications for being a moral parent.

Notes

1. In this case, disability is certain. Similar arguments apply even when it is uncertain or even unlikely—see Savulescu and De Crespigny (2014) for the case of avoiding unlikely person-affecting harm.
2. For a discussion of other issues relating to selecting against disability, see David Wasserman, this volume, Chapter 20.
3. It is currently very demanding for lay people to obtain and assess this scientific information because genetic selection is now widely seen as deeply wrong. Once PB or something close would be more widely accepted, it is almost certain that the relevant evidence and considerations will be compiled in an accessible way, reducing the demandingness of the decision process.
4. Here we follow W. D. Ross in describing this as a prima facie obligation (Ross 1930), though others prefer to speak instead of pro tanto moral obligations to avoid the mistaken impression that when such an obligation is outweighed by other considerations, this means that it does not still have genuine moral force (see Kagan 1989, 17).
5. Moreover, once procreative decisions have been made, they are typically irreversible, making some forms of blame pointless. This is not true of many parenting decisions where blame can pressure parents to better behavior. However, it would be self-defeating to deliberately create a child with a disadvantageous condition that *could* be corrected after conception or birth (see Kahane 2009).
6. http://emedicine.medscape.com/article/1181570-overview.
7. This is not to say that knowingly conceiving an anencephalic child by natural means is defensible.
8. Barnes (2014) suggests (but does not fully endorse) that it may be wrong to interfere with a child's natural endowment. If this was correct, then reasons to preserve a feature need not immediately imply that this feature is beneficial or that we should select for it. For some criticism of this idea, see Kahane and Savulescu (2016).
9. Of course, we must take account of gene–environment interactions, which may modify or even flip the effect of a particular gene. Though fascinating, such considerations are beyond the scope of this chapter.
10. Subjectivist accounts of well-being are often driven by subjectivist accounts of value more generally. When this is so, they have their roots in a metaethical view about the nature of value. In principle, however, even a metaethical realist could still hold that what makes a life go best is the satisfaction of our desires. Such a view combines objectivism at the metaethical level with a substantive view of well-being that is subjectivist in character. We will ignore this complication in what follows.
11. Thanks to Leslie Francis for drawing these considerations to our attention.

12. Notice that we have shifted here to general criticism of desire-based theories of value and reasons. On a preference-satisfaction theory of well-being, Jahi's life would not contain either positive or negative well-being since in her brain-dead state she has no preferences.

13. James Griffin (1986) proposes a "prudential value theory" that is also a form of objective list theory. His list of prudential values includes accomplishment, "the components of human existence" (including autonomy, basic capabilities, and liberty), understanding, enjoyment, and deep personal relations.

14. Thanks to Leslie Francis for this objection. Notice that even those who are strongly objectivist about well-being can hold such a pluralist view.

15. On a stronger version of the objection, we cannot compare the lives of the deaf and of the hearing because certain goods are incommensurable. But even if you hold such a view, the point remains that a hearing life can contain more of the relevant kinds of values than a life that gives no access to sound. Of course, a hearing musician might also be extremely lonely and unhappy. Her well-being would be poorer to that of most deaf people who enjoy deep relationships with others. But that some deaf lives are better than some hearing lives does not change the point that before conception we can expect that, in current circumstances, hearing lives have greater prospects by offering access to a wider range of goods.

16. Even if there were a single best genome, it is highly unlikely that we would ever be in a position to identify it, and there will therefore still be a range of genomes we would be equally justified in selecting.

17. For the seminal discussion of what is now known as the "nonidentity problem," see Parfit (1984). This issue is also discussed in this volume in the chapters by Cohen, de Grazia, Malek, and Orentlicher and, less directly, in the chapter by Wasserman. See Malek's chapter for an attempt to reject the consensus view that a person cannot be harmed by being brought into existence so long as their life is worth living.

18. Various authors have tried to propose alternative ways to impersonal reasons to account for the couple's reason to wait in cases such as Medical Consultation I. In Savulescu and Kahane (2009), we pointed out that in principle PB could be also grounded in any of these alternative views. But since we are not ourselves persuaded by any of these alternative accounts, we shall focus here only on impersonal reasons.

19. Leaving aside the person-affecting reasons that may also exist, for example that a child with a disability will be more difficult for the parents to care for, more expensive, and so on. The chapter by David Wasserman in this volume addresses these considerations.

20. Notice that for those, like Elizabeth Barnes, who think of disability as merely a difference from the normal, there would be no good reasons to support *either* program, if prejudice against the disabled were removed (Barnes 2014).

21. If there were a gene therapy available to cure deafness, then it would be wrong not to administer it to Doris. In our view, this would be as wrong (or nearly as wrong) as deafening David.

22. An important complication, however, is that in time deafness might become part of David's sense of self so that, looking back at his parents' action, he may not regret it. But this, of course, hardly shows that his parents did not act wrongly.

23. Whether such decisions are wrong cannot be determined without attention to the details of specific cases. It would matter to what extent the disadvantageous condition in question is actually expected to reduce well-being, to what extent its presence will benefit the parents or others (and thus constitute person-affecting benefit) and to what extent there might be significant reasons of justice not to select against the condition.

Bibliography

Agar, Nicholas. 2014. A question about defining moral bioenhancement. *Journal of Medical Ethics* 40: 369–370.

Argyle, M. 2001. *The psychology of happiness*. Hove, East Sussex: Routledge.

Bennett, Rebecca. 2009. The fallacy of the principle of procreative beneficence. *Bioethics* 23, no. 5: 265–273.

Bentham, Jeremy. 1830. *The rationale of reward*. London: Robert Heward.

Boorse, Christopher. 1975. On the distinction between disease and illness. *Philosophy & Public Affairs* 5, no. 1: 49–68.

Bostrom, Nick, and Toby Ord. 2006. The reversal test: Eliminating status quo bias in applied ethics. *Ethics* 116, no. 4: 656–679.

Brandt, Richard B. 1979. *A theory of the good and the right*. Amherst, NY: Prometheus Books.

Brickman, P., Coates, D. and Janoff-Bulman, R. 1978. "Lottery winners and accident victims: is happiness relative?" *Journal of Personality and Social Psychology*, 36, no. 8: 917–927.

Buchanan, Allen, Dan W. Brock, Norman Daniels, and Daniel Wikler. 2001. *From chance to choice: Genetics and justice*. New York: Cambridge University Press.

Davis, Dena S. 1997. Genetic dilemmas and the child's right to an open future. *Hastings Center Report* 27, no. 2: 7–15.

Diener, E. 2000. Subjective well-being: The science of happiness and a proposal for a national index. *American Psychologist* 55, no. 1: 34–43.

Douglas, Thomas, and Katrien Devolder. 2013. Procreative altruism: Beyond individualism in reproductive selection. *Journal of Medicine and Philosophy* 38, no. 4: 400–419.

Dunlop, Mikael, and Julian Savulescu. 2014. Distributive justice and cognitive enhancement in lower, normal intelligence. *Monash Bioethics Review* 32, no. 3–4: 189–204.

Dworkin, Ronald. 1977. *Taking rights seriously*. Cambridge, MA: Harvard University Press.

Elster, Jakob. 2011. Procreative beneficence–cui bono? *Bioethics* 25, no. 9: 482–488.

Griffin, James. 1986. *Well-being: Its meaning, measurement, and moral importance*. Oxford: Clarendon Press.

Habermas Jurgen. 2003. *The future of human nature*. Cambridge, UK: Polity Press.

Harris, J. 1996. What is the good of health care? *Bioethics* 10, no. 4: 269–291.

Heyd, D. 1994. *Genethics: Moral issues in the creation of people*. Berkeley, CA: University of California Press.

Holm, Søren. 1998. A life in the shadow: One reason why we should not clone humans. *Cambridge Quarterly of Healthcare Ethics* 7, no. 2: 160–162.

Hotke, Andrew. 2014. The principle of procreative beneficence: Old arguments and a new challenge. *Bioethics* 28, no. 5: 255–262.

Hume, D., 1978. *A treatise on human nature*, 2nd ed. Oxford: Clarendon Press.

Kagan, Shelly. 1989. *The limits of morality*. Oxford: Clarendon Press.

Kahane, Guy. 2009. Non-identity, self-defeat, and attitudes to future people. *Philosophical Studies* 145, no. 2: 193–214.

Kahane, Guy. 2011. Mastery without mystery: Why there is no promethean sin in enhancement. *The Journal of Applied Philosophy* 28, no. 4: 355–368.

Kahane, Guy, and Julian Savulescu. 2016. Disability and mere difference," *Ethics* 126, no 3: 774–788.

Kahane, Guy, and Julian Savulescu. 2015. Normal human variation: Refocusing the enhancement debate. *Bioethics* 29, no. 2: 133–143.

Kahane, Guy, and Julian Savulescu. 2009. The welfarist account of disability. In K. Brownlee and A. Cureton, eds., *Disability and disadvantage*, 14–53. Oxford: Oxford University Press.

Kahneman, D., and C. Varey. 1991. Notes on the psychology of utility. In J. Elster and J. E. Roemer, eds. *Interpersonal comparisons of well-being*, 127–163, New York: Cambridge University Press.

Kass, L. 2003. Ageless bodies, happy souls: Biotechnology and the pursuit of perfection. *The New Atlantis* 1 (Spring): 9–28.

Konrath, Sara H., Edward H. O'Brien, and Courtney Hsing. 2011. Changes in dispositional empathy in American college students over time: A meta-analysis. *Personality and Social Psychology Review* 15, no. 2: 180–198.

de Lazari-Radek, Katarzyna, and Peter Singer. 2014. *The point of view of the universe: Sidgwick and contemporary ethics*. Oxford: Oxford University Press.

de Melo-Martín, Inmaculada. 2004. On our obligation to select the best children: A reply to Savulescu. *Bioethics* 18, no. 1: 72–83.

Minerva, Francesca. Forthcoming. How should we tackle financial and prosocial biases against unattractive people? *Behavioral and Brain Sciences*.

Moller, Dan. 2007. Love and death. *The Journal of Philosophy* 104, no. 6: 301–316.

Narveson, Jan. 1973. Moral problems of population. *The Monist* 57, no. 1: 62–86.

Overall, Christine. 2012. *Why have children? The ethical debate*. Boston, MA: MIT Press.

Parfit, Derek. 1984. *Reasons and persons*. Oxford: Oxford University Press.

Parfit, Derek. 2011. *On what matters*. Oxford: Oxford University Press.

Parfit, Derek. Can we avoid the repugnant conclusion? Unpublished paper. Accessed February 2014.

Persson, Ingmar, and Julian Savulescu. 2012. *Unfit for the future: The need for moral enhancement*. Oxford: Oxford University Press.

Pope, T. M. McMath family sues Oakland Children's Hospital; Alleges Jahi is alive. Medical futility blog. March 3, 2015. http://medicalfutility.blogspot.co.uk/2015/03/mcmath-family-sues-oakland-childrens.html. Accessed August 6, 2015.

Railton, Peter. 1986. Facts and values. *Philosophical Topics* 14, no. 2: 5–31.

Ross, W. D. 1930. *The right and the good*. Reprinted with an introduction by Philip Stratton-Lake. 2002. Oxford: Oxford University Press.

Sandel, Michael. 2007. *The case against perfection*. Cambridge, MA: Belknap Press,

Savulescu, Julian. 1999. Desire-based and value-based normative reasons, *Bioethics* 13, no. 5: 405–413.

Savulescu, Julian. 2002. Deaf lesbians, "designer disability," and the future of medicine. *British Medical Journal* 32, no. 7367: 771–773.

Savulescu, Julian. 2007. Genetic interventions and the ethics of enhancement of human beings. In B. Steinbock, ed. *The Oxford handbook of bioethics*, 516–535. Oxford: Oxford University Press.

Savulescu, Julian. 2014. The nature of the moral obligation to select the best children. In *The future of bioethics: International dialogues*, ed. A. Akayabashi, 170–182. Oxford: Oxford University Press.

Savulescu, Julian. 2016. The unfairness of unattractives. *Practical Ethics in the News*. http://blog.practicalethics.ox.ac.uk/2016/07/the-unfairness-of-unattractiveness/. Accessed 26 July 2016.

Savulescu, Julian. 2015a. Procreative beneficence, diversity, intersubjectivity, and imprecision, *The American Journal of Bioethics* 15, no. 6: 16–18.

Savulescu, Julian. 2015b. Bioethics: Why philosophy is essential for progress. *Journal of Medical Ethics* 41, no. 1: 28–33.

Savulescu, Julian, and Lachlan de Crespigny. 2014. Homebirth and the future child. *Journal of Medical Ethics* 40, no. 12: 807–812.

Savulescu, Julian, and Guy Kahane. 2009. The moral obligation to create children with the best chance of the best life, *Bioethics* 23, no. 5: 274–290.

Savulescu, Julian, and Guy Kahane. 2011. Disability: A welfarist approach, *Journal of Clinical Ethics* 6, no. 1: 45–51.

Savulescu, Julian, and Richard W. Momeyer. 1997. Should informed consent be based on rational beliefs? *Journal of Medical Ethics* 23, no. 5: 282–288.

Savulescu, Julian, Anders Sandberg, and Guy Kahane. 2011. Well-being and enhancement." In Julian Savulescu, Ruud ter Meulen, and Guy Kahane, eds., *Enhancing human capacities*, 3–18. Oxford: Wiley-Blackwell.

Schaefer, G. Owen, Guy Kahane, and Julian Savulescu. 2014. Autonomy and enhancement, *Neuroethics* 7, no. 2: 123–136.

Sidgwick, Henry. 1907. *The methods of ethics*. Cambridge, MA: Hackett Publishing.

Singer, Peter. 2011. *Practical ethics*. Cambridge, UK: Cambridge University Press.

Smith, Michael. 1994. *The moral problem*. Oxford: Wiley-Blackwell.

Sparrow, Robert J. 2007. Procreative beneficence, obligation, and eugenics. *Genomics, Society and Policy* 3, no. 3: 43–59.

Sparrow, Robert J. 2011. A not-so-new eugenics: Harris and Savulescu on human enhancement. *Hastings Center Report* 41, no. 1: 32–42.

Sparrow, Robert J. 2014a. Ethics, eugenics and politics, In *The Future of Bioethics: International Dialogues*, edited by Akira Akabayashi, 139–153. Oxford: Oxford University Press.

Sparrow, Robert J. 2014b. The real force of procreative beneficence. In *The future of bioethics: International dialogues*, edited by Akira Akabayashi, 183–192. Oxford: Oxford University Press.

Sparrow, Robert J. 2015. Imposing genetic diversity. *The American Journal of Bioethics* 15, no. 6: 2–10.

Wilkinson, Dominic J. 2010. Antenatal diagnosis of trisomy 18, harm and parental choice. *Journal of Medical Ethics* 36, no. 11: 644–645.

CHAPTER 27

OPTING FOR TWINS IN IN VITRO FERTILIZATION

What Does Procreative Responsibility Require?

BONNIE STEINBOCK

AN unfortunate side effect of assisted reproductive technology (ART) has been the dramatic increase in the number of multiple births. When a woman gives birth to eight children, as in the case of Nadya Suleman, the 33-year-old infertility patient dubbed "Octomom" in the media, it is front-page news and there are outraged calls for increased surveillance over and limits to ART (Caplan 2009). However, a focus on extreme cases is misplaced, both because they are extremely rare and because the physician in the case, Dr. Michael Kamrava, was guilty of gross negligence. Although he originally claimed to have replaced only six embryos into Ms. Suleman's uterus, in fact, he replaced twelve. Guidelines from the Society for Reproductive Medicine and the American Society for Reproductive Medicine (ASRM/SART) at the time called for no more than three embryos to be transferred to women under 35. Kamrava was expelled from the American Society for Reproductive Medicine (ASRM) in 2009, and his medical license was revoked by the California Medical Board two years later (Rong-Gong Lin II 2011).

The real problem is not the rare cases of septuplets and octuplets, or cowboys, like Kamrava, but the dramatic rise in the births of twins and triplets, which are far more common. The rate of high-order multiple births (triplets and more) rose more than 400% in the 1980s and 1990s, while the rate of twin births increased 76% (Martin et al. 2012, p. 12). There has been a significant decrease in the rate of high-order multiple births in recent years, due to improvements in infertility treatment, combined with a widespread consensus among fertility physicians that triplets and more are a bad outcome. There is less agreement among practitioners about whether twin births are also a bad outcome, with some regarding twins as an acceptable outcome, and even a minority who maintain that a twin pregnancy and birth is a desirable outcome for patients who want more than one child (Gleicher and Barad 2009). Despite numerous statements by various professional organizations that the essential aim of in vitro fertilization (IVF) is the birth of one single healthy child (Land and Evers 2003; ASRM Practice Committee report 2012), the rate of twin births has continued to rise (Blickstein 2004), although it may have plateaued (Martin et al. 2012, p. 12). In 2010, the most recent year for which data are available, the rate of twin births in assisted reproduction was slightly over than 33 per 1,000 births (Martin et al. 2012, p. 12), much higher than the rate of twins in natural conception, which is about 1 in 250 pregnancies (ASRM 2012b, p. 4).

While some of the increase in multiple births can be explained by the greater number of older women (who face an increased risk of multiple births) having more babies, the primary reason for the increase in multiple births is infertility treatment (Dickey 2007, p. 1554). It is often assumed that the increase in multiple births is due to the widespread practice in IVF of transferring multiple embryos. However, some fertility experts think that the focus on IVF is misplaced. They believe that that the increase in multiple births is due, not to IVF, but to a different fertility technique known as controlled ovarian stimulation (COS). COS is responsible for close to 50% of all triplet and higher births, much higher than that associated with IVF. To see why, a brief discussion of these two techniques is in order.

In both COS and IVF, the woman is given superovulatory drugs, drugs that cause her to ovulate and produce multiple eggs. The difference between the two treatments is that in IVF, the eggs are surgically removed from the woman's body, fertilized in a petri dish, and one or more is replaced in her uterus. The decision to transfer only one embryo is known as single-embryo transfer (SET).[1] SET almost always results in a singleton pregnancy, although a twin pregnancy is still possible, though unlikely, since a single embryo can split after transfer. In a double-embryo transfer (DET), the risk of a twin pregnancy is much greater. Despite recommendations from several professional groups, SET is not widely used in the United States. In 2012, American doctors transferred single embryos in only 14.8% of cycles, even for the women with the best chances of getting pregnant, those under 35 years old (SART Clinic Summary Report, 2012).

In COS, by contrast, the eggs are not removed from the woman's body. After the drugs are administered, and ovulation occurs, the woman is artificially inseminated or engages in timed intercourse. If fertilization takes place, it occurs within the woman's body. Although most women who get pregnant taking fertility drugs have singletons, COS may result in a multiple pregnancy because once the eggs are released, it is impossible to control how many get fertilized. To some extent, the number of eggs released can be controlled by the dosage of the medications, but it is not possible to control this with precision. An ultrasound can be done to check if too many eggs are likely to be released, in which case, the cycle can be called off before the woman is inseminated. However, monitoring is difficult, because the eggs develop inside follicles: "the eggs themselves are not visible, not all follicles contain eggs, occasionally one follicle may contain more than one egg, and not all follicles will mature in time for ovulation" (Johnston et al. 2013, p. 13).

COS is more commonly performed than IVF. It is less invasive and less expensive, so it is usually the first treatment for infertility, with IVF being used when COS fails or in cases whether COS is not indicated. Moreover, it can be done by general practitioners, who may be less experienced in determining the correct dosage of ovulatory drugs than board-certified reproductive endocrinologists. These factors lead some experts to think that it is COS, not IVF, that is primarily responsible for the failure to reduce the rate of multiple births. In light of this, some have suggested limiting the use of COS and fast-tracking patients to IVF (Johnston et al. 2013, p. 47).

In any event, even if IVF is not the only or primary reason for the increase in twin births, IVF accounts for 16.2% of them in the United States (Janvier et al. 2011, p. 409). If SET became the norm for good-prognosis patients, this rate would likely be significantly reduced. Sweden managed to reduce its rate of twins from about 35% to about 5%, without reducing the birth rate, after adopting a policy of SET in almost all cases (Orentlicher 2010). Continued research on COS may also reduce the twin birth rate. However, IVF uniquely offers the choice of a technique—SET—that virtually eliminates the possibility of a twin pregnancy. IVF thus provides a good lens for assessing individual procreative choices. Is DET a choice IVF patients are morally permitted to make, or ought they to choose SET?

Fertility doctors often note that many, even most, infertility patients express a desire for twins, and this has been confirmed by numerous studies (Ryan et al. 2004; Gleicher and Barad 2009; Levens and Hill 2013). Some practitioners regard this all by itself as a justification for DET, arguing that depriving patients of the option of DET or SET would violate patient autonomy. This suggests a particular model of the physician–patient relationship (Emanuel and Emanuel 1992), the informative model, in which physicians are supposed simply to provide patients with all the facts and then to let them make their own decisions, without attempting to discover, much less influence, the patients' values. I agree with Emanuel and Emanuel that the informative model rests on an overly simplistic view of autonomy and the doctor–patient relationship. The deliberative model they propose, which includes dialogue between doctor and patient regarding the patient's values, is an improvement. But even if the informative model is the correct one and patients are entitled to make their own treatment choices, their choices must be fully informed in order to be autonomous. Many patients do not know the risks of multiple births, and research shows that patients who are educated about the risks of multiple pregnancies are less likely to regard twin pregnancies as desirable and more likely to be accepting of SET (Stillman et al. 2013, p. 2601). Finally, the right of patients to decide on treatment choices does not make those choices immune from moral evaluation, which is the topic of this chapter. Such an evaluation requires an examination of the reasons for the choice of DET over SET, and the nature and magnitude of the risks incurred.

Critics of multiple births sometimes portray the reasons for wanting twins as frivolous. Due to the glamorization of twins in the media (Schumann 2013), prospective parents may want twins because they think it will be fun to dress them alike or to get attention from passersby. This is probably a mistaken view. As my obstetrician, Naomi Bloomfield, herself a mother of twins, told a patient who discovered late in pregnancy that she was having twins, "Twins are special; they're not fun." In any event, finding twins adorable is hardly a morally good reason for exposing one's offspring to additional risks.

However, there are reasons in favor of DET that are not frivolous and deserve to be taken seriously. The most important reason given by infertility patients for wanting DET is that they believe it increases their chance of achieving a pregnancy. They regard having a child with disabilities, even serious disabilities, as more desirable than having no child at all (Scotland et al., 2007). Another consideration in favor of DET is that it enables people who want more than one child to complete their family in one round of fertility treatment, sparing them the expense and burdens of multiple rounds. This is often referred to as "getting two for the price of one" or a "2-for-1 mentality" (Levens and Hill 2013). Older patients have an additional reason for wanting a twin pregnancy: they are afraid that they may not be able to get pregnant a second time.

Some of the risks of multifetal pregnancy are increased risks to the women themselves: "multifetal pregnancies are associated with an increased risk of morbidity for the mother, including increased rates of preeclampsia, cardiac morbidity, amniotic fluid or thromboembolism, the need for obstetric intervention, postpartum hemorrhage, hysterectomy, blood transfusion, prolonged hospital stay, and pregnancy-related death" (MacKay et al. 2006, p. 563). There are also psychosocial consequences of multiple births, such as increased risk for postpartum depression (Stillman et al. 2013, p. 2603). I will not consider such risks, because while they are clearly relevant to the decision for SET or DET, they are not directly relevant to a moral evaluation of the decision. Taking additional risks with one's own physical or psychological health may be imprudent, but it is not immoral. Informed women can decide for themselves what health risks they are willing to undergo to fulfill their procreative goals. It is a very different matter when they impose additional health risks on others (their future children) in order to fulfill those goals.

Nor will I consider the additional economic costs to society as a whole that are incurred by multiple pregnancies, primarily from premature infants who typically need longer hospital stays, including expensive stays in neonatal intensive care units (NICUs). These costs are quite high. It has been estimated that a mandatory SET policy would save Canada $40 million a year, by reducing the number of infants in NICUs (Janvier et al. 2011, p. 413). Canada might use these savings to cover IVF, which it currently does not.

However, while cost is clearly relevant to social policy, I would argue that it is not directly relevant to the patient's choice of treatment. That is, patients are not obligated to choose treatments based on the cost to society. They may choose any treatment offered to them on the basis that it furthers their own goals. The central moral issue raised by multiple pregnancies is the potential for conflict between the fertility patient's desire to get pregnant and have a live birth, and the increased risks imposed on offspring.

HEALTH RISKS TO OFFSPRING
FROM TWIN PREGNANCIES

About 60% of IVF twins are born prematurely, at an average of 35 weeks; more than half are low birth weight, weighing less than five and a half pounds (ASRM 2012b). Preterm birth and low birth weight put twins at increased risk of death, respiratory disorders, cerebral palsy, eye and ear impairments, and learning disabilities (Johnston et al. 2013). At the same time, most twin pregnancies result in the birth of two healthy children (van Wely et al. 2006, p. 2737). However, the riskiness of a choice is not solely determined by how likely a bad outcome is to occur. For example, most children born to women who smoke are also born healthy. Yet obstetricians recommend against smoking during pregnancy because of the increased risks. So, how risky are twin pregnancies? One problem in answering this question is that the experts do not agree.

Consider the increased risk of mortality. The infant mortality rate for twins compared to singletons has been estimated at fourfold to sevenfold greater (Dickey 2007, p. 1559), nearly five times greater (Mathews and MacDorman 2013, p. 6), or more than twice as high (Stillman et al. 2013, p. 2603). Bradley Van Voorhis, an obstetrician/gynecologist and reproductive endocrinologist, puts the additional risk in context by comparing it to other risks of dying. He estimates that DET has an excess iatrogenic mortality rate per newborn of 0.8%. While that is considerably lower than some of the aforementioned estimates, Van Voorhis claims that it is 80 times the risk of dying in surgery under general anesthesia, and about the same risk a US soldier in Iraq or Afghanistan has of dying within a year. He refers to DET as the "riskiest procedure in OB-GYN," and among the riskiest in medicine generally (Van Voorhis 2012). However, Swedish researchers found no difference in mortality at all in IVF twins compared to IVF singletons, despite significantly higher rates of preterm birth and low birth weight (Sazonova et al. 2013).

What explains this disagreement among the experts? There may be multiple reasons, including the date of the studies and the location. Another factor is making the correct comparison. Some argue that it is unfair to compare IVF twins with non-IVF singletons, since IVF imposes more risks than non-medically assisted births (Helmerhorst et al. 2004, p. 3). For example, if one compares the risk of cerebral palsy in twins as compared with singletons, twins are four times as likely to have cerebral palsy as singletons. However, that figure comes from comparing naturally conceived twins and singletons. It fails to take into account the increased risk all IVF-conceived children, singletons and twins, have of cerebral palsy and other neurological sequelae (van Wely et al. 2006, p. 2737). In addition, it is argued that the correct comparison is not between one twin pregnancy and one singleton pregnancy, but rather between one twin pregnancy and *two* singleton pregnancies, given that most infertility patients want more than one child. Gleicher and Barad argue that IVF twin pregnancies do not impose higher overall outcome risks per newborn than IVF singleton pregnancies (Gleicher and Barad 2009).

Stillman et al. call this claim "demonstrably false" (Stillman et al. 2013, p. 2602). They cite studies that show that when the comparison is between one twin IVF pregnancy and two singleton IVF pregnancies, each child born in a twin pregnancy is three times as likely to require assisted ventilation, more than three times as likely to suffer from respiratory disorders or have intercranial bleeding, and four times as likely to have jaundice. Each IVF twin is more than twice as likely to be admitted to the NICU and, once admitted, will spend nearly twice as long there. Even adjusting for the increased risk of cerebral palsy that IVF singletons face, the risk that IVF twins will have cerebral palsy is twice as high as IVF singletons. Moreover, the delivery of twins at 29 weeks gestation is "a too common phenomenon in twin gestations and the consequences to two fetuses delivered at 29 weeks in a twin gestation can be catastrophic and life-long for either or both, should they survive at all" (Stillman et al. 2013, p. 2603). By contrast, they note, the likelihood of two separate singleton pregnancies both delivering at 29 weeks is extremely unlikely.

While there is disagreement about precisely how risky twin pregnancies are, it seems reasonable to conclude that twin IVF pregnancies do impose additional risks on off-spring, compared with singleton IVF pregnancies. The question of risk must be separated from how things actually turn out. Leaving one's toddler alone in the bathtub is unjustifiably risky and irresponsible, even if the child does not drown, and even if the absolute numbers of children who drown each year are low. For this reason, it misses the point to say that "a twin pregnancy that *results in the birth of two healthy children* does not necessarily deserve to be condemned as an adverse outcome" (van Wely et al. 2006, p. 2738; my emphasis). The question is whether the choice of a twin pregnancy, when a singleton pregnancy is a possibility, is irresponsible because it imposes significantly increased risks on the resulting offspring.

If the only issue were the additional risks to offspring, DET would not be a morally responsible choice. However, it is not the only factor. We must also consider the possibility that DET improves the chance of achieving pregnancy. Given the high priority they place on getting pregnant, most fertility patients are not willing to reduce their chances of getting pregnant, even if this means some increase in the risk of disabling conditions.

DOES SINGLE-EMBRYO TRANSFER REDUCE THE CHANCES OF GETTING PREGNANT?

As noted earlier, Sweden managed to reduce its rate of twins from about 35% to about 5%, without reducing the birth rate, after adopting a policy of SET in almost all cases (Orentlicher 2010). However, some researchers maintain that adopting SET for all or most IVF patients would result in a decrease in the pregnancy rate (Joint SOGC-CFAS Clinical Practice Guideline 2010). Most randomized clinical trials (RCTs) comparing single transfers of either one or two embryos have demonstrated that pregnancy rates are higher when two embryos are transferred (Stillman et al. 2013, p. 2602). However, RCTs by definition do not distinguish between favorable- and unfavorable-prognosis patients. For this reason, many practitioners favor a more flexible approach that involves identifying favorable-prognosis patients and either offering them SET, or even, in the case of one clinic, mandating SET for such patients (Kresowik et al. 2011). This clinic defined "favorable-prognosis patients" as those less than 38 years of age without a history of failed fresh cycle at their institution, with seven zygotes for culture, and at least one good- or excellent-quality blastocyst available for transfer. After studying the results of this policy during the five years before and after it was instituted, they found "improved live birth rates, unchanged clinic volume, and a dramatic decrease in multiple births" (Kresowik et al. 2011, p. 1368). According to Dr. Bradley Van Voorhis, director of the clinic, "good-prognosis patients who qualify for the mandatory SET policy have a very high birthrate in the fresh cycle and a cumulative pregnancy rate that exceeds 80%" (Van Voorhis 2013, p. 3).

The ability to identify good-quality embryos also plays a role in keeping up pregnancy rates. American infertility experts often complain that restrictions on federal funding for embryo research hamper their attempts to improve techniques for determining the quality of blastocysts. Despite such obstacles, techniques are improving. Combined with the ability to identify which patients are at greater risk of having multiple births (Lannon et al. 2012), this should result in improved pregnancy rates. A third factor is cryopreservation of good-quality embryos that can be used at a later date in a subsequent SET. Steady improvement in cryopreservation techniques has led to an improvement in implantation, pregnancy, and delivery rates, leading to equality, or near equality, between SET and DET in cumulative pregnancy rates.

> Thus, this apparent choice between singleton transfer and higher pregnancy rates represents a false dichotomy, as RCT and non-randomized studies have consistently shown that the cumulative chances of pregnancy and birth per cycle are no lower with eSET than with multiple embryo transfer when the subsequent transfer of additional cryopreserved embryos is included. (Stillman et al. 2013, p. 2602)

A group of Scandinavian researchers report a similar finding. In women under 36 years of age, transferring one fresh embryo and then, if needed, one frozen-and-thawed embryo "dramatically reduces the rate of multiple births while achieving a rate of live births that is not substantially lower than the rate that is achievable with double-embryo transfer" (Thurin 2004, p. 2392).

In fact, it may be that a "freeze-all policy" actually produces a higher pregnancy rate than the transfer of a fresh embryo, followed, if necessary, by the transfer of a frozen and thawed embryo. A press release from ESHRE (European Society of Human Reproduction and Embryology) in 2012 reported that "the first meta-analysis on this subject indicates that the chance of a clinical pregnancy is around 30% higher when all embryos are frozen for later transfer than with fresh embryo transfer." The results are considered "preliminary" although statistically robust (ESHRE 2012). The reason for the improvement is presumably that cryopreserving all embryos generated in a stimulated IVF cycle for later transfer in a nonstimulated natural cycle avoids the adverse effects that ovarian stimulation might have on endometrial receptivity during the treatment cycle.

It seems, then, that SET need not reduce the chances of getting pregnant in good- or favorable-prognosis patients. I say "need not" because obviously the skill of the physicians in the program will affect cumulative pregnancy rates. Less skilled practitioners may not be able to get as good pregnancy rates with SET as with DET, and there are wide variations between practices. Another factor to be considered concerns patient characteristics: the claim of comparable cumulative pregnancy rates is made only for favorable-prognosis patients. This qualification is important. Some of those who oppose the movement toward SET, and especially legally mandated SET, do so because they fear a slippery slope. Norbert Gleicher notes that the Finnish group that initially introduced SET to the world for favorable-prognosis patients now proposes it for women up to age 44. Gleicher asks, "Can one responsibly suggest to a patient to have an eSET at age 44 because she always can have another child 12 to 18 months later? I don't think so" (Gleicher 2013, p. 4). However, even if there is no moral obligation for *all* IVF patients to choose SET, there may be a moral obligation on the part of favorable-prognosis patients, as a way of reducing the risks in offspring.

One of the increased risks in twin pregnancies is mortality. Whether prenatal or perinatal death is a harm to the infant is a complicated issue, beyond the scope of this paper.[2] By contrast, imposing a disabling condition on a child, when this could have been avoided, may seem obviously harmful. However, in recent years, disability advocates have argued that the able-bodied overemphasize the badness of disability. This would appear to have clear implications for evaluating the riskiness of twin pregnancies. If the possible outcomes for twins are not so bad, then imposing such risks on offspring may not be irresponsible after all. Moreover, many IVF patients would prefer to give birth to a child with a chronic disability than never give birth at all (Scotland et al. 2007, p. 979). They are willing to accept greater risks of disability for two children than lowering even slightly their chances of giving birth. Is that a permissible, or even praiseworthy, attitude to take toward the risk of disability? To answer this question, we need to examine the disability critique.

THE DISABILITY CRITIQUE

The disability critique emphasizes that the lives of people with disabilities, even severe disabilities, are usually well worth living. Indeed, as disability advocates remind us, people living with disabilities are usually as happy as those who are not disabled (Asch 1999). On this view, the belief that disability is always a serious disadvantage, and incompatible with life satisfaction, stems from prejudice and ignorance about the lives of people with disabling conditions. The disability critique also criticizes the "medical model" of disability, which sees deviations from "normal" functioning as inherently disadvantageous. This ignores the fact that the problems people with disabilities face usually stem not from the disabling condition itself, but from prejudiced attitudes of the nondisabled toward them, combined with an absence of accommodations and services that would enable those with disabilities to participate fully in society.

Some derive conclusions from the disability critique about the morality of prenatal testing, which, if the fetus is found to have, or be at serious risk for, a genetic disease, is most often followed by selective abortion. Adrienne Asch and David Wasserman think that such abortions usually reflect the unwillingness to be the parent of a child with a disability, an attitude they regard as "a morally impoverished conception of parenthood and family" (Asch and Wasserman 2005, p. 173). The mistake, they contend, is to think that the one piece of information that is given by prenatal testing—the likelihood of genetic disease or disability—can provide the prospective parents with good information about whether raising a child with a disabling condition can meet their parental expectations. Moreover, they maintain that the belief that the lives of children with disabilities and those of their parents are inevitable painful and burdensome is "false or greatly exaggerated . . . "

> The most that can plausibly be claimed is that being or having a child with a disability is at times different and more difficult than being or having a "normal" child, and that specific impairments are very unlikely to meet specific parental expectations (e.g., a child with Down syndrome is not likely to become a great mathematician like her mother). (Asch and Wasserman 2005, p. 175)

Asch and Wasserman think that the false beliefs and prejudices that give rise to prenatal testing and selective abortion not only reflect problematic attitudes toward parenting. Prenatal testing also harms existing people with impairments by contributing to their stigmatization and stereotyping (Asch and Wasserman 2005, p. 183).

What follows from the disability critique about opting for twins in IVF? Does the claim that parents morally ought to choose SET to avoid disability in their offspring reflect morally problematic attitudes toward disability? Does it express the wrong view of parenting? While Asch and Wasserman do not directly discuss opting for twins in IVF,[3] they make it clear that the morality of trying to avoid a child with a particular characteristic, such as a disability, depends in part on the strength of the preference not to have a child with that characteristic. They write:

> In general, a person appears to reject a parental relationship with an impaired child more emphatically if she sees herself as choosing between an impaired child and no child than if she sees herself as choosing between an impaired child and an unimpaired child. In the latter case, she may be expressing a preference that is less hurtful than the categorical rejection involved in the former case. (Asch and Wasserman 2005, p. 196)

This suggests that they would not consider it necessarily *wrong* for IVF patients to opt for SET to reduce the risk of disability in offspring. However, it seems unlikely they would regard the choice *for* twins, given the increased risk of disability, to be an impermissible or irresponsible choice. Consider what they say about measures to prevent disability before pregnancy:

> For example, taking folic acid before conception may express concern for the capacities of any potential child, but need not express a refusal or even a strong reluctance to have a child with the impairment that folic acid is intended to prevent. A prospective parent who tries to preserve her child's capacity for unimpeded mobility

by taking folic acid in order to prevent spina bifida may be willing, or committed, to having the child even if the preventative regiment [*sic*] fails. (Asch and Wasserman 2005, pp. 196–197)

The primary moral argument in favor of SET is the avoidance of the increased risk of disability. If the choice of SET reflects a "strong reluctance" to have any child with a disability, Asch and Wasserman clearly regard the choice as morally problematic. However, they would also see opting for SET, which is done before a pregnancy begins, as morally different from selective abortion, which involves rejecting a particular fetus because of its disability. It seems, therefore, that they would regard the choice of SET as permissible, but not obligatory.

I reject the analysis given by Asch and Wasserman on several grounds. First, I think they underestimate the difficulties that accompany having and raising a child with certain disabilities, especially cognitive disabilities. Undoubtedly, the difficulties have been exaggerated. For example, children born with Down syndrome can have lives that are happy and satisfying. Their parents love them fiercely and do not regret their presence in their lives for a moment. And yet, the difficulties are real and not limited to their example of being unlikely to become a great mathematician. As one parent of a child with Down syndrome acknowledges, "It is at best uncertain whether she will go to college or get married, and very unlikely that she could have children of her own. She may not be able to fully support herself financially. She has a high likelihood of developing Alzheimer's at an early age" (Becker, 2010). It is not unreasonable, in my opinion, to wish to have children who will not face such obstacles. If abortion is permissible to avoid other burdens, such as loss of employment or educational opportunities, I cannot see why it is not equally permissible to avoid the extra burdens that come with having a child with significant disability.

But even if they are right about the morality of prenatal testing and selective abortion, I think they are wrong about preconception and preimplantation measures to avoid disability in offspring. In my view, a woman who refuses to take folic acid before pregnancy, for no good reason, harms and wrongs her child if the child is born with spina bifida, as much as a woman who binge-drinks and has a child with fetal alcohol syndrome. This is a harm to a particular child, a harm that could have been prevented. Preventing disability, including an increased risk of disability, in one's children and future children is not merely permissible. It is morally obligatory, unless there are pressing countervailing moral considerations.

It has been suggested that respect for patient autonomy is a countervailing moral consideration. I will return to that issue in the last section. However, first I need to address a claim that is related to the disability critique. It is the claim that even if both twins are born with severe disabling conditions, they have not been harmed by their parents' choice of DET, because had the parents chosen SET, only one of them would have been born. Since the disabilities are unlikely to be so bad as to make their lives not worth living, and since DET is a condition of their both being born at all, we cannot say that either one would have been better off, had SET been chosen. The choice of SET would not have made both twins healthy and whole, but rather would have prevented one of them from being born at all. This argument is known as the nonidentity problem, and it arises in numerous procreative contexts, including women deemed to be too young or too old to have children, surrogate motherhood (contract pregnancy), and couples who may transmit genetic diseases to offspring. It also arises in the question of how many embryos to transfer.

THE NONIDENTITY PROBLEM

John Robertson has argued that banning risky procreative technologies or arrangements *out of concern for the welfare of offspring* makes no sense because "But for the technique in question, the child never would have been born" (Robertson 1994, p. 122). If the child will have a life worth living, despite whatever disability is caused by the technique in question, and that child could not have been born except by using the technique, then it seems nonsensical to say that we are protecting *that child* by preventing his or her birth.

Thus, a fertility patient who wants DET, either because she thinks it will improve her chances of getting pregnant, or because she wants to avoid the burden and expense of an additional round of treatment, could utilize Robertson's argument as follows: "Yes, I realize that I am imposing extra health risks on one or both of my twins, if twins should result from DET. But I want very much to have two children, and I am willing to take on the extra burdens of raising children who may have disabilities. The children, once born, cannot complain that I disadvantaged them by choosing DET, since if I had chosen to have a singleton pregnancy, one of them would not have been born. Moreover, neither twin can be sure that, had I chosen SET, she would have been born in a healthier condition; she might not have been born at all. Therefore, so long as the disability is not so horrific as to make their lives not worth living, neither twin has justifiable complaint against me for choosing DET. And if opting for twins does not harm or wrong the resulting offspring, on what grounds can anyone criticize my choice?"

To answer this question, we need to explore the concept of procreative liberty and its companion concept, procreative responsibility.

PROCREATIVE LIBERTY/
PROCREATIVE RESPONSIBILITY

The principle of procreative liberty supports the notion that patients should be able to make their own decisions about whether or not to have offspring (Robertson 1994, p. 4). The United Nations has proclaimed that the right to decide the number, timing, and spacing of children is a fundamental human right (UNFPA). The principle of patient autonomy might also be thought to support the idea that informed patients should be able to make their own decisions about what treatment options they find acceptable or desirable. Some argue that, while risks to offspring matter, it is equally important to consider patient preferences (van Wely et al. 2006, p. 2738). They maintain that it is not the physician's place to try to dissuade IVF patients from having twins, but only to provide them with accurate information about the risks and benefits.

However, virtually no one thinks that patient choice should be unlimited, in fertility treatment or other medical specialties. Dr. Michael Kamrava cited patient autonomy as his reason for transferring all of Ms. Suleman's available embryos into her uterus in one cycle, saying, "the ultimate decision should be largely driven by the patient's wishes" (*In the Matter of Michael Kamrava* 2009). He was drummed out of ASRM and lost his medical license as a result. The right of patients to make their own decisions about medical treatments, to weigh the risks and benefits according to their own values, is not absolute. The duty of physicians to respect patient autonomy is balanced against their ethical and professional responsibility to avoid harming their patients (Stillman et al. 2013). Moreover, procreative autonomy is limited by what I have elsewhere called procreative responsibility (Steinbock 2011, p. 206).

Procreative liberty—the right of individuals to make their own decisions about when and whether and how many children to have—is certainly important, but it is not the only important factor. As I argued in *Life Before Birth*, "Becoming a parent is not solely, or even primarily, a right. It is also, and primarily, an awesome responsibility. Prospective parents must think not simply of their own reproductive interests but also of the welfare of their offspring . . . " (Steinbock 2011, p. 92). Their procreative liberty ought to be restricted to reasonable and defensible choices. Such a restriction is captured by the idea of procreative responsibility, which includes concern for the welfare of children who are brought into the world. This means that parents and prospective parents have an obligation to prevent avoidable harm to offspring.

However, the nonidentity problem challenges the notion that children *can* be harmed, if they have no other way of being born except with the harmful condition. Admittedly, nonidentity cases are, in an important respect, different from cases of straightforward prenatal harming. Smoking, drinking to excess, and using illegal drugs during pregnancy are all examples of risking harm to the fetus and future child. If the child is adversely affected, this will be a case of straightforward prenatal harming. Abstaining from smoking, binge-drinking, and using illegal drugs during pregnancy improves the chances that *this child* will be born healthy. By contrast, in nonidentity cases, there is no way to improve the chances for *this child*. The only way to avoid the harm is not to have the child at all. But how can not getting born *protect* a child or *be good for* him or her? The claim that it can seems paradoxical.

And yet the idea that responsible people sometimes ought to delay procreation, for the sake of the child, is a very common one. Consider the 2012 teen pregnancy prevention campaign in New York City. Posters on the subway showed a little girl saying, "Honestly, Mom . . . chances are he won't stay with you. What happens to me?" The clear message is that, for the sake of the child, young women should delay pregnancy until they are older, in more stable relationships, financially better off, and generally more prepared to care for a child. How can we explain this, in light of the fact that if the teenager takes the advice to delay pregnancy, she will not have the adorable little girl on the poster. She will not have the *same* child she would have had as a teenager. If she postpones pregnancy until she is older, she will have a *different* child, arising from different egg and sperm.

Delaying pregnancy is different from not smoking in that it protects the child by substituting a different child. It is not the same as harming in the straightforward sense, yet I maintain that there can be a moral obligation to substitute. Although the teenager cannot protect *this child* (the one she would have if she became pregnant now) by waiting to become pregnant, she can choose to bring another child into the world, under better conditions. She can delay pregnancy in order to give *some child* a better start in life. Unless there is some overwhelming reason for her not to wait, the responsible procreative choice is to delay pregnancy and have a different child later on.[4]

The possibility of substitution differentiates the case of the young teenager from that of a postmenopausal woman who wants to use assisted reproduction to have a child. The teenager can avoid the increased risks to her child by delaying pregnancy and having a different child. This is obviously not an option for the older woman. If being born to an elderly mother would be very bad for the child (an empirical question), pregnancy would be an irresponsible procreative choice. However, this means she is morally required to forego pregnancy altogether. This imposes a greater burden on the older woman than on the teenager. Depending on the answer to the empirical question, "How bad is it?" the older woman might be more justified in having a child than the teenager for whom substitution is an option.

It would appear that the choice between SET and DET poses a nonidentity problem, and one that has substitution as a possible solution. Choosing SET in effect substitutes one healthy child (or more accurately, one that has a better chance of being healthy) for two children with a higher risk of health problems. Admittedly, the numbers change in the SET/DET choice, differentiating the case from that of the teenager who delays pregnancy. This might be thought to have moral significance, since most infertility patients want two children, and there is no guarantee that the infertile woman will be able to become pregnant a second time. Opting for SET may deprive her of the chance to have the number of children she wants. However, her procreative interests are not the whole story. She must balance her desire for two children against the increased risks to offspring. The question then is whether having only one child constitutes an unreasonable restriction on her procreative liberty. It does not seem that it is. After all, she is not being asked to give up parenthood altogether. Depending on the magnitude and likelihood of the risks, being satisfied with one child is arguably required by procreative responsibility.

However, does opting for SET over DET really pose a nonidentity problem? That is, does it achieve the reduction of risk by preventing the birth of one of the twins? If the woman's embryos are cryopreserved, she can have two pregnancies, and both children will be born as singletons. So both children will get born *and* incur lower health risks than if they were born in a twin pregnancy. SET, it seems, need not pose a choice between an increased risk of disability and not getting born at all. Because both children have a better chance of being born "healthy and whole" with SET than with DET, the choice of SET by favorable-prognosis patients is more like standard cases of prenatal harming and less like a nonidentity problem. This strengthens the moral obligation of good-prognosis patients to accept SET and have two singleton pregnancies.

Factors that Make it Difficult to Make Good Choices

It may be argued that even if the health outcomes of offspring are improved with two singleton pregnancies, this may not be a realistic option for individuals who cannot afford two cycles. For those who have to pay the full cost of IVF, because they do not live in a country that pays for it, or because their insurance does not cover it, a single round of treatment, with DET, may be the only way they can accomplish their goal of having two children.

Although one-child families are becoming increasingly popular, for both social and economic reasons, many people want more than one child, and this is not a frivolous or unreasonable desire. Respect for procreative liberty does preclude putting limits on the number of children a person may have, for example, by mandatory sterilization after a certain number of offspring. However, the rejection of mandatory sterilization does not imply that the number of embryos transferred in IVF is, or should be, solely a matter of patient preference. Physicians, both as individuals and as members of professional societies, are morally required to develop reasonable professional guidelines restricting the number of embryos transferred where this is aimed at, and likely to achieve, the important goal of promoting maternal and fetal health. Patients are morally required to consider the information they are given about the increased health risks imposed by twin pregnancies and to make responsible procreative choices. While some patients—those who are older or have had repeated IVF failures—can responsibly decide to transfer two or even three embryos—SET is the responsible choice for favorable-prognosis patients.

At the same time, procreative choices are not made in a vacuum. The economic reasons that lead patients to prefer DET must be addressed. This is beginning to be recognized in the literature, with calls for expanding insurance coverage for IVF (Janvier et al. 2011; Stillman et al. 2013; Johnston et al. 2014), as well as investing in research to improve fertility treatments (Johnston et al. 2013, pp. 51–53).

Economic constraints are not the only pressures patients face. I know a woman, a mother of twins, who had planned to have SET when she was called on a weekend and told to get over to the clinic right away as they had two good-quality embryos. When she mentioned that she had planned to transfer only one embryo, the response was, "Well, you want to get pregnant, don't you?" The pressures on clinicians to keep up pregnancy rates are a significant part of this story and also need to be addressed.

CONCLUSION

Although I have not addressed the case for legally mandating SET, there are compelling arguments against it, at least in a country like the United States, which has no oversight body (like the HFEA in the United Kingdom) regulating infertility treatment (Robertson 2009). However, the increasing awareness of both practitioners and professional societies of the importance of reducing multiple births, including twin pregnancies, has led to professional guidelines intended to reduce twin pregnancies, and some clinics have adopted their own mandatory SET policies for good-prognosis patients. Practices that emphasize their "dedication to achieve both a high pregnancy rate *and* a safe, healthy pregnancy outcome" have found their patients to be "not only accepting but indeed excited about qualifying for SET" (Van Voorhis 2013). Better patient education, including data about the increased risks from multiple pregnancies, is clearly necessary, but so are better insurance coverage and more research to improve fertility treatment, so that patients can make morally responsible procreative choices without sacrificing their goal to become parents.

NOTES

1. Often SET is referred to in the literature as elective single-embryo transfer (eSET), to emphasize that a choice has been made to transfer only one embryo out of several available good-quality embryos. However, not all clinicians follow this usage, and for simplicity's sake, I will use the term "SET" when a single embryo is transferred.
2. Those who maintain that dying in infancy is bad for the infant include Marquis and Sumner, 119–120. For an opposing view, see McMahan, 162–174; 338–362.
3. They do note that, unlike children with disabilities, multiples are not stigmatized: "the birth of sextuplets and septuplets, let alone of twins or triplets, is generally regarded as cause for celebration, not grieving (Asch and Wasserman 2005, 179). This may be no longer the case as regards supermultiples, but they are undoubtedly right about twins.
4. Of course, this assumes that the teenager has meaningful procreative choices, and that she is not forced or coerced into sexual activity and has access to birth control.

BIBLIOGRAPHY

Asch, A. 1999. Prenatal diagnosis and selective abortion: A challenge to practice and policy. *American Journal of Public Health* 89, no. 11: 1649–1657.

Asch, A., and D. Wasserman. 2005. Where is the sin in synecdoche? Prenatal testing and the parent-child relationship. In *Quality of life and human difference: Genetic testing, health care, and disability*, ed. D. Wasserman, J. Bickenbach, and R. Wachbroit. Cambridge: Cambridge University Press.

ASRM. 2012a. Practice Committee report. Elective single-embryo transfer. *Fertility and Sterility* 97, no. 4: 835–842.

ASRM. 2012b. Multiple pregnancy and birth: Twins, triplets, and high-order multiples: A guide for patients. http://www.reproductivefacts.org/uploadedFiles/ASRM_Content/Resources/Patient_Resources/Fact_Sheets_and_Info_Booklets/multiples.pdf (accessed March 29, 2014).

Becker, A. 2010. Is it harder to have a child with Down syndrome? http://parenting.blogs.nytimes.com/2010/09/21/is-it-harder-to-have-a-child-with-down-syndrome/?_php=true&_type=blogs&_r=0 (accessed April 27, 2014).

Blickstein, I., and L. G. Keith. 2005. The decreased rates of triplet births: Temporal trends and biologic speculations. *American Journal of Obstetrics & Gynecology* 193: 327–331.

Caplan, A. 2009. Ethics and octuplets: Society is responsible. Mega-multiple births must be discouraged. If needed, government must get involved. http://articles.philly.com/2009-02-06/news/25282602_1_fertility-treatment-renowned-fertility-specialist-nadya-suleman.

Dickey, R. P. 2007. The relative contribution of assisted reproductive technologies and ovulation induction to multiple births in the United States 5 years after the society for assisted reproductive technology/American Society for Reproductive Medicine recommendation to limit the number of embryos transferred. *Fertility and Sterility* 88, no. 6: 1554–1561.

Emanuel, E. J., and L. L. Emanuel. 1992. Four models of the physician-patient relationship. *Journal of the American Medical Association* 267, no. 16: 2221–2226.

ESHRE. 2012. Freezing all embryos in IVF with transfer in a later non-stimulated cycle may improve outcome. http://www.eshre.eu/Press-Room/Press-releases/Press-releases-ESHRE-2012/Frozen-vs-fresh-embryos.aspx (accessed May 1, 2014).

Gleicher, N., and D. Barad. 2009. Twin pregnancies, contrary to consensus, is a desirable outcome in infertility. *Fertility and Sterility* 91, no. 6: 2426–2431.

Gleicher, N. 2013. For some infertility patients, twins are the best outcome. *Contemporary Ob/Gyn.* September. http://contemporaryobgyn.modernmedicine.com/contemporary-obgyn/news/some-infertility-patients-twins-are-best-outcome?page=full (accessed April 19, 2014).

Helmerhorst, Frans M., D. Perquin, D. Donker, and M. Keirse. 2004. Perinatal outcome of singletons and twins after assisted conception: A systematic review of controlled studies. *British Medical Journal*, doi:10.1136/bmj.37957.560278.EE.

Janvier, A., B. Spelke, and K. J. Barrington. 2011. The epidemic of multiple gestations and neonatal intensive care unit use: the cost of irresponsibility. *Journal of Pediatrics* 159, no. 3: 409–413.

Johnston, J., M. K. Gusmano, and P. Patrizio. 2013. Multiple births following fertility treatment: Causes, consequences and opportunities for change. Available from The Hastings Center.

Johnston, J., M. K. Gusmano, and P. Patrizio. 2014. Preterm births, multiples, and fertility treatment: Recommendations for changes to policy and clinical practices. *Fertility and Sterility*. http://www.fertstert.org/article/S0015-0282%2814%2900260-X/fulltext

Joint SOGC-CFAS Clinical Practice Guideline. 2010. Elective single embryo transfer following in vitro fertilization. *Journal of Obstetrics and Gynaecology Canada* 32, no. 4: 363–377.

Kamrava, Michael. 2009. Matter of the Accusation Against. http://www.latimes.com/includes/misc/kamravaaccusation.pdf (accessed May 1, 2014).

Kresowik, J. D., B. J. Stegmann, A. E. Sparks, G. L. Ryan, and B. J. Van Voorhis. 2011. Five years of a mandatory single-embryo transfer (mSET) policy dramatically reduces twinning rates without lowering pregnancy rates. *Fertility and Sterility* 96, no. 6: 1367–1369.

Land, J. A., and J. L. Evers. 2003. Risks and complications in assisted reproduction techniques: report of an ESHRE consensus meeting. *Human Reproduction* 18: 455–457.

Lannon, B. M., B. Choi, M. R. Hacker, L. E. Dodge, B. A. Malizia, C. B. Barrett, W. H. Wong, M. W. Yao, and A. S. Penzias. 2012. Predicting personalized multiple risks after in vitro fertilization—double embryo transfer. *Fertility and Sterility* 98, no. 1: 69–76.

Levens, E. D., and M. J. Hill. 2013. Should single-embryo transfer be mandatory in patients undergoing IVF? CON: Regulation is not the best way to reduce multifetal gestations. *Contemporary Ob/Gyn.* http://contemporaryobgyn.modernmedicine.com/contemporary-obgyn/news/should-single-embryo-transfer-be-mandatory-patients-undergoing-ivf?contextCategoryId=26 (accessed March 27, 2014).

MacKay, A., C. J. Berg, J. C. King, C. Duran, and J. Chang. 2006. Pregnancy-related mortality among women with multifetal pregnancies. *Obstetrics & Gynecology* 107, no. 3: 563–568.

Marquis, D. 1989. Why abortion is immoral. *The Journal of Philosophy* 76, no. 4: 183–202.

Martin, J. A., B. E. Hamilton, S. J. Ventura, and M. J. K. Osterman. 2012. Births: Final data for 2011. *National Vital Statistics Reports* 62, no. 1.

Mathews, T. J., and MacDorman, M. 2013. *National Vital Statistics Reports* 61, no. 8: 1–27.

McMahan, J. 2002. *The ethics of killing: Problems at the margins of life.* New York: Oxford University Press.

Orentlicher, D. 2010. Multiple embryo transfers: time for policy. *Hastings Center Report* 40, no. 3: 12–13.

Robertson, J. A. 1994. *Children of choice: Freedom and the new reproductive technologies.* Princeton, NJ: Princeton University Press.

Robertson, J. 2009. The octuplet case—why more regulation is not likely. *Hastings Center Report* 39, no. 3: 26–28.

Rong-Gong Lin II. 2011. Accusations against "Octomom" fertility doctor: Michael Kamrava's medical license revoked. http://documents.latimes.com/michael-kamrava-disciplinary-decision/ (accessed April 29, 2014).

Ryan, G., S. Zhang, A. Dokras, C. H. Syrop, and B. J. Van Voorhis. 2004. The desire of infertile patients for multiple births. *Fertility and Sterility* 81: 500–504.

SART. 2010. Clinic summary report. https://www.sartcorsonline.com/rptCSR_PublicMultYear.aspx?ClinicPKID=0 (accessed April 29, 2014).

Sazonova, A., K. Källen, A. Thurin-Kjellberg, Ulla-Britt Wennerholm, and C. Bergh. 2013. Neonatal and maternal outcomes comparing women undergoing two in vitro fertilization (IVF) singleton pregnancies and women undergoing one IVF twin pregnancy. *Fertility and Sterility* 99, no. 3: 731–737.

Schumann, R. 2013. Kim Zolciak and four other celebrities who have announced twin pregnancies. http://www.ibtimes.com/kim-zolciak-4-other-celebrities-who-have-announced-twin-pregnancies-photos-1392151 (accessed March 28, 2014).

Scotland, G. S., P. McNamee, V. L. Peddie, and S. Bhattacharya. 2007. Safety versus success in elective single embryo transfer: women's preferences for outcomes of in vitro fertilization. *British Journal of Gynecology* 114: 977–983.

Steinbock, B. 2011. *Life before birth: The moral and legal status of embryos and fetuses,* 2nd ed. New York: Oxford University Press.

Stillman, R. J., K. S. Richter, and H. W. Jones, Jr. 2013. Refuting a misguided campaign against the goal of single-embryo transfer and singleton birth in assisted reproduction. *Human Reproduction* 28, no. 10: 2599–2607.

Stillman, R. J., K. S. Richter, and H. W. Jones, Jr. 2013. Refuting a misguided campaign against the goal of single-embryo transfer and singleton birth in assisted reproduction. *Human Reproduction* 28, no. 10: 2599–2607.

Sumner, L. W. 2011. *Assisted death: A study in ethics & law*. New York: Oxford University Press.

Thurin, A., J. Hausken, T. Hillensjő, B. Jablonowska, A. Pinborg, A. Strandell, and C. Bergh. 2004. Elective single-embryo transfer versus double-embryo transfer in in vitro fertilization. *New England Journal of Medicine* 351: 2392–2402.

United Nations Fund for Population Activities (UNFPA). 2014. Reproductive rights. http://www.unfpa.org/rights/rights.htm (accessed April 17, 2014).

Van Voorhis, B. J. 2012. SET in the good prognosis patient—the case for professionalism. Presentation in the Ken Ryan Ethics Symposium: Multiple pregnancy and ART, annual ASRM meeting, San Diego, October 23.

Van Voorhis, B. J. 2013. Should single-embryo transfer be mandatory in patients undergoing IVF? Pro. *Contemporary Ob/Gyn*. http://contemporaryobgyn.modernmedicine.com/contemporary-obgyn/news/should-single-embryo-transfer-be-mandatory-patients-undergoing-ivf?contextCategoryId=26 (accessed March 27, 2014).

Van Wely, M., M. Twisk, B. W. Mol, and F. van der Veen. 2006. Is twin pregnancy necessarily an adverse outcome of assisted reproductive technologies? *Human Reproduction* 21: 2736–2738.

CHAPTER 28

PROCREATIVE RESPONSIBILITY IN VIEW OF WHAT PARENTS OWE THEIR CHILDREN

DAVID DEGRAZIA

LIKE other animals, human beings procreate. Yet, among terrestrial species, humans are presumably unique in bearing moral responsibilities regarding their procreative choices. In this chapter I will address only those procreative acts—by which I mean sexual intercourse and later decisions and actions that permit the continuation of pregnancy—that are undertaken *voluntarily*, rather than accidentally or through coercion, *with the intention of raising the offspring*. Such acts (or series of actions) may be described as "procreation with the intention of parenting." The question I will address is fairly specific: *In view of what parents owe their children, under what conditions is it morally responsible to procreate with the intention of parenting?* For ease of reference, I will hereafter refer to procreation with this intention simply as "procreation." And by asking whether certain acts are "morally responsible," I mean to ask whether they are morally permissible—that and nothing more.[1]

It is important to clarify the scope of our question, which does not cover all significant moral issues concerning procreation. Our question does not address the matter of how a morally responsible person should take into account the expected impact of procreation on the environment, limited resources, and the like. Nor does it ask about the responsibility of deciding to procreate in view of the importance of finding homes for the many children who stand to be adopted. Because of the qualification "in view of what parents owe their children," our question does not—as explained later—engage the impersonal, consequentialist considerations that arise in connection with what has been called the *nonidentity problem*, although I will, in passing, briefly address this problem and adduce such considerations. By contrast, the question does engage the value of reproductive freedom, a factor that may partly determine when procreation is morally responsible.

The discussion that follows will be organized primarily around three conditions that I submit as necessary and jointly sufficient for procreation to be morally responsible in view of what parents owe their children. (Because there may be additional necessary conditions that address other factors such as environmental impact and the importance of adoption, I do not claim that the conditions I present are sufficient for morally responsible procreation, all things considered.) The first condition is a *worthwhile-life condition*, discussion of which will require us to consider wrongful-life cases and their conceptual basis. An examination of the interests of children-to-be and procreative freedom will vindicate the commonsense judgment that while some procreative acts are wrongful or impermissible, some are permissible. Further reflection will reveal that the wrongful-life condition is not sufficient for responsible procreation, motivating a *doing-more condition*: that parents do more for their children than provide a worthwhile life if they can do so without undue sacrifice. Because it will become apparent that these two conditions are not jointly sufficient for responsible procreation in view of what parents owe their children, I will defend a *basic-needs condition*, providing an approximate list of basic needs and considering whether exceptions to the requirement of meeting particular basic needs are tolerable. Next, I consider several case scenarios that could motivate the addition of an intention-based condition and explain why I do not think such a condition is warranted. I then consider whether freedom from avoidable disability should count as a basic need, taking us to the nonidentity problem. Exploration of this problem demonstrates how procreative ethics involves not only what parents owe their children but also the factor of foreseeable impersonal consequences. The discussion will conclude with a provisional classification of types of irresponsible procreation.[2]

A WORTHWHILE-LIFE CONDITION

One necessary condition for morally responsible procreation is that the child to be is reasonably expected to have a life worth living. It would be wrong to procreate when one could reasonably expect that the child would have a life so awful that it would not be worth living. Indeed, to do so is sometimes thought to wrong the child who is brought into being. This idea draws us into conceptually puzzling terrain.

The Concept of Wrongful Life

Intuitively, it seems that some lives are not worth living. Either they were never worth starting in the first place, or they were worth starting but are now so miserable and hopeless that they are not worth continuing, or both. Because our topic is procreation, which involves starting a life, I will focus on lives that are not worth starting.[3]

Consider, for example, Lesch-Nyhan syndrome (LNS), a recessive genetic disorder that is caused by the buildup of uric acid in body fluids and is generally passed on only to sons. Symptoms of LNS that appear in a child's first year include kidney stones, bladder stones, severe gout, arthritis, limited muscle control, and moderate mental retardation. In his second year, an affected child will begin such self-mutilating behaviors as head banging and biting of lips and fingers. Neurological symptoms include involuntary flailing and writhing, facial grimacing, and repetitive movements. Most LNS children cannot walk. Although some neurological symptoms can be alleviated with medications, there is no effective treatment for LNS, whose victims usually die in their first two decades from renal failure.

LNS is a condition that—at least today, in the absence of effective treatment—appears to be so awful for its victims that it makes an affected life not worth starting.[4] Moreover, it would seem morally irresponsible to procreate with the intention of creating a child with LNS, or even with the negligent willingness—say, knowing that at least one parent carried the disease gene and not getting genetic testing—of creating such a child. If one does intentionally or negligently create such a child, the moral (and legal) charge of *wrongful life* seems appropriate. The idea of wrongful life is that one wrongs an individual by intentionally or negligently bringing him into existence with a condition that makes the affected life not worth living. This idea seems to apply here.

Yet it raises a puzzle. The child with LNS has a genetic disorder. He could not have existed without this condition. Even if someday genetic therapy in vitro or in utero will permit repairing the genetic defect, enabling the continuing existence of someone who will live free of the disorder, this is not presently possible. So how, today, could an affected child—or, more realistically given the cognitive deficits associated with LNS, an advocate for the child—claim that the child was wronged? How could *that child* have been treated better? Not causing *him* to exist with LNS would have required not permitting *him* to exist at all.

One might not initially realize that there is a puzzle here, because it may seem obvious that nonexistence would have been better for the child than existing with LNS. What is tricky is the qualification "for the child." Nonexistence is not some state the child can be in. Rather, the word "nonexistence" informs us (in a slightly misleading, reifying way) that *there would be no child* had he not been conceived and brought to term with LNS. It is puzzling to think that someone might have been wronged, even though there was no way for *him* to have been treated better or even differently.

At the same time, this way of stating the puzzle ignores the possibility that the boy could have existed briefly, in utero, and then aborted. His life, by hypothesis, was not worth living—neither starting nor continuing. But, if he could have been aborted at any time before acquiring the capacity for suffering (which apparently emerges only in the third trimester of pregnancy), he could have avoided suffering. Failure to abort, one might argue, wronged the boy by failing to spare him of terrible, uncompensated misery. The charge of wrongful life, then, applies not necessarily to the creation of the life in question but to the decision to allow it to continue beyond the presentient stage of life during which suffering is impossible. (It is worth noting that my present remarks make the assumption—which is sometimes challenged—that we come into existence as human organisms long before we acquire any mental life.[5])

Although the charge of wrongful life, directed to a failure to terminate pregnancy, seems relatively straightforward and conceptually coherent, matters are trickier when the charge of wrongful life is directed at procreation itself. For, in this case, the child could not have been treated better because the child could not have existed without the genetic disorder. Again, how can one have been wronged if one couldn't have been treated differently, much less better?

One might suppose that this conceptual challenge is best developed by emphasizing that our ordinary concept of harm is comparative. A harms B, as harm is ordinarily understood, only if A makes B *worse off* than (1) B was before A's intervention (a historical conception of harm) or (2) B would have been without A's intervention (a counterfactual conception). In the case under consideration, the only alternative to the boy's having LNS is his never existing at all, so bringing him into existence is not harmful according to the ordinary concept, which does not apply in this case. The present way of developing the challenge raises interesting questions about the nature of harm, but it misses the deeper point that the victim of wrongful life is claimed to have been *wronged*—whether or not she was *harmed*. (Here I am making a point about wrongful life from a moral perspective, setting aside what the law may require for a successful tort action.[6]) One can wrong someone without harming her, for example, by violating her rights in a nonharmful way.[7] For example, a doctor might wrong a competent adult patient by neglecting to mention reasonable alternatives to the recommended medical treatment—violating the patient's right to adequate disclosure—even if the recommended treatment proves to be highly beneficial and not at all harmful. So, our most basic question is not whether the LNS child was harmed, but whether he was wronged—even though he could not have existed without the disorder.

It seems to me that the most cogent approach to this issue accepts that one can be wronged by being brought into an existence that is *noncomparatively bad for the subject.*[8] Such a life is bad for the subject in the sense of containing much that is bad for her—suffering, dysfunction, and/or deprivation—without being compensated for by whatever good the life may contain. This way of understanding wrongful life as applied to procreation (as opposed to failure to abort) need not claim that any harm is done, a claim that would be doubted by those who think harm is necessarily comparative (a matter of making one worse off). Rather, one is wronged by the intentional or negligent procreation of a child with a condition that makes life not worth living, even though the victim could not have been treated better because he could not have existed had the action considered wrongful not been performed.

An alternative to understanding wrongful procreation in terms of imposing lives that are noncomparatively bad for their subjects is an approach that may seem attractive to some thinkers, but I find it very strange logically and metaphysically. The alternative is to assert that the individual conceived with LNS *existed prior to conception as a mere possible person* and, as a preexisting individual, could have been treated better by being allowed to remain forever only possible and never actual. Although there are thoughtful people who take such metaphysical conceits seriously, here I simply report that I find such thinking objectionably divorced from reality. Readers may regard my rejection of possible people as real entities as a premise of the remainder of this discussion.

Might All Procreation Involve Wrongful Life?

Some acts of procreation constitute wrongful life. These acts involve the intentional or negligent imposition of a life not worth starting. Ordinary thinking about procreation makes room for the possibility that some procreative acts are wrongful while maintaining that most, or at least many, procreative acts are morally responsible. Two scholars, however, have advanced significant arguments that challenge this congenial assumption. David Benatar explicitly argues that all deliberate procreation is wrongful while Seanna Shiffrin, without explicitly defending this thesis, advances arguments that can be reasonably understood to lead to this thesis.[9] Having responded to their arguments in detail elsewhere, I will not recapitulate my responses here.[10] Instead, I will cut to the chase and briefly explain why I think that many procreative acts are morally responsible.

But, first, very briefly, why would anyone doubt this? The strongest reason, in my estimation, is connected with the imposition of harm. We tend to believe that it is wrong to harm someone, without her consent, for the sake of her own good unless doing so involves the prevention of worse harm to her. Pulling someone out of a car with the foreseeable result of breaking her arm may be justified in an emergency in which there is no opportunity to obtain consent and death is the expected consequence of inaction. Here the harm of breaking an arm is imposed in order to prevent the worse harm of death. But breaking someone's arm without his consent in order to win a bet, the earnings from which will allow you to pay him a large sum of money, is likely to be considered wrong. Here the unconsented harm is not justified by the "pure benefits"[11]: the benefit of cash as opposed to the prevention of a harm worse than a broken arm.

Considering that procreation involves the imposition of unconsented harm for pure benefits, one might doubt that procreation is ever justified. Clearly, the individual brought into being does not consent to being created. Surely, if harm is involved in being brought into being, it cannot be claimed that the harm is justified by the prevention of greater harm, for the alternative of nonexistence cannot involve any harm. So, if procreation entails the imposition of unconsented harm, it cannot be justified by the prevention of greater harm to the individual brought into being; a justification must appeal to the creation of pure benefits (the goods that the life will contain) for that individual. Finally, and crucially, a proponent of the present line of reasoning claims that *bringing someone into existence imposes harm on that individual because every human life includes the experience of harm.*

Now it is true, setting aside the possible and very rare exception of never-sentient human beings (e.g., anencephalic infants), that every human life includes the experience of harm, including at least some of the following: pain, distress, sadness, sickness, and injury. I am also comfortable in granting, at least for the sake of argument, that bringing someone into existence in some sense involves harming (and/or benefiting) that individual. Even though, prior to existing, there is no individual who can be benefited or harmed, once someone comes into being there is an individual who is the subject of harm (and/or benefit). And bringing someone into existence guarantees that the individual will undergo harm—to which she did not consent and not for the purpose of preventing worse harm to her.

If I am willing to grant all this, one might wonder, how can I claim that procreation is often morally justified? Isn't it just a case of imposing unconsented harm for the sake of procuring pure benefits? And isn't doing so always wrong?

In response to these questions, first, I doubt that it is *always* wrong to impose unconsented harm for the sake of pure benefits. But, even if it is, the relationship between procreating in favorable circumstances and whatever harms the created life will inevitably include is often not best characterized as *imposing* the harm. Consider an example.

Let's say I get my elementary school child involved in basketball or soccer and strongly encourage her to stick with it for several seasons. The kid is too young and my encouragement too strong for consent to be a realistic possibility. I know that my child will experience some harm over the course of several seasons: probably some minor injuries, surely some bitter disappointment, and so on. The best reason for encouraging her involvement in the sport is not to prevent some greater harm—she could avoid obesity, for example, without taking the risks involved in these sports—but to create the opportunity and likelihood of procuring the benefits of physical discipline, improved skills, camaraderie with teammates, the learning of sportsmanship, probably some pride, and possibly some glory. But, significantly, my directing my kid to play basketball or soccer does not *impose* whatever harms eventually occur. Rather, I am *exposing* her to these harms.[12] I do so as part of the price of creating opportunities for the aforementioned benefits. It is a reasonable price.

Similarly, while human life inevitably involves some harm, in most if not all cases it also features benefits. Often the benefits, the good experiences of human life, are very considerable and outweigh the harms of a particular life. If a couple procreates in circumstances in which they have every reason to expect that their child will have a life that is well worth living, and they meet other necessary conditions (to be discussed) for responsible procreation, then exposing their child to harm is justified (in part) by the opportunity they afford him to have a good life. This thesis will be fleshed out further in later sections. For now, it is enough to clarify the cogent basis for denying that all procreation involves wrongful life.

Why the Worthwhile-Life Condition Is not Sufficient

As noted earlier, one necessary condition for morally responsible procreation is that the child to be is reasonably expected to have a life worth living. Although it seems impossible to draw a clear, nonarbitrary line dividing all cases of such worthwhile lives from all cases of lives not worth living, it is sufficiently clear that some lives are worth living and some lives are not. We can therefore tolerate the gray, ambiguous area between the clear cases on each side and maintain that the distinction is useful insofar as procreation is irresponsible when it is reasonably expected that the resulting life will not be worth living, an idea that motivates the worthwhile-life condition. Are there are other necessary conditions for responsible procreation?

A negative answer would permit a simple criterion for determining when procreation is responsible (once again, in terms of what parents owe their children): "As long as a couple can reasonably expect that their future child will have a life worth living, they may procreate responsibly." But further reflection suggests the inadequacy of this position. Imagine a wealthy, self-indulgent, lazy couple who decide to have a child because "That's what people our age do," yet have no interest in putting much care into childrearing. They will make sure their child gets a couple of meals a day and gets to a hospital if seriously hurt or sick, and will have the child attend school. But the school district is terrible and the prospective parents are too cheap to send their child to a good private school; meanwhile, their reason for living in that particular school district is simply that it is near some beautiful mountains in which they like to hike; if they moved ten miles away, their child could attend a good public school. As for stimulation at home, the child will be allowed to watch television during most of his free time and will not receive any encouragement to cultivate his talents. Even with this patchy description of the prospective parents' intentions, one is struck by *how much more they could do for their child.* Materially, even if not psychologically, the parents are well positioned as prospective parents. They can reasonably expect that, despite their negligence, their child will have a life worth living. Yet they are not doing nearly enough.

The worthwhile-life condition is insufficient. One might propose that parents owe their children (1) *worthwhile lives* and (2) *whatever other benefits they, in view of their circumstances, can provide them.* This analysis would plausibly condemn the parenting sloth of the aforementioned couple, who would flunk the second condition. Yet this second condition is excessively demanding.

Imagine that a couple devotes a great deal of attention to their young child while assuring that her basic needs are taken care of. The father has a job outside the house, but works the minimum he can get away with, so he can be home more and present for his child. The mother is presently staying at home as the primary caregiver. (The lesson of this thought experiment will be equally clear if the roles are reversed and it is the father who is the stay-at-home parent, or if the parents are a same-sex couple.) Suppose that the mother feels a strong identity-based need to resume her career outside the house. With some creative scheduling of their work hours, and some use of day care and babysitting, their psychologically healthy child, it seems, will fare well. Yet the child, it is expected, would admittedly do a little better if her mother stayed home, full-time, for several more years. If the parents are required to do as much as possible for their child, then either the woman should sacrifice her career (at least for a few more years) or the man should quit his job and let his wife return to work. It seems obvious to me that the couple may responsibly decide to take neither of these drastic steps. They do not owe it to their child to do so, since she will be fine with both parents working, and one of her parents would have to make a massive sacrifice to do what is optimal for the child.

In many other sorts of family situations, parents can do right by their children without literally maximizing their welfare. The previous example featured an important interest of the parents as competing (a bit) with their child's interests. In other situations, a child's interests may compete with those of another sibling, or an important community or charity endeavor. In a family with more than one child, it may be logistically impossible to maximize the welfare of each child because doing so for one will prevent doing so for another; here, the children's competing interests must be balanced in some reasonable way. Or consider a parent who donates funds in an effort to help save the lives of children at risk of an early death due to starvation or easily treated illness. Suppose these noble donations have the consequence that the child, now ready for college, must attend a university that, while good, is not the very best she could have attended had her parent not contributed to the charity. The failure to maximize the child's welfare does not seem sufficient to judge that the parent owed the child more, especially if the parent is loving and attentive to the child's most important needs, including getting a good education.

"Doing the best for one's child" and similar phrases have a nice ring, perhaps because children throughout the world are more often neglected than overindulged—and neglect may generally pose a greater threat to children's welfare than overindulgence does. In addition, since most people tend to be less literal-minded than philosophers and other highly analytical scholars, most people might interpret "doing the best for one's child" not as literally *maximizing* the satisfaction of the child's interests but as doing a great deal for the child and addressing his or her most important and legitimate interests. This looser understanding of the phrase gets us closer to the normative mark. Accordingly, we should reject condition (2), as stated earlier, and focus on children's most important interests. As we will see, some remnant of (2) will survive the analysis.

A CHILD'S BASIC NEEDS
OR ESSENTIAL INTERESTS

Parents owe their children a lot, but not literally everything they can do for a particular child because this exacting standard would sometimes demand excessive sacrifice of the parents' interests, other family members' interests, or other important values. Much of what parents owe their children can be captured in the idea of their children's *basic needs* or *essential interests*. Although "basic needs" is a familiar term, "essential interests" suggests the point that "best interests" is an exaggerated standard for implying a requirement to maximize children's welfare. In any case, I will use the terms "basic needs" and "essential interests" interchangeably.

Parents owe their children an effort to ensure that their basic needs are met. It would be excessive to demand that parents *guarantee* that children's basic needs are met, because parents have too little control over their children's lives for this to be a reasonable expectation. If parents do all they reasonably can to protect their child, yet he proves very unlucky and is assaulted, the parents have not failed their child. There is only so much they can do to provide protection—without overly constricting their child's life (e.g., never letting him play outside), which would thwart other basic needs.

Perhaps, then, parents owe their children whatever is necessary for a reasonable expectation that their basic needs will be met. In view of our discussion about well-positioned parents owing their children more than worthwhile lives, but not to the point of excessive sacrifice, let us consider the following tripartite analysis: *Parents owe their children (1) worthwhile lives, (2) in which their basic needs are reasonably expected to be met, and (3) doing more for them if they can without undue sacrifice.* I find this analysis intuitively satisfying, at least at first glance. Indeed, I think that in a just world this tripartite standard might be exactly correct. At least in large part because our world is not just, we will have to confront a difficult issue: whether to permit some exceptions to condition (2).

Before doing so, let us add content to that condition by enumerating a list of children's basic needs. Of course, any list will be somewhat arbitrary, but a list that presents a reasonable approximation is far better than no list at all. In addition to helping to fill in an account of what parents owe their children, basic needs can be understood as *general conditions for the prospect of living a decent human life*—where "decent" gestures farther in the direction of flourishing than "minimally worthwhile" without going so far in that direction as to present unreasonable demands on parents and social institutions. Although I will not emphasize rights in this discussion, it is worth noting that at least some rights theorists (including this one) will find basic needs to be plausible objects of children's rights.

Here, then, is a proposed list of children's basic needs:

- nutritious food, clean water, safe shelter, protective clothing, and competent medical care when medical care is needed;
- freedom from slavery, other forms of wrongful coercion, and physical abuse;
- education and adequate stimulation;
- opportunities to play and experience enjoyment;
- the opportunity to develop independent interests and gradually find one's own path; and
- the love, kindness, and attention of at least one committed, reasonably competent parent.[13]

The second condition, as it stands, would require as a condition of responsible procreation that it be reasonably expected that all of these basic needs will be met in the case of one's child.

From the standpoint of a child's interests, this demand seems excellent. But consider now prospective parents who live in circumstances of social injustice. More specifically, these individuals, who would be loving and attentive parents, are economically disadvantaged Blacks in contemporary (postapartheid) South Africa who do not have reliable access to medical services. Although it can be expected that, if they have a child, most of her basic needs will be met, it cannot be expected that she will receive needed medical care whenever such care is needed. Unless we qualify the second condition, our tripartite standard will imply that the South African couple in question would choose irresponsibly if they decided to have a child. This verdict seems harsh. After all, it is not the couple's fault that medical care might be out of reach. More generally, the second condition, if not qualified, would imply that many disadvantaged prospective parents would act irresponsibly if they procreated—whereas their advantaged counterparts, who may be no more disposed to be good parents, would act responsibly if they procreated. We find, therefore, an uncomfortable tension between being demanding enough for children and being fair and compassionate toward disadvantaged persons who could be loving, resourceful parents.

My inclination is to permit *some* exceptions to the expectation to meet basic needs where failure to meet them is due to external circumstances beyond the parents' control. For example, parents who can expect to meet the basic needs of their child with the exception of competent medical care whenever it is needed may, if they meet other relevant conditions, responsibly choose to procreate. Admittedly, this is a very difficult issue, and I can easily understand how one might take a harder line, such as: "It's not the child's fault that her parents live in a society that doesn't provide reliable access to health care to all its members, so the child shouldn't have to bear the burden of this deprivation." In reply, it is of course not the child's fault, just as it is by hypothesis not the parents' fault, yet the child is expected to have a worthwhile life and to have other basic needs met. Moreover, *the parents' interest in procreative freedom should count for something*. Taking that factor into account, along with the parents' lack of control over access to medical care and the overall good life they can expect for their child, supports a policy of allowing some exceptions to the basic-needs requirement.

I do not favor tolerating many exceptions. For one thing, if parents have a child when the only reasonable expectation is that many of their basic needs will go unmet, it is somewhat unlikely that even the worthwhile-life condition will be met. For me, an especially hard case is one in which loving, resourceful parents could be expected to meet nearly all of a child's basic needs, but not freedom from slavery. Here I am deeply conflicted. Slavery, the institutional ownership of some persons by other persons, is a monstrous injustice. At the same time, slave couples may consider the prospect of becoming loving parents as among the only true joys life can offer them. Maybe an exception to the basic need of freedom from slavery would be tolerable if the conditions in which the slaves lived were relatively good (consistent, that is, with being slaves) and there appeared to be a strong chance that the family could escape from slavery either through successfully running away, being bought out by a benefactor, or the termination of the institution itself. But maybe not. Importantly, here, the parents could be described as *imposing* the condition of slavery on their child—rather than just *exposing* her to it—not because they themselves are slaveowners, but because they are freely procreating in circumstances that directly include the imposition of this legal status. I leave this issue open, while leaning in the direction of taking a hard line against any exceptions to this basic need.

Returning to the tripartite analysis articulated earlier, we may modify it by adding a parenthetical phrase, like so: *(2) in which their basic needs are reasonably expected to be met (some exceptions being justified only when the expected failure to meet a basic need is due to external circumstances beyond the parents' control).*

What underlies the stipulation that circumstances beyond the parents' control must be *external* in order for an exception to be eligible for consideration? Consider that one might not be able to meet a child's basic need to be free of abuse due to the internal factor of one's compulsion—one ineradicable by medication or therapy—to abuse young children. In my view, such a person should not become a parent, period, even though the internal factor may be no more within a prospective parent's control than, say, the external circumstance of entrenched poverty or slavery. What might justify this double standard between internal and external factors? My suggestion is that *someone who is constitutionally incapable of being a good parent—incapable, even, of being a neutral, benign parent—should not become a parent, whereas someone who is constituted to be a good parent, but hamstrung by certain external circumstances, should be afforded some flexibility.* I do not know how to provide deeper support for this assertion. However, it is highly plausible on its face.

The assertion is also related to another claim: that the last basic need on the list is nonnegotiable. In other words, if a prospective parent is incapable of being a kind, loving, attentive, and reasonably competent parent, and is not with a partner who makes this grade, then he or she should not become a parent. (This allows for the possibility that one member of a couple who would be an inadequate single parent may become a parent so long as he or she is not abusive or otherwise highly destructive and is partnered with someone who would be a loving, committed, and capable parent.) Note, however, that by singling out this basic need for its nonnegotiable status, I do not mean to suggest that all other basic needs are negotiable. Access to medical care may be negotiable, but, for example, access to nutritious food, clean water, and clothing is not.

Does this suggest that some basic needs are more important than others? I think it does. While maintaining that access to competent medical care when it is needed is a basic need, I believe that it is less central to the prospect of a decent life than are nutritious food, clean water, clothing, freedom from abuse, and the presence of at least one loving, competent parent. (Admittedly, I have no evidence for this claim beyond reflection on people's life experiences.) Maybe education shares this status of being slightly less central with access to medical care. If so, then one implication is that it could have been morally responsible for Afghani parents to procreate even when the Taliban prevented girls from receiving an education.

This is the modified tripartite standard that was defended in the previous section:

> *Parents owe their children (1) worthwhile lives, (2) in which their basic needs are reasonably expected to be met (some exceptions being justified only when the expected failure to meet a basic need is due to external circumstances beyond the parents' control), and (3) doing more for them if they can without undue sacrifice.*

The reference to basic needs here is vague, so we considered a rough list of basic needs. In addition, it was argued that the last item on the list—and at least a few others—were nonnegotiable.

One notable aspect of the tripartite standard is that it makes no mention of the prospective parents' intentions, a factor that might be thought to bear on the permissibility of procreation. A few case scenarios can motivate the issue.[14]

Suppose a couple has a child with leukemia and considers having a second child who could serve as a histocompatible bone marrow donor for the older sibling, thereby saving her life. One might feel that the parents intend, immorally, to use the second child as a means to saving the first, and that therefore their procreative plan is irresponsible. Accordingly, one might believe that the tripartite standard needs to be supplemented with some sort of intention-based condition. I disagree. Parents may decide to have a second child with an eye toward her being a "savior sibling" while committing themselves, and reasonably expecting, to be good, loving parents to both children. Wanting the second child as a means to saving the first does not preclude *also* loving the second child for her own sake. What the tripartite standard requires—appropriately—is not the absence of any motive for procreating that refers to interests other than those of the created child, but rather that parents do right by the child. So far, we find no reason to add an intention-based condition.

Consider a second couple, A and B, in which A wants them to procreate in order to punish B. B doesn't want a child, but A knows B won't favor abortion if the couple becomes pregnant. This, to be sure, is a terrible reason to bring a child into the world. In another couple, C and D, C wants them to procreate in order to induce D to remain in the relationship. D doesn't want a child, but C knows D won't favor abortion if the couple conceives. This case, too, features a dreadful reason to procreate. Both cases suggest the possibility that procreative ethics partly concerns an agent's behavior toward a procreating partner: treating the partner with respect rather than, say, manipulating him or her. Such a requirement of partnering respect would give one's intentions a role in procreative ethics because whether conduct is respectful or disrespectful toward another person has much to do with the agent's intentions.

But remember this paper's topic: the conditions of morally responsible procreation *in view of what parents owe their children*. The topic is not the conditions of responsible procreation, *all things considered*. What parents owe their children includes love, attention, and kindness, but (for all I know) fulfilling that need once a child comes into the world may be consistent with one or both partners having had very dubious reasons for wanting to procreate. Indeed, it might be possible for someone to decide to procreate for a bad reason yet be in a position to expect that the future child's basic needs (and the other conditions of the tripartite standard) will be met. It seems reasonable to suppose that the worse the motive, other things being equal, the less likely it is that a parent has the sort of character needed for good parenting, but there may be exceptions. In any case, what is immediately problematic in these two cases is procreative intentions that evince disrespect for one's partner, so I understand the cases to raise issues beyond the scope of this paper. At the same time, the cases remind us that the tripartite standard is unlikely to be sufficient for responsible procreation, *all things considered*. Maybe a condition regarding appropriate intentions would be needed for a comprehensive account of responsible procreation.[15]

Is Freedom from Avoidable Disability a Basic Need?

At this point in the investigation, it will be instructive to consider a candidate for another basis need: freedom from avoidable disability. The qualification *avoidable* is motivated by the recognition that, generally speaking, disabilities do not preclude, or even much diminish, the prospects for living a decent human life, at least where discrimination is minimal or absent and social accommodations are adequate. So consider this case:

> *Neonatal Neglect.* A doctor informs a couple under her care that their newborn has a rare condition that, if left untreated, will probably cause paralysis from the waist down. The doctor prescribes a safe medicine that is effective in treating this condition. Although the parents could easily fill this prescription and administer the medicine, they neglect to do so with the result that their child becomes paraplegic.

In Neonatal Neglect, it is clear that the parents' passivity is wrong and that, in particular, that they wrong their child by failing to prevent a major, avoidable disability. One might think that a case like this motivates adding to the list of basic needs freedom from avoidable disability. But the way to avoid the relevant disability in this case is by providing needed medical care, which is already on the list of basic needs. Of course, disabilities can come about in other ways. For example, a person might become brain-damaged due to severe physical abuse. But freedom from abuse has already been identified as a basic need. Perhaps there is no need to add freedom from avoidable disability to the list of basic needs.

But now consider this case:

> *Preconception Neglect.* A physician informs a couple under her care that they should delay attempts to conceive because the woman has a medical condition that would likely cause any child she has to be paralyzed from the waist down. If she takes a safe medicine for a month, however, she can later get pregnant and give birth to a healthy child. Because the couple (for no particularly good reason) ignores this advice, they achieve pregnancy a week later, leading to the birth of a paraplegic child.

As in the case of Neonatal Neglect, the parents in Preconception Neglect act wrongly in neglecting the doctor's sound advice and taking a risk that predictably leads to the birth of a child with a substantial disability. But the two cases are very different in one respect that provokes what has been called "the nonidentity problem." The crucial way in which the two cases differ is that in Preconception Neglect there is no identifiable victim of the parent's negligence. That is because, had the parents acted responsibly and delayed conception, they would have conceived through the uniting of different gametes than did in fact unite in leading to the birth of the child with paraplegia. The latter child, in other words, is *not identical to* (not the same child as) the child who would have been born had the parents responsibly conceived later. Therefore, the actual child could not have been better off had the parents done the right thing, because he would not have existed at all had they done so. And the actual child, let us assume, has a life worth living and is therefore not the victim of "wrongful life," as discussed earlier.

So the actual child in Preconception Negligence is not a victim of the parent's wrongful behavior. Nor is anyone else directly harmed or wronged by their behavior. The parents act wrongly, it seems, without wronging anyone in particular. In my view, the wrongdoing in nonidentity cases such as this must be understood in the impersonal, consequentialist terms of making the world a slightly worse place than it would have been had they acted responsibly. The world, given their action, includes an individual who must face the challenges associated with paraplegia, whereas the world, had they acted responsibly, would have been the same except that, instead of the paraplegic child, there would have been a child who did not have to face the challenges associated with that condition.

Looking retrospectively over what happened given what the parents did, and what would have happened had the parents acted as they should have, one might say that the cost of their negligent behavior was an avoidable disability. Accordingly, one might recommend adding to the list of basic needs freedom from avoidable disability. But this addition would be based on a conceptual error: conflating the actual, paraplegic individual with the merely possible child who would have existed had the parents taken the doctor's advice, and on the basis of this conflation judging that the actual individual has an avoidable disability. The disability was not avoidable *for him*. True, it was avoidable for the world, so to speak, but only an individual—not the world—can have basic needs.

Conclusion

We arrive at the interesting point that the kind of wrong that characterizes nonidentity cases cannot be understood in terms of what parents owe their children. We are looking in the wrong place if we look at our tripartite standard of parental obligations and the appended list of basic needs. Ethics does not involve only what we moral agents owe each other.[16] Indeed, ethics is not even limited to what we moral agents owe each other and what we owe individuals—such as infants and dogs—who are not moral agents. For ethics also involves the impersonal project of making the world a better place.

This means that there are several types of wrongful life that are worth distinguishing. Or, if we don't want to use the term "wrongful life" for all of these categories because it is too closely associated with the paradigm cases in which a life was predictably not worth living, we might coin a new term for our purposes. Let's use the term *wrongful* (or *irresponsible*) *procreation*.

One type of wrongful procreation, again, includes the paradigm wrongful-life cases in which parents violate the worthwhile-life standard. A second type of wrongful procreation we might call *wrongful, personal disadvantage*. In these cases, the created child's life is expected to be worth living, but some part of the tripartite standard—involving either basic needs or doing more for a child—is violated. Note that both wrongful life and wrongful, personal disadvantage involve moral failings in terms of what parents owe their children. Not so in nonidentity cases such as Preconception Neglect, which we may term *wrongful, impersonal disadvantage*. This sort of lapse is understood not in personal terms but in the impersonal terms of failing to make things better when one could reasonably have been expected to do so.

As noted earlier in this chapter, however, I have left open certain other issues in procreative ethics. I have not addressed how the expected environmental impact of one's choice to procreate might affect whether it is morally responsible; nor have I addressed whether at least some prospective parents, in view of their circumstances, might have an obligation to adopt a child (or remain childless) rather than bringing a new child into the world. Furthermore, the question of whether and how one's intentions or motivations in choosing to procreate bear on procreative ethics was found to lie beyond the scope of this chapter. I therefore leave it up to other thinkers to help determine whether, in addition to the three types of wrongful procreation identified here, there might also be *wrongful, impersonal resource depletion, wrongful nonbeneficence*, where the latter refers to an irresponsible choice not to adopt, and/or *wrongful procreative intention*.

ACKNOWLEDGMENT

My thanks to Leslie Francis for helpful feedback on an earlier draft.

NOTES

1. Some authors, by contrast, seem to hold that responsible acts are not only permissible but also decent. See, e.g., Judith Jarvis Thomson, "A Defense of Abortion," *Philosophy and Public Affairs* 1 (1971): 47–66.
2. My discussion will both draw significantly and diverge from my *Creation Ethics: Reproduction, Genetics, and Quality of Life* (New York: Oxford University Press), chaps. 5 and 6.
3. David Benatar helpfully underscores the distinction between lives (not) worth starting and those (not) worth continuing (*Better Never to Have Been* [Oxford: Oxford University Press, 2006], chap. 2).
4. Some people believe that any human life is worth starting and continuing irrespective of its experiential quality. This belief, which is highly counterintuitive as applied to such cases

as LNS, is likely to derive from a religious dogma. In this discussion, I set aside beliefs that depend on religious dogma.

5. For a defense of this assumption, appealing to a view of what we essentially are, see my *Human Identity and Bioethics* (Cambridge: Cambridge University Press, 2005), chap. 2. A discussion of this topic that significantly influenced my own is Eric Olson, *The Human Animal* (Oxford: Oxford University Press, 1998). By contrast, Jeff McMahan argues that we, who are essentially embodied minds, necessarily do not come into existence prior to the emergence of mental life in the human organism *(The Ethics of Killing* [Oxford: Oxford University Press, 2002], chap. 1).

6. In fact, I am fairly sure the law would require demonstration of harm to the wronged party.

7. It seems commonsensical to me that there are some harm-independent rights, as the example that follows suggests. Anyone who disagrees, however, can nevertheless agree that the fundamental question is whether the putative victim in a possible wrongful life situation has been wronged. The person who disagrees with me would simply understand the issue of wrong through the lens of harm: Was the putative victim harmed?

8. See Jeff McMahan, "Wrongful Life: Paradoxes in the Morality of Causing People to Exist," in Jules Coleman and Christopher Morris (eds.), *Rational Commitment and Social Justice* (Cambridge: Cambridge University Press, 1998).

9. Benatar, *Better Never to Have Been,* and Shiffrin, "Wrongful Life, Procreative Responsibility, and the Significance of Harm," *Legal Theory* 5 (1999): 117–148.

10. See my "Is It Wrong to Impose the Harms of Human Life," *Theoretical Medicine and Bioethics* 31 (2010): 317–331 and *Creation Ethics*, chap. 5.

11. The term is Shiffrin's ("Wrongful Life, Procreative Responsibility, and the Significance of Harm").

12. Admittedly, the distinction between exposing to and imposing harm is not very sharp. But the more closely tied the harm is to the activity itself, the stronger the case for conceptualizing the instance at hand as involving the imposition of harm. Thus, parents who have their young children take up boxing could be thought of as imposing head trauma on their youngsters, and for this reason I believe the parental push toward boxing to be misguided. With what we know about tackle football and head injuries today—that there is a higher risk of head injury than we used to believe, although the risks are far short of those associated with boxing—parents' choice to have their child play tackle football may lie somewhere between clear cases of imposing and clear cases of exposing a child to harm.

13. Lest there be any misunderstanding, the *parent* mentioned here need not be a genetic, gestational, or even legal parent, but she or he must *function socially* as the child's parent and undertake a commitment to parent the child. Ordinarily, this social parent will also be the legal parent, but I leave open the possibility of exceptions in which legal status does not, for some reason, track the social role. And how long must such a parent be around to fulfill the basic need for parenting as I understand it? I suggest that responsible parenting requires the reasonable expectation that such a parent will be alive and able to function as a parent long enough for the child to enter adulthood.

14. Thanks to Leslie Francis for raising this issue and suggesting roughly the cases I address in this section.

15. Another case mentioned by Leslie Francis (see previous note) features a rebellious teenager who wants to have a baby simply to defy her parents. Although we can stipulate that this teenager intends to give up the baby for adoption and knows that excellent adoptive parents are available, so that the tripartite standard would probably be met, it would seem

wrong for this teenager to procreate with the stated intention. But, as mentioned at the outset, my analysis concerns procreation *with the intention of parenting*. So this case lies outside the scope of my analysis. It does, however, add to the sense that some intention-based condition may be needed for a comprehensive account.

16. What moral agents owe each other would include the respect procreative partners owe each other, as discussed earlier in connection with procreative intentions.

INDEX